a LANGE medical book

CURRENT

Rheumatology
Diagnosis
& Treatment

first edition

Edited by

John B. Imboden
Professor of Medicine
University of California
Chief, Division of
San Francisco General

David B. Hellmann
Mary Betty Stevens
Department of Medicine
Johns Hopkins Bayview
Hopkins University
Baltimore, Maryland

Hopkins University

Vasculitis Center

Lange Medical
Medical Publishing

New York   Chicago
San Juan   Seoul   Singapore   Sydney   Toronto

Current Rheumatology Diagnosis & Treatment

1 2 3 4 5 6 7 8 9 0 DOC/DOC 0 9 8 7 6 5 4

ISBN: 0-07-141027-9
ISSN: 1547-8998

Notice

Medicine is an ever-changing science. As new research and clinical experience broaden our knowledge, changes in treatment and drug therapy are required. The authors and the publisher of this work have checked with sources believed to be reliable in their efforts to provide information that is complete and generally in accord with the standards accepted at the time of publication. However, in view of the possibility of human error or changes in medical sciences, neither the authors nor the publisher nor any other party who has been involved in the preparation or publication of this work warrants that the information contained herein is in every respect accurate or complete, and they disclaim all responsibility for any errors or omissions or for the results obtained from use of the information contained in this work. Readers are encouraged to confirm the information contained herein with other sources. For example and in particular, readers are advised to check the product information sheet included in the package of each drug they plan to administer to be certain that the information contained in this work is accurate and that changes have not been made in the recommended dose or in the contraindications for administration. This recommendation is of particular importance in connection with new or infrequently used drugs.

This book was set in Adobe Garamond by Pine Tree Composition, Inc.
The editors were Isabel Nogueira, Harriet Lebowitz, and Barbara Holton.
The production supervisor was Catherine Saggese.
The illustration manager was Maria T. Magtoto.
The index was prepared by Katherine Pitcoff.
RR Donnelley was the printer and binder.

This book is printed on acid-free paper.

In this, as in all of our endeavors, we are grateful
for the love and support of our wives and children:
Dolores Shoback and Tom and Elizabeth Imboden;
Linda, Matthew, and Jessica Hellmann;
and Martha, Sarah, and William Stone.

Contents

Authors

Jeffrey S. Alderman, MD
Assistant Professor of Medicine, Department of
   Medicine, University of Oklahoma College
   of Medicine, Tulsa
jeffrey-alderman@ouhsc.edu
*Pseudogout: Calcium Pyrophosphate Dihydrate Crystal
Deposition Disease*

Sharon E. Banks, DO
Assistant Professor of Medicine, Division of Rheuma-
   tology, Penn State Milton S. Hershey Medical
   Center, Hershey, Pennsylvania
sbanks@psu.edu
*Rheumatic Manifestations of Acute & Chronic Viral
Arthritis*

Ralf Baron, MD
Professor, Vice-Director, Neurology Clinic, Christian-
   Albrechts-University, Kiel, Germany
r.baron@neurologie.uni-kiel.de
*Complex Regional Pain Syndromes: Reflex Sympathetic
Dystrophy & Causalgia*

Linda K. Bockenstedt, MD
Harold W. Jockers Associate Professor, Section of
   Rheumatology, Yale University School of Medicine,
   New Haven, Connecticut
linda.bockenstedt@yale.edu
Lyme Disease

Phyllis N. Bonaminio, MD
Rheumatology Fellow, Northwestern University/
   The Feinberg School of Medicine, Chicago, Illinois
pnbonaminio@aol.com
Pregnancy & Rheumatic Diseases

David Borenstein, MD
Clinical Professor of Medicine, the George Washington
   University Medical Center, Washington, DC
dborenstein715@aol.com
Approach to the Patient with Neck Pain

Calvin R. Brown, Jr., MD
Associate Professor of Medicine and Orthopaedic
   Surgery, Rush Medical College, Chicago, Illinois
cbrown@rush.edu
Common Injuries from Running

Victor R. Cotton, MD, JD
Adjunct Professor of Law, Widener University School
   of Law, Hummelstown, Pennsylvania
cottonmdjd@aol.com
Legal Issues

Jeff Critchfield, MD
Assistant Clinical Professor of Medicine, University
   of California, San Francisco; Vice-Chief of
   Medicine, San Francisco General Hospital
jeff@itsa.ucsf.edu
*Evaluation of Rheumatic Complaints in Patients with
HIV*

David I. Daikh, MD, PhD
Assistant Professor of Medicine, University of Califor-
   nia, San Francisco and Veterans Affairs Medical
   Center, San Francisco, California
daikh@itsa.ucsf.edu
*Practical Guide to the Use of Assistive Devices,
Physical Therapy, & Occupational Therapy*

E. Gene Deune, MD
Assistant Professor, Division of Plastic Surgery, and
   Co-Director, Section of Hand Surgery, The Johns
   Hopkins University School of Medicine, Baltimore,
   Maryland
egdeune@jhmi.edu
The Patient with Hand, Wrist, or Elbow Pain

Rajiv K. Dixit, MD
Associate Clinical Professor of Medicine, University of
   California, San Francisco; Director, Northern Cali-
   fornia Arthritis Center, Walnut Creek, California
ncarthritiscenter@hotmail.com
Approach to the Patient with Low Back Pain

Fiona A. Donald, MD, FRCP(C)
Attending Physician, Department of Medicine,
   Division of Rheumatology, University of California,
   San Francisco
fdonald@itsa.ucsf.edu
*Rheumatic Manifestations of Malignancy; Medications:
Intravenous Immune Globulin (IVIG)*

Kenneth H. Fye, MD
Clinical Professor of Medicine, Division of Rheumatology, University of California, San Francisco
kenfye@itsa.ucsf.edu
Aspiration & Joint Injection; Sjögren Syndrome

Monica Gandhi, MD, MPH
Assistant Professor, Division of Infectious Diseases, Department of Medicine, University of California, San Francisco
mgandhi@itsa.ucsf.edu
Septic Arthritis & Disseminated Gonococcal Infection

Allan C. Gelber, MD, MPH, PhD
Associate Professor of Medicine, Division of Rheumatology, The Johns Hopkins University School of Medicine, Baltimore, Maryland
agelber@jhmi.edu
Osteoarthritis

Jennifer D. Gorman, MD, MPH
Assistant Adjunct Professor of Medicine, Division of Rheumatology, University of California, San Francisco
gormanj@itsa.ucsf.edu
Spondyloarthropathies

Jonathan Graf, MD
Assistant Adjunct Professor of Medicine, Department of Medicine, University of California, San Francisco; Division of Rheumatology, San Francisco General Hospital
grafj@itsa.ucsf.edu
Endocrine & Metabolic Disorders; Medications: Anti-Tumor Necrosis Factor Agents: Etanercept (Enbrel), Infliximab (Remicade), and Adalimumab (Humira)

Ilksen Gurkan, MD
Fellow, Department of Orthopedic Surgery, The Johns Hopkins University/Johns Hopkins Bayview Medical Center, Baltimore, Maryland
ilksen@doctor.com
The Patient with Hip Pain

David B. Hellmann, MD
Mary Betty Stevens Professor of Medicine and Chairman, Department of Medicine, Johns Hopkins Bayview Medical Center, The Johns Hopkins University School of Medicine, Baltimore, Maryland
hellmann@jhmi.edu
Introduction to Vasculitis: Classification & Clinical Clues; Giant Cell Arteritis & Polymyalgia Rheumatica; Takayasu Arteritis; Behçet Disease; Vasculitis of the Central Nervous System; Medications: Allopurinol; Medications: Colchicine

Laura K. Hummers, MD
Instructor of Medicine, Division of Rheumatology, The Johns Hopkins University School of Medicine, Baltimore, Maryland
lhummers@jhmi.edu
Scleroderma

John B. Imboden, MD
Professor of Medicine, University of California, San Francisco; Chief, Division of Rheumatology, San Francisco General Hospital
imboden@itsa.ucsf.edu
Laboratory Diagnosis; The Approach to the Patient with Arthritis; Mycobacterial & Fungal Infections of Bone & Joints; Medications: Nonsteroidal Anti-Inflammatory Drugs; Medications: Systemic Glucocorticoid Therapy: Prednisone, Prednisolone, & Methylprednisolone; Medications: Methotrexate (MTX); Medications: Leflunomide (Arava); Medications: Sulfasalazine (SSA); Medications: Antimalarial Drugs: Hydroxychloroquine (Plaquenil) & Chloroquine

Richard Jacobs, MD, PhD
Clinical Professor of Medicine and Clinical Pharmacy, University of California, San Francisco
jacobsd@medicine.ucsf.edu
Septic Arthritis & Disseminated Gonococcal Infection

William M. Jenkin, DPM
Professor and Chair, Department of Podiatric Surgery, California School of Podiatric Medicine at Samuel Merritt College, Oakland, California
bjenkin@samuelmerritt.edu
Approach to the Patient with Ankle & Foot Pain

Carl A. Johnson, MD
Associate Professor of Orthopaedic Surgery, The Johns Hopkins University School of Medicine, Baltimore, Maryland
cjohnsoa@jhmi.edu
Approach to the Patient with Knee Pain

Sharon L. Kolasinski, MD
Chief of Clinical Service and Assistant Professor of Medicine, Division of Rheumatology, University of Pennsylvania School of Medicine, Philadelphia
sharonk@mail.med.upenn.edu
Complementary & Alternative Therapies

Jon D. Levine, MD, PhD
Professor of Medicine, University of California, San Francisco
levine@itsa.ucsf.edu
Complex Regional Pain Syndromes: Reflex Sympathetic Dystrophy & Causalgia

Steven A. Lietman, MD
Department of Orthopaedic Surgery, The Cleveland Clinic Foundation, Cleveland, Ohio
lietmans@ccf.org
The Approach to the Patient with a Painful Prosthetic Joint

David R. Moller, MD
Associate Professor, Division of Pulmonary and Critical Care Medicine, Department of Medicine, The Johns Hopkins University School of Medicine, Baltimore, Maryland
dmoller@jhmi.edu
Sarcoidosis

Daniel Most, MD
Chief Resident, Division of Plastic Surgery, The Johns Hopkins University School of Medicine, Baltimore, Maryland
danmost@yahoo.com
The Patient with Hand, Wrist, or Elbow Pain

Paul S. Mueller, MD, MPH
Assistant Professor of Medicine, Mayo Clinic College of Medicine and Consultant, Division of General Internal Medicine, Mayo Clinic, Rochester, Minnesota
mueller.pauls@mayo.edu
Amyloidosis

Stanley J. Naides, MD
Thomas B. Hallowell Professor of Medicine; Professor of Microbiology & Immunology, and Pharmacology; Chief, Division of Rheumatology, Department of Medicine, Penn State Milton S. Hershey Medical Center, Hershey, Pennsylvania
snaides@psu.edu
Rheumatic Manifestations of Acute & Chronic Viral Arthritis

Meg Newman, MD
Associate Professor of Clinical Medicine, University of California, San Francisco; Director, HIV Clinical Scholars Program and AIDS Eduction Program, University of California, San Francisco Positive Health Program at San Francisco General Hospital
mnewman@php.ucsf.edu
Evaluation of Rheumatic Complaints in Patients with HIV

James R. O'Dell
Professor and Vice-Chairman, Section of Rheumatology, Department of Internal Medicine, University of Nebraska Medical Center, Omaha
jrodell@unmc.edu
Rheumatoid Arthritis

Irina Petrache, MD
Assistant Professor of Medicine, Division of Pulmonary and Critical Care Medicine, Department of Medicine, The Johns Hopkins University School of Medicine, Baltimore, Maryland
ipetra@jhmi.edu
Sarcoidosis

Michelle Petri, MD, MPH
Professor of Medicine, Division of Rheumatology, Department of Medicine, The Johns Hopkins University School of Medicine, Baltimore, Maryland
mpetri@jhmi.edu
Systemic Lupus Erythematosus; Antiphospholipid Antibody Syndrome

Rosalind Ramsey-Goldman, MD, DrPH
Professor of Medicine, Northwestern University, The Feinberg School of Medicine, Chicago, Illinois
rgramsey@northwestern.edu
Pregnancy & Rheumatic Diseases

Mark W. Rodosky, MD
Chief, Division of Shoulder and Elbow Surgery, University of Pittsburgh Center for Sports Medicine; Assistant Team Physician, Pittsburgh Penguins, Pittsburgh, Pennsylvania
rodoskymw@msx.upmc.edu
Approach to the Painful shoulder

Kenneth E. Sack, MD
Professor of Clinical Medicine, Department of Rheumatology, University of California, San Francisco
kensac@medicine.ucsf.edu
Physical Examination of the Musculoskeletal System

Sherri Sanders, MD
Assistant Professor, Department of Internal Medicine University of Oklahoma College of Medicine, Tulsa
sherri-sanders@ouhsc.edu
Gout

Peggy Schlesinger, MD
Clinical Associate Professor, University of Washington School of Medicine
p.schlesinger@earthlink.net
Approach to the Adolescent with Arthritis; Adult Still Disease

Philip Seo, MD
Post-Doctoral Fellow, The Johns Hopkins University School of Medicine, Baltimore, Maryland
seo@jhmi.edu
Miscellaneous Forms of Vasculitis; Medications: Azathioprine (AZA; Imuran); Medications: Mycophenolate Mofetil (MMF; CellCept)

Dolores Shoback, MD
Professor of Medicine, University of California, San
  Francisco; Staff Physician, San Francisco Veterans
  Affairs Medical Center
dolores@itsa.ucsf.edu
*Endocrine & Metabolic Disorders; Osteoporosis & Gluco-
corticoid-Induced Osteoporosis; Medications: Bisphosphonates: Etidronate (Didronel), Pamidronate (Aredia), Alendronate (Fosamax), Risedronate (Actonel), Zoledronic
acid (Zometa)*

John H. Stone, MD, MPH
Associate Professor of Medicine, Division of Rheumatology, The Johns Hopkins University School of
  Medicine; Director, The Johns Hopkins University
  Vasculitis Center, Baltimore, Maryland
jstone@mail.jhmi.edu
*Relapsing Polychondritis; Wegener Granulomatosis; Mi-
croscopic Polyangiitis; Churg-Strauss Syndrome; Pol-
yarteritis Nodosa; Mixed Cryoglobulinemia; Hypersensi-
tivity Vasculitis; Henoch-Schönlein Purpura; Buerger
Disease; Miscellaneous Forms of Vasculitis; Medications:
Cyclophosphamide(CYC; Cytoxan); Medications: Chlo-
rambucil (CHL; Leukeran); Medications: Azathioprine
(AZA; Imuran); Medications: Mycophenolate Mofetil
(MMF; CellCept)*

Sangeeta Dileep Sule, MD
Instructor in Rheumatology and Pediatrics, The Johns
  Hopkins University School of Medicine, Baltimore,
  Maryland
ssule@jhmi.edu
Raynaud Phenomenon

James F. Wenz, MD†
Chairman, Department of Orthopaedic Surgery, The
  Johns Hopkins University/Johns Hopkins Bayview
  Medical Center, Baltimore, Maryland
The Patient with Hip Pain

Robin V. West, MD
Assistant Professor, University of Pittsburgh, UPMC
  Sports Medicine; Head Team Physician, The University of Pittsburgh Men's Basketball Team; Assistant Team Physician, The Pittsburgh Steelers, Pennsylvania
westrv@msx.upmc.edu
Approach to the Painful shoulder

Fredrick M. Wigley, MD
Professor of Medicine, Johns Hopkins University
  School of Medicine; Associate Director, Division of
  Rheumatology, and Director, The Johns Hopkins
  Scleroderma Center, Baltimore, Maryland
fwig@jhmi.edu
Raynaud Phenomenon; Scleroderma

John B. Winfield, MD
Herman & Louise Smith Distinguished Professor of
  Medicine, and Attending Physician, University of
  North Carolina School of Medicine, Chapel Hill
john_winfield@med.unc.edu
The Patient with Diffuse Pain

Robert L. Wortmann, MD
Professor of Medicine and Chair, Department of Internal Medicine, University of Oklahoma College of
  Medicine, Tulsa
robert-wortmann@ouhsc.edu
*Polymyositis & Dermatomyositis; Gout; Pseudogout: Cal-
cium Pyrophosphate Dihydrate Crystal Deposition Disease*

Carol M. Ziminski, MD
Associate Professor of Medicine, Division of Rheuma-
  tology, The Johns Hopkins University School of
  Medicine; Deputy Director, Johns Hopkins
  Rheumatology at Good Samaritan Hospital, Balti-
  more, Maryland
ziminski@jhmi.edu
Osteonecrosis

Preface

Current Rheumatology Diagnosis and Treatment is the only rheumatology textbook written with the practicing physician foremost in mind. The book is a practical guide to the diagnosis and management of the complete range of rheumatological problems encountered in clinical medicine, from common musculoskeletal complaints to complex, multi-organ system inflammatory diseases.

DISTINGUISHING FEATURES

• Chapters devoted to the evaluation of common musculoskeletal symptoms.

• Concise, authoritative reviews of specific rheumatic diseases.

• Consistent format that facilitates access to clinical information.

• Practical guide to medications used in the treatment of rheumatic disease.

• Unique chapters on clinical topics of special interest, including: pregnancy and rheumatic disease, the recognition of vasculitis, common running injuries, pain in a prosthetic joint, the adolescent with arthritis, the patient with diffuse pain, the evaluation of rheumatic complaints in the HIV-infected patient, and the use of complementary and alternative therapies.

• Guidance in minimizing lawsuits and other legal entanglements.

INTENDED AUDIENCE

• Primary care physicians will appreciate the book's problem-oriented approach to musculoskeletal symptoms and its emphasis on the clinical features, laboratory findings, differential diagnosis, and treatment of specific rheumatic diseases.

• Rheumatologists will find the book to be a quick, reliable, and up-to-date reference.

• For other specialists the book will serve as a primary textbook in rheumatology.

• Fellows, house officers, and medical students will appreciate this engaging introduction to clinical rheumatology.

• The book will prove to be invaluable for those studying for board certification or recertification in rheumatology.

Acknowledgments

We are deeply grateful to Isabel Nogueira whose sound advice, always leavened with good cheer and delivered with tact, kept us on track and made this book possible. The final version of the text benefited greatly from the careful, expert copyediting of Jennifer Bernstein.

John B. Imboden, MD
David B. Hellmann, MD
John H. Stone, MD, MPH

San Francisco and Baltimore
May 2004

SECTION I

Approach to the Patient With Rheumatic Disease

<table>
<tr><td>

Physical Examination of the Musculoskeletal System

</td><td>

1

</td></tr>
</table>

Kenneth E. Sack, MD

The physical examination begins when the physician meets the patient. The physician can assess posture, gait, skin texture, and gross muscle strength by shaking hands, accompanying the patient into the office, and watching him or her move. A comprehensive assessment of the musculoskeletal system includes inspection and palpation of joints and soft tissues as well as evaluation of joint range of motion and neuromuscular function.

INSPECTION

Joint swelling, color, and alignment, as well as skin rashes and muscle wasting, are usually obvious in a glance. Comparing similar joints and muscle groups on opposite sides of the body helps detect subtle abnormalities.

Swelling

The hallmark of inflammation is swelling, which, when present in a joint, indicates that **arthralgia** has become **arthritis.** An increase in synovial fluid causes generalized joint swelling unless fluid accumulates in a contiguous synovial pouch (eg, suprapatellar space) or bursa (eg, gastrocnemius-semimembranous popliteal bursa [Baker cyst]). Inflammation of a tendon sheath may cause soft, localized para-articular swelling. Soft tissue edema tends to be more diffuse.

Well-defined swelling over a bony prominence such as the olecranon process or patella may represent an inflamed subcutaneous bursa, a rheumatoid nodule, a gouty tophus, or rarely, a xanthoma or an amyloid deposit. Bony enlargements (osteophytes) adjacent to

joints are typical of osteoarthritis and occur as a result of cartilage damage. Occasionally, such overgrowths are a product of chronic inflammation. Osteophytes may be palpable and visible at the distal interphalangeal (DIP) and proximal interphalangeal (PIP) joints, where they are called Heberden and Bouchard nodes, respectively.

Color Changes

Acute inflammation of a joint may impart an erythematous hue to the overlying skin, reflecting vasodilation of cutaneous vessels. In some cases of crystal-induced disease, such as gout, the joint and surrounding areas have an intense red-violet color mimicking that seen in infectious cellulitis and septic arthritis.

Deformity

Inflamed joints tend to assume positions that maximize intrasynovial volume, thereby minimizing intrasynovial pressure and reducing pain. In chronic arthritis, when such positions are held for prolonged periods, flexion deformities may ensue. Chronic arthritis can also lead to destruction of supporting structures with consequent malalignment of adjacent bones.

Muscle Wasting

Atrophy of muscles may result from lack of use, neurologic disease, inflammation of an adjacent joint, or myositis associated with an underlying disease. Thus, atrophy of the intrinsic muscles of the hand commonly accompanies inflammation of the fingers or wrists and is visible as depressions between the extensor tendons on the dorsum of the hand. Similarly, synovitis of the knee typically causes atrophy of the quadriceps muscles, resulting in a concavity just above the knee, particularly on the medial aspect.

PALPATION

A "hands on" examination is vital to the detection of inflammation and structural damage in a joint.

Tenderness

Joint tenderness is the most sensitive but the least specific indicator of inflammation. During examination, apply similar pressure to all joint groups and surrounding structures. (Some experts suggest exerting pressure sufficient to blanch the examiner's fingernail bed.) When indicated, test normal structures to determine the patient's baseline pain threshold. Remember that the joint capsule and periosteum are pain-sensitive structures, but the articular cartilage and meniscus are not.

Swelling

A tense synovial effusion has the consistency of a hollow rubber ball, whereas synovial hypertrophy feels more doughy. Inflammation of a tendon sheath results in soft, para-articular swelling in the distribution of the tendon, and the associated subcutaneous edema tends to be more diffuse. Osteophytes produce the bony swelling typical of Heberden and Bouchard nodes. Simultaneous swelling of different joint components can confuse even the most experienced examiner.

Temperature

An increase in the surface temperature of the joint usually indicates underlying inflammation. By using the dorsum of the hand to palpate the same joint on each side of the body, temperature changes as small as 0.5 °C can be detected. Note that surface temperatures of superficial joints such as the knee are normally *lower* than the surrounding tissue (unless there is extra subcutaneous fat overlying the joint). Thus, an equalization of temperatures often indicates joint inflammation.

Crepitus

Joint motion may produce a "crackling" sound or a "crunching" sensation on palpation. This phenomenon, called crepitus, occurs when the surfaces of degenerated cartilage rub together or when bone rubs against bone after extensive loss of cartilage. Inflammation of tendon sheaths also can cause crepitus. In normal joints, crepitus usually reflects motion of tendon over bone.

RANGE OF MOTION

A number of mechanisms can reduce joint motion (Table 1–1). Excessive joint motion may result from destruction of supporting structures or subchondral bone or from joint dislocation. Active range of motion (by the patient) allows rapid assessment of joint mobility, while passive range of motion (by the examiner) permits a more complete evaluation of joint function.

Normal range of joint motion varies according to age and gender. Flexibility tends to diminish with age, and women are typically more flexible than men.

NEUROLOGIC TESTING

A complete musculoskeletal evaluation includes a neurologic examination with specific attention to the sensorimotor components. Inflammatory myopathies typically cause weakness or wasting of proximal muscles. Immune-mediated diseases tend to affect the central or peripheral nervous systems. Degenerative processes affecting the spine or extremities may lead to impingement on nerve roots or various portions of peripheral nerves.

THE PHYSICAL EXAMINATION

Having a consistent routine facilitates thoroughness without sacrificing speed, but the nature of the patient's problem will dictate emphasis on any given aspect of the examination. Evaluating the back and the neuromuscular system of the lower extremity is a reasonable starting point.

Back & Neuromuscular System of the Lower Extremity

Begin with the patient seated in a chair. Ask him or her to stand without using the arms. This gives you a good idea of the patient's proximal lower extremity strength. If the patient has trouble rising, ask whether it is because of pain or weakness. If a psychogenic reason is suspected, ask the patient to sit down slowly without using the arms. Because the same muscles that facilitate rising allow sitting, the person with true weakness will

Table 1–1. Factors that reduce joint motion.

Damage to articular cartilage or bone
Large synovial effusions
Loose bodies within the joint cavity
Joint subluxation
Fibrous or bony ankylosis
Contracture of the capsule or contiguous tendons
Irritation of pain-sensitive structures in and about the joint

fall into the chair early in the process. Now have the patient take one or two steps on the heels and then on the toes. This indicates strength in the distal muscles and gives some idea of coordination.

With the patient standing comfortably, evaluate the configuration of the spine and lower extremities from the front and back. This is the best way to look for structural abnormalities in the back (eg, scoliosis, kyphosis), legs (eg, genu valgum or varum), and feet (eg, pes planus). Prominence of one shoulder or scapula suggests **scoliosis.** If this asymmetry vanishes when the patient bends forward, the vertebral column is probably normal, and the scoliosis is "functional" (ie, caused by such processes as hip disease, leg-length discrepancy, or nerve root irritation). Structural scoliosis results from abnormalities of the vertebral column and rib cage consequent to disorders of bone, nerve, or muscle. It may also have no obvious cause (idiopathic). Associated skin lesions, such as café-au-lait spots, patches of hair, dimpling, or lipomata, may be clues to an underlying causative abnormality. The direction of spinal convexity defines the scoliosis—compensated (first thoracic vertebra is centered over the sacrum) or uncompensated (first thoracic vertebra is to the right or left of the sacrum). To quantitate the degree of list, drop a plumb line from the first thoracic vertebra and measure the distance from this line to the midgluteal crease.

Check whether the iliac crests are level. Asymmetry may reflect real or apparent leg-length discrepancy. The relationship of the hip to the pelvis affects functional leg length. Thus, an adducted hip raises the pelvis and makes the leg appear shorter. Conversely, an abducted hip lowers the pelvis and "lengthens" the leg. Fixed obliquity of the pelvis also causes relative changes in leg length. Measuring the distance from the anterior superior iliac spine to the ipsilateral medial malleolus detects real differences in leg length. (This measurement can also be performed later when the patient is lying supine.)

Note the mobility of the thoracolumbar spine by asking the patient to bend forward as far as possible with the knees straight; also determine the amount of lumbar extension and lateral bending. Limited motion or pain consequent to these maneuvers may indicate disease of spinal articulations or supporting structures, as well as irritation of a muscle or nerve root. To quantify the amount of lumbar mobility, use the **modified Schober maneuver** (Figure 1–1). Mark a spot in the midline 5 cm below the level of the buttock dimples. Using a tape measure, place a mark 15 cm directly above the first mark and ask the patient to bend forward as far as possible. The distance between the two marks should increase at least 5 cm. Periodic measurements are useful in monitoring patients with inflammatory back disease, such as ankylosing spondylitis. Test thoracolumbar function by having the patient rotate the upper torso from side to side. Determine **chest expansion** by holding the tape measure at approximately nipple level and measuring the difference between full expiration and inspiration. Chest expansion, which is normally at least 5 cm, diminishes with

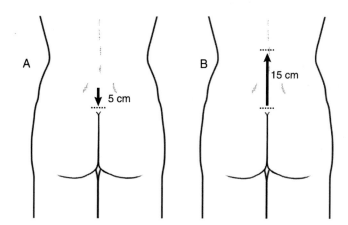

Figure 1–1. Modified Schober test of flexion of the lumbar spine. With the patient standing upright, the examiner makes a mark on the skin 5 cm below an imaginary line drawn between the buttock dimples that overlie the posterior superior iliac spines (**A**). A second mark is made 15 cm above the first (**B**). The distance between the two marks is then measured while the patient bends over and attempts to touch his or her toes while keeping the knees fully extended. The distance between the marks increases to at least 20 cm if there is normal flexion of the lumbar spine. In the original Schober test, the first mark is placed between the buttock dimples and a second mark is made 10 cm above that; the distance between these marks should increase to at least 15 cm when the patient bends over.

costovertebral disease, a frequent early component of ankylosing spondylitis.

Press firmly over the spinous processes and interspinous ligaments for areas of tenderness or bony defects. Full palpation of the coccyx requires a rectal examination. Although it is possible to palpate the lower portion of the sacroiliac (SI) joint between the posterior inferior iliac spine and the sciatic notch, tenderness in this area may represent irritation of a bursa or the sciatic nerve. Therefore, indirect maneuvers (performed later in the examination) are necessary to elicit pain in the SI joint. When indicated, palpate the ischial tuberosities or the posterior portions of the greater trochanters for bursal tenderness.

Analysis of the patient's **gait** can localize a neurologic or musculoskeletal disorder in the lower extremities. Have the patient walk several steps in a straight line and then return. The normal gait is narrow-based (2–4 inches between the feet) with a shift in the pelvis of no more than 1–2 inches in the vertical or horizontal direction. Table 1–2 outlines the causes of several common gait abnormalities.

Upper Extremities

A. HANDS

With the patient seated at the end of the examination table, examine the hands. Look closely at the fingernails for clubbing, discoloration, dilated periungual capillaries, and pitting or other dystrophic changes. Palpate the DIP, PIP, and metacarpophalangeal (MCP) joints for swelling, tenderness, and warmth (Figures 1–2 and 1–3). Have the patient make a full fist for gross evaluation of hand function. Test separately any abnormal joints, and palpate the flexor tendons for nodules or crepitance.

Inability to flex the fingers may result not only from a damaged joint but also from abnormalities in tendons or supporting structures. When active flexion is diminished but passive flexion remains, consider adhesions between the flexor profundus and sublimus digitorum tendons. Also, when flexion of a PIP joint is difficult, attempt to flex the joint while at the same time flexing the MCP joint. If PIP flexion *increases* during this maneuver, suspect tightening of the intrinsic muscles (lumbricales and interossei). If flexion of the MCPs *decreases* flexion of the PIPs, tightness of the extrinsic extensor tendons may be the culprit. Examine the palm for skin lesions, soft tissue nodules, and muscle atrophy.

B. WRISTS

Palpate the dorsum of the wrist. Thickened tissue occupying the normal depression just distal to the radial styloid may indicate early synovitis. Swelling, tenderness, or increased mobility of the ulnar styloid is typical of

Table 1–2. Common gait abnormalities and their causes.

Gait	Description	Cause
Antalgic	Rapid shift from painful extremity (short stance phase)	Pain in foot, knee, or hip
Abductor (gluteus medius)	Shift of thorax over involved hip	Weakened gluteus maximus unable to fully extend hip
Extensor (gluteus maximus)	Excessive shift of thorax posteriorly	Weakened gluteus maximus unable to fully extend hip
Quadriceps weakness	Shift of trunk anteriorly (sometimes with patient pushing knee manually into extension)	Weakened quadriceps unable to extend knees
Excessive lateral foot contact	Diminished pronation of foot during stance phase	Weakened peroneus or painful medial foot
Excessive medial foot contact	Diminished supination of foot during stance phase	Weakness of invertors or tight peroneus
Hip hiking	Vertical lifting of hip during swing phase	Increased leg length, hamstring weakness, or fused knee
Steppage	Excessive flexion of knee to enable foot to clear ground (may be accompanied by foot slap)	Weakened dorsiflexors
Insufficient push-off	Entire foot leaves ground at once	Weakness of gastrocnemius or painful foot

rheumatoid arthritis. Flex and extend the wrist to determine range of motion. These maneuvers also may bring into prominence a ganglion cyst on the dorsal or volar aspects of the wrist.

Pain and tenderness along the radial aspect of the wrist are characteristic of tenosynovitis of the abductor pollicis longus and extensor pollicis brevis, both of which conjoin to form the volar aspect of the "snuff box." To distinguish this process from degenerative disease of the first carpometacarpal joint, have the patient make a fist with the thumb tucked inside the fingers. Then, deviate the wrist in the ulnar direction (**Finkelstein maneuver**) (Figure 1–4). A sharp pain along the distal radial border confirms tenosynovitis.

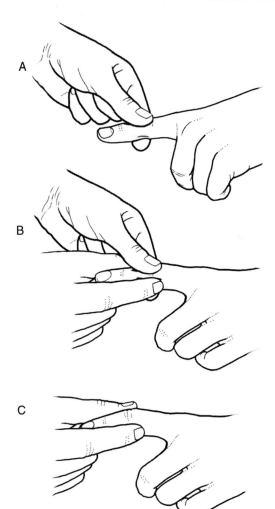

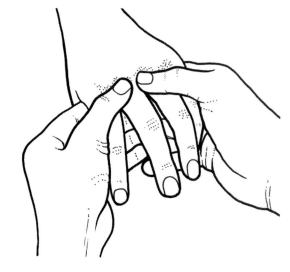

Figure 1–3. Examination of the metacarpophalangeal joints. With the metacarpophalangeal joints partially flexed to approximately 60 degrees, the joint lines should be easily palpable just below the heads of the metacarpals.

Figure 1–2. Method for detecting subtle synovitis of the proximal interphalangeal joints. The examiner firmly compresses the proximal interphalangeal joint with the thumb and forefinger of one hand (**A**) and then palpates the lateral aspects of the joint with the thumb and forefinger of the other hand (**B**). Palpation of the lateral aspect of the joint is repeated without compression (**C**). When synovitis is present, there is a sensation of "bogginess" overlying the lateral surface of the joint that is more pronounced when the joint is compressed.

To test for carpal tunnel syndrome, hold the wrist in slight extension and tap the volar aspect at the distal end of the palmaris longus tendon. A tingling feeling either up the arm or in any of the first three digits indicates irritation of the median nerve (a positive **Tinel sign**). If this test is negative or equivocal, hold the wrist in full flexion for at least 1 minute (**Phalen test**) to elicit similar symptoms.

C. ELBOWS

Palpate along the proximal ulna and over the olecranon process for nodules. Synovial thickening or joint effusions are easily palpable in the groove between the olecranon process and the lateral epicondyle. Bursitis manifests as swelling directly over the olecranon process. Tenderness along the medial epicondyle usually indicates injury to the tendinous origins of the flexors of the wrist (**medial epicondylitis**). Confirm this by attempting to reproduce the pain on resisted flexion of the wrist. Conversely, tenderness along the lateral epicondyle usually reflects inflammation at the tendinous origins of the extensors of the wrist (**lateral epicondylitis**); resisted extension of the wrist usually elicits pain. Assess maximum flexion and extension of the elbow; test pronation and supination with the elbow held at 90 degrees flexion and close to the waist to prevent shoulder motion.

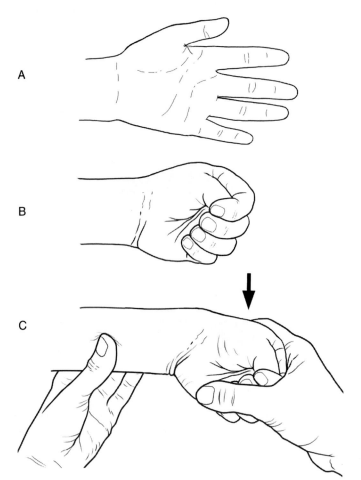

A

B

C

Figure 1–4. Finkelstein maneuver. After the patient makes a fist with the thumb inside the fingers (**A, B**), the examiner forces the wrist in an ulnar direction (**C**). This maneuver elicits pain along the distal radial aspect of the wrist when there is tenosynovitis of the abductor pollicis longus. (From Hoppenfeld S. *Physical Examination of the Spine and Extremities.* Appleton-Century-Crofts, 1976, Figure 49. With permission.)

D. SHOULDERS

Test active shoulder abduction by having the patient touch his or her outstretched palms over the head. Similarly, test internal rotation and adduction by having the patient reach behind the back to touch the opposite scapula, and test external rotation and abduction by having the patient reach behind the head for the opposite scapula (Figure 1–5). Pursue abnormalities noted on active motion by performing passive tests of glenohumeral motion. Place hand firmly on the upper border of the scapula to prevent scapulothoracic motion, and with the patient's palm facing down and elbow held at approximately 90 degrees flexion, abduct the arm. With the flexed arm abducted at shoulder level, assess external and internal rotation by raising and lowering the forearm. Pain on these maneuvers may arise from an inflamed bursa or an injured rotator cuff tendon. To evaluate glenohumeral motion, have the patient relax his or her arm at the side with the elbow held at 90 degrees flexion; the forearm should externally rotate about 90 degrees.

Palpate for tender areas, particularly under the lateral acromion (near the subacromial bursa and the insertion of the supraspinatus tendon), and over the acromioclavicular joint, the anterior capsule overlying the humeral head, and the long head of the biceps tendon lying in the bicipital groove. Search for tender areas that may serve as "trigger points" for pain that is difficult to localize. Such areas include the medial border of the scapula and the upper trapezius as well as the ligaments joining the transverse processes of the lower cervical vertebrae.

E. STERNUM

Palpate along the sternal border at the sternoclavicular and costosternal junctions, as well as over the sternomanubrial junction.

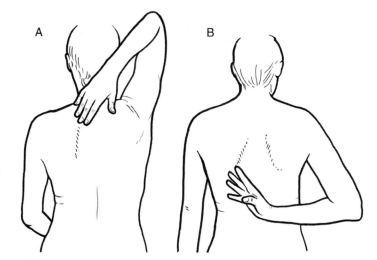

Figure 1–5. Examination of the shoulder. To test external rotation and abduction of the shoulder, ask the patient to reach behind the back and touch the top of the opposite scapula (**A**). To examine internal rotation and adduction ask the patient to reach behind the back and touch the inferior aspect of the shoulder (**B**).

F. TEMPOROMANDIBULAR JOINTS

Place index fingers in front of the patient's ears below the zygomatic arch (or insert the tips of the fifth fingers in the ear canals) and have the patient open and close his or her mouth. Assess for asymmetric or painful motion, tenderness, or crepitus. Inability to fully open the jaw (about three fingerbreadths or 5 cm between the teeth) may reflect tightening of the skin (as in scleroderma), dysfunction of muscles of mastication, or an abnormality of the temporomandibular joint.

G. NECK

Palpate the cervical spinous processes and paraspinal muscles for tenderness and assess range of motion in all directions. Approximately 50% of cervical flexion and extension occurs at the atlantooccipital joint; 50% involves the remaining lower vertebrae. Normal flexion brings the chin to within a fingerbreadth of the chest. Normal extension permits an imaginary vertical line to be drawn between the outer canthus of the eye, the ear lobe, and the shoulder (Figure 1–6). The atlantoaxial articulation and the lower cervical vertebrae contribute equally to cervical rotation, normally about 75 degrees. Lateral bending, normally about 45 degrees, involves all of the cervical vertebrae.

H. HIPS

With the patient supine and the leg extended, check abduction and adduction of the hip. Test flexion by bringing the patient's fully flexed knee as close as possible to the abdomen. To assess rotation, position the leg vertically with the knee directly over the hip and flexed to about 90 degrees. Swing the foot from right to left; normal rotation is approximately 45 degrees (Figure 1–7). It is important to compare both hips; remember that women tend to be more flexible than men and that flexibility tends to diminish with age. To bring out a subtle flexion contracture of the hip, have the patient grasp his or her opposite knee and bring it to the chest. This flattens the lumbar lordosis, and the thigh on the affected side will rise from the table. Palpate for tender areas, particularly over the anterior hip and along the posterior aspect of the greater trochanter. Tenderness in this latter region may arise from the trochanteric bursa or from nearby tendons. To elicit pain in the SI joint, press down on the supine patient's iliac crests, or fully abduct and externally rotate the flexed hip. These maneuvers will cause pain in the buttock on the affected side.

I. KNEES

Examine the knee for swelling, being careful not to mistake infrapatellar fat for hypertrophied synovium. Look for an effusion by alternately squeezing the suprapatellar and infrapatellar aspects of the knee with each hand. To demonstrate a small effusion, rub several times along the medial patellofemoral junction in a cephalad direction to "milk" the fluid into the lateral side. Then, gently press the superolateral aspect of the knee and watch for fluid to bulge out on the medial aspect. Check the popliteal fossa for swelling of the gastrocnemius-semimembranous bursa (Baker cyst).

Look for atrophy of the distal quadriceps muscle, an early indicator of inflammation or pain in the knee. Test flexion and extension while placing a hand on the patella to detect crepitus. With the knee flexed, check for tenderness medially and laterally over the femoral condyles and tibial plateaus and tubercle and along the

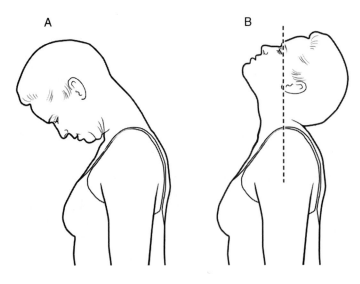

Figure 1–6. Flexion and extension of the cervical spine. Normal flexion brings the chin to within a fingerbreadth of the chest (**A**). With normal extension of the neck, an imaginary line should connect the eye, ear lobe, and shoulder (**B**).

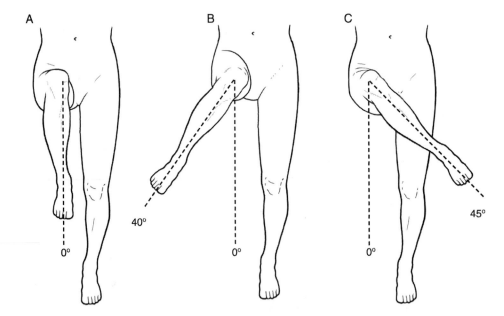

Figure 1–7. Internal and external rotation of the hip. The patient is positioned supine with the both the hip and knee flexed to 90 degrees (**A**). To test internal rotation, the examiner swings the foot outward with one hand while keeping the knee positioned over the hip with the other hand (**B**). Normal external rotation is approximately 40 degrees. To test external rotation, the examiner swings the foot inward while keeping the knee positioned over the hip (**C**). Normal external rotation is 45 degrees. (From Polley HF, Hunder GS. *Rheumatologic Interviewing and Physical Examination of the Joints.* 2nd ed. WB Saunders, 1978, Figure 12–8. With permission.)

joint articulations, collateral ligaments, and infrapatellar tendon. Tenderness 2–3 cm inferior to the medial tibial plateau may indicate inflammation in the anserine bursa.

With the knee extended and relaxed, move the patella from side to side while applying firm pressure downward toward the table; pain or crepitus indicates patellofemoral disease. However, a more sensitive indicator of such disease is the **patellar inhibition test,** performed by pressing downward on the upper patellar border while at the same time pushing the patella toward the feet. Even with mild patellofemoral arthritis, pain will occur when the patient contracts his or her quadriceps muscle (elicited by asking the patient to lift the leg while keeping the knee extended) and the patella moves under the examiner's fingers.

For suspected recurrent patellar subluxation, push the relaxed patella laterally and note whether the patient actively resists or appears anxious (positive "anxiety sign"). Check for laxity of the medial and lateral collateral ligaments by first having the patient flex the knee slightly to loosen the posterior joint capsule. Then, press the lateral femoral condyle while applying valgus force to the lower leg. Excessive motion or a palpable gap along the medial joint line indicates laxity of the medial collateral ligament. Repeat this maneuver in the opposite direction to test the lateral collateral ligament. Finally, with the knee in slight flexion, check for laxity of the anterior cruciate ligament by pulling the upper tibia in the anterior direction; push backward to test the posterior cruciate ligament. Excessive motion in either direction is a positive **drawer sign.**

J. FEET AND ANKLES

Evaluate these areas first with the patient standing (ie, during the initial part of the examination). From behind the patient, check for excessive pronation (outward turning) of the foot by noting the amount of lateral slope of the heel. Note also any loss of the normal longitudinal arch. With the patient supine, palpate the areas around the malleoli for tenderness, synovial thickening, or effusion. Check the calcaneal insertion of the Achilles tendon for nodules or tenderness. Also, look for tenderness at the insertion of the plantar aponeurosis into the medial plantar surface of the calcaneus. Dorsiflex and plantarflex the ankle. Pain or limitation of motion indicates disease in the tibiotalar joint. To test the subtalar joint, bring the foot into the neutral position to stabilize the talus; then invert and evert the ankle.

Palpate the midfoot for tarsal tenderness. Squeeze the forefoot at the level of the metatarsal heads. If this causes pain, press each metatarsal head from above and below to elicit tenderness. Metatarsophalangeal swelling is sometimes manifested by widening of the space between adjacent toes. For a suspected Morton neuroma, press between the metatarsal heads from the plantar surface with a blunt object, such as a pencil eraser. Such lesions occur most commonly between the third and fourth metatarsals.

REFERENCES

Hoppenfeld S. *Physical Examination of the Spine and Extremities.* Appleton-Century-Crofts, 1976. (A superbly illustrated treatise on physical examination of the musculoskeletal system. Contains countless "pearls.")

McCarty D. Differential diagnosis of arthritis: analysis of signs and symptoms. In: Koopman W, ed. *Arthritis and Allied Conditions.* 14th ed. Lippincott Williams and Wilkins, 2001:39-50. (An easy-to-read description of important symptoms and physical findings in rheumatic diseases by a master rheumatologist. Includes illustrations of normal joint range of motion.)

Polley H, Hunder G. *Rheumatologic Interviewing and Physical Examination of the Joints.* 2nd ed. WB Saunders, 1978. (A timeless, well-illustrated textbook describing the musculoskeletal examination.)

Sack K, Miller C. Examining adults and children for rheumatic disease. *J Musculoskel Med.* 1986;3(5):19-30; 3(6):14-20. (A step-by-step approach to the musculoskeletal examination.)

Aspiration & Joint Injection

2

Kenneth H. Fye, MD

ESSENTIAL FEATURES

- *Joint aspiration and synovial fluid analysis are essential to the diagnoses of microcrystalline and infectious forms of arthritis.*
- *Glucocorticoid injections are often the swiftest means of providing relief to patients with inflamed joints.*
- *Aspiration should be performed with the joint positioned to maximize intra-articular pressure, allowing easier withdrawal of synovial fluid.*
- *The four major components of synovial fluid analysis are assessment of fluid clarity and color, cell count, crystals, and culture.*
- *Culture is more sensitive than Gram stain for identifying an infection. Thus, sending fluid for culture takes priority over Gram stain when a limited quantity of synovial fluid is available.*

Joint aspiration and synovial fluid analysis are essential tools in the diagnosis of arthritic conditions. Local injection of therapeutic agents into articular or periarticular structures can lead to rapid decreases in pain and inflammation without many of the side effects associated with systemic medications. The removal of inflammatory cells and destructive enzymes from an inflamed joint may decrease the likelihood of permanent articular damage. As with any diagnostic or therapeutic procedure, success depends on the expertise of the clinician.

Diagnostic Indications for Aspiration

Aspiration and synovial fluid analysis are most crucial in the initial evaluation of an acute monarticular arthritis because of the importance of ruling out septic arthritis. A septic joint signals the presence of a life-threatening illness. Without immediate and aggressive antibiotic therapy, a bacterial infection can lead rapidly to joint destruction and long-term disability. Analysis of synovial fluid from a septic joint usually reveals white blood cell (WBC) counts of 100,000/µL or higher,

with greater than 95% polymorphonuclear leukocytes. Gram stain, culture, and sensitivity studies are essential to the selection of appropriate antibiotic therapy.

A. DIFFERENTIAL DIAGNOSIS

The major differential diagnoses in patients with monarticular arthritis are the crystal-induced arthropathies, particularly gout. In gout, examination of synovial fluid with a polarized light microscope will reveal uric acid crystals in 80–90% of patients; gout can also—albeit rarely—result in WBC counts of up to 100,000/µL. Even when crystals are identified, it is important to obtain culture and sensitivity studies because superinfections can occur in patients with gouty arthropathy. Severe trauma can lead to an acute monoarthritis as a result of bleeding into a joint. In such cases, arthrocentesis will reveal a hemarthrosis.

Even degenerative arthritis can sometimes appear clinically as a monarticular process. Although the monoarthritis in these cases is not usually inflammatory, arthrocentesis may be necessary to exclude indolent infections. Arthrocentesis plays a significant diagnostic role in other, less common causes of monarticular disease, including malignancy (either primary in the joint or as a result of metastasis), pigmented villonodular synovitis, and clotting disorders with recurrent hemarthrois.

Synovial fluid analysis is often the only way to make the distinction between a noninflammatory polyarticular disease, such as osteoarthritis, and inflammatory polyarticular conditions, such as rheumatoid or psoriatic arthritis. In addition, some crystal-induced arthritides, such as calcium pyrophosphate dihydrate deposition disease (CPPD) or oxalosis, may present as polyarticular disease.

B. CLASSES OF SYNOVIAL FLUID

The four classes of synovial fluid are described in Table 2–1. The classes are differentiated by characteristics that define inflammation.

Class I (noninflammatory) fluid is transparent with a color ranging from clear to yellow, has a high viscosity, and has a normal string test. The WBC count is 2000/µL (normal synovial fluid has < 200/µL), and < 25% are polymorphonuclear leukocytes. Gram stain and culture and sensitivity studies are all negative. Class I synovial fluid is typical of osteoarthritis.

Table 2–1. Classes of synovial fluid.

	Class I (Noninflammatory)	Class II (Inflammatory)	Class III (Septic)	Class IV (Hemorrhagic)
Color	Clear/yellow	Yellow/white	Yellow/white	Red
Clarity	Transparent	Translucent/opaque	Opaque	Opaque
Viscosity	High	Variable	Low	NA
Mucin clot	Firm	Variable	Friable	NA
White blood cell count	< 2000/μL	2000–75,000/μL[a]	> 100,000/μL	NA
Differential	< 25% PMNs	> 50% PMNs	> 95% PMNs	NA
Culture	Negative	Negative	Positive	Variable

[a]In rare instances the count may be as high as 100,000/μL.
NA, not applicable; PMNs, polymorphonuclear leukocytes.
Reprinted from *The Primer on the Rheumatic Diseases,* 12th ed., with permission of the Arthritis Foundation.

Class II (inflammatory) synovial fluid ranges from translucent to opaque and is yellow or white. The WBC count generally ranges from 2000 to 75,000/μL although in rare instances counts may range up to 100,000/μL. More than 50% are polymorphonuclear leukocytes. Gram stain and culture and sensitivity studies are negative. Class II synovial fluid is characteristic of all of the autoimmune arthropathies, such as rheumatoid arthritis and systemic lupus erythematosus; the spondyloarthropathies; the crystal-induced arthropathies; postinfectious arthropathies; indolent infections; and a variety of noninfectious arthropathies that are not easily categorized (Table 2–2).

Class III (septic) synovial fluid is opaque and yellow (sometimes white) with a low viscosity. WBC counts are generally > 100,000/μL, although counts as low 50,000/μL are not uncommon. Gram stain, culture, and sensitivity studies may all be positive. Class III synovial fluid is typical of bacterial joint infections.

Class IV (hemorrhagic) fluid is red and opaque. Culture is negative except in patients with tuberculosis. Class IV synovial fluid is typical of trauma, tuberculo-

Table 2–2. Diagnosis by synovial fluid class.

Class I	Class II	Class III	Class IV
Osteoarthritis	RA	Bacterial arthritis	Trauma
Traumatic	SLE		Pigmented villonodular synovitis
Osteonecrosis	Poly/dermatomyositis		Tuberculosis
Charcot arthropathy	Scleroderma		Tumor
	Systemic necrotizing vasculitides		Coagulopathy
	Polychondritis		Charcot arthropathy
	Gout		
	CPPD		
	Hydroxyapatite deposition disease		
	Juvenile RA		
	Ankylosing spondylitis		
	Psoriatic arthritis		
	Reactive arthritis		
	Chronic inflammatory bowel disease		
	Hypogammaglobulinemia		
	Sarcoidosis		
	Rheumatic fever		
	Indolent/low virulence infections (viral, mycobacterial, fungal, Whipple disease, Lyme arthritis)		

RA, rheumatoid arthritis; SLE, systemic lupus erythematosus; CPPD, calcium pyrophosphate dihydrate deposition disease.
Reprinted from *The Primer on the Rheumatic Diseases,* 12th ed., with permission of the Arthritis Foundation.

sis, pigmented villonodular synovitis, neoplasia, coagulopathies, and Charcot arthropathy.

Therapeutic Indications for Aspiration or Injection

The response to joint injection can have diagnostic implications. For example, in patients with equivocal low back or hip pain, injection of lidocaine into the hip or epidural space will enable the clinician to determine the source of the pain. If injection of the hip alleviates the pain, the hip is probably the source of the problem. If an epidural injection alleviates the symptoms, the pain is probably the result of back disease.

A. ASPIRATION

The removal of synovial fluid from an acutely inflamed joint may provide significant benefit. This is particularly true in infected joints, from which removal of synovial fluid will decrease intra-articular synovial pressure, the number of activated inflammatory cells, and the concentration of destructive enzymes and cytokines that can damage articular and periarticular structures. Septic joints may need to be aspirated daily to prevent reaccumulation of inflammatory synovial fluid. Removing blood from a hemarthrosis may also be beneficial. A significant collection of blood may increase intra-articular pressure, thereby stretching periarticular supporting structures and resulting in subsequent joint laxity. Intra-articular blood can also lead to the development of adhesions, eventually resulting in decreased range of motion.

B. INJECTION

A number of locally injected pharmacologic agents have been used in the treatment of rheumatic disorders. Local glucocorticoids in conjunction with lidocaine are valuable in the treatment of the arthritic conditions. Joints, tenosynovium, bursae, soft tissue tender points (such as the medial and lateral epicondyles in tennis or golfer elbow or the lateral thigh in meralgia paresthetica), and even the epidural space can be injected with a reasonable expectation of benefit. Although most target tissues can be injected without radiographic help, it is always wise to inject the hip or the epidural space under computed tomographic guidance to ensure that the medication is delivered to the proper tissue space. In refractory septic arthritis that does not respond to systemic antibiotics and serial aspirations, surgical drainage and washing with local antibiotics are indicated. The injection of any of a variety of hyaluronic acid preparations into a joint, although expensive, has been shown to be of short-term benefit in the treatment of osteoarthritis.

Technique

A. EQUIPMENT

The specific procedure and size of the joint will determine the size of the syringe needed for aspiration. Syringes 3 mL and smaller are usually adequate for injecting lidocaine and glucocorticoids into a peripheral target. Three- to 10-mL syringes are preferred for aspiration of small joints, and 10- to 20-mL syringes are best for intermediate joints, such as the elbow or ankle (Figure 2–1). For larger joints, such as the knee or glenohumeral joint, or when copious amounts of synovial fluid must be aspirated, a 60-mL syringe may be more appropriate. When using a large syringe, it is important to break the vacuum in the syringe before introducing it into the joint. Aspiration should be performed slowly to avoid generating significant negative pressure that can draw synovial tissue into the opening of the needle and actually prevent adequate withdrawal of fluid. To aspirate ≥ 100 mL from an arthritic joint, several large syringes or a stopcock on the end of a syringe may be used. If using several syringes, a Kelly clamp can stabilize the needle (which can be left in place) while the syringes are changed.

The size of the needle also depends on the procedure. Needles as small as 25 or 30 gauge are most appropriate for injecting lidocaine into articular or periarticular structures before aspiration or for injecting glucocorticoids into small joints. A 25-gauge needle also can be used to aspirate synovial fluid or periarticular interstitial fluid from small, acutely inflamed joints, such as the first metatarsophalangeal joint in podagra. A 1.5-inch, 22-gauge needle is useful for injecting large joints, such as the knee, or deep structures, such as the supraspinatus tendon (see Figure 2–1) and trochanteric bursa. These 22-gauge needles also can be used to aspirate small joints, but 19- or 20-gauge needles are indicated for the aspiration of large joints, joints with large amounts of synovial fluid, or joints or cysts with inspissated synovial fluid.

Gloves are important in protecting the clinician from the patient's body fluids. With proper antiseptic technique, the likelihood of an infection after an aspiration or injection is so low that sterile gloves are not generally necessary. Usually the clinician simply marks the injection target with a ballpoint pen, applies appropriate antisepsis, and then proceeds using nonsterile gloves. Sterile gloves are indicated only if the anatomy is equivocal and the clinician must reexamine the procedure site after prepping the area with povidone-iodine.

Joint infection after aspiration or injection is extremely rare, but the possibility of complication must always be minimized. Povidone-iodine should be applied to the arthrocentesis site and allowed to dry. An alcohol swab then should be used to wipe off the excess

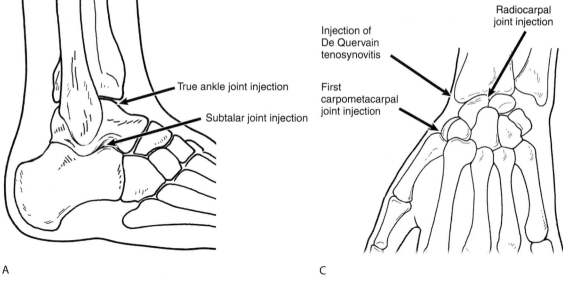

True ankle joint injection

Subtalar joint injection

A

Radiocarpal joint injection

Injection of De Quervain tenosynovitis

First carpometacarpal joint injection

C

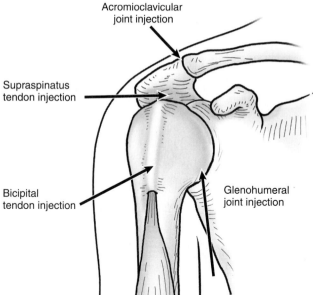

Acromioclavicular joint injection

Supraspinatus tendon injection

Bicipital tendon injection

Glenohumeral joint injection

B

Figure 2–1. **A:** Lateral view of the ankle. **B:** Anterior view of the shoulder. **C:** Dorsum of the left wrist.

to prevent skin irritation in those patients sensitive to iodine or iodine derivatives. It is also appropriate to use an alcohol swab for hemostasis after the procedure.

B. MEDICATIONS

Many clinicians use ethyl chloride to numb the skin before the procedure. However, this technique is somewhat cumbersome and of equivocal benefit. The value of ethyl chloride is its cooling effect on cutaneous pain

fibers. A similar effect may be achieved with the use of refrigerated needles, which in plastic surgery has been reported to be less painful for the injection of local anesthesia.

Lidocaine (1–2%, without epinephrine) is a safe and effective local anesthetic, and 5–10 mg should be injected into the capsule and periarticular supporting structures before aspiration is attempted. Aspiration without benefit of anesthesia can be quite painful. Because serial aspirations may be necessary in the treatment of arthritic conditions, the clinician should attempt to make the first aspiration as painless as possible. A similar amount of lidocaine should be drawn up with the glucocorticoids to be injected. This will provide anesthesia as the glucocorticoids are being injected into the target tissue. Single-dose vials of lidocaine, although more costly, are less likely to be contaminated.

Local injections are an efficient way to administer high concentrations of glucocorticoids directly into target tissues, maximizing the desired anti-inflammatory effects of the medication and minimizing the many unpleasant side effects associated with systemic glucocorticoids. Glucocorticoids can be injected with reasonable expectation of clinical benefit into joints, synovial cysts, peritendinous structures, bursal sacs, ligamentous attachments, tender points, and periarticular tissues. Patients should be aware that injection of local glucocorticoids, although frequently helpful, is not always curative. The long-term efficacy of the procedure depends in large part on the nature of the underlying problem.

Several preparations of glucocorticoids are available. Dexamethasone can be obtained in a crystalloid solution, dissolved in lidocaine. It is short acting and less likely to lead to atrophy, even when injected into soft tissues. Both dexamethasone and triamcinolone are available as colloidal suspensions. These suspensions remain in target tissues longer and may be more effective in the treatment of chronic inflammatory processes. However, they are more likely to lead to atrophy or cutaneous pigment changes when injected into superficial structures, such as the lateral epicondyle in the treatment of lateral epicondylitis. Some very stable (and therefore extremely long-acting) agents, such as triamcinolone, should be used only for the injection of large joints or deep structures, because of the possibility of atrophy of superficial tissues. Repeat glucocorticoid injections should be administered judiciously. Too many injections sometimes lead to laxity of the periarticular supporting structures, soft tissue atrophy, or bone dissolution. No solid data provide guidance on which to base definitive recommendations. However, a single joint or soft tissue target probably should not be injected more than three times a year.

Several preparations of injectable hyaluronic acid are available. Evidence suggests that a series of three injections of hyaluronic acid into an affected joint (particularly the knee) in a patient with degenerative arthritis can give short-term relief of pain equal to the response observed in patients receiving glucocorticoid injections into the joint. However, 6 months after injection, no significant difference in pain or function was noted among groups of patients receiving hyaluronic acid, glucocorticoids, or placebo. Although no difference has been reported in the long-term clinical benefits of hyaluronic acid and glucocorticoid injections, the cost difference is significant. The prohibitive expense of a series of hyaluronic acid injections makes glucocorticoid injection the preferable therapeutic modality.

C. APPROACH

Aspiration of a joint should be performed with the joint positioned to maximize intra-articular pressure, allowing easier withdrawal of synovial fluid. Intra-articular pressure is usually highest at maximum extension or flexion. For example, in the knee, the intra-articular pressure is highest when the knee is in full extension (Figure 2–2). Conversely, joint injection (without aspiration) is performed most easily with the joint semi-flexed to minimize intra-articular pressure. The simplest approach for a knee injection is to seat the patient on an examining table, with the leg dangling down and the knee flexed at a 90-degree angle. This flexed position minimizes intra-articular pressure. Gravity pulls the lower leg down, thus opening the joint and facilitating introduction of the needle. The best position for aspiration alone or with injection depends on the anatomy of the specific target joint.

The best approach for aspiration or injection of soft tissues also depends on the anatomy of the target. Aspiration or injection of the olecranon or prepatellar bursae is performed most effectively with the elbow or knee in full flexion, thereby maximizing intrabursal pressure. Positioning is less important when injecting ligaments or tendinous attachments, such as the lateral epicondyle in tennis elbow (Figure 2–3), because the target is a tissue plane or area of swelling, nodularity, tenderness, or pain, rather than a distinct structure. When treating tendinitis, the target tissue is the tendon sheath, not the tendon itself.

Care must be taken *not* to inject against resistance, because an unusual degree of resistance may indicate that the tip of the needle is in the tendon. Injection directly into an inflamed tendon may increase the likelihood of tendon rupture.

D. DIFFICULTY IN OBTAINING ADEQUATE SAMPLES

On occasion, initial efforts at aspiration may fail to produce an adequate sample of synovial fluid. This may occur because the needle is not in the joint space, and simple repositioning of the needle may result in a successful aspiration. If the needle is properly positioned but the synovial fluid is too viscous to be withdrawn easily, a larger-gauge needle must be used.

Sometimes chronic inflammatory arthritis results in the formation of loculations that make adequate joint

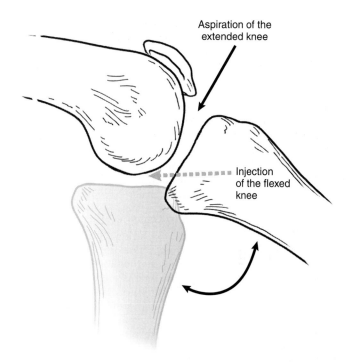

Figure 2–2. Lateral view of the knee.

drainage difficult. In such cases, arthroscopic surgery should be considered.

In some attempts at aspiration, synovial fluid flows easily at first and then stops. This may be the result of too much negative pressure and can be resolved either by slowing the rate of fluid withdrawal or by using a smaller syringe.

Synovial fluid debris can easily clog the needle. The needle can be cleared by reinjecting a small amount of synovial fluid from the syringe; aspiration is then resumed.

When enough synovial fluid has been removed to significantly lower intra-articular pressure, aspiration becomes increasingly difficult. In aspiration from the

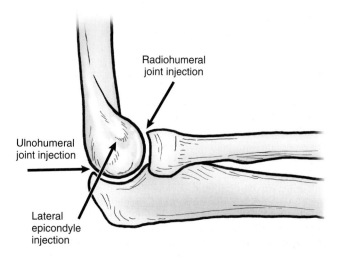

Figure 2–3. Lateral view of the elbow flexed to 90 degrees.

knee, an assistant can apply external pressure to the joint, thereby increasing intra-articular pressure and facilitating the aspiration.

Synovial Fluid Analysis

A. CLARITY AND COLOR

Examination of the synovial fluid begins with a visual determination of clarity and color. Although various crystals (such as monosodium urate, calcium pyrophosphate dihydrate, and hydroxyapatite), lipids, and even cellular debris may affect clarity, the major determinant of synovial fluid clarity and color is the cell count. Noninflammatory fluid, such as that associated with osteoarthritis, has a low cell count and is clear. Synovial fluid from moderately inflammatory forms of arthritis, such as systemic lupus erythematosus or mild rheumatoid arthritis, has higher cell counts and is translucent and yellow. Fluid from intensely inflammatory processes, such as septic joints or crystal-induced arthropathies, has very high cell counts and is opaque and white to yellow. Bleeding into a joint leads to a hemarthrosis with characteristic opaque, red synovial fluid (see Table 2–1).

The physical characteristics of synovial fluid depend largely on the integrity of the hyaluronan and lubricin produced by synoviocytes. The WBCs in inflammatory arthritis release activated enzymes that digest the hyaluronan, decreasing the high viscosity typical of normal synovial fluid. A single drop of normal synovial fluid expressed from a needle will form a "tail" or "string" that will stretch to 10 cm before surface tension is broken. Increasing degrees of inflammation lead to higher cell counts, greater concentrations of activated enzymes in the synovial fluid, lower concentrations of intact hyaluronan, and shorter strings. Inflammatory synovial fluid may have a string test of only 5 cm or shorter.

B. CELL COUNT

The WBC count and differential are among the most valuable pieces of information derived from synovial fluid. Normal synovial fluid has < 200 cells/μL, most of which are mononuclear. In contrast, synovial fluid from patients with noninflammatory arthritis may contain up to 2000 cells/μL, almost half of which may be polymorphonuclear leukocytes. Cell counts in mildly inflammatory synovial fluid, such as that from a patient with systemic lupus erythematosus or mild reactive arthritis, generally range from 2000 to 30,000 cells/μL.

Cell counts may be as high as 50,000 cells/μL in rheumatoid arthritis or a destructive seronegative arthropathy such as psoriatic arthritis. In crystal-induced arthropathies, cell counts of 30,000–50,000 cells/μL are typical, but ≥ 100,000 cells/μL are sometimes observed. Early or partially treated bacterial or chronic infections, such as those caused by mycobacteria or fungi, may have cell counts as low as 50,000 cells/μL. Patients with chronic inflammatory arthritides, such as rheumatoid or psoriatic arthritis or the crystal-induced arthropathies, are more susceptible to bacterial superinfection. A Gram stain and culture and sensitivity studies should be performed on synovial fluid from any patient in whom infection is suspected, even when accompanied by a history of known nonseptic chronic inflammatory arthritis.

C. CRYSTALS

Crystal analysis is best performed with a fresh wet preparation with a clean slide and cover slip. Synovial fluid analysis for crystals is performed under polarized light. The strength of birefringence and shape of the crystals are helpful in distinguishing among the different forms of microcrystalline disease.

- Monosodium urate crystals are needle-shaped and strongly birefringent (ie, bright and easily seen under the microscope). In rare instances, monosodium urate crystals will form negatively birefringent spherules.
- Calcium pyrophosphate dihydrate crystals are rhomboid and weakly birefringent (ie, dim and sometimes difficult to detect even under the polarized microscope).
- Calcium oxalate crystals can be seen in patients with primary oxalosis or in renal failure. These crystals are rod- or tetrahedron-shaped and positively birefringent.
- Cholesterol crystals are rectangular and tend to have notched corners. Lipids form spherules with birefringence in the shape of a Maltese cross. Because the arms of the cross that parallel the slow axis of vibration of the red compensator are blue, these spherules are positively birefringent.
- Hydroxyapatite crystals are not birefringent and form amorphous clumps that stain red with alizarin red S.
- Glucocorticoids from previous joint injections, talc from gloves, and even debris can form birefringent crystals and lead to mistaken diagnoses of microcrystalline disease.

The presence of intracellular crystals in synovial fluid inflammatory cells is diagnostic of a crystal-induced arthropathy. However, this diagnosis does not rule out infection, so it is always wise to culture the fluid from an acute monarticular arthritis even when crystals are identified. In addition, a patient may have more than one crystal-induced arthropathy. Fifteen percent of patients with gout also have CPPD. Appropriate short- and long-term therapies depend on proper diagnosis. A superinfected gouty joint will require aggressive antibiosis as well as anti-inflammatory therapy. A patient with gout and CPPD may require long-term anti-inflammatory therapy and a hypouricemic agent.

When aspirating a small joint, such as the first metatarsophalangeal joint, it is important to remember that monosodium urate crystals can be identified in interstitial fluid. Even when synovial fluid cannot be drawn into the syringe, negative pressure maintained as the needle is withdrawn will allow enough interstitial fluid for crystal analysis to be pulled into the needle. The needle is then removed, the syringe is filled with air, the needle is replaced, and the air is used to express the contents of the needle onto a slide. The small amount of material obtained is often enough to allow detection of monosodium urate crystals.

D. CULTURE

Any inflammatory monarticular arthritis must be considered infectious until proven otherwise. The best way to rule out infection is Gram stain and culture and sensitivity studies of synovial fluid. Microbiologic analysis usually is performed on fluid collected into a sterile tube. However, if the aspiration is difficult, material in the needle may be expressed onto a swab and sent for culture and sensitivity studies. It is important to remember that many significant pathogens are difficult to culture. For example, two thirds of patients with gonococcal arthritis have negative cultures, even when the specimen is cultured directly onto chocolate agar. Tuberculosis and other mycobacterial infections, fungal infections, and anaerobic infections are difficult to detect from synovial fluid analysis, and diagnosis may depend on synovial biopsy. Because septic arthritis can be so quickly destructive, it is wise to initiate antibiotic therapy based on the clinical picture, WBC count, differential, and Gram stain and, if necessary, make subsequent appropriate adjustments in therapy based on culture and sensitivity study results.

Synovial Biopsy

Sometimes an arthritic condition cannot be diagnosed by synovial fluid analysis. Diagnoses of indolent infections or noninfectious forms of granulomatous arthritis (such as sarcoidosis) usually require synovial biopsy. Although synovial fluid cytologic studies can sometimes reveal the presence of malignant cells, neoplastic arthritic conditions are usually diagnosed by histologic analysis of synovial biopsy material. Finally, a host of infiltrative, metabolic, or presumably infectious disorders, such as amyloidosis, ochronosis, hemochromatosis, Wilson disease, and Whipple disease, that can affect the joints are difficult to detect by synovial fluid analysis but easily recognized by synovial biopsy.

REFERENCES

American College of Rheumatology Ad Hoc Committee on Clinical Guidelines. Guidelines for the initial evaluation of the adult patient with acute musculoskeletal symptoms. *Arthritis Rheum.* 1996;39:1. [PMID: 8546717]

Gatter RA, Schumacher HR Jr. *A Practical Handbook of Joint Fluid Analysis.* 2nd ed. Lea & Febiger, 1991.

Shmerling RH. Synovial fluid analysis: a critical reappraisal. *Rheum Dis Clin North Am.* 1994;20:503. [PMID: 8016423]

Laboratory Diagnosis

John B. Imboden, MD

3

■ AUTOANTIBODIES

METHODS OF DETECTION

A variety of basic assays are used to detect autoantibodies. More than one type of assay may be available for any given autoantibody, and the particular test used may vary from institution to institution. In general, there has been a trend away from labor-intensive tests, such as agglutination assays and countercurrent immunoelectrophoresis, and toward assays amenable to automation, such as nephelometry and enzyme-linked immunoabsorbent assay (ELISA).

Indirect immunofluorescence assays identify autoantibodies reactive with antigens in particular tissues or subcellular compartments (eg, nuclear antigens). Fixed tissue samples or cells are overlaid with patient sera, and the presence of autoantibodies is revealed by staining with a fluorescein-labeled antiserum to human immunoglobulin (Ig).

Agglutination assays identify autoantibodies through the aggregation of particles (eg, latex beads) coated with a defined autoantigen.

Immunodiffusion assays detect the formation of immune complexes in a semisolid support, such as an agar gel. Patient sera and antigen, placed in separate wells in the gel, diffuse toward one another and form a line of precipitation when insoluble immune complexes form. Placing the gel in an electrical field (**countercurrent immunoelectrophoresis**) increases the rate of diffusion and facilitates complex formation.

Nephelometry measures the interaction of antibodies and antigens in solution, detecting immune complex formation by monitoring changes in the scattering of an incident light.

In **ELISA,** sera are incubated with antigens immobilized on a surface. After extensive washing, a detecting antibody (eg, an antiserum to human immunoglobulin) conjugated to an enzyme is added. In the final step, substrate is added, and the product of the enzymatic reaction is measured. There are several modifications of the basic ELISA, but all take advantage of the remarkable sensitivity imparted by the enzymatic readout.

RHEUMATOID FACTOR

Rheumatoid factor is an autoantibody, usually IgM, directed against the Fc region of IgG. The most commonly used methods of detecting rheumatoid factor are latex fixation (using latex beads coated with human IgG) and nephelometry (using human IgG as the target antigen). Both assays primarily detect IgM rheumatoid factors. The results of latex fixation assays are reported as the greatest dilution that retains agglutination activity; in most laboratories, sera with titers of > 1:40 are considered abnormal. Rheumatoid factor measured by nephelometry is quantified in international units, with ≥ 20 IU reported as abnormal in most laboratories. ELISAs for rheumatoid factor are also available but are not in wide use. ELISAs can measure IgG, IgA, and IgM rheumatoid factors.

A. ASSOCIATED CONDITIONS

Despite its name, rheumatoid factor is not specific for rheumatoid arthritis. Positive tests for rheumatoid factor occur in a wide range of autoimmune disorders, inflammatory diseases, and chronic infections (Table 3–1). Also, the prevalence of positive rheumatoid factor tests increases with age; as many as 25% of persons over the age of 65 may test positive. In the absence of disease, the titer for rheumatoid factor is usually low (≤ 1:160). High titer for rheumatoid (≥ 1:640) almost always reflect an underlying disease.

B. INDICATION

Rheumatoid factor should be ordered when there is clinical suspicion of rheumatoid arthritis.

C. INTERPRETATION OF RESULTS

Most series report that 70–90% of patients with rheumatoid arthritis have a positive test for rheumatoid factor. Early in disease, however, the prevalence of a positive rheumatoid factor test is substantially lower (in the range of 50%). Therefore, the sensitivity of the test is lowest when the diagnosis is most likely to be in doubt. A negative test for rheumatoid factor should never be the only reason to rule out the possibility of rheumatoid arthritis, even in the patient with long-standing disease. Because of the large number of disor-

Table 3–1. Disorders associated with a positive test for rheumatoid factor.

Autoimmune Disorders
    Rheumatoid arthritis[a]
    Primary Sjögren syndrome[a]
    Mixed connective tissue disease[a]
    Polymyositis/dermatomyositis
    Scleroderma
    ANCA-associated vasculitis[a]
    Polyarteritis nodosa
    Primary biliary cirrhosis[a]
Chronic Infections
    Subacute bacterial endocarditis[a]
    Tuberculosis
    Leprosy
    Syphilis
    Hepatitis C[a] (with or without mixed cryoglobulinemia)
    Hepatitis B[a]
    Other viral infections
    Parasitic infections
Miscellaneous conditions
    Sarcoidosis
    Idiopathic pulmonary fibrosis
    Silicosis
    Asbestosis
    Malignancy
    Age $\geq$ 65

[a]Prevalence of rheumatoid factor >50% in most series.
ANCA, antineutrophilic cytoplasmic antibodies.

ders associated with rheumatoid factor (see Table 3–1), the value of a positive test for rheumatoid factor depends on the pretest probability of the disease. The combination of arthritis and a positive test for rheumatoid factor is not specific for rheumatoid arthritis and can be seen in patients with systemic lupus erythematosus (SLE), mixed connective tissue disease, systemic vasculitis, polymyositis, dermatomyositis, sarcoidosis, subacute bacterial endocarditis, and viral infections, particularly hepatitis C.

ANTINUCLEAR ANTIBODIES

Antinuclear antibodies (ANA) are autoantibodies directed against histones, double-stranded and single-stranded DNA, ribonucleoprotein (RNP) complexes, and other nuclear components. Current indirect immunofluorescence assays for ANA use HEp-2 cells, a human epithelial cell line, as the source of nuclei and are more sensitive than older tests that used rodent liver and kidney.

Indirect immunofluorescence assays for ANA report the titer of the ANA and the pattern of nuclear staining. In most laboratories, ANA with titers $\geq$ 1:40 are consid-

ered positive. The staining patterns are diffuse or homogeneous (due to antibodies to histone), rim (an uncommon pattern due to antibodies to nuclear envelope proteins and to double-stranded [ds] DNA), speckled (due to antibodies to Sm, RNP, Ro/SS-A, La/SS-B, and other antigens), nucleolar (see the section, Antibodies to Nucleolar Antigens, below), and centromeric. In general, there is a poor correlation between the pattern of the ANA and the identity of the underlying disease. An exception is the centromeric pattern, which has considerable specificity for limited scleroderma (see the section, Anticentromere Antibodies, below). Patients often have antibodies to multiple nuclear components, and the staining pattern of certain autoantibodies (eg, antihistone antibodies) can prevent detection of others. The pattern of the ANA should not preclude, or substitute for, the ordering of more specific tests that are otherwise indicated.

A. Associated Conditions

Positive tests for ANA occur in wide range of conditions, including SLE and other rheumatic diseases, organ-specific autoimmune diseases, lymphoproliferative diseases, and chronic infections (Table 3–2). A

Table 3–2. Conditions associated with positive ANA detected by indirect immunofluorescence assays.

Rheumatic Diseases
    Systemic lupus erythematosus
    Mixed connective tissue disease
    Scleroderma
    Sjögren syndrome
    Rheumatoid arthritis
    Polymyositis
    Dermatomyositis
    Discoid lupus
Organ-Specific Autoimmune Diseases
    Autoimmune thyroid disease
    Autoimmune hepatitis
    Primary biliary cirrhosis
    Autoimmune cholangitis
Other
    Drug-induced lupus[a]
    Asymptomatic drug-induced ANA[a]
    Chronic infections
    Idiopathic pulmonary fibrosis
    Primary pulmonary hypertension
    Lymphoproliferative disorders

[a]Drugs that can induce lupus or positive tests for ANA include procainamide, hydralazine, minocycline, antitumor necrosis factor agents, interferon-α, isoniazid, quinidine, methyldopa, chlorpromazine, quinidine, penicillamine, and anticonvulsants.
ANA, antinuclear antibodies.

number of drugs induce ANA and, less commonly, a lupus-like syndrome (Table 3–2). Low-titer ANA are relatively common among healthy adults; in one analysis, an ANA titer of ≥ 1:40 was seen in 32% of healthy adults and ≥ 1:160 was seen in 5%.

B. INDICATIONS

Testing for ANA by indirect immunofluorescence is a very useful initial laboratory investigation when there is clinical suspicion of SLE, drug-induced lupus, mixed connective tissue disease, or scleroderma. The ANA may provide useful prognostic information for patients with isolated Raynaud phenomenon, identifying those at greater risk for systemic rheumatic disease.

C. INTERPRETATION OF RESULTS

The sensitivity of the immunofluorescent ANA for SLE is very high (> 95%). A negative result, therefore, is very strong evidence against this diagnosis and usually precludes the need to pursue tests for antibodies to specific nuclear antigens (eg, dsDNA, Sm, RNP). A positive ANA test is one of the diagnostic criteria for drug-induced lupus and mixed connective tissue disease. The sensitivity of the ANA for scleroderma is approximately 85%.

In general, the probability of an underlying autoimmune disease increases with the titer of the ANA. Nonetheless, because the specificity of the ANA is limited, the value of a positive test depends on the pretest probability of disease. In the proper clinical context, a positive ANA by immunofluorescence provides supportive evidence of disease and should prompt tests for antibodies to specific nuclear antigens (Table 3–3).

Serial determinations of ANA by immunofluorescence are not useful for monitoring disease activity.

ANTIBODIES TO DEFINED NUCLEAR ANTIGENS

Antibodies to Double-stranded DNA

Antibodies to dsDNA recognize its base pairs, its ribose-phosphate backbone, and the structure of its double helix. ELISA is the most commonly used method to detect antibodies to dsDNA and has largely supplanted the Farr radioimmunoassay and the crithidia immunofluorescence assay, which measures binding to the dsDNA of the protozoan *Crithidia lucilae*.

A. ASSOCIATED CONDITIONS

Antibodies to dsDNA occur in SLE and are rare in other diseases and in healthy persons. When detected outside the context of SLE, antibodies to dsDNA are almost always of low titer. Antibodies to dsDNA do not occur in most forms of drug-induced lupus but have been observed during treatment with penicillamine, minocycline, and antitumor necrosis factor agents.

B. INDICATIONS

Antibodies to dsDNA should be measured when there is clinical suspicion of SLE and the ANA is positive. The yield of testing for anti-dsDNA antibodies is extremely low when ANA are not detected by indirect immunofluorescence on HEp-2 cells. Longitudinal determinations of the levels of antibodies to dsDNA may aid in the analysis of disease activity for patients with known SLE.

Table 3–3. Selected autoantibodies with high sensitivity or specificity for rheumatic diseases.

Condition	High Sensitivity[a]	High Specificity[b]
SLE	ANA	Anti-dsDNA, anti-Sm
Drug-induced lupus	ANA, antihistone[c]	—
Neonatal cutaneous lupus	Maternal anti-Ro/SS-A (90%)	—
Congenital complete heart block	Maternal anti-Ro/SS-A	—
Mixed connective tissue disease	ANA, anti-RNP[d]	—
1° Sjögren	Anti-Ro/SS-A (75%)	—
Limited and diffuse scleroderma	ANA (85%)	Anticentromere
		Anti-Scl-70 and other antinucleolar antibodies
Myositis	—	AntiJo-1 and other antisynthetase antibodies
		Anti-signal recognition particle
		Anti-Mi-2

[a]Sensitivity (probability of a positive test result in a patient with the disease) > 95% except where noted.
[b]Specificity (probability of a negative test result in a patient without the disease) > 95%.
[c]Antihistone antibodies occur in only a minority of cases of minocycline-induced lupus.
[d]The presence of antibodies to RNP is required for diagnosis.
SLE, systemic lupus erythematosus; ANA, antinuclear antibodies.

C. INTERPRETATION OF RESULTS

The specificity of anti-dsDNA antibodies for SLE is 97% overall and approaches 100% when the antibody titer is high. A positive test, therefore, is a very strong argument for the diagnosis of SLE.

Antibodies to dsDNA occur in 60–80% of patients with SLE. Because titers can fluctuate in and out of the normal range over time, the sensitivity of an isolated test for anti-dsDNA antibodies is probably in the range of 50% for SLE. A negative test, therefore, does not argue strongly against the diagnosis of SLE.

Studies of patient populations indicate that the level of anti-dsDNA antibodies correlates with certain manifestations of SLE activity, such as lupus nephritis, but not others, most notably lupus cerebritis. The strength of this relationship, however, varies from patient to patient. For most patients, a rise in antibody titer often precedes—or occurs concomitantly with—a disease flare. However, there are subsets of patients who manifest disease flares in the absence of anti-dsDNA antibodies and others whose disease is quiescent despite elevated levels of this autoantibody.

Antibodies to Sm & RNP

Smith (Sm) and RNP were initially identified as extractable nuclear antigens. Antibodies to Sm recognize nuclear proteins that bind to small nuclear RNAs, forming complexes involved in the processing of messenger RNA. Antibodies to RNP recognize a complex of protein and the small nuclear RNA designated U1. ELISA has largely replaced immunodiffusion assays for the measurement of antibodies to Sm and RNP. Antibodies to Sm or to RNP produce a speckled pattern on indirect immunofluorescence assays for ANA.

A. ASSOCIATED CONDITIONS

Antibodies to Sm are specific for SLE. Antibodies to RNP occur in SLE and mixed connective tissue disease. The prevalence of these autoantibodies in other conditions is very low.

B. INDICATIONS

Antibodies to Sm and RNP should be determined when there is clinical suspicion of SLE or mixed connective tissue disease and the ANA are positive by indirect immunofluorescence.

C. INTERPRETATION OF RESULTS

Antibodies to Sm are highly specific for SLE but occur in only 10–40% of patients. The prevalence of anti-Sm antibodies appears to be lower in white patients than in African American and Asian patients.

Antibodies to RNP occur in 30–40% of patients with SLE. The diagnosis of mixed connective tissue disease requires the presence of antibodies to RNP; by definition, therefore, 100% of patients with this disease have anti-RNP antibodies.

Serial determinations of antibodies to Sm and RNP are not useful for monitoring disease activity.

Antibodies to Ro (SS-A) & La (SS-B)

The Ro (also known as Sjögren syndrome A or SS-A) and La (SS-B or Sjögren syndrome B) antigens are distinct RNP particles. ELISA and immunoblot assays are supplanting the older immunodiffusion assays for detection of anti-Ro and anti-La antibodies. Antibodies to Ro and La produce a speckled pattern on immunofluorescence assays for ANA. When rodent tissues were used for this assay, antibodies to Ro often went undetected and were a cause of "ANA-negative" lupus if these were the dominant autoantibody system. The use of HEp-2 cells enhances detection of anti-Ro antibodies and has led to a decline in the prevalence of ANA-negative lupus.

A. ASSOCIATED CONDITIONS

Antibodies to Ro are uncommon in the normal population and in patients with rheumatic diseases other than Sjögren syndrome and SLE. Antibodies to Ro are present in 75% of patients with primary Sjögren syndrome but only in 10–15% of patients with rheumatoid arthritis and secondary Sjögren syndrome. In SLE, anti-Ro antibodies are present in up to 50% of patients and are associated with photosensitivity, subacute cutaneous lupus, and interstitial lung disease. Transfer of maternal anti-Ro antibodies across the placenta appears to be important in the pathogenesis of neonatal cutaneous lupus and congenital complete heart block (see Table 3–3).

Antibodies to La occur, almost always in association with anti-Ro antibodies, in primary Sjögren syndrome (40–50%), SLE (10–15%), congenital complete heart block (90%), and neonatal cutaneous lupus (70%).

B. INDICATIONS

Antibodies to Ro and La should be measured when there is clinical suspicion of primary Sjögren syndrome or SLE. Even when ANA are not detected by indirect immunofluorescence, testing for anti-Ro antibodies is still indicated for patients with suspected subacute cutaneous lupus or with recurrent photosensitive rashes. Mothers of children with neonatal cutaneous lupus and congenital complete heart block should be tested for antibodies to Ro and La; many of these women are asymptomatic. Testing is also indicated for patients with

SLE who become pregnant or who are planning to become pregnant.

C. INTERPRETATION OF RESULTS

The presence of antibodies to Ro, or to Ro and La, is a strong argument for the diagnosis of Sjögren syndrome in a patient with sicca symptoms. Although not a sensitive test for SLE, a positive test for anti-Ro antibodies can facilitate a diagnosis of subacute cutaneous lupus. Chapter 27 reviews the monitoring of pregnancy in the setting of maternal antibodies to Ro and the evaluation of asymptomatic mothers found to have anti-Ro antibodies.

Anticentromere Antibodies

Antibodies to centromere proteins produce a characteristic pattern of staining in indirect immunofluorescence assays using HEp-2 cells. Anticentromere antibodies can be measured by ELISA, but indirect immunofluorescence is the most commonly used method of detection.

A. ASSOCIATED CONDITIONS

Anticentromere antibodies occur in limited scleroderma and scleroderma. They are very rare in other rheumatic conditions and in healthy persons.

B. INDICATIONS

Anticentromere antibodies should be determined when there is clinical suspicion of scleroderma or its CREST variant (calcinosis, Raynaud phenomenon, esophageal dysmotility, sclerodactyly, telangiectasias).

C. INTERPRETATION OF RESULTS

Anticentromere antibodies occur in approximately 60% of patients with CREST and in 15% of those with scleroderma. The specificity of this test is remarkable (> 98%). A positive test for anticentromere antibodies, therefore, is a very strong argument for the presence of CREST or scleroderma. The presence of anticentromere antibodies early in the course of disease predicts limited cutaneous involvement and a decreased likelihood of interstitial lung disease. Anticentromere antibodies and antibodies to Scl-70 rarely coexist. Serial determinations of anticentromere antibodies are not useful for monitoring disease activity.

ANTIBODIES TO NUCLEOLAR ANTIGENS

Antibodies to Scl-70 (Topoisomerase-I)

Antibodies to Scl-70 (or topoisomerase I) produce nucleolar staining on indirect immunofluorescence and are measured by immunodiffusion assays, immunoblotting, and ELISA.

A. ASSOCIATED CONDITIONS

Antibodies to Scl-70 occur in scleroderma and are rare in patients with other systemic rheumatic diseases and in healthy persons.

B. INDICATIONS

Antibodies to Scl-70 should be measured when there is clinical suspicion of scleroderma.

C. INTERPRETATION OF RESULTS

Immunodiffusion assays identify antibodies to Scl-70 in 20–30% of patients with scleroderma; approximately 40% of patients have antibodies to Scl-70 detectable by immunoblotting or ELISA. The specificity of anti-Scl-70 antibodies approaches 100% for the immunoblotting and immunodiffusion assays. A positive test by these assays, therefore, is a very strong argument for the diagnosis of scleroderma. The specificity of ELISA is not certain but may be lower. The presence of antibodies to Scl-70 has prognostic value in scleroderma and carries an increased likelihood of diffuse skin involvement and of interstitial lung disease. Serial determinations of anti-Scl-70 antibodies are not useful for monitoring the disease.

Antibodies to Other Nucleolar Antigens

Antibodies to nucleolar antigens other than Scl-70 occur in scleroderma. Antibodies with high specificity for scleroderma include anti-RNA polymerase I, anti-RNA polymerase III, anti-U3 small nucleolar RNP (or antifibrillarin), and anti-Th small nucleolar RNP. The low sensitivity of these antibodies limits their usefulness in the diagnosis of scleroderma. Antibodies to RNA polymerase II are present in scleroderma, SLE, and overlap syndromes. Antibodies to PM-Scl occur in scleroderma and in an overlap syndrome of myositis and scleroderma.

ANTIBODIES TO HISTONES

Antibodies to histones usually produce a homogeneous staining on indirect immunofluorescence assays for ANA. Antihistone antibodies are almost always present in lupus induced by drugs such as procainamide, hydralazine, and isoniazid (sensitivity > 95%). An important exception is minocycline-induced lupus; antihistone antibodies are present in only a minority of patients with this disorder. Antibodies to histones are common in SLE (prevalence 50–70%) and occur at low frequency in a range of rheumatic and nonrheumatic disorders. The clinical usefulness of testing for antibodies to histones is limited. Antihistone antibodies are nonspecific and do not distinguish drug-induced lupus from SLE. Although the absence of antihistone antibodies is strong evidence against most forms of drug-induced lupus, the clinical diagnosis of drug-induced lupus is based on the clinical manifestations, a positive test for ANA by indirect immunofluorescence, and resolution of symptoms following withdrawal of the implicated drug.

MYOSITIS-ASSOCIATED ANTIBODIES (See Chapter 25)

Anti-Jo-1 & Other Antisynthetase Antibodies

Autoantibodies against amino acyl-tRNA synthetases occur almost exclusively in inflammatory myositis and can cause cytoplasmic staining when sera are analyzed for ANA by indirect immunofluorescence. The most common of these autoantibodies (anti-Jo-1) is directed against histidyl-tRNA synthetase and is present in 20–30% of the patients with polymyositis. Patients with antisynthetase antibodies tend to have interstitial lung disease, arthritis, mechanic's hands, and Raynaud phenomenon as well as myositis.

Antibodies to Signal Recognition Particle

These antibodies recognize a cytoplasmic RNP, occur in 4% of myositis patients, and are associated with acute onset and severe disease.

Anti-Mi-2 Antibodies

These antibodies are directed against helicase activities and produce homogeneous nuclear staining on indirect immunofluorescence assays for ANA. Anti-Mi-2 antibodies have high specificity for dermatomyositis and occur in 15–20% of patients with that disorder.

ANTINEUTROPHILIC CYTOPLASMIC ANTIBODIES

Antineutrophilic cytoplasmic antibodies (ANCA) are reviewed in Chapter 31.

■ MEASUREMENT OF THE ACUTE PHASE RESPONSE

The acute phase response develops in the setting of a wide range of acute and chronic inflammatory conditions: severe bacterial, viral, or fungal infections; rheumatic and other inflammatory diseases; malignancy; and tissue injury or necrosis. These conditions elicit a response in which interleukin-6 and other cytokines trigger the synthesis by the liver of a variety of plasma proteins, including C-reactive protein (CRP) and fibrinogen. The detection and monitoring of this response can be clinically useful and is accomplished by measuring the level of CRP or by determining the erythrocyte sedimentation rate (ESR), which is influenced by the binding of fibrinogen to erythrocytes. As a general rule, CRP is a more sensitive and accurate reflection of the acute phase response than the ESR.

C-REACTIVE PROTEIN

CRP likely has a physiologic role in the innate immune response to infection and may participate in the clearance of necrotic and apoptotic cells. The availability of highly sensitive assays of CRP has allowed accurate determination of baseline CRP levels and has revealed a correlation between baseline CRP and cardiovascular disease. The median baseline level for young adults is 0.8 mg/L, and the 90th percentile is 3.0 mg/L. The baseline levels of CRP increase with age and with body mass index. Laboratories often offer a choice between a routine CRP assay (suitable for the detection and monitoring of inflammatory disease) and a highly sensitive CRP assay for the determination of cardiac risk.

During the acute phase response, levels of CRP rapidly increase up to 1000-fold, reaching a peak at 48 hours. With resolution of the acute phase response, CRP declines with a relatively short half-life of 18 hours. Because there are a large number of disparate conditions that can induce CRP production, an elevated CRP level does not have diagnostic specificity. An elevated CRP level, however, can provide support for the presence of a clinically suspected inflammatory disease, such as polymyalgia rheumatica or giant cell arteritis, when other objective findings are absent. Values > 10 mg/L are generally thought to indicate clinically significant inflammation. Monitoring CRP levels can provide useful information on the activity of diseases such as rheumatoid arthritis and giant cell arteritis.

Despite their apparent inflammatory nature, scleroderma, polymyositis, and dermatomyositis often elicit little or no CRP response. CRP levels also tend not to be elevated in SLE unless serositis or synovitis is present.

Elevations of CRP in the absence of clinically important inflammation can occur in renal failure.

ERYTHROCYTE SEDIMENTATION RATE

The ESR is determined by allowing anticoagulated blood to sediment for 1 hour in a glass tube (200 mm in length for the commonly used Westergren method; 100 mm for the Wintrobe method). Normal ranges for the ESR are 0–10 mm/h and 0-15 mm/h for men and women, respectively, but the upper limit of normal increases with age and with obesity.

Because fibrinogen and certain other acute phase proteins (not including CRP) bind to erythrocytes and increase their sedimentation rate, the ESR is a measure of the acute phase response. The ESR responds slower (over days) to the onset and resolution of an acute phase response than does the level of CRP, and the dynamic range of the ESR is less than that of CRP. More so than CRP, the ESR can be influenced by factors other than the acute phase response.

The ESR is a useful diagnostic test when there is clinical suspicion of polymyalgia rheumatica or giant cell arteritis; it also is commonly used to monitor the activity of these conditions as well as rheumatoid arthritis. Due to the wide range of disorders associated with an acute phase response, elevations of the ESR have little diagnostic specificity. Transient mild to moderate elevations, moreover, can occur in the absence of other indications of disease. Marked elevations of the ESR (> 100 mm/h by the Westergren method), however, are almost always due to a clinically significant condition, usually infection, malignancy, or rheumatic disease.

The ESR is of very limited value in patients with the nephrotic syndrome or end-stage renal disease because virtually all have an elevated ESR (some > 100 mm/h), probably due to high levels of fibrinogen. Elevations of the ESR in the absence of clinically important inflammation also occur in pregnancy, anemia, erythrocyte macrocytosis, and hypercholesterolemia. Conversely, hypofibrinogenemia, polycythemia, microcytosis, sickle cell disease, and congestive heart failure lower the ESR.

■ MEASUREMENTS OF COMPLEMENT

The Complement System

Complement is a complex system of at least 30 proteins that play key roles in the innate and adaptive immune responses. Effector functions of complement include opsonization, chemotaxis and activation of leukocytes, lysis of bacteria and cells, promotion of antibody responses, and clearance of immune complexes and apoptotic cells. Three enzymatic complement cascades (the classical pathway, the alternative pathway, and the mannose-binding lectin pathway) lead to the generation of a convertase that cleaves C3, releasing C3a (an anaphylatoxin) and producing C3b, which binds to the target surface. C3b, a potent opsonin, forms a complex

that cleaves C5 to C5a (another anaphylatoxin) and C5b, which sequentially binds C6, C7, C8, and C9 to form the membrane attack complex, a channel that can induce osmotic lysis of the target cell.

Indications for Measurements of Complement

Complement should be measured when there is clinical suspicion of a disease that is associated with hypocomplementemia (Table 3–4) or an inherited or acquired abnormality of the complement system (Table 3–5). Complement levels also can be used to monitor the activity of diseases such as SLE. Some components of the complement system, including C3 and C4, are acute phase proteins, and their synthesis increases during the acute phase response. Because the liver synthesizes many complement components, severe hepatic failure can produce hypocomplementemia.

There are three commonly used measurements of complement in clinical practice: the CH50 and determination of the levels of C3 and C4.

A. CH50

The CH50 is a functional assay for the classical pathway (components C1 through C9) of complement activation (Figure 3–1). The test measures the complement-dependent lysis of sheep red blood cells, using patient sera as a source of complement and rabbit antibodies to sheep red blood cells. Units are standardized with a known source of complement and may vary from laboratory to laboratory if the standard reagents differ. Immune complex diseases (see Table 3–4) can lead to the activation of the classical pathway, the depletion of complement components, and a depressed CH50. In general, a reduction in the CH50 requires at least a 50% reduction of one or more components. Because each component of the classical pathway has an essential role in this assay, the CH50 is an excellent screen for defi-

Table 3–4. Immune complex diseases associated with hypocomplementemia.

Systemic lupus erythematosus
Vasculitis
   Hypocomplementemic urticarial vasculitis
   Polyarteritis nodosa (especially hepatitis B-associated)
Glomerulonephritis
   Post-streptococcal
   Membranoproliferative
Cryoglobulinemia (types II and III)
Subacute bacterial endocarditis
Serum sickness

Table 3–5. Clinical syndromes associated with deficiences of components of the classical pathway of complement activation.

Component	Syndrome
Pathway components	
C1q, C4, C2	Lupus-like syndromes
C3	Recurrent pyogenic infections; immune complex glomerulo-nephritis
C5, C6, C7, C8	Recurrent neisserial infections
Regulatory proteins	
C1 inhibitor	Angioedema

ciencies of the classical pathway (Table 3–5). The CH50 is undetectable when there is complete deficiency of any individual component, and a persistently undetectable CH50 should raise the possibility of such a deficiency. Conversely, a detectable CH50 rules out complete deficiency of components of the classical pathway.

B. C4 LEVELS

The concentration of C4 is determined by immunoassay, usually by rate nephelometry. Low levels of C4, or of both C4 and C3, usually reflect activation of the classical pathway by immune complex disease. Deficiency in C1 inhibitor leads to unregulated C1 esterase activity and to depression of C4 levels. Thus, C4 is an excellent screen for C1 inhibitor deficiency and should be performed before more specific (and costly) determinations of C1 inhibitor protein levels and enzymatic activity. Two tandem genes on chromosome 6 encode C4. Although null alleles for these genes are relatively common, complete deficiency of C4 is rare, because four genes encode C4 protein. Partial deficiencies (due to the presence of one, two, or three null alleles) can produce persistently low levels of C4 and predispose to SLE.

C. C3 LEVELS

The concentration of C3 is determined by immunoassay, usually by rate nephelometry. The classical and alternative pathways converge on C3. Depression of both C4 and C3 indicates activation of the classical pathway. A depressed C3 with normal C4 suggests activation of the alternative pathway. Complete deficiency of C3 is rare and usually manifests in childhood as severe, recurrent infections with pyogenic organisms. C3 nephritic factor, an autoantibody associated with membranoproliferative glomerulonephritis and partial lipodystrophy, stabilizes the alternative pathway C3 convertase, leading to dysregulated cleavage of C3 and low levels of C3.

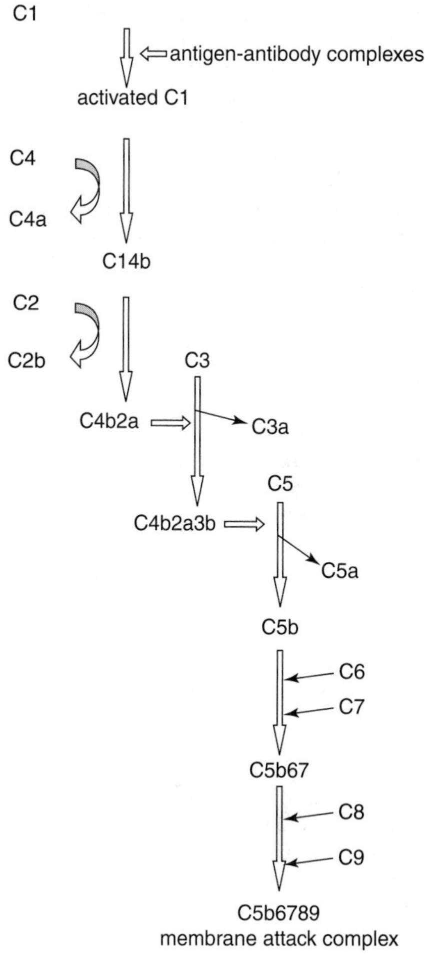

Figure 3–1. Classical pathway of complement activation. Antigen-antibody complexes activate C1 esterase, which acts on C4 and then C2, forming the C3 convertase (C4b2a) that cleaves C3. C4b2a3b acts on C5, releasing C5a and generating C5b, which interacts with C6, C7, C8, and C9 to form the membrane attack complex. (Adapted from Parslow T, Stites D, Terr A, Imboden J, eds. *Medical Immunology.* McGraw-Hill, 2001.)

■ CRYOGLOBULINS

CLASSIFICATION

Cryoglobulins are cold-insoluble immunoglobulins that dissolve on rewarming. The Brouet classification describes three categories.

Type I is a monoclonal immunoglobulin that precipitates in the cold. Type I cryoglobulins are often associated with underlying lymphoproliferative disorders and may cause cold-induced hyperviscosity symptoms if the monoclonal immunoglobulin precipitates at physiologically relevant temperatures.

Type II cryoglobulins are immune complexes composed of a monoclonal immunoglobulin (usually IgMκ) with rheumatoid factor activity and polyclonal IgG. Most cases of type II cryoglobulinemia are associated with chronic hepatitis C infection and manifest clinically as an immune complex–mediated vasculitis with palpable purpura (see Chapter 36).

Type III cryoglobulins are immune complexes composed of polyclonal rheumatoid factor and polyclonal IgG. Type III cryoglobulinemia occurs in hepatitis C, other chronic infections including subacute bacterial endocarditis, and autoimmune diseases such as SLE and rheumatoid arthritis.

MEASUREMENT

Blood to be tested for cryoglobulins is drawn in prewarmed tubes, is allowed to clot at 37 °C, and then is centrifuged at 37 °C; exposure to temperatures lower than 37 °C during these steps can result in a false-negative test due to premature precipitation of the cryoglobulin. The resulting serum is placed at 4 °C for 2–7 days (usually 2–3) and then is examined for a precipitate. A "cryocrit" provides a crude estimate of quantity of cryoglobulin. The highest levels are usually seen in type I cryoglobulinemia, but in general the cryocrit correlates poorly with clinical severity. Analysis of resolubilized cryoglobulins by immunofixation electrophoresis permits classification as type I, II, or III. Positive tests for serum rheumatoid factor are seen in types II and III cryoglobulinemia unless handling of the sample at lower than 37 °C produces a false-negative test. The levels of C4 are frequently low in type II cryoglobulinemia.

REFERENCES

Bathon J, et al. The erythrocyte sedimentation rate in end-stage renal failure. *Am J Kidney Dis.* 1987;10:34. [PMID: 3605082]

Kavanaugh AF, Solomon DH, and the American College of Rheumatology Ad Hoc Committee on Immunologic Testing Guidelines. Guidelines for immunologic laboratory testing in the rheumatic diseases: anti-DNA antibody tests. *Arthritis Rheum.* 2002;47:546. [PMID: 12382306]

Pepys MB, Hirschfield GM. C-reactive protein: a critical update. *J Clin Invest.* 2003;111:1805. [PMID: 12813013]

Reveille JD, Solomon DH, and the American College of Rheumatology Ad Hoc Committee of Immunologic Testing Guidelines. Evidence-based guidelines for the use of immunologic tests: anticentromere, Scl-70, and nucleolar antibodies. *Arthritis Rheum.* 2003;49:399. [PMID: 12794797]

Solomon DH, et al, and the American College of Rheumatology Ad Hoc Committee on Immunologic Testing Guidelines. Evidence-based guidelines for the use of immunologic tests: antinuclear antibody testing. *Arthritis Rheum.* 2002;47:434. [PMID: 12209492]

Sox HC Jr, Liang MH. The erythrocyte sedimentation rate. Guidelines for rational use. *Ann Intern Med.* 1986;104:515. [PMID: 3954279]

Walport MJ. Complement. *N Engl J Med.* 2001;344:1140,1058. [PMID: 11297706, 11287977]

Approach to the Patient with Arthritis

John B. Imboden, MD

4

When evaluating a patient with arthritis, it is important to determine whether the process is acute (presenting within days) or chronic (persisting for weeks or more) and whether it is monarticular, oligoarticular (two to four joints involved), or polyarticular (five or more affected joints). If more than one joint is involved, the arthritis should be characterized as symmetric or asymmetric and as additive or migratory. The distinction between inflammatory and noninflammatory arthritis is critical for accurate diagnosis. The presence of constitutional signs or symptoms and the involvement of other organ systems can be important clues to the correct diagnosis.

INFLAMMATORY VERSUS NONINFLAMMATORY ARTHRITIS

The most reliable means for distinguishing between inflammatory and noninflammatory arthritis is analyzing the white blood cell (WBC) count in the synovial fluid. In inflammatory arthritis, the WBC count is > 2000/μL; in noninflammatory arthritis, the WBC count is < 2000/μL. Arthrocentesis should be performed whenever feasible because, although clinical features and other laboratory investigations also help distinguish inflammatory from noninflammatory arthritis, no single finding is definitive. Patients with an inflammatory arthritis usually complain of pain and stiffness in involved joints; typically these symptoms are worse in the morning or after periods of inactivity (the so-called "gel phenomenon") and improve with mild to moderate activity. On examination, the larger joints can be warm and, when severely inflamed, can have erythema of the overlying skin. Laboratory studies often reveal an elevated erythrocyte sedimentation rate (ESR) and a high C-reactive protein (CRP) level. In contrast, patients with noninflammatory arthritis have pain that worsens with activity and improves with rest. Stiffness is generally mild and usually not a prominent symptom. The ESR and CRP are usually normal.

ACUTE MONOARTHRITIS

 ESSENTIAL FEATURES

- *Bacterial infection, crystal-induced arthritis, and trauma are leading causes of acute monoarthritis.*
- *Septic arthritis is a major concern and must be ruled out.*
- *Arthrocentesis is the most important diagnostic test.*

Initial Clinical Evaluation

The history and physical examination should determine whether the process is acute (onset over hours to days), involves the joint rather than surrounding tissues or bone, and is truly monarticular.

The most common causes of acute monoarthritis are infection, crystal-induced arthritis, and trauma (Table 4–1). In cases of suspected trauma, it is important to ascertain whether the reported trauma is sufficiently severe to account for the joint findings. (Patients with new-onset joint effusions often attribute the joint abnormality to incidental bumps, turns, or other minor trauma.) The foremost concern in evaluating a patient with acute pain and swelling in a single joint that is not

Table 4–1. Common causes
of acute monoarthritis.

• Bacterial infection of the joint space
  Nongonococcal: Especially, *Staphylococcus aureus,*
  β-hemolytic streptococci, *Streptococcus pneumoniae,*
  gram-negative organisms
  Gonococcal: Often preceded by a migratory tenosyno-
  vitis or oligoarthritis associated with characteristic skin
  lesions
• Crystal-induced arthritis
  Gout (monosodium urate crystals)
  Pseudogout (calcium pyrophosphate dihydrate crystals)
• Trauma

---

clearly due to trauma is the possibility of a joint space
infection.

A. Laboratory Evaluation

Arthrocentesis is indicated for all cases of unexplained
acute monoarthritis. Synovial fluid should be sent for
culture (bacterial, mycobacterial, and fungal), WBC
count, and Gram stain and examined for crystals by polarized light microscopy. Determining whether the synovial fluid is inflammatory, noninflammatory, or bloody
guides the initial differential diagnosis.

Polarized light microscopy is a sensitive test for urate
crystals. Calcium pyrophosphate dihydrate crystals are
somewhat more difficult to visualize because of their
weaker birefringence, but their detection should not
present difficulties for the experienced clinician. On the
other hand, Gram staining for bacteria is relatively insensitive (false-negative rates range from 25% to 50%
for nongonococcal septic arthritis and are substantially
higher for gonococcal infections). Thus, the absence of
crystals is a strong argument against microcrystalline
disease, but a negative Gram stain does not exclude infection. Occasionally, infection and microcrystalline
disease coexist; therefore, the finding of crystals in the
synovial fluid does not exclude the possibility of infection.

Properly performed cultures of synovial fluid are a
sensitive test for nongonococcal septic arthritis (positive
in up to 90% of cases). However, synovial fluid cultures
are positive in only 20–50% of cases of gonococcal
arthritis. The diagnosis often depends on identifying
Neisseria gonorrhoeae on culture from the pharynx,
urethra, cervix, or rectum (in aggregate, positive in
80–90%) or, in some cases, on the patient's response to
appropriate antibiotic therapy.

Routine laboratory tests (eg, complete blood cell
count, serum electrolytes and creatinine, and urinalysis)
can provide helpful ancillary information. Blood cultures should be obtained if septic arthritis is suspected.

B. Imaging Studies

Radiographs can demonstrate fractures in cases of trauma
but usually contribute little to the diagnosis of acute
nontraumatic monoarthritis. Occasionally, imaging studies can be misleading. In cases of septic arthritis, for example, radiographs may show evidence of osteoarthritis
or other chronic conditions that predispose to infection
but are not the cause of the acute joint inflammation.

Differential Diagnosis

A. Inflammatory

Differentiating between arthritis caused by infection
and crystal-induced arthritis can be difficult without results from synovial fluid analysis and culture. Patients
with septic arthritis may be afebrile and may not manifest a peripheral leukocytosis. Conversely, patients with
crystal-induced arthritis can have fever and an elevated
peripheral blood WBC count. An elevated serum uric
acid level does not establish a diagnosis of gout, and patients with gout can have a normal serum uric acid level
at the time of an acute attack.

Septic arthritis indicates the presence of a potentially
life-threatening infection. Delaying treatment of nongonococcal septic arthritis can cause substantial morbidity due to the rapid destruction of articular cartilage.
Therefore, acute inflammatory monoarthritis should be
considered septic arthritis until there is compelling evidence either against bacterial infection or in favor of an
alternative diagnosis. When the synovial fluid is highly
inflammatory (WBC count > 50,000/μL) but the
Gram stain and the polarized light microscopy findings
are negative, empiric treatment with antibiotics is prudent until the results of synovial fluid and other cultures are known. Depending on the clinical context,
empiric antibiotic coverage also may be indicated for
unexplained acute inflammatory monoarthritis with
synovial fluid WBC count < 50,000/μL. Although
nongonococcal septic arthritis often generates very high
synovial fluid WBC counts (> 100,000/μL), there are
exceptions to this rule. Septic arthritis can present with
synovial fluid WBC counts as low as 3000/μL. The
synovial fluid WBC count in gonococcal arthritis is
generally lower than in nongonococcal septic arthritis
(mean synovial fluid WBC count as low as 34,000/μL
in some series).

The differential diagnosis of acute inflammatory
monoarthritis not due to septic arthritis, gout, or pseudogout is broad. Many of these diseases present more
commonly as subacute or chronic processes (Table
4–2). Diseases that are typically oligoarticular or pol-

Table 4–2. Differential diagnosis of chronic inflammatory monoarthritis.

- Infection
    - Nongonococcal septic arthritis
    - Gonococcal
    - Chronic Lyme disease and other spirochetal infections
    - Mycobacterial
    - Fungal
    - Viral[a]
- Crystal-induced arthritis
    - Gout
    - Pseudogout
    - Calcium apatite crystals[b]
- Monarticular presentation of an oligoarthritis or polyarthritis
    - Spondyloarthropathy
    - Rheumatoid arthritis
    - Lupus and other systemic autoimmune diseases
- Sarcoidosis[a]
- Uncommon or rare
    - Familial Mediterranean fever
    - Amyloidosis[a]
    - Foreign-body synovitis due to plant thorns, sea urchin spikes, wood fragments, etc
    - Pigmented villonodular synovitis[c]

[a]Also can cause noninflammatory synovial fluid.
[b]Not detected by polarized light microscopy.
[c]Commonly associated with bloody, or blood-tinged brown, synovial fluid.

yarticular, such as the spondyloarthropathies and adult-onset Still disease, occasionally begin as an inflammatory monoarthritis.

B. NONINFLAMMATORY

Noninflammatory synovial fluid can be seen with internal derangements (eg, torn meniscus of the knee). Osteoarthritis of a single joint usually presents as a chronic condition, but occasionally, the onset of pain may be acute. Similarly, neuropathic arthropathy, amyloidosis, and osteonecrosis usually cause chronic noninflammatory arthritis of one or several joints, but acute symptoms are sometimes present.

C. HEMARTHROSIS

Frank blood on arthrocentesis can be indicative of a fracture or other joint trauma and should prompt appropriate imaging studies and referral to an orthopedic surgeon. Hemarthrosis also occurs in patients receiving anticoagulant therapy or who have a clotting factor deficiency such as hemophilia. Bloody synovial fluid can be seen in pigmented villonodular synovitis, a rare prolifer-

ative disorder of the synovium that presents as a chronic monoarthritis, typically of the knee, in young adults.

CHRONIC MONOARTHRITIS

 ESSENTIAL FEATURES

- *Chronic inflammatory monoarthritis may be caused by infection, crystal-induced arthritis, sarcoidosis, or a monarticular presentation of an oligoarthritis or polyarthritis.*
- *Chronic noninflammatory monoarthritis may be caused by osteoarthritis, internal derangements, chondromalacia patellae, and osteonecrosis.*
- *Arthrocentesis and imaging studies are important diagnostic tests.*

Initial Clinical Evaluation

Infections, particularly indolent infections, are a concern with inflammatory monoarthritis that lasts from weeks to months. The particular joint involved influences the differential diagnosis.

A. LABORATORY EVALUATION

A critical step is to determine whether the monoarthritis is inflammatory or noninflammatory, preferably by analyzing synovial fluid. Synovial fluid should be sent for culture (bacterial, mycobacterial, and fungal), WBC count, and Gram stain and examined for crystals by polarized light microscopy.

Routine laboratory studies (eg, complete blood cell count, serum electrolytes and creatinine, and urinalysis) and determinations of the ESR or CRP level can provide helpful information. Patients with inflammatory monoarthritis and negative bacterial cultures should be tested for reactivity to purified protein derivative (PPD).

B. IMAGING STUDIES

Unlike in acute monoarthritis, radiographs can be helpful in evaluating chronic monoarthritis and can point to the correct diagnosis in cases of infection, osteoarthritis, osteonecrosis, neuropathic joints, and other disorders.

Differential Diagnosis

A. INFLAMMATORY

A wide range of diseases can cause inflammatory arthritis in a single joint for several weeks or longer (Table 4–2). Most patients with septic arthritis and gonococcal arthritis experience significant pain in the infected joint and seek medical attention within hours to days of the onset of symptoms. However, some patients may delay in seeking treatment for several weeks, particularly if symptoms have been partially masked by the use of nonsteroidal anti-inflammatory drugs, antibiotics, or corticosteroids (systemic or intra-articular).

Patients with untreated indolent infections commonly have symptoms for weeks or longer before seeking medical attention. In these types of infections, synovial fluid culture is negative for bacteria, and additional diagnostic tests and cultures are required to establish the correct diagnosis. Chronic Lyme disease can cause an inflammatory monoarthritis, often of the knee, with synovial fluid WBC count typically in the 10,000–25,000/μL range. Tuberculous infection of a joint can present after days, weeks, or months of symptoms. Smears for acid-fast bacilli are positive in only 20% of cases; cultures for mycobacteria are positive in 80%, but test results take weeks. Synovial biopsy can expedite the diagnosis of tuberculous arthritis and is also indicated in suspected cases of fungal arthritis.

B. Noninflammatory

Osteoarthritis is the leading cause of chronic noninflammatory monoarthritis, particularly when the hip, knee, first carpometacarpal joint, or acromioclavicular joint is involved (Table 4–3). Internal derangements, such as a torn meniscus in the knee, often produce mechanical symptoms and characteristic findings on physical examination (see Chapter 12). Pain is frequently a prominent feature of osteonecrosis, which can produce large knee effusions when the distal femur is involved. Radiographs are often normal early in the course of osteonecrosis, and diagnosis may require magnetic resonance imaging. Hip pain with a normal radiograph should raise the possibility of early osteonecrosis, particularly if the patient is relatively young or has a risk

Table 4–3. Differential diagnosis of chronic noninflammatory monoarthritis.

- Osteoarthritis
- Internal derangements (eg, torn meniscus)[a]
- Chondromalacia patellae[a]
- Osteonecrosis[a]
- Uncommon or rare
    Neuropathic (Charcot) arthropathy
    Sarcoidosis[a,b]
    Amyloidosis[a,b]

---

[a]Radiograph of the affected joint often normal at presentation.
[b]Can also cause inflammatory synovial fluid.

factor for osteonecrosis (see Chapter 54). Diabetes mellitus is the most common underlying cause of neuropathic arthropathy, which should be considered in a diabetic patient with foot, ankle, or knee arthritis. The involved joint may be warm and painful, but the joint fluid is typically noninflammatory. Radiographs usually show characteristic neuropathic changes (see Chapter 51).

ACUTE OLIGOARTHRITIS

 ESSENTIAL FEATURES

- *Disseminated gonococcal infection, nongonococcal septic arthritis, and the spondyloarthropathies are leading causes of acute inflammatory oligoarthritis.*
- *Arthrocentesis and appropriate cultures are important diagnostic tests.*

Initial Clinical Evaluation

Acute oligoarthritis is usually due to an inflammatory process. Infectious causes of the arthritis need to be ruled out. Disseminated gonococcal infection is the most common cause of acute oligoarthritis in sexually active young people. Nongonococcal septic arthritis is usually monarticular but involves more than one joint in up to 20% of cases.

Spondyloarthropathies typically cause an asymmetric oligoarthritis. Of these, reactive arthritis is most likely to present with acute onset of arthritis and, early in its course, can be difficult to distinguish from disseminated gonococcal infection.

The use of four joints as a dividing line between oligoarthritis and polyarthritis is somewhat arbitrary, and there is overlap between disorders that cause oligoarthritis and polyarthritis. For example, parvovirus B19 infection usually causes a true polyarthritis but on occasion produces an oligoarthritis. Many of the disorders listed in Table 4–4 sometimes involve more than four joints.

A. Laboratory Evaluation

Analysis and culture of the synovial fluid are critical in the evaluation of acute oligoarthritis. The pharynx, urethra, cervix, and rectum should be tested for *N gonorrhoeae* by culture. Urethral and cervical swabs should be

Table 4–4. Differential diagnosis of acute inflammatory oligoarthritis.

- Infection
    - Disseminated gonococcal infection[a]
    - Nongonococcal septic arthritis
    - Bacterial endocarditis[b]
    - Viral[c]
- Postinfection
    - Reactive arthritis[b]
    - Rheumatic fever (post-streptococcal arthritis)[d]
- Spondyloarthropathy
    - Reactive arthritis[b]
    - Ankylosing spondylitis[b]
    - Psoriatic arthritis[b]
    - Inflammatory bowel disease[b]
- Oligoarticular presentation of rheumatoid arthritis, systemic lupus erythematosus,[a] adult-onset Still disease, or other polyarthritis
- Gout and pseudogout

[a]Often migratory.
[b]Can be associated with back pain.
[c]Usually causes polyarthritis but occasionally oligoarticular and sometimes noninflammatory.
[d]Migratory in children but not in adults.

performed for *Chlamydia trachomatis.* If bacterial endocarditis is a possibility, at least three blood cultures should be obtained, and a transesophageal echocardiogram may be indicated. Complete blood cell count, serum electrolytes and creatinine, and urinalysis should be obtained.

B. IMAGING STUDIES

Radiographs usually are of little help if the onset of the oligoarthritis is truly acute.

Differential Diagnosis

Disseminated gonococcal infection usually presents as a migratory tenosynovitis, often with characteristic skin lesions; meningococcemia can cause a similar syndrome but is much less common. Bacterial endocarditis can cause an oligoarthritis with either septic joints (due to hematogenous spread) or sterile inflammatory synovial fluid (likely due to immune complex disease); back pain is common, particularly in acute bacterial endocarditis (Table 4–4). Reactive arthritis classically follows within 1 to 4 weeks of enteric or genitourinary infections, but the triggering infection is sometimes subclinical. In its presenting phase, reactive arthritis can be associated with significant constitutional signs and symptoms including prominent weight loss and fever. Most patients with new-onset psoriatic arthritis either have, or have

had, psoriasis; however, the arthritis precedes the skin disease in about 15% of patients. Acute rheumatic fever produces a migratory arthritis in children; in adults, however, post-streptococcal arthritis is usually not migratory and is rarely associated with the other distinctive manifestations of rheumatic fever (eg, rash, subcutaneous nodules, carditis, and chorea).

CHRONIC OLIGOARTHRITIS

 ESSENTIAL FEATURES

- *Careful description of the arthritis and detection of extra-articular disease facilitate accurate diagnosis.*
- *Radiographs are often of diagnostic value.*

Initial Clinical Evaluation

Spondyloarthropathies are the most common cause of chronic inflammatory oligoarthritis (Table 4–5). However, distinguishing spondyloarthropathies from early-onset rheumatoid arthritis may be difficult, taking months or longer. Osteoarthritis commonly presents as a noninflammatory oligoarthritis of the hips or knees and usually does not present diagnostic difficulties.

A. LABORATORY EVALUATION

Synovial fluid should be analyzed for crystals and cultured. The distinction between inflammatory and noninflammatory chronic oligoarthritis often can be made on clinical grounds but is confirmed by the synovial fluid WBC count.

A positive test for serum rheumatoid factor is seen in 70–80% of patients with rheumatoid arthritis and, although not a specific test for this disease, can help establish the diagnosis in the proper clinical context. Testing for HLA-B27 is usually of limited value (see Chapter 18).

B. IMAGING STUDIES

Radiographs can be of considerable value. An experienced radiologist or rheumatologist can often distinguish among the erosions of the spondyloarthropathies, rheumatoid arthritis, and gout. Radiographic evidence of sacroiliitis indicates a spondyloarthropathy and narrows the differential diagnosis considerably.

Table 4–5. Differential diagnosis
of chronic oligoarthritis.

- Inflammatory causes
  Common
      Spondyloarthropathy
        Reactive arthritis[a]
        Ankylosing spondylitis[a]
        Psoriatic arthritis[a]
        Inflammatory bowel disease[a]
      Atypical presentation of rheumatoid arthritis
      Gout
  Uncommon or rare
      Subacute bacterial endocarditis
      Sarcoidosis[b]
      Behçet disease
      Relapsing polychondritis
      Celiac disease[a]
- Noninflammatory causes
  Common
      Osteoarthritis
  Uncommon or rare
      Hypothyroidism
      Amyloidosis

---

[a]Can be associated with involvement of the axial skeleton.
[b]Can be a migratory arthritis and have either inflammatory or
noninflammatory synovial fluid.

Differential Diagnosis

Although spondyloarthropathies typically cause an asymmetric oligoarthritis and rheumatoid arthritis is usually a symmetric polyarthritis, it can be difficult to differentiate these disorders in a subset of patients with relatively early disease. Several features are helpful in making this distinction. Inflammatory axial skeleton disease with sacroiliitis that causes pain and stiffness in the low back, particularly in the morning, is always seen in ankylosing spondylitis and often seen in other spondyloarthropathies (Table 4–5). Sacroiliitis is not a feature of rheumatoid arthritis, which involves the cervical spine but no other part of the axial skeleton. The prominent tenosynovitis of the spondyloarthropathies can produce dactylitis ("sausage digits") of the toes or fingers. Dactylitis is not seen in rheumatoid arthritis. (Dactylitis is not specific for the spondyloarthropathies; it may also occur in sarcoidosis and gout.) Reactive arthritis and the arthritis of inflammatory bowel disease have a predilection for the lower extremities. Rheumatoid arthritis invariably involves the hands, and > 90% of cases eventually have wrist arthritis.

Many of the disorders that cause chronic oligoarthritis have extra-articular manifestations that point to the correct diagnosis but that are easily overlooked. For example, psoriasis may be subtle; the patient may be un-

aware of psoriatic lesions, particularly in the umbilicus, the external auditory canal, the scalp, and the anal cleft. The oral ulcers of reactive arthritis are painless and usually not detected unless specifically looked for by the examining physician. Patients with inflammatory bowel disease may not volunteer that they have chronic diarrhea, particularly if bowel symptoms are intermittent. Antecedent anterior uveitis can be an important clue to the presence of a spondyloarthropathy, but patients generally do not associate ocular inflammation with arthritis and may not mention a past episode of anterior uveitis unless asked directly.

ACUTE POLYARTHRITIS

 ESSENTIAL FEATURES

- *Viral infections and rheumatoid arthritis are the leading causes of acute polyarthritis.*
- *Observation to distinguish persistent from self-limited polyarthritis is critical.*

Initial Clinical Evaluation

Although rheumatoid arthritis often has an insidious onset and patients have symptoms for months before seeking medical attention, it begins abruptly in some patients. Acute-onset rheumatoid arthritis can be difficult to distinguish from virally induced acute polyarthritis, and many rheumatologists are hesitant to make a diagnosis of rheumatoid arthritis in the acute setting. Viral polyarthritis usually resolves over days to a few weeks (but can persist for months). Thus, the longer the polyarthritis persists, the less likely viral polyarthritis becomes.

A. LABORATORY EVALUATION

Routine laboratory studies (including complete blood cell count, serum electrolytes and creatinine, liver function tests, and urinalysis) and determinations of the ESR or CRP levels should be done. Tests for serum rheumatoid factor, antinuclear antibodies (ANA), and hepatitis B are indicated.

Rheumatoid factor is an autoantibody with specificity for the Fc region of immunoglobulin (Ig) G. Despite its name, rheumatoid factor is neither a specific nor a sensitive test for rheumatoid arthritis. Positive tests for rheumatoid factor are seen in a variety of infectious and inflammatory conditions, some of which also cause arthritis (see Chapter 3). Eventually, 70–80% of patients with rheumatoid arthritis test positive for rheumatoid factor, but this figure is substantially lower (about 50%) early in the course of the disease.

Testing for ANA is essentially 100% sensitive for systemic lupus erythematosus (SLE) but has low specificity. A positive assay for ANA should prompt a careful evaluation for other clinical signs of SLE and additional serologic tests (see Chapters 3 and 19).

The likelihood of exposure and clinical features such as fever or characteristic rash should guide the decision of whether to perform serologic tests for Lyme disease and parvovirus B19. The immunoglobulin class (IgM vs IgG) is crucial to interpret the antibody tests for parvovirus B19. Patients with polyarthritis due to acute infection with parvovirus B19 have IgM antibodies that wane in titer over several months. Detection of IgM antibodies to parvovirus B19, therefore, is indicative of recent infection and strongly suggests that the acute polyarthritis is due to parvovirus B19. In the absence of an IgM response, IgG antibodies to parvovirus B19 simply reflect past infection with this common virus and are not likely to be a causative factor in acute polyarthritis. Indeed, most healthy adults have detectable IgG to parvovirus B19.

B. IMAGING STUDIES

Radiographs are rarely of value in acute polyarthritis and should be deferred until it is clear whether the polyarthritis is persistent.

Differential Diagnosis

Many acute viral infections cause joint symptoms, with polyarthralgias being considerably more common than true polyarthritis. The prevalence of polyarthritis is high, however, in adults who have acute parvovirus B19, hepatitis B, or rubella infections (Table 4–6). The pattern of viral polyarthritis often mimics that of rheumatoid arthritis. Adults with acute parvovirus B19 infection, the cause of "slapped cheek fever" in children, usually have only a faint rash on the trunk or no rash at all. IgM antibodies to parvovirus B19 are generally present at the onset of joint symptoms and persist for approximately 2 months. Acute hepatitis B causes an immune complex–mediated arthritis, often with urticaria or maculopapular rash, during the preicteric phase of infection; tests for hepatitis B surface antigen are positive. Joint symptoms with rubella generally precede the onset of rash. Polyarthritis due to rubella vaccination is less common with the currently used strain of attenuated virus.

Fever can be an important diagnostic clue. Patients with virally induced polyarthritis often have a flu-like illness; fever is common and may precede the onset of

Table 4–6. Differential diagnosis of acute polyarthritis.

- Common
  - Acute viral infections, especially parvovirus B19, hepatitis B, rubella, and rubella vaccines
  - Early disseminated Lyme disease
  - Rheumatoid arthritis
  - Systemic lupus erythematosus
- Uncommon or rare
  - Paraneoplastic polyarthritis
  - Remitting seronegative symmetric polyarthritis with pitting edema (RS3PE)
  - Acute sarcoidosis, usually with erythema nodosum and hilar adenopathy
  - Adult-onset Still disease
  - Secondary syphilis
  - Systemic autoimmune diseases and vasculitides
  - Whipple disease

the arthritis. Rheumatoid arthritis, in contrast, rarely causes fever higher than 38 °C. SLE can cause fever of up to 40 °C, but fever is unusual when polyarthritis is the major manifestation of the disease. Intermittent high fever is a common feature of adult-onset Still disease. Fever can accompany polyarthritis due to drug-induced lupus, secondary syphilis, acute sarcoidosis, and systemic vasculitis.

CHRONIC POLYARTHRITIS

 ESSENTIAL FEATURES

- *Rheumatoid arthritis and osteoarthritis are the leading causes of chronic polyarthritis.*
- *Careful delineation of the joints involved, particularly in the hands, can help point to the correct diagnosis.*

Initial Clinical Evaluation

Rheumatoid arthritis is the leading cause of chronic inflammatory polyarthritis, and osteoarthritis is the most common cause of chronic noninflammatory polyarthritis. Nonetheless, polyarthritis that persists for weeks or more has many possible causes and warrants careful diagnostic evaluation (Table 4–7). As is the case with

Table 4–7. Differential diagnosis of chronic polyarthritis.

- **Inflammatory**
  Common
  Rheumatoid arthritis
  Systemic lupus erythematosus
  Spondyloarthropathies (especially psoriatic arthritis)
  Chronic hepatitis C infection
  Gout
  Drug-induced lupus syndromes
  Uncommon or rare
  Paraneoplastic polyarthritis
  Remitting seronegative symmetric polyarthritis with pitting edema (RS3PE)
  Adult-onset Still disease
  Systemic autoimmune diseases and vasculitides
  Sjögren syndrome
  Viral infections other than hepatitis C
  Whipple disease
- **Noninflammatory**
  Primary generalized osteoathritis
  Hemochromatosis
  Calcium pyrophosphate deposition disease

other forms of arthritis, the distinction between inflammatory and noninflammatory processes is critical.

A. LABORATORY EVALUATION

If arthrocentesis is feasible, synovial fluid should be obtained and tested for cell count and analyzed for crystals. Routine laboratory investigations (complete blood cell count, serum electrolytes and creatinine, and urinalysis) should be done. When the process appears inflammatory, the ESR or CRP level should be determined and tests for serum rheumatoid factor, ANA, and hepatitis B and C should be done.

B. IMAGING STUDIES

Radiographs are indicated in most cases of chronic polyarthritis of the hand. Radiographs of the hand usually show characteristic changes at the time of presentation of primary generalized osteoarthritis, hemochromatosis, calcium pyrophosphate deposition disease, and chronic tophaceous gout. In cases of rheumatoid arthritis and the spondyloarthropathies, however, the likelihood of radiographic joint erosions and other characteristic findings increases with the duration of the polyarthritis; hand radiographs may be normal or demonstrate nonspecific changes only for months or longer. The polyarthritis of SLE, drug-induced lupus, and chronic hepatitis C is usually nonerosive and does not produce characteristic radiographic findings.

Differential Diagnosis

Osteoarthritis and rheumatoid arthritis have different patterns of joint involvement in the hand. Osteoarthritis involves the distal interphalangeal (DIP) and proximal interphalangeal (PIP) joints and the first carpometacarpal joint. Rheumatoid arthritis, in contrast, involves the PIPs, the metacarpophalangeal (MCP) joints, and the wrists.

Osteoarthritis and rheumatoid arthritis typically spare certain joints. Osteoarthritis usually does not involve the MCP joints, wrists, elbows, glenohumeral joints, and ankles; degenerative arthritis of these joints raises the possibility of antecedent trauma, calcium pyrophosphate deposition disease, underlying osteonecrosis, or neuropathic arthropathy. Rheumatoid arthritis usually spares the DIP joints, thoracic and lumbosacral spine, and sacroiliac joints.

In generalized osteoarthritis, interphalangeal joints, particularly the DIPs, may appear to be inflamed ("inflammatory osteoarthritis"), thus causing some uncertainty about the diagnosis. Radiographs, however, usually show typical degenerative changes (irregular joint space narrowing, sclerosis, and osteophytes). Psoriatic arthritis also commonly involves the DIP joints, usually with radiographic changes distinct from those of osteoarthritis. Psoriatic changes of the fingernail on the same digit usually occur concomitantly with psoriatic involvement of a DIP joint.

Many diseases can mimic rheumatoid arthritis, but several warrant particular emphasis (Table 4–8). Features that distinguish rheumatoid arthritis and the spondyloarthropathies are discussed above. Chronic infection

Table 4–8. Some mimics of chronic rheumatoid arthritis.

Arthritis with radiographic erosions
Spondyloarthropathies, especially psoriatic arthritis
Gout
Arthritis with positive rheumatoid factor
Chronic hepatitis C infection
Systemic lupus erythematosus
Sarcoidosis
Systemic vasculitides
Polymyositis/dermatomyositis
Subacute bacterial endocarditis
Arthritis with nodules
Chronic tophaceous gout
Hyperlipoproteinemia (rare)
Multicentric reticulohistiocytosis (rare)
Arthritis of metacarpophalangeal joints or wrists, or both
Hemochromatosis
Calcium pyrophosphate deposition disease

with hepatitis C is associated with a symmetric polyarthritis and a positive test for rheumatoid factor. The polyarthritis of SLE is nonerosive but can lead to reducible "swan neck" deformities of the fingers. On occasion, chronic tophaceous gout is a remarkable mimic of rheumatoid arthritis, with tophi mistaken for rheumatoid nodules. Gout is not associated with rheumatoid factor (virtually all cases of nodular rheumatoid arthritis are seropositive), and the erosions of gout and rheumatoid arthritis have different radiographic characteristics. Analysis of synovial fluid for urate crystals is the definitive diagnostic test. Hemochromatosis and other causes of calcium pyrophosphate deposition disease lead to arthritis of the MCPs (especially the second and third) and wrists; radiographs often reveal "hook-like" osteophytes of the MCPs and degenerative changes, usually with chondrocalcinosis, of the wrist.

Although rheumatoid arthritis is the leading cause of chronic inflammatory polyarthritis, physicians must be certain that rheumatoid arthritis accounts for the full clinical picture. Rheumatoid arthritis is not a plausible explanation for the following: fever greater than 38 °C, substantial weight loss, significant adenopathy, rashes (apart from subcutaneous nodules), hematuria, and proteinuria. Failure to account for these additional clinical findings can lead to a failure to diagnose such diseases as SLE, Still disease, subacute bacterial endocarditis, paraneoplastic syndromes, and vasculitides.

REFERENCES

Baker DG, Schumacher HR. Acute monoarthritis. *N Engl J Med.* 1993;329:1013. [PMID: 8366902] (Thorough discussion of the differential diagnosis and evaluation of acute monoarthritis.)

Pinals RS. Polyarthritis and fever. *N Engl J Med.* 1994;330:769. [PMID: 8107744] (Clinically useful guide to the important problem of fever in the setting of arthritis.)

Relevant World Wide Web Sites

[Johns Hopkins Arthritis Center]
http://www.hopkins-arthritis.som.jhmi.edu/

Approach to the Adolescent with Arthritis

Peggy Schlesinger, MD

ESSENTIAL FEATURES

- *Inflammatory and noninflammatory conditions can cause joint pain in adolescents.*
- *Juvenile rheumatoid arthritis (JRA) encompasses five subgroups/subtypes: systemic-onset (Still disease); juvenile-onset spondylitis; pauciarticular, polyarticular seronegative, and polyarticular seropositive arthritis.*
- *Type of JRA subgroup is determined by age of the child; the number and type of joints involved; the presence of associated symptoms, such as rash, fever, iritis, fatigue, and significant morning stiffness; and the course of the illness during the first 6 months after the diagnosis is confirmed.*
- *Effective therapy for adolescents requires attention to developmental needs and school and vocational issues.*

General Considerations

There are many causes of joint pain occurring in childhood and adolescence. Diagnostic accuracy is very important to ensure that the patient receives appropriate treatment.

The first step in caring for a young patient with musculoskeletal discomfort is to make the distinction between **arthritis with true synovitis** (persistent joint swelling) and **arthralgia** (pain in and around joints). Pain in and around the joints without synovitis is usually caused by trauma, mechanical factors, or soft tissue syndromes. Excruciating joint pain and swelling, often with erythema, may indicate malignancy. A careful history of recent infections and exposures, as well as immunizations, can highlight possible infection-related causes of joint swelling and pain in adolescents (Table 5–1). Other conditions such as metabolic syndromes and connective tissue diseases are rare; however, chronic arthritis is one of the five most common chronic diseases of childhood, occurring with a frequency greater than diabetes or cystic fibrosis. Juvenile rheumatoid arthritis (JRA), including psoriatic arthritis and the spondyloarthropathies, is the most common cause of chronic arthritis in childhood and adolescence.

Evaluation

The initial evaluation of an adolescent with rheumatic disease includes a complete history and physical examination. Information that is important to obtain during history taking includes the following:

- Age at menarche
- Is the patient skeletally mature? (A rough guide: Is shoe size changing with every new pair?)
- Is the patient sexually active?
- Have there been prolonged or recurrent school absences?
- Has there been uninterrupted participation in physical education?
- Is there a history of participation in athletics?
- Are there barriers at school that make participation or attendance difficult?
- In what way does the patient make accommodations to compensate for his or her disability (wearing elastic waist sweat pants instead of jeans with buttons and zippers, avoiding going to the bathroom at school because of difficulty getting on and off the toilet, etc)?
- Does the patient have a best friend with whom to share arthritis-related concerns?
- Is there a receptive teacher or school counselor to contact if a Section 504 or an individualized education plan (IEP) is needed?
- Have vocational and career goals been identified?
- Has a disability/SSI application been filed?

Juvenile Rheumatoid Arthritis

JRA is a heterogeneous group of disorders affecting children younger than 17 years. The common thread in all five types of JRA is the presence of persistent synovitis in affected joints lasting 6 weeks or longer. This

Table 5–1. Differential diagnosis of arthritis in adolescents.

Infection-related	Metabolic/genetic
Lyme disease	Cystic fibrosis
Septic arthritis	Diabetes
Gonococcal arthritis	Sickle cell disease
Parvovirus	**Connective tissue diseases**
Mononucleosis	Systemic lupus
Cytomegalovirus	erythematosus
HIV	Dermatomyositis
Varicella	Mixed connective tissue
Endocarditis	disease
Streptococcal-associated	Sarcoidosis
arthritis	Vasculitis
Acute rheumatic fever	**Noninflammatory conditions**
Hepatitis	Chondromalacia patellae
Toxic synovitis	Hypermobility syndrome
Malignancy	Avascular necrosis
Bone tumors	Skeletal dysplasias
Leukemia	Slipped capital-femoral
Lymphoma	epiphysis
Neuroblastoma	Osgood-Schlatter disease
Juvenile rheumatoid	Sever disease
arthritis (JRA)	Scheuermann disease
Polyarticular JRA	Osteochondritis dessicans
Systemic-onset JRA	Synovial chondromatosis
Pauciarticular JRA	Synovial hemangioma
(recurrent)	Pigmented villonodular
Juvenile-onset spondylitis	synovitis
-Ankylosing spondylitis	
-Psoriatic arthritis	
-Arthritis of inflammatory	
bowel disease	
-Reactive arthritis	

alone distinguishes JRA from many of the other causes of joint pain in childhood. The majority of other causes of arthritis in childhood are associated with joint pain or swelling that is intermittent but not persistent. The five types of JRA are systemic-onset (Still disease), juvenile-onset spondylitis, pauciarticular, polyarticular seronegative, and polyarticular seropositive. Seronegative and seropositive refer to the presence or absence of rheumatoid factor in the blood. This test can have prognostic but not diagnostic significance. The systemic-onset, spondylitis, and polyarticular seropositive subgroups are more commonly seen in the adolescent age group. The determination of which subgroup of JRA a patient has is based on clinical criteria: the age of the child, the number and type of joints involved, and the presence of associated symptoms such as rash and fever or iritis. The subgroup of JRA is also determined by the course of the illness during the first 6 months after the diagnosis of arthritis is confirmed. Laboratory testing and radiologic imaging are helpful more often to rule out other possible causes of arthritis in children. There is no definitive laboratory test or imaging finding that can confirm the diagnosis of JRA.

Systemic-onset JRA can present at any age and recur at any age through adulthood. The symptoms of this disorder include a spiking daily fever in a "rabbit ears" pattern in association with an evanescent, salmon-colored macular rash on trunk and extremities. The rash typically appears with the fever and disappears when the child is afebrile. Joint and muscle pain are prominent features, although specific synovitis may be absent at presentation. Enlargement of lymph nodes, hepatosplenomegaly, pleuropericarditis, and marked leukocytosis can occur with fever and underscore the need to differentiate this entity from malignancy and infection.

The **juvenile-onset spondylitis** subgroup includes the family of HLA-B27–related diseases, such as Reiter syndrome, reactive arthritis, ankylosing spondylitis, psoriatic arthritis, and the arthritis associated with inflammatory bowel disease. These disorders commonly present in prepubertal boys with painful swelling of lower extremity joints, in association with heel pain, iritis or conjunctivitis, and enthesitis (pain at tendon insertion sites). Back pain is not always present at the time of diagnosis; however, widening and irregularity of the sacroiliac joints (which can be seen on plain films) with subsequent fusion can develop over time. The prognosis for children with this disorder and the HLA-B27–related diseases is much better than the prognosis for adults with spondylitis that begins in the third and fourth decade. Although some patients continue to have recurring symptoms throughout adulthood, progression to spinal fusion is not seen as often among patients in whom disease onset occurred at a younger age.

Polyarticular seronegative JRA begins in the prepubertal years (ages 8–12) and usually involves synovitis of large joints in a symmetric pattern. These patients do not get rheumatoid nodules and the rheumatoid factor is not present in the serum. The prognosis for this subgroup is excellent because this type of arthritis is persistent but usually nonerosive, with remission often occurring before adulthood. Disease-modifying antirheumatic drugs (DMARDs), other than hydroxychloroquine, are not often needed since these patients usually respond well to treatment with anti-inflammatory medication and therapeutic exercise.

Polyarticular seropositive JRA is the subgroup that most closely resembles the classic rheumatoid arthritis seen in adults. These patients are usually teenagers with typical aggressive, nodular, erosive arthritis involving both small and large joints. Symptoms include significant morning stiffness, gelling phenomenon, and fatigue, in addition to swollen joints in hands and feet.

Significant functional limitations occur all too frequently, especially in teenage girls. These patients have persistent and often aggressive disease that warrants early treatment with DMARDs (Table 5–2). This type of JRA usually persists into adulthood.

Pauciarticular JRA affects very young children of preschool age with swelling of up to five total joints in an asymmetric pattern. Painless iridocyclitis occurs in 75% of children with this type of JRA, usually girls, in whom an antinuclear antibody test was positive. Rarely, an occasional patient who has experienced this disease during preschool years may have a recurrence of joint swelling and painless iridocyclitis during his or her teenage years. Both the arthritis and iritis of pauciartic-

ular JRA can recur in later childhood or can evolve into a polyarticular JRA pattern. Regular slit lamp examinations until age 18 are recommended for patients with pauciarticular disease to minimize the risk of complications from unrecognized and untreated inflammation in the anterior chamber of the eye. Unrecognized, untreated iridocyclitis can lead to scarring and loss of vision. The major cause of morbidity in children with this type of JRA is visual impairment and *not* arthritis.

Psoriatic arthritis can present in adolescents with active arthritis that closely resembles either the polyarticular or juvenile-onset spondylitis types of JRA. The distinguishing characteristics of psoriatic arthritis include the presence of a typical psoriatic rash, nail pit-

Table 5–2. DMARDs used in pediatric patients.[a]

Drug	Dose	Formulation	Route / Frequency	Special Considerations
Methotrexate	15 mg/m² per dose	Pills: 2.5 mg Liquid: 2.5 mg = 0.1 mL 25 mg/mL	PO, IM, or SQ once a week	• Higher doses well tolerated in children • Poor absorption can cause decreased clinical response; try same dose SQ • Avoid concomitant sulfonamides and tetracycline • Liquid can be taken PO or SQ • This is the **least expensive** DMARD
Hydroxychloroquine	6 mg/kg/d	200-mg pills	qd or bid daily	• Periodic eye examinations; retinal toxicity rare at these doses
Sulfasalazine	30–50 mg/kg/d	500-mg tablets	tid or bid daily	• Contraindicated in patients who are allergic to sulfonamides or sensitive to aspirin • Useful in polyarticular or spondylitis subgroups • Not for use in systemic-onset JRA • Enteric-coated formulation is often better tolerated
Cyclosporine	3 mg/kg/d	Pills: 25-mg and 100-mg capsules Liquid: 100 mg/mL	qd or bid	• Grapefruit juice increases absorption • **Most effective in systemic-onset JRA** • Monitor kidney function and blood pressure frequently • Many drug interactions
Etanercept	0.4 mg/kg/dose	Powder reconstituted with water in pre-filled syringe; refrigerate	SQ twice a week	• Avoid live virus immunization during therapy • **Approved and indicated for polyarticular JRA** • Combination with methotrexate prolongs effect • Serious infection can occur

[a]Leflunomide, anakinra, infliximab, and adalimumab are currently under investigation regarding usefulness in the pediatric age group. No pediatric dosing information is available.
DMARDs, disease modifying antirheumatic drugs; JRA, juvenile rheumatoid arthritis.

ting, arthritis of distal interphalangeal joints, and sausage digits. These clues may be present at the onset of arthritis symptoms or develop later. Sometimes a history of psoriasis in a first-degree relative is enough to raise the suspicion that a psoriatic arthritis diagnosis will develop. In some patients, it can take years from the onset of arthritis until the typical skin lesions or other distinguishing characteristics of psoriasis appear to confirm the diagnosis.

Infections

Rubella, mononucleosis, hepatitis B and C, and varicella infections have all been associated with transient joint swelling (< 6 weeks) and should be considered in the differential diagnosis of arthritis in this age group (see Table 5–1). Immunization for varicella and the measles, mumps, rubella vaccine may be given to teenagers who did not receive their full complement of vaccinations as children; vaccination with these attenuated viruses has been associated with transient arthritis symptoms. Lyme disease, caused by *Borrelia burgdorferi,* can initially present with a rash followed by migratory, large joint arthritis. It is important to distinguish Lyme disease from JRA so that proper antibiotic therapy can be given. Although rheumatic fever is rare today, the syndrome of streptococcal-associated arthritis is much more common and usually self-limited. True synovitis can develop within 7 to 10 days among adolescents with antecedent streptococcal infection as a result of the molecular mimicry involved in the immune response to the infection. In this syndrome of streptococcal-associated arthritis, the chorea and carditis of rheumatic fever are absent. Joint symptoms resolve completely but can recur with subsequent streptococcal infections. Bloody diarrheal illnesses caused by *Campylobacter, Salmonella, Shigella, Yersinia,* and toxigenic *Escherichia coli* can be associated with postinfectious reactive arthritis in HLA-B27–positive teenagers. Sexually active teenagers may contract chlamydia infection, which has also been associated with a reactive arthritis pattern, or gonococcal infection with immune complex–mediated vasculitis and arthritis.

Mechanical Mimics

Noninflammatory conditions can cause joint swelling in adolescent patients, which can be confusing diagnostically. The hallmark of this group of disorders is the absence of signs and symptoms of inflammation; joints have no morning stiffness, little if any swelling, and normal acute phase reactants such as the erythrocyte sedimentation rate and C-reactive protein. Chondromalacia, Osgood-Schlatter disease, osteochondritis dessicans, Sever disease, Scheuermann disease, and hyper-

mobility syndromes represent the most common causes of noninflammatory joint pain in this age group.

Chondromalacia patellae, or patellofemoral syndrome, is commonly seen in teenage girls as a cause of unilateral or bilateral knee pain that worsens with activity. Any activity that involves weight bearing on a bent knee can aggravate the pain of this condition. Climbing stairs, using the clutch in a car, standing up after prolonged sitting, participation in gym class, and competitive athletic activities can be particularly troublesome. A minority of girls with chondromalacia patellae (approximately 10%) will have knee swelling in addition to knee pain, and even fewer of these patients will have persistent knee swelling lasting more than 6 weeks. When this does occur, chondromalacia patellae is easily confused with JRA.

The diagnosis of chondromalacia patellae is confirmed by the absence of morning stiffness, activity as the main aggravating factor, a positive patellar inhibition test on examination, and the lack of other affected joints even in patients with prolonged knee swelling. Isometric quadriceps strengthening exercises (Figure 5–1) will reduce pain and swelling and allow for a return to normal activity, even if this includes competitive athletics. Nonsteroidal anti-inflammatory drugs (NSAIDs) (Table 5–3), ice, and occasionally joint injection with 20–40 mg of methylprednisolone mixed with 1–2 mL of a long-acting local anesthetic will help manage the patient's knee pain and reduce swelling, allowing them to continue making progress in the exercise program. Often knee pain with or without swelling returns when the patient becomes less compliant with the exercise program of regular isometric quadriceps strengthening exercises. The pain can be a good reminder to teenagers to make daily isometric quadriceps exercises a part of their routine. Chondromalacia patellae is very common in adolescent girls, and the symptoms can last for several years. Despite several years of knee pain as teenagers, most of these patients do not develop degenerative patellofemoral joint disease as adults.

Osteochondritis dessicans and Osgood-Schlatter disease are common causes of knee or ankle pain in adolescent boys. In osteochondritis dessicans, a piece of cartilage fractures, producing pain and swelling in the affected joint. Knees (femoral condyles) and ankles (dome of the talus) are the most commonly affected joints. There is often a history of trauma to the area, and the recommended treatment is orthopedic consultation. Osgood-Schlatter disease is caused by apophysitis at the patellar tendon insertion on the tibial tubercle with localized pain in this area just below the knee. True synovitis is rare; however, the presence of painful swelling in close proximity to the knee joint can be easily confused with true arthritis.

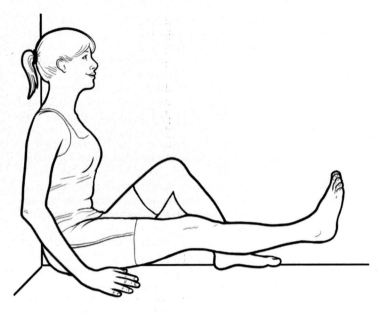

Figure 5–1. Isometric quadriceps strengthening exercise.

Table 5–3. NSAIDs used in pediatric patients.[a]

Drug	Dose	Formulation
Naproxen	20 mg/kg/d up to 1000 mg/d 10 mg/kg/dose bid	Liquid: 125 mg/5 mL Tablet: 220 mg, available over the counter Twice daily dosing is convenient
Ibuprofen	40 mg/kg/d up to 2400 mg/d 10 mg/kg/dose qid	Liquid: 100 mg/5 mL Tablet: 200 mg, available over the counter
Tolmetin	30 mg/kg/d up to 1800 mg/d 10 mg/kg/dose tid	Tablets: 200 mg, 400 mg, 600 mg
Indomethacin	4 mg/kg/d up to 200 mg/d tid or qid	Liquid: 25 mg/5 mL Approved for patients younger than 14 years Used in younger patients with systemic-onset JRA or spondylitis

[a]As of this writing, other NSAIDs have not been approved by the Food and Drug Administration for use in the pediatric age group. NSAIDs, nonsteroidal anti-inflammatory drugs; JRA, juvenile rheumatoid arthritis.

Sever disease is a syndrome of similar etiology with apophysitis occurring at the growth plate of the heel. This disorder is commonly seen in soccer players, and treatment may include the use of a heel cup, ice, and NSAIDs (see Table 5–3). Sever disease is self-limited and unrelated to any of the HLA-B27–related spondyloarthropathies, although the occurrence of heel pain in the adolescent boy may be misleading to practitioners.

Joint hypermobility syndrome is familial and can be troublesome in adolescents. Some teenagers are "double jointed," with ligamentous laxity and freely subluxing shoulders, patellae, and hips. The increased joint range of motion often leads to pain that is aggravated by continued use or repetitive activity, especially when they participate in competitive athletics. Weight lifting and strength training can help offset the tendency to subluxation in these patients by building tight, bulky muscles to help provide internal stability to the affected joint. This is particularly helpful for shoulder and knee joints, where increasing muscle bulk and tone in the rotator cuff mechanism and the quadriceps can help reduce pain and bring useful joint excursion back to normal levels.

Slipped capital-femoral epiphysis is a common cause of hip pain in teenage boys. Typically, the adolescent will complain of groin pain or referred pain in the knee, worsening with activity. Obesity is a predisposing factor in the development of this idiopathic disorder. Once the diagnosis is confirmed radiographically, orthopedic consultation should be obtained.

Scheuermann disease, or vertebral apophysitis, can cause back pain in adolescents. It typically involves three contiguous vertebrae with involvement of the end plates at each level; lower thoracic vertebrae are most commonly affected, and complications such as thoracic kyphosis can develop in later life. This condition is easily confused with juvenile-onset spondylitis because both can be a cause of back pain in teenagers.

Rheumatic Diseases & Syndromes

Other rheumatic syndromes that are well known in adults, such as Raynaud phenomenon and fibromyalgia, can present initially in adolescence. The majority of teenagers who have Raynaud phenomenon have *no* associated rheumatic disease, and reassurance regarding the prognosis can be given liberally. Although an antinuclear antibody test result may be positive in these patients, it is not as useful as nail fold capillaroscopy in predicting in which patients a systemic rheumatic disease will eventually develop. In young adults with Raynaud phenomenon, abnormal nail fold capillaroscopy showing the typical pattern of dilation and dropout of capillary loops has been strongly correlated with the development of systemic disease, either progressive systemic sclerosis or juvenile dermatomyositis. Normal nail fold capillaries are seen in adolescents with Raynaud phenomenon alone and Raynaud phenomenon associated with other rheumatic diseases.

Treatment of Raynaud phenomenon is directed at reducing the frequency of vasospastic episodes by keeping the hands and feet warm. Unfortunately, asking teenagers to wear socks and gloves to keep their extremities warm can be as effective as asking them to turn in homework early. Fortunately, treatment with biofeedback, solid-fuel hand warmers, and medications such as extended-release niacin tablets, diltiazem, and transdermal nitroglycerin can be used when needed, giving the patients some control over their symptoms.

Sleep issues loom large in adolescence. Teenagers seem to require much more sleep than adults and younger children do. The growth spurt and pubertal changes at this age are fueled by hormones such as growth hormone that are secreted in a circadian rhythm with the highest output during the night. Sleep disorders can present in early adolescence with fibromyalgia-like arthralgias and myalgias. The good news is that these symptoms are amenable to therapeutic intervention. Treatment with low-dose amitriptyline (10–30 mg at bedtime) or cyclobenzaprine (10–30 mg at bedtime) can correct a nonrestorative sleep pattern. Once the sleep cycle has been reset, a gradually increasing exercise program will help build specific muscle strength and improve endurance, thus allowing the patient to return to normal activity. As in adults, the disability from this fibromyalgia-like syndrome can be extreme. However, with proper treatment the outlook for a return to normal activity is excellent.

Regional pain syndromes and soft tissue rheumatism present special challenges when they occur in the adolescent age group. Treatment is focused on returning the patient to normal activity as quickly as possible and addressing the accompanying psychosocial issues that can complicate recovery.

Systemic lupus erythematosus (SLE) can present in adolescence as a cause of arthritis in this age group. The incidence of SLE is approximately 2:1 girls:boys before puberty, but 8:1 after puberty. The changing hormonal milieu of teenage girls can be incendiary, causing flares of this disease during these difficult years. Neuropsychiatric involvement with SLE can be particularly challenging to diagnose and treat in adolescent girls with frequent mood swings.

Vasculitis, including Wegener granulomatosis, microscopic polyangiitis, polyarteritis nodosa, Henoch-Schönlein purpura, and leukocytoclastic vasculitis, among others, is also seen in the adolescent age group with signs and symptoms at presentation very similar to the adult form of the disease.

School Issues

The goal of treatment should be to help the teenager return to normal function, which in most cases involves regular school attendance as well as participation in after-school activities. Under Public Law 94-142, students with disabling conditions are guaranteed access to an education in the public schools. Modification of the school program may be needed to accomplish the goal of regular attendance. Examples of common modifications that can be done in public school include scheduling core classes later in the day to accommodate morning stiffness, arranging classes all on one level of the building to avoid stairs, offering an adaptive physical education program, and providing an extra set of textbooks to keep at home. The necessary changes can be made on either an individual basis or by utilizing the Section 504 or IEP process. Parent advocacy programs are in place in many states to help educate parents on the rights of disabled students and on how to work within the public school system to ensure a quality education for their child.

Developmental Stages of Adolescence

During the teenage years, the adolescent begins to establish relationships outside the family, with the ultimate goal of achieving independence from the nuclear family. In the process, teenagers deconstruct and reconstruct their self-image, finding an identity that encompasses their new experiences. During this period, the parents' roles change from primary caregivers to advocates, allowing and encouraging more independence in their offspring.

It is important that these changes be incorporated into the medical setting as well. Adolescents want to be taken seriously in the physician-patient encounter. Adolescents may be more comfortable transitioning from a pediatrician to an internal medicine physician for their primary care. They may prefer to see the doctor by themselves, without a parent present. The physician can use this time alone with the young person to talk over feelings about many sensitive subjects such as body image concerns, sexuality, worries about the future, and the impact of disability on everyday activities. Parents must be heard as well, often in a separate session, so that the physician has an accurate picture of the situation as a whole. Parental concerns can overwhelm both the patient and the physician; parents tend to be overprotective toward teens with a chronic illness. Opportunities will arise when the physician can point out to parents how appropriately their teenager is responding to his or her illness. This will help parents begin to see their teenagers as capable managers of their illness. Summer camps for children of all ages with arthritis are another good place to encourage independence and appropriate self-care, while also building self-esteem.

The task of adolescents is to put together a healthy self-concept as they near adulthood, ideally one that incorporates their illness but is not solely defined by it. They must also take on the responsibility of caring for themselves and their disease. The physician's job is to encourage this development in the adolescent patient, while helping parents transition comfortably into their secondary roles as patient advocates. The physician can facilitate these changes by commenting when the patient takes appropriate care of himself or herself and thus modeling encouragement for parents for such behaviors. For a time, it may feel as if the physician has two patients in each family—the adolescent patient and the parents—until such time as the adolescent can feel comfortable in the role of primary caregiver to himself or herself. This transition is absolutely necessary if the patient is to become an effective self-advocate and a responsible member of the healing partnership.

Vocational Issues

There are approximately 200 transition planning programs in this country that address the vocational needs of teenagers with chronic and potentially disabling conditions, but they cannot reach everyone who needs assistance. Vocational rehabilitation services can begin career counseling and the employment identification process with teenagers during their senior year in high school. Case management services may continue depending on whether the patient qualifies for Social Security disability benefits. Working with the patient to identify specific career goals and individual strengths can help adolescents focus their studies and make appropriate plans for their future. Physician involvement in this process is essential to making this transition to adulthood a success.

REFERENCES

Burgos-Vargas R. The juvenile-onset spondyloarthritides. *Rheum Dis Clin North Am.* 2002;28:531. [PMID: 12380369] (Volume 28 of this journal gives the best overall update of pediatric rheumatology.)

Cassidy JT. *Textbook of Pediatric Rheumatology.* John Wiley & Sons, 1995.

Emery HM. Juvenile rheumatoid arthritis and the spondyloarthropathies. *Adolesc Med.* 1998;9:45. [PMID: 10961251]

Isenberg DA, Miller JJ. *Adolescent Rheumatology.* Martin Dunitz, 1999.

McDonaugh JE, et al. Bridging the gap in rheumatology. *Ann Rheum Dis.* 2000;59:86. [PMID: 10666161]

Milojevic DS, Ilowite NT. Treatment of rheumatic diseases in children: special considerations. *Rheum Dis Clin North Am.* 2002;28:461. [PMID: 12380365]

Rabinovich CE. Bone metabolism in childhood rheumatic disease. *Rheum Dis Clin North Am.* 2002;28:655. [PMID: 12380374]

Schneider R, Passo MH. Juvenile rheumatoid arthritis. *Rheum Dis Clin North Am.* 2002;28:503. [PMID: 12380368]

White PH. Success on the road to adulthood. Issues and hurdles for adolescents with disabilities. *Rheum Dis Clin North Am.* 1997;23:697. [PMID: 9287383]

White PH. Transition: a future promise for children and adolescents with special health care needs and disabilities. *Rheum Dis Clin North Am.* 2002;28:687. [PMID: 12380376]

The Patient with Hand, Wrist, or Elbow Pain

6

Daniel Most, MD, & E. Gene Deune, MD

Pain in the hand, wrist, and elbow usually falls into three broad categories: neurologic, musculoskeletal, and vascular. A careful history often distinguishes among these categories. However, patients may be unable to accurately describe their symptoms. For example, a patient may refer to numbness or the lack of sensation as "painful" rather than conveying the perception of numbness. A disorder in the hand may produce pain referred proximally to the elbow, the axilla, or the neck. Conversely, disease in the cervical spine and proximal nerve roots can produce pain in the distal upper extremity. A full physical and neurologic examination of both upper extremities is therefore important to help isolate the cause of symptoms. Often, the history and examination are sufficient to establish a diagnosis. In selected cases, however, diagnostic tests such as radiographs, nerve conduction tests and electromyography, computed tomography scans, and magnetic resonance imaging (MRI) are needed to confirm the diagnosis.

■ NEUROLOGIC CAUSES OF PAIN

Pain due to peripheral nerve dysfunction can present with varying symptoms, ranging from pure sensory dysfunction to pure motor paralysis or a combination of both. Most commonly, the dysfunction is due to external compression. As peripheral nerves travel from the vertebral foramina to their end organs, they pass through several anatomic sites where compression can occur. Compression produces localized ischemia of the nerve and interferes with the axonal transport of metabolic products. The level of compression determines the clinical symptoms. Proximal compression of a nerve root as it exits the vertebral bodies will produce symptoms in a dermatome distribution, whereas distal nerve compression will produce symptoms in the defined region of the specific nerves. Peripheral neuropathies, in contrast, tend to manifest in multiple limbs and are more global within each limb. After the physical examination, the next step in the evaluation should be an electrodiagnostic examination. Nerve conduction studies reveal the level and sever-

ity of compression. Electromyography reveals whether the compression has led to denervation of muscle.

COMPRESSION OF THE MEDIAN NERVE AT THE WRIST (CARPAL TUNNEL SYNDROME)

 ESSENTIALS OF DIAGNOSIS

- *Paresthesias of the volar aspect of the thumb, index and long fingers, and radial side of the ring fingers.*
- *Positive Phalen maneuver or Tinel sign at the wrist.*
- *Thenar atrophy and weakened pinch with long-standing compression.*

General Considerations

Carpal tunnel syndrome, the most common nerve entrapment in the upper extremity, occurs most often in the fourth to the sixth decades of life and affects more women than men. Most cases are idiopathic. There may be an association with activities that produce repetitive motion of the wrist, such as keyboarding. Idiopathic carpal tunnel syndrome is frequently associated with the inflammation of the tenosynovium of the nine tendons within the carpal tunnel. Synovitis of the wrist (due to rheumatoid arthritis or any other inflammatory arthritis of the wrist) can result in the compression of the median nerve, as the space within the carpal tunnel is limited. Pregnancy, diabetes, and hypothyroidism can also be associated with carpal tunnel syndrome. Rare causes may include amyloidosis and acromegaly. Occasionally, compression of the median nerve is due to a giant cell tumor, lipoma, or ganglion cyst in the carpal tunnel.

Clinical Findings

A. SYMPTOMS AND SIGNS

Symptoms include burning in the volar thumb, index and long fingers, and the radial side of the ring fingers. Dysesthesias may be felt along the volar surface of the forearm as well. Shaking or flicking the hand can sometimes relieve the pain; this is called the "flick test." Patients may say that lowering the hand or gravity dependency helps with the pain or that the hand feels cold, perceiving vascular insufficiency as the cause. Symptoms are commonly nocturnal but also can occur during the day, especially when the wrist is hyperflexed or hyperextended, such as during driving or typing.

There is usually decreased sensation in digits innervated by the median nerve (thumb, index and long fingers, and radial side of the ring fingers). With long-standing compression, there is thenar atrophy and weakness of grip and pinch. A Tinel sign, elicited by tapping over the median nerve at the wrist, triggers radiating paresthesias in the median nerve distribution. Active hyperflexing of the wrist for 60 seconds may reproduce the patient's symptoms (Phalen maneuver). In the provocative Phalen maneuver, the examiner exerts finger or thumb pressure over the median nerve at the distal forearm while passively flexing the patient's wrist. Some clinicians use the cuff compression test; a blood pressure cuff is placed on the patient's forearm and inflated for 60 seconds to the midpoint pressure between the patient's systolic and diastolic pressures. It is positive if symptoms occur.

B. IMAGING STUDIES AND SPECIAL TESTS

Imaging studies are not necessary unless a compressing tumor or mass is suspected, in which case an MRI should be ordered. If the diagnosis is in doubt or if symptoms persist despite conservative management (see following Treatment section), electrodiagnostic testing should be performed.

Treatment

The initial management for idiopathic carpal tunnel syndrome should be conservative and should aim to reduce inflammation and swelling within the carpal tunnel. Splinting and nonsteroidal anti-inflammatory drugs (NSAIDs) usually are the first-line therapy. The patients are fitted with prefabricated wrist splints that maintain the wrist at 5 to 10 degrees of extension. The patients are instructed to wear the splints during the most symptomatic times of the day, which often is during the night when the patients flex their wrist during the fetal sleeping position. These wrist splints are available either in the hand surgeon's office or over the counter as "carpal tunnel splints." Splints can also be custom fabricated by the hand therapists. The patients are also instructed on proper ergonomics during the awake and sleeping hours to avoid any positions that cause compression of the median nerve. Approximately one-third of patients who are treated with these noninvasive methods respond favorably.

Glucocorticoid injections into the carpal tunnel can alleviate the symptoms but can cause median nerve injury if done incorrectly. The relief of symptoms is often short-lived because patients who require steroid injection generally have severe enough symptoms to warrant surgical decompression. Steroid injections, however, may be the only effective treatment for the patient who is unwilling or unable to have surgery.

If symptoms persist after 2–3 months of splinting, NSAIDs, and perhaps steroid injections, surgical intervention is indicated to avoid permanent damage to the median nerve and the muscles that it innervates. Surgical release can be done by either an open procedure or endoscopically.

COMPRESSION OF THE ULNAR NERVE AT THE WRIST IN THE GUYON CANAL

 ESSENTIALS OF DIAGNOSIS

- *Paresthesias of the volar aspect of the ring finger and small finger.*
- *Absence of numbness on the dorsal ulnar aspect of the hand.*

Clinical Findings

A. SYMPTOMS AND SIGNS

Numbness that occurs primarily in the volar aspect of the small and ring fingers, with or without weakness in the hypothenar muscles, is most likely due to compression of the ulnar nerve in the Guyon canal at the base of the hypothenar region. The Guyon canal is triangular in dimension. The roof is defined by the volar palmar fascia. The lateral wall is formed by the hook of the hamate and the insertion of the transverse carpal ligament. The medial wall is formed by the pisiform bone. It is through this small space that the ulnar nerve and the ulnar artery pass from the forearm to the hand. The lack of numbness on the dorsal ulnar aspect of the hand isolates the compression to the wrist rather than to the elbow. This is because the dorsal ulnar sensory nerve separates from the main trunk of the ulnar nerve 9 cm proximal to the Guyon canal. Therefore, dorsal ulnar sensation is not affected by ulnar nerve compression within the Guyon canal. Lipomas and ganglion cysts in the canal can cause ulnar nerve compression. Manual labor with repeated trauma to the hypothenar region can lead to scar adhesions of the ulnar nerve or the development of an ulnar artery pseudoaneurysm causing ulnar nerve compression (the hypothenar hammer syndrome).

B. SPECIAL TESTS

Electrodiagnostic studies may show slowing of the ulnar nerve conduction across the canal but are often normal. The diagnosis is based on the clinical presentation and normal ulnar nerve conduction velocity at the elbow through the cubital tunnel. If hypothenar hammer syndrome is suspected, an upper extremity vascular Doppler examination and an arteriogram should be ordered.

Treatment

Because the tortuosity of the Guyon canal precludes glucocorticoid injections and splinting is often ineffective, surgical decompression is recommended.

COMPRESSION OF THE SUPERFICIAL RADIAL NERVE AT THE DISTAL FOREARM

ESSENTIAL OF DIAGNOSIS

- *Paresthesias of the dorsal aspects of the thumb as well as index and long fingers.*

The superficial branch of the radial nerve provides sensation to the dorsal thumb and index and long fingers, and the radial dorsum of the hand and wrist. Its proximity to the bony prominence of the radius makes it vulnerable to extrinsic compression, such as from a tight wristwatch, splint, or other constrictive band.

Clinical Findings

Presenting symptoms include numbness and paresthesias in the radial sensory distribution. Lancinating pain may indicate a traumatic cause of the compression.

Differential Diagnosis

The differential diagnosis includes DeQuervain tenosynovitis and arthritis of the thumb carpometacarpal (CMC) joint. Occasionally, radial sensory neuritis can be caused by DeQuervain tenosynovitis with adjacent inflammation.

Treatment

Injection of a short-acting local anesthetic into the area of most severe pain can be both diagnostic and therapeutic. The treatment is directed at alleviating the compression either from the adjacent extensor tendons or from scar tissue resulting from previous trauma. If the symptoms persist after several weeks, referral to a hand surgeon should be made for potential exploration and neurolysis.

COMPRESSION OF THE ULNAR NERVE AT THE ELBOW

ESSENTIALS OF DIAGNOSIS

- *Pain in the proximal forearm.*
- *Paresthesias of the small finger and the ulnar side of the ring finger.*
- *Positive Tinel sign with percussion of the ulnar nerve at the elbow.*
- *Weakness and atrophy of the intrinsic muscles with long-standing compression.*

Clinical Findings

A. SYMPTOMS AND SIGNS

Compression of the ulnar nerve within the cubital tunnel at the elbow produces an extreme aching or lancinating pain in the proximal forearm and paresthesias radiating distally to the small finger and ulnar side of the ring finger. These symptoms are exacerbated by elbow flexion because the cubital tunnel is below the pivot point of the compression. Percussion of the ulnar nerve at the elbow will produce discomfort and paresthesia (a positive Tinel sign). Weakness and intrinsic muscular atrophy are usually late manifestations.

B. SPECIAL TESTS

Electrodiagnostic studies help establish the diagnosis and assess the severity of the compression.

Treatment

Conservative therapy is indicated in patients with minimal compression. Patients are advised against maintaining postures that involve elbow flexion, such as arm crossing while awake and the fetal position during sleep. To prevent elbow flexion during sleep, the patients wear custom-made long arm splints to maintain the elbow at about 5 degrees of flexion. For those with coexisting carpal tunnel syndrome, the splint is extended beyond the wrist to keep the wrist at neutral. If both sides are affected, bilateral splints are made, and the patients are instructed to alternate the splints nightly so that one arm is free to function in its normal capacity such as removing eyeglasses, turning the light off at night, and reaching for the clock. The patients are referred to the occupational therapists for ergonomic exercises and posture modifications. The use of NSAIDs is recommended. If symptoms do not improve over 2–3 months, then surgical decompression may be indicated.

RADIAL TUNNEL SYNDROME

ESSENTIALS OF DIAGNOSIS

- Dysesthesias and paresthesias that radiate to the dorsal radial surface of the forearm and the hand.
- Aching pain in the extensor and supinator muscle mass in the proximal forearm.

Clinical Findings

A. SYMPTOMS AND SIGNS

Radial tunnel syndrome results from compression of the nerve in the region from the radius head to the supinator. Patients describe aching pain in the extensor and supinator muscle mass in the proximal forearm. Involvement of the superficial branch of the radial nerve produces dysesthesias and paresthesias that radiate to the dorsal radial surface of the forearm and the hand. Physical findings include tenderness of the radial nerve upon palpation along its path. Although not entirely reliable, radial tunnel syndrome should be strongly suspected if the symptoms are reproduced by (1) resisted supination, (2) elbow flexion with the forearm in supination and the wrist in neutral position, or (3) passive pronation with the wrist in full flexion.

B. SPECIAL TESTS

Neurodiagnostic studies are usually not helpful unless there is evidence of muscle denervation, which is usually a late symptom of chronic compression.

Differential Diagnosis

Differential diagnosis of this relatively rare condition should include lateral epicondylitis. Although much has been written about the various maneuvers used to differentiate the symptoms between lateral epicondylitis and radial tunnel syndrome, this diagnosis can sometimes still be very difficult because both conditions can exist in the same patient. Often, therapeutic and diagnostic injections with lidocaine at the lateral epicondyle or within the radial tunnel can determine the cause of proximal forearm pain.

Treatment

A 2–3-month course of NSAIDs, splinting, and muscle stretching exercises is often helpful. Refractory cases should be referred for surgical exploration and decompression.

REFLEX SYMPATHETIC DYSTROPHY

Reflex sympathetic dystrophy (RSD) is a severe and often disabling condition that can occur after minor trauma, surgery, or stroke. In stage 1, there is burning spontaneous pain felt in the distal upper extremity, edema, hyperhydrosis, and hypothermia. These symptoms can occur either immediately or several weeks after an injury to the limb. Skin paleness and coolness characterize stage 2. The edematous tissues become indurated, and the patient has constant pain. In stage 3, the skin becomes atrophic, and pain spreads proximally. There are fixed joint contractures because the pain limits the use of the extremity. Patchy osteoporosis can be seen on radiographs. Diagnosis and management of RSD are discussed in Chapter 14.

■ UPPER EXTREMITY PAIN DUE TO MUSCULOSKELETAL CAUSES

FLEXOR & EXTENSOR TENDINITIS

ESSENTIALS OF DIAGNOSIS

- Inflammation of the tenosynovium in the hand and wrist causes pain and limitation of motion, typically in one or two fingers, that is worse upon awakening.

- *Inflammation can occur in any region where tendons traverse underneath a retinacular pulley.*
- *Thickened, tender volar tendon sheaths on palpation, with limited active but normal passive motion of the affected digits.*

Clinical Findings

Dorsal wrist tenosynovitis can produce an hourglass-shaped swelling, as soft tissues bulge on either side of the extensor retinaculum. Many cases are idiopathic; identifiable causes include rheumatic disease, diabetes, sports-related or occupational trauma, and repetitive motion injury. Trigger finger and DeQuervain tenosynovitis are two classic examples of flexor and extensor tendinitis.

Treatment

Many patients respond to a 1–2-week course of NSAIDs and splinting. After this, hand therapy may be helpful in increasing strength and range of motion. Refractory cases may require glucocorticoid injections into the tendon sheaths or surgical decompression and synovectomy.

TRIGGER FINGER (STENOSING TENOSYNOVITIS)

ESSENTIALS OF DIAGNOSIS

- *Ratcheting motion during flexion of the finger.*
- *Locking of the finger.*

Clinical Findings

Triggering of the finger is caused by irritation and subsequent swelling of the flexor tendon tenosynovium at the proximal edge of the A1 pulley. The flexor tendons are then unable to glide smoothly within the A1 pulley, resulting in the classic triggering or ratcheting motion during finger flexion. The constant motion of the inflamed tenosynovium causes intense pain. Further swelling results in locking of the finger in extension or more commonly in flexion, as the swollen tendon can no longer glide through the A1 pulley. Once the finger is locked, the patient needs to passively extend or flex the finger to make it mobile. Acquired trigger fingers can be associated with rheumatoid arthritis and diabetes mellitus, although most cases are idiopathic and thought to be due to minor trauma such as that from repetitive motion or minor blunt force.

Treatment

Conservative therapy is initially indicated in trigger finger. Patients are educated about possible etiology such as the preferential use of the finger during typing or forceful grasping of objects that causes minor direct blunt trauma to the proximal edge of the A1 pulley. Finger splints and NSAIDs are recommended as initial treatment for a trial of several weeks. If the patient has already tried this or the triggering is severe, steroid injections are given into the potential space between the A1 pulley and the flexor tendon. Steroid injections may be repeated several times, but usually should not exceed three injections, unless there are medical contraindications to surgery. If triggering recurs, surgical release of the A1 pulley is indicated. This can be accomplished quite easily under local anesthetic with low morbidity, although digital nerve laceration, stiffness, and infection with delayed wound healing have been reported.

DEQUERVAIN TENOSYNOVITIS

ESSENTIALS OF DIAGNOSIS

- *Radial wrist pain.*
- *Pain with extension and abduction of the thumb.*
- *Positive Finkelstein sign.*

Clinical Findings & Differential Diagnosis

A common cause of radial-sided wrist pain is tendinitis of the first dorsal extensor compartment. The dorsal compartments act as pulleys for the wrist and finger extensors. Within the first dorsal compartment are the extensor pollicis brevis and the abductor pollicis longus. When the first dorsal compartment and the tenosynovium around these two tendons are inflamed, there can be severe pain with thumb extension and abduction. There is usually pain on direct palpation of the compartment when the patient "hitchhikes" the thumb against resistance. There can also be pain with passive ulnar deviation of the wrist with a clasped thumb. The elucidation of pain is referred to as a positive Finkelstein sign. Occasionally, palpable crepitance is present in the compartment when the patient ranges the thumb, and a radial osteophyte may also be visible on radiographs. Differential diagnoses include thumb basilar joint arthritis and compression of the dorsal radial sensory nerve.

Treatment

Conservative treatment is the first-line therapy, consisting of NSAIDs, a thumb spica splint, and glucocorticoid injections into the first dorsal compartment. Care must be taken to infiltrate over both the extensor pollicis brevis and the abductor pollicis longus tendons, which are often separated by a septum within the first dorsal extensor compartment. Failure of conservative treatment will necessitate surgical first compartment release, which can be performed as an outpatient procedure under local anesthesia and intravenous sedation, with a very low rate of morbidity and a high rate of success.

GANGLION CYSTS

ESSENTIALS OF DIAGNOSIS

- *Firm cystic masses adjacent to joints.*
- *Usually painless.*

Clinical Findings

Despite the name, a ganglion cyst is not related to a nerve. Ganglion cysts arise when synovial lining and joint fluid herniate through a weakness in the joint capsule. The inciting factor may be a tear or localized degenerative change in the tenosynovium. A localized check-valve effect occurs at the base of the stalk, allowing ingress but not egress of synovial fluid from the joint into the protrusion. As fluid accumulates, a cyst forms. With partial resorption of the fluid by the cyst lining, the fluid inside becomes more concentrated and viscous, making aspiration of the fluid difficult. The most common location is at the dorsal wrist with the origin at the scapholunate joint. The second most common location is at the volar radial wrist. Cysts can also occur in the fingers, elbow, and shoulder. Ganglion cysts are generally painless but can cause pain resulting from compression of the overlying nerve or the joint space. An occult ganglion cyst is a very common cause joint pain.

Treatment

Aspirating ganglion cysts with a wide-gauge needle, such as an 18 or 20 gauge, is sometimes successful, but the recurrence rate is high. Surgical exploration is the most effective means of long-term control if the entire cyst, check-valve, and underlying cause of the localized synovial degeneration (such as an osteophyte) are resected.

MEDIAL & LATERAL HUMERAL EPICONDYLITIS

ESSENTIALS OF DIAGNOSIS

- *Pain and tenderness over the involved epicondyle.*
- *Medial epicondyle pain made worse by wrist flexion.*
- *Lateral epicondyle pain made worse by wrist extension.*

The forearm flexors originate from the medial humeral epicondyle, and the extensors originate from the lateral humeral epicondyle. Inflammation at the insertions of these muscles is referred to as epicondylitis, either lateral or medial. The term "tennis elbow" is still used to refer to lateral epicondylitis although the great majority of patients with this condition do not play tennis.

Clinical Findings

Clinically, there is pain at the epicondyle, which is worsened with contraction of the involved muscles. Wrist extension exacerbates the pain of lateral epicondylitis, and the pain of medial epicondylitis is made worse by wrist flexion. There may be weakness of the associated muscles. Epicondylitis is seen more commonly in the fourth and fifth decades of life. Younger patients should be examined for other causes of pain, such as elbow instability, tumors, or osteochondritis dissecans.

Treatment

A substantial majority (85–95%) of patients respond to conservative therapy in the form of a 2–3-week course of rest, splinting, and NSAIDs, followed by gentle strengthening exercises and the use of a commercially available forearm support band. Steroid injections (no more than three) are given for severe discomfort. Because of the risk of damage to the ulnar nerve, only experienced clinicians should attempt injections at the medial epicondyle. Surgery is indicated if conservative measures fail. Surgical options include (1) the repair of the flexor or extensor tendon origins at the epicondyle; (2) lengthening or fasciotomy of the tendon origin if there is tension; (3) decompression of the radial sensory branches around the elbow; or (4) elbow joint arthroplasty with ligament division, synovectomy, or epicondylectomy. Results of surgery can be good, but patients should expect a long period of physical rehabilitation afterward.

■ OSSEOUS CAUSES OF PAIN

Hand and wrist pain can be due also to the underlying skeletal structures. Usually, the most common cause of pain among middle-aged and elderly persons is osteoarthritis. Again, history and physical examination are important, and three-view radiographs of the hand and wrist should be obtained. Other osseous causes of pain include minor trauma or bony tumors. Subtle joint changes, hairline fractures, and tumors are in the spectrum of lesions detectable on a radiograph but may not be apparent on physical examination. Inflammatory arthritis as a cause of hand pain is reviewed elsewhere (see Chapter 4).

BASILAR THUMB OSTEOARTHRITIS (FIRST CARPOMETACARPAL JOINT OSTEOARTHRITIS)

ESSENTIALS OF DIAGNOSIS

- *Pain at the base of the thumb made worse by pinching activity.*
- *Pain and crepitance with passive rotation and compression of the first carpometacarpal (CMC) joint.*
- *Degenerative changes of the first carpometacarpal joint on radiographs.*

The base of the thumb is the area in the hand most commonly affected by osteoarthritis. The thumb is a long lever, and the power of the thumb pinch can be more than 30 pounds. Pinch power at the tip of the thumb is amplified 25 times at the base of the thumb, because of the long lever arm (ie, up to 750 pounds of force).

Clinical Findings

Physical examination findings include pain and crepitance on passive rotation and compression of the first CMC joint. This is referred to as the "grind test." Radiographs usually show degenerative changes involving the first CMC joint. DeQuervain tendinitis must be ruled out because the two entities have similar symptoms.

Treatment

Osteoarthritis of the first CMC joint is treated initially with NSAIDs and a wrist-based thumb splint to immobilize the CMC joint. Should this not work, glucocorticoids can be injected into the joint to temporarily relieve the pain and the inflammation. It is important that patients understand that the injections are given to relieve the pain and do not reverse the degenerative process. With few exceptions, patients should not receive more than three steroid injections into the joint. As cartilage and joint destruction progress, pain and stiffness may eventually necessitate surgical intervention. Surgical options include tendon interpositional arthroplasty, with removal of both the proximal articular surface of the thumb metacarpal and the trapezium followed by a tendon interpositional grafting and ligament reconstruction of the joint. Silicone interposition arthroplasties have been performed in the past but are no longer advised because of prosthetic failure and silicone synovitis. Arthrodesis between the thumb metacarpal and the trapezium is another option in CMC joint arthritis, but this limits the range of motion in the thumb.

■ VASCULAR CAUSES OF PAIN

Ischemic symptoms range from mild (such as cold intolerance, decreased digital temperature, or intermittent color changes) to severe (such as excruciating ischemic pain, fingertip ulceration, or necrosis). If vascular insufficiency is suspected, it is important to identify predisposing medical condition such as hypercoagulable disorder, atherosclerosis, embolic disorder, connective tissue diseases, malignancy, or diabetes mellitus. The patient should be asked about occupational and recreational exposure to vibration or other repetitive hand trauma that could cause hypothenar hammer syndrome. It is important to ask about exposure to tobacco and toxic chemicals, such as vinyl chloride and epoxy resins. Symptoms that change with arm position or exercise may indicate thoracic outlet syndrome or proximal occlusive disease. The patient may also point out the presence of a mass that could be an aneurysm or an arteriovenous malformation.

The upper extremity vascular examination begins with a thorough inspection of the skin for discoloration, scars, rashes, hair pattern, and ulceration. The fingernails may have chronic infection, hyponychial skin breakdown and scarring indicating chronic ischemia, or splinter hemorrhages from microemboli. Careful palpation detects temperature differences between digits, the presence of vascular masses, thrills, and the presence and strength of brachial, radial, and ulnar pulses. Unilateral vascular findings suggest embolic disease.

Hand perfusion should be assessed with the Allen test, testing for perfusion through either the ulnar or the radial artery. Although there are false-positive and false-negative results, the Allen test is easy and useful. To increase sensitivity and specificity, Doppler should be used to evaluate the radial and ulnar arteries, as well as the digital arteries on both the ulnar and radial sides of the finger. Magnetic resonance angiography is noninvasive and can image a vessel as small as 1 mm with good resolution. However, the gold standard in evaluating the vascular anatomy in the hand is still the upper extremity arteriogram, which can image the entire vascular tree from the aortic root to the distal finger. A comprehensive survey of the many vascular disorders of the upper extremity is beyond the scope of this chapter.

(See Chapter 21, Raynaud Phenomenon; Chapter 30, Takayasu Disease; and Chapter 40, Buerger Disease.)

REFERENCES

Chumbley EM, et al. Evaluation of overuse elbow injuries. *Am Fam Physician.* 2000;61:691. [PMID: 10695582]

Deune EG, Mackinnon SE. Endoscopic carpal tunnel release. The voice of polite dissent. *Clin Plast Surg.* 1996;23:487. [PMID: 8826685]

Drucker WR, et al. Pathogenesis of post-traumatic sympathetic dystrophy. *Am J Surg.* 1959;97:454.

Ekstrom RA, Holden K. Examination of and intervention for a patient with chronic lateral elbow pain with signs of nerve entrapment. *Phys Ther.* 2002;82:1077. [PMID: 12405872]

Foley AE. Tennis elbow. *Am Fam Physician.* 1993;48:281. [PMID: 8342481]

Goergen T, et al. Chronic elbow pain. American College of Radiology. ACR Appropriateness Criteria. *Radiology.* 2000;215:339. [PMID: 11037446]

Kalb RL. Evaluation and treatment of wrist and hand pain. *Hosp Pract.* 1998;33:129. [PMID: 9522837]

Urbaniak JR, Roth JH. Office diagnosis and treatment of hand pain. *Orthop Clin North Am.* 1982;13:477. [PMID: 7099585]

Viegas SF. Atypical causes of hand pain. *Am Fam Physician.* 1987; 35:167. [PMID: 3814245]

Watrous BG, Ho G Jr. Elbow pain. *Prim Care.* 1988;15:725. [PMID: 3068691]

Approach to the Patient with Ankle & Foot Pain

7

William M. Jenkin, DPM

Motion of the ankle and foot occurs primarily at the "essential" joints: the ankle (the joint between the talus and the distal ends of the fibula and tibia), the subtalar (talocalcaneal) joint, the midtarsal (talonavicular and calcaneal-cuboid) joints, and the metatarsophalangeal (MTP) joints (Figure 7–1). Each region of the distal lower extremity has its specific disorders. Therefore, the diagnostic approach to chronic pain in the foot and ankle begins with identifying the location of the problem (ie, the ankle, heel, midfoot, or forefoot).

■ ANKLE PAIN

The ankle joint allows the foot to dorsiflex and to plantarflex. An **ankle equinus** exists when there is inadequate dorsiflexion (less than 10 degrees) with the leg extended. The first step in the evaluation of a patient with ankle pain is to determine whether the pain is due to intra-articular or extra-articular causes.

Intra-articular pain is often felt anteriorly, but some patients complain of a dull aching discomfort that is difficult to localize. Motion of the ankle joint (ie, dorsiflexion and plantar flexion of the foot) elicits pain. An ankle effusion may be present (Table 7–1).

INTRA-ARTICULAR CAUSES OF ANKLE PAIN

ESSENTIALS OF DIAGNOSIS

- Ankle pain with dorsiflexion and plantar flexion of the foot.
- Tenderness or swelling or both of the ankle joint.

Clinical Findings

A. SYMPTOMS AND SIGNS

Ankle effusions, if present, can be palpated anteriorly, just medial and lateral to the extensor tendons as they cross the joint line. Ankle motion may be limited and may demonstrate crepitation. If the process is isolated to the tibiotalar joint, the pain occurs with ankle motion (dorsiflexion and plantar flexion of the foot) but not with motion of the subtalar joint (inversion and eversion of the foot). Occasionally, determining whether the tibiotalar joint or the subtalar joint is the source of the discomfort is difficult; in these cases, symptomatic relief following injection of a local anesthetic into the tibiotalar joint defines it as the cause of symptoms.

B. IMAGING STUDIES

Radiographs of the ankle are obtained to evaluate for talar dome lesions and arthritic changes. When necessary, magnetic resonance imaging (MRI) further defines the pathology noninvasively and provides information about the soft tissue around and within the joint. Arthroscopic evaluation provides definitive diagnosis as well as treatment.

Differential Diagnosis

The approach to acute onset of inflammatory arthritis in one ankle is the same as the approach to acute monoarthritis elsewhere; infection and crystal-induced arthritis are leading causes, and the major priority is to exclude the possibility of septic arthritis (see Chapter 4). The spondyloarthropathies, particularly reactive arthritis, can cause acute or subacute onset of inflammatory arthritis of the ankle joint, usually as a component of an oligoarthritis. Sarcoidosis also can cause acute inflammatory arthritis of the ankles, often in association with erythema nodosum.

Rheumatoid arthritis and the spondyloarthropathies are the leading causes of chronic inflammatory arthritis of the ankles, almost always with evidence of arthritis in other joints.

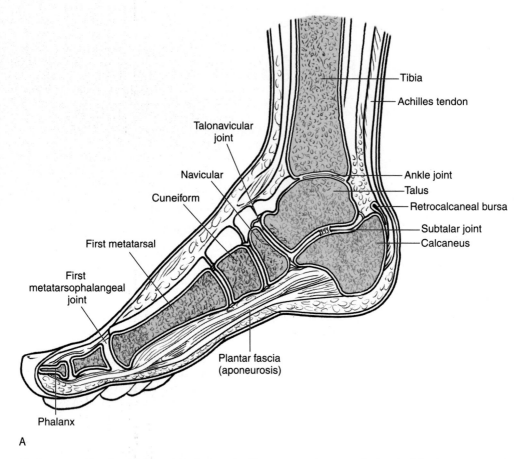

Figure 7–1. Anatomic relationships of the foot and ankle. **A:** Sagittal view at the level of the first metatarsal. (From Polley HF, Hunder GS. *Rheumatologic Interviewing and Physical Examination of the Joints.* 2nd ed. WB Saunders, 1978, Figure 14–5. With permission.)

Persistent ankle pain following an injury raises the possibility of a talar dome injury (eg, osteochondritis dissecans and transchondral "fractures"). Osteoarthritis of the tibiotalar joint is uncommon and, when present, is usually the result of significant trauma. Severe degenerative disease of the tibiotalar joint suggests neuropathic arthropathy, particularly if the patient is diabetic. Neuropathic changes in the subtalar and talonavicular joints usually accompany neuropathic arthropathy of the tibiotalar joint.

Treatment

Symptomatic anti-inflammatory measures are instituted. Once an infectious, traumatic, or neoplastic cause has been eliminated, an intra-articular glucocorticoid injection often provides lasting relief. Exterior support is helpful but must extend above the ankle. Various types of ankle braces or ankle foot orthoses can be used.

In severe cases, immobilization in a BK walker for 1 month is necessary. In recalcitrant cases, especially when the diagnosis is questionable, referral for arthroscopic evaluation and treatment is often definitive.

Table 7–1. Causes of intra-articular ankle pain.

Arthritis: inflammatory, infectious, DJD
Synovitis
Synovial impingement
Meniscoid body
Adhesive capsulitis
Ligament pathology
Talar dome injury ("fracture")
Osteochondritis dissecans
Loose bodies
Anterior ankle impingement

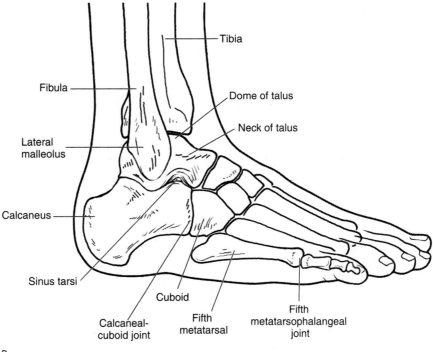

B

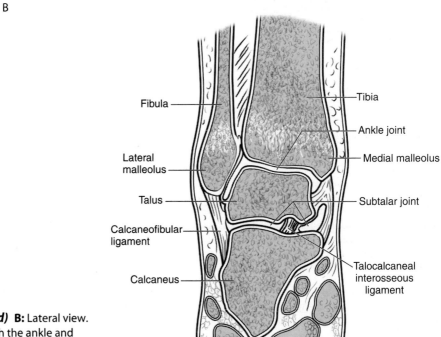

***Figure 7–1. (Continued)* B:** Lateral view. **C:** Frontal section through the ankle and subtalar joint. (From Polley HF, Hunder GS. *Rheumatologic Interviewing and Physical Examination of the Joints.* 2nd ed. WB Saunders, 1978, Figure 14–1. With permission.)

C

POSTERIOR MEDIAL ANKLE PAIN

Extra-articular causes of ankle pain (Table 7–2) tend to localize to the posterior medial, the posterior lateral, or the anterolateral aspects of the ankle and produce characteristic findings as described below.

1. Flexor Hallucis Longus Dysfunction

ESSENTIALS OF DIAGNOSIS

- *Pain with deep palpation of flexor hallucis longus (FHL) posterior to the talus.*
- *Pain with ankle and hallux dorsiflexion.*
- *Triggering of the hallux.*

Clinical Findings

A. SYMPTOMS AND SIGNS

FHL dysfunction is a repetitive use injury resulting in inflammation of the FHL tendon and, in more severe cases, stenosing tenosynovitis with nodule development and triggering of the great toe. FHL dysfunction occurs in both genders at all ages. Hypertrophy of the FHL muscle may contribute to development of the syndrome (placing ballet dancers at risk), but FHL dysfunction occurs in nonathletic persons as well.

FHL dysfunction causes pain or crepitation or both posterior medial to the ankle and is reproduced by passive or active motion of the FHL tendon. The pain may radiate along the medial arch and may be mistaken for distal plantar fasciitis. The pain improves with inactiv-

Table 7–2. Extra-articular causes of ankle pain.

Posterior medial ankle pain
  Flexor hallucis longus dysfunction
  Tibialis posterior tendon dysfunction
  Tarsal tunnel syndrome
Posterior lateral ankle pain
  Posterior talar impingement syndrome
  Peroneal tendon dysfunction
  Subtalar joint coalition
  Sural nerve entrapment
Anterior lateral ankle pain
  Sinus tarsi syndrome
  Superficial peroneal nerve entrapment
  Lateral ankle ligament disorder
  Coalition of the talocalcaneal or calcaneal-navicular joints

ity and may not be apparent when the patient first stands after sitting for a prolonged period. On examination, palpation of the FHL tendon at the posterior medial ankle (Figure 7–2) or the distal medial arch (or both) reproduces the pain, which is further exacerbated by dorsiflexion of the ankle and hallux.

B. IMAGING STUDIES

If the diagnosis is in doubt, tenography under fluoroscopy is the imaging study of choice.

Treatment

Initial measures include rest with avoidance of repetitive ankle motion, the use of nonsteroidal anti-inflammatory drugs (NSAIDs), and physical therapy. Recalcitrant cases should be treated with a glucocorticoid injection into the tendon sheath and a period of immobilization in a below-the-knee walker. If these measures fail, referral for surgical intervention in the form of a synovectomy and release of the retinaculum is indicated.

2. Tibialis Posterior Tendon Dysfunction

ESSENTIALS OF DIAGNOSIS

- *Early disease: pain and tenderness along the tibialis posterior tendon.*
- *Severe disease: ankle equinus, pes plano valgus.*

Clinical Findings

A. SYMPTOMS AND SIGNS

Progressive degenerative changes in the tibialis posterior tendon occur below the medial malleolus, producing posterior medial ankle pain and a series of foot deformities. In the early phase (stage 1), the patient complains of pain along the posterior tibial tendon either as it courses around and below the medial malleolus or at its insertion into the navicular bone. There is no gross deformity at this stage. Pain is reproduced with palpation and with resisted abduction of the foot. A gastrocnemius equinus (less than 10 degrees of ankle dorsiflexion with the leg extended while holding the foot neutral to supinated) is present. The tibialis posterior muscle and tendon are still functional, as evidenced by the patient's ability to lift the heel off the ground when standing on one foot (single heel raise) and to subtly invert

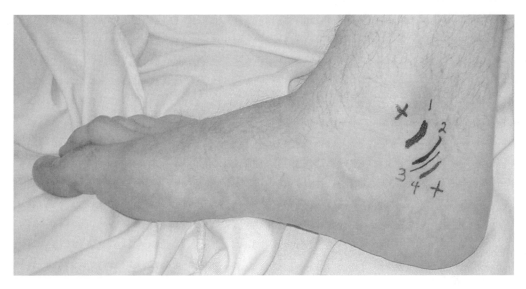

Figure 7–2. Photograph of the medial aspect of the foot demonstrating the relationships of the anatomic structures of the ankle and heel. The flexor retinaculum or laciniate ligament stretches between the medial malleolus (**X**) and the medial process of the tuberosity of the calcaneus (X). Passing below the flexor retinaculum are the tibialis posterior tendon (**1**), the flexor digitorum longus tendon (**2**), the neurovascular bundle containing the posterior tibial artery and nerve (**3**), and the flexor hallucis longus tendon (**4**).

the heel during the heel raise test. As the problem progresses, the tibialis posterior tendon becomes elongated, thin, and weakened and is no longer able to stabilize the midtarsal joint. The medial arch begins to sag as the forefoot begins to abduct upon the rearfoot, developing a pes plano valgus foot deformity (stage 2). This stage is associated with little to no muscle strength, depending on whether the tendon is weakened or ruptured. When the affected side is bearing weight and is viewed from behind, a maximum eversion (valgus) of the calcaneus is noted and more toes are visible as the forefoot abducts upon the rearfoot ("too many toes" sign) (Figure 7–3). The patient is unable to lift the heel off the ground when standing on one foot. The deformity is flexible and the arch can still rise as the hallux is dorsiflexed. In chronic situations, secondary problems, such as lateral sinus tarsi syndrome, hammertoe, and hallux valgus deformity, result. Eventually, degenerative changes

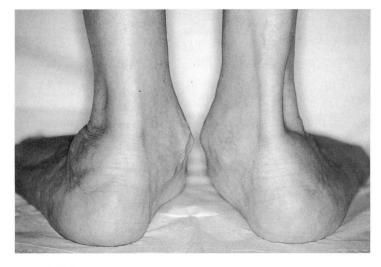

Figure 7–3. Pes planus. A posterior view photograph of severely pronated feet reveals a maximum eversion of the calcaneus (heel valgus). Abduction of the forefoot upon the rearfoot produces the "too many toes" sign. Bilateral pes planus can be congenital or acquired. Tibialis posterior tendon dysfunction can lead to unilateral pes planus.

occur in the subtalar and midtarsal joints, resulting in pain in these joints and a nonreducible or fixed deformity that is severely disabling (stage 3).

B. IMAGING STUDIES

Weight-bearing anteroposterior and lateral radiographs of the foot aid in evaluating biomechanical relationships and detecting secondary arthritic changes.

Treatment

Early recognition of this problem improves the likelihood for success of nonoperative intervention in the form of custom rigid foot orthotics. Patients with stage 2 disease, however, should be referred to a foot and ankle surgeon for consideration of tendoachilles lengthening, tibialis posterior repair and augmentation, and medial column fusions as necessary. Triple arthrodesis is usually necessary for stage 3 disease. Regardless of stage, NSAIDs provide some symptomatic relief.

3. Tarsal Tunnel Syndrome (TTS)

ESSENTIALS OF DIAGNOSIS

- Entrapment of the posterior tibial nerve within the tarsal tunnel produces medial ankle pain and dysesthesias on the sole of the foot.
- Tapping over the tarsal tunnel just posterior to the medial malleolus elicits symptoms (Tinel sign).

Clinical Findings

A. SYMPTOMS AND SIGNS

Entrapment of the posterior tibial nerve must be considered in the differential diagnosis of any plantar rearfoot or forefoot pain. The tarsal tunnel is a compartment located posteromedial to the ankle and bounded superficially by the laciniate ligament. In this compartment, the posterior tibial nerve lies just anterior to the tendon of the FHL. The nerve can be compressed by a space-occupying lesion within the tunnel such as a ganglion, by inflammation of the tendons that pass through the tunnel, or by an os trigonum and trigonal process. Excessive pronation of the foot can stretch the nerve against the laciniate ligament and also result in an entrapment.

B. IMAGING STUDIES AND SPECIAL TESTS

Electromyography and nerve conduction studies should be performed but can be normal early in the entrapment. MRI provides excellent visualization of the tarsal tunnel and is indicated if there is suspicion of a space-occupying lesion within the tunnel.

Treatment

Treatment consists of activity modification, anti-inflammatory modalities and, if there is abnormal pronation, a trial of mechanical control. Recalcitrant cases or cases demonstrating abnormal electrodiagnostic testing should be referred for possible surgical intervention.

LATERAL ANKLE PAIN

1. Posterior Talar Impingement Syndrome

ESSENTIALS OF DIAGNOSIS

- Pain with forced ankle plantar flexion.
- Radiographic demonstration of os trigonum, a trigonal process, or fracture of a trigonal process (Shepherd fracture).

Clinical Findings

A. SYMPTOMS AND SIGNS

Posterior talar impingement syndrome is a painful symptom complex caused by impingement of the ankle joint capsule by the posterior lateral aspect of the talus. Os trigonum, trigonal process, and Shepherd fracture predispose the patient to posterior talar impingement (Figure 7–4). An os trigonum is a secondary ossicle attached to the posterior lateral tubercle of the talus by fibrous tissue. A trigonal process is an elongation of the posterior lateral tubercle. A fracture of the trigonal process (Shepherd fracture) can be difficult to distinguish radiographically from an os trigonum.

There may be a history of trauma. Symptoms consist of a dull aching pain localized to the posterior lateral aspect of the ankle. The pain is often worse with increased activity, especially forceful, repetitive plantar flexion at the ankle joint. The acute injury is of a plantar flexion inversion type. The patient often relates a history of an audible "popping" sound at the time of injury. In the chronic condition, the patient describes a

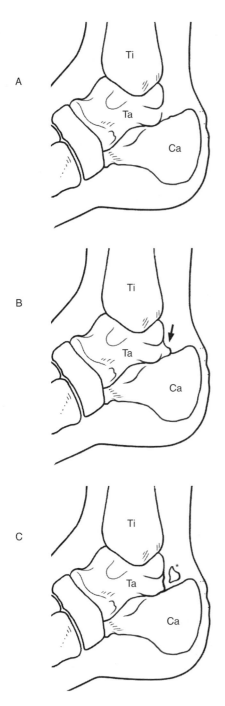

Figure 7–4. Trigonal process and os trigonum. Schematic representations of a lateral view of the tibia (Ti), talus (Ta), and calcaneus (Ca) of a normal foot (**A**), an elongated posterior lateral process of the talus or a trigonal process (arrow) (**B**), and an os trigonum (∗)(**C**).

history of repetitive plantar flexion associated with pain and swelling that increases with activities. Shepherd fracture should be suspected when "ankle sprains" fail to respond to treatment after 6–8 weeks.

On examination, pain often can be reproduced by direct palpation laterally over the posterior process, just anterior to the Achilles tendon at the ankle/subtalar joint level. Pain is inevitably reproduced by the forceful plantar flexion of the foot at the ankle. Edema is common. When evaluating the chronic injury, it is imperative to also closely evaluate for FHL dysfunction.

B. Imaging Studies

Lateral radiographs of the ankle often reveal the presence of os trigonum, trigonal process, and Shepherd fracture. Computed tomography can detect fractures missed by plain radiography as well as other injuries to the lateral talus, including osteochondritis dissecans. An MRI of the area should be obtained if tendon involvement is suspected.

Treatment

Treatment of the Shepherd fracture consists of a weight-bearing, below-the-knee cast for 4–6 weeks. In the chronic condition, symptomatic anti-inflammatory therapies are instituted. If these treatments fail, it may be necessary to resort to night splints or injection of a glucocorticoid into the area in conjunction with casting. Patients with recalcitrant cases should be referred for possible surgical excision.

2. Sinus Tarsi Syndrome

 ESSENTIAL FEATURES

- *History of inversion injury.*
- *Pain over the sinus tarsi and sensation of rearfoot instability.*
- *Relief of symptoms following injection of local anesthetic into the sinus tarsi.*

Clinical Findings

A. Symptoms and Signs

The sinus tarsi (a sulcus between the neck of the talus and the distal calcaneus) is located just anterior to, and slightly below, the lateral mallelolus (Figures 7–1B and 7–5). Sinus tarsi syndrome is a result of damage to the tarsal canal ligaments. An inversion ankle injury is the most common cause, and sinus tarsi syndrome is often

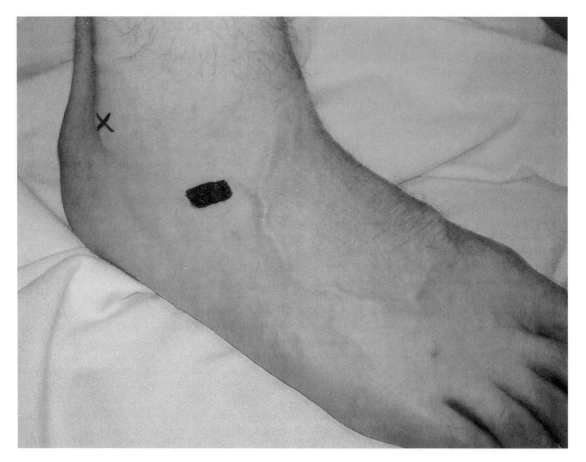

Figure 7–5. Sinus tarsi. The photograph demonstrates the location of the sinus tarsi (rectangle) anterior to, and slightly below, the lateral malleolus (**X**).

misdiagnosed as a chronic ankle sprain. Abnormal biomechanics resulting in chronic strain on the lateral talocalcaneal interosseous ligament induced by either pes planus or pes cavus also can cause sinus tarsi syndrome.

Patients complain of diffuse, deep aching pain on the dorsal-lateral aspect of the foot that increases on ambulation and is relieved by rest. There is a sensation of rearfoot instability, especially when walking on uneven terrain. The pain is reproduced by direct pressure over the sinus tarsi as well as with forced inversion and plantar flexion of the foot. Subtalar joint motion may be painful; despite the ligamentous injury and sensation of instability, the range of motion of the subtalar joint is not increased. Injection of local anaesthetic deep into the sinus tarsi should cause transient relief of pain and is a helpful diagnostic tool. If care is taken to avoid skin anesthesia, a response to sinus tarsi injection excludes the possibility of entrapment of the superficial peroneal nerve, which can cause similar symptoms and can occur secondary to ankle sprain.

B. IMAGING STUDIES

Plain radiographs are normal but are indicated to rule out fractures and coalitions between the talus and calcaneus or calcaneus and navicular bones. MRI is a sensitive means for detecting disease in the sinus tarsi but is only indicated in those cases where the diagnosis cannot be made on clinical grounds alone.

Treatment

Most cases respond to symptomatic anti-inflammatory measures, including injection of glucocorticoid into the sinus tarsi. Recalcitrant cases can respond to immobilization for 3–4 weeks. If a biomechanical fault exists, the patient should be fitted with custom foot orthotics.

If all other therapies fail, the patient should be referred for sinus tarsectomy.

■ HEEL PAIN

A range of disorders cause heel pain (Table 7–3). The initial approach to the patient with isolated heel pain should focus on identifying factors that exacerbate and ameliorate the pain and locating pain and tenderness within the heel.

Post-static dyskinesia (pain is worse on first standing and diminishes with walking) is characteristic of plantar fasciitis. The pain of Achilles tendinitis also subsides during activity. Conversely, patients with entrapment of the infracalcaneal nerve have pain that worsens with activity. Shoes with stiff counters exacerbate pain in patients with Haglund deformity (enlargement of the posterior superior aspect of the calcaneus) and retrocalcaneal bursitis.

The pain and tenderness of plantar fasciitis localize just anterior to the weight-bearing area of the heel. Palpation of the plantar fascia can elicit paresthesias when there is entrapment of the infracalcaneal nerve. In retrocalcaneal bursitis, tenderness is maximal over the posterior superior portion of the heel just anterior to the Achilles tendon. Patients with Achilles tendinitis have tenderness along the tendon or at the insertion of

Table 7–3. Causes of heel pain.

Infracalcaneal pain
  Plantar fasciitis
  Infracalcaneal nerve entrapment
  Fat pad atrophy
  Infracalcaneal bursitis
  Calcaneal stress fracture
  Tarsal tunnel syndrome
  Radiculopathy
  Spondyloarthopathy
  Infection
  Tumor
Retrocalcaneal heel pain
  Achilles tendinitis
  Haglund deformity
  Pre-Achilles bursitis
  Retrocalcaneal bursitis
  Posterior lateral calcaneal exostosis
  Lateral calcaneal adventitious bursitis
Tenderness with lateral compression of the heel
  Stress fracture of the calcaneus
  Osteomyelitis (especially in children)
  Calcaneal apophysitis (especially in boys ages 8–15 years)

the Achilles tendon, and ankle dorsiflexion often reproduces the pain. Tenderness with lateral compression of the heel suggests a stress fracture of the calcaneus.

PLANTAR FASCIITIS

ESSENTIALS OF DIAGNOSIS

- *Pain and tenderness anterior-inferior to the calcaneus.*
- *Significant improvement with mechanical control.*

Clinical Findings

A. SYMPTOMS AND SIGNS

Plantar fasciitis is the most common cause of heel pain. It is the consequence of a biomechanical fault that causes tension of the intrinsic muscles and of the plantar fascia at its insertion to the calcaneus. Plantar fasciitis is aggravated by using flexible sole shoes, by walking or standing on hard surfaces, and, in the athlete, by poor training.

Classically, the patient complains of heel pain on first arising and after a period of rest. Symptoms diminish with walking. Pain and tenderness are maximal at the point of insertion of the fascia into the medial tubercle just anterior to the weight-bearing area of the heel (proximal plantar fasciitis) or extend distally along the fascia as it courses to the toes (Figure 7–6). The foot usually appears to be normal; occasionally, pes planus or pes cavus is present.

B. IMAGING STUDIES

The diagnosis of plantar fasciitis is based on the history and examination. Radiographs are of little value in the diagnosis of plantar fasciitis but are important to rule out other disorders. The presence of infracalcaneal heel spurs on radiographs correlates poorly with symptoms.

Treatment

Treatment consists of activity modification, anti-inflammatory measures, Achilles and plantar fascial stretching, and addressing biomechanical faults. The patient is advised to avoid wearing slippers or walking barefoot. Tape immobilization, temporary over-the-counter supports, and custom foot orthotics are used to neutralize

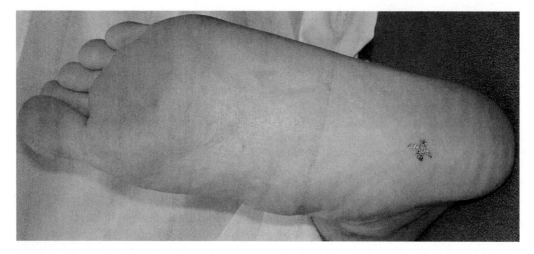

Figure 7–6. Plantar fasciitis. Photograph of the plantar aspect of the foot demonstrating the area where the clinician palpates for the pain of proximal plantar fasciitis.

abnormal mechanical forces. After biomechanical control has been instituted, injections with a local anesthetic and glucocorticoid can be of benefit. Surgical release of the plantar fascia is an option in recalcitrant cases.

ENTRAPMENT NEUROPATHY OF THE INFRACALCANEAL NERVE (DISTAL TARSAL TUNNEL SYNDROME)

 ESSENTIALS OF DIAGNOSIS

- *Burning pain along the rim of the heel.*
- *Paresthesias with palpation medial to the fascia insertion.*

Clinical Findings

A. SYMPTOMS AND SIGNS

Entrapment of the infracalcaneal nerve (a branch of the posterior tibial nerve) accounts for up to 20% of chronic infracalcaneal heel pain. It produces a sensation of burning along the rim of the heel that worsens with activity. There may be a history of post-static dyskinesia because the nerve entrapment is often the sequela of plantar fasciitis. The point of maximal tenderness is medial and just dorsal to the insertion of the plantar fascia; palpation in this area can elicit paresthesias.

B. SPECIAL TESTS

Nerve conduction studies and electromyography are normal but help exclude tarsal tunnel syndrome and radiculopathy.

Treatment

The initial treatment for this condition is the same as for plantar fasciitis. If symptoms persist after 6-12 months of treatment, neurolysis is performed.

FAT PAD ATROPHY

 ESSENTIALS OF DIAGNOSIS

- *Diffuse, central plantar heel pain aggravated by standing and activity on hard surfaces.*
- *Palpable atrophy of heel pad.*

Clinical Findings

The fat pad of the heel consists of irreplaceable, specialized, separate hydraulic fat chambers designed to absorb shock and transmit mechanical forces to the calcaneus. The fat pad atrophies with age, certain rheumatologic diseases, vascular disease, multiple glucocorticoid injections, and trauma. The heel pain is central and diffuse. In severe cases, the underlying bone is palpable.

Treatment

The initial treatment consists of shoes and flexible heel cups that cushion and absorb shock.

HAGLUND DEFORMITY & RETROCALCANEAL BURSITIS

ESSENTIALS OF DIAGNOSIS

- *The posterior superior aspect of the calcaneus is prominent, painful, and tender.*
- *Radiographic evidence of Haglund deformity of the calcaneus.*

Clinical Findings

Haglund deformity (posterior superior enlargement of the calcaneus) predisposes to shoe counter irritation, producing inflammation of the bursae located between the Achilles tendon and the calcaneus (retrocalcaneal bursitis). In some presentations, there is also an adventitious bursitis between the Achilles tendon and skin (pre-Achilles bursitis) as well as an insertional Achilles tendinitis. The patient typically complains of posterior heel pain and tenderness exacerbated by wearing shoes with enclosed stiff counters. Weight-bearing lateral radiographs reveal an enlarged retrocalcaneal bursal prominence.

Treatment

Avoidance of shoes with stiff counters is mandatory. Soft-counter shoes with a heel lift or shoes without counters (eg, clogs, sandals) should be worn. NSAIDs, contrast baths, and ice massage can be used in the acute management. Pressure-off silicone sheet pads can be used long term when wearing shoes with counters. Glucocorticoid injections are to be used prudently and only as a last resort. They are best delivered in conjunction with cast immobilization. In recalcitrant cases, the patient should be referred for surgical intervention.

ACHILLES TENDINITIS

ESSENTIALS OF DIAGNOSIS

- *Posterior heel pain with the initiation of activity and with ankle dorsiflexion.*

- *Tenderness at the insertion of the Achilles tendon onto the calcaneus (insertional tendinitis) or 4–5 cm proximal to the insertion (noninsertional tendinitis).*

Clinical Findings

A. SYMPTOMS AND SIGNS

Achilles tendinitis is usually mechanical in origin but can be a manifestation of reactive arthritis and the other spondyloarthropathies. Pain from Achilles tendinitis presents at the initiation of activity and often subsides during the activity, only to recur more intensely after the activity. Squeezing the Achilles tendon between the thumb and forefinger determines the degree of the disorder. With insertional tendinitis, tenderness is maximal where the Achilles inserts onto the middle third of the calcaneus. Noninsertional tendinitis occurs 4–5 cm proximal to the insertion in an area where the tendon torques upon itself. Ankle dorsiflexion often reproduces the pain of Achilles tendinitis. The examination should determine whether ankle equinus is present.

B. IMAGING STUDIES

Radiographs (lateral weight-bearing and calcaneal axial views) can reveal an enlarged retrocalcaneal prominence (when insertional tendinitis is associated with Haglund deformity), insertional spurring, and tendon calcifications (Figure 7–7). MRI can detect the extent and location of intratendinous linear tears and is essential prior to any surgical intervention.

Treatment

Treatment should begin with anti-inflammatory measures, stretching exercises, modification of activity (avoiding running and walking up hills and stairs), and biomechanical control in the form of temporary heel lifts, tape immobilization and, if abnormal pronation is present, custom foot orthotics. Immobilization in night splints or a cast for 4–6 weeks is indicated for recalcitrant cases. If the above measures fail, the patient should be referred for debridement and tendon lengthening.

■ SUBTALAR JOINT & MIDFOOT DISORDERS

When a person is walking, subtalar joint motion correlates with hip motion and causes the foot to pronate with internal rotation of the hip and to supinate with external

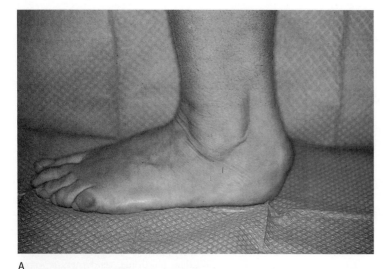

A

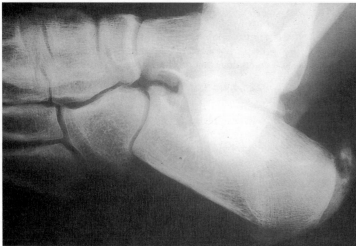

B

Figure 7–7. Achilles tendinitis. **A:** Lateral view photograph of a patient with a prominence in the area of the posterior superior aspect of the calcaneus. **B:** Lateral view radiograph of same patient demonstrating that an insertional calcific Achilles tendinitis, not Haglund deformity, is the cause of this deformity.

rotation of the hip. The motion of pronation unlocks the joints of the foot and occurs at heel contact as the foot strikes the ground, thereby absorbing shock and allowing the foot to adapt to uneven surfaces. Approaching mid stance (as the upper body moves over the foot), the hip externally rotates while the foot supinates. The motion of supination raises the arch, locks the joints of the foot, and creates a rigid lever for propulsion.

Inflammatory arthritis (eg, rheumatoid arthritis) and talocalcaneal coalitions can compromise subtalar motion.

A **pes planus** exists if the foot remains pronated beyond mid stance when subtalar joint motion produces maximal eversion of the heel. Pes planus often produces a heel valgus as the midtarsal joints unlock and collapse and as the forefoot abducts upon the rearfoot (see Figure 7–3). A pes planus is also often associated with an ankle equinus. Pes planus can be congenital or can be acquired as the result of rheumatoid arthritis, hypermobility syndromes, neuropathic arthropathy, and biomechanical disorders such as dysfunction of the tibialis posterior tendon.

Pes cavus is a rigid, excessively supinated foot that lacks "shock" absorption and has a high medial arch. Pes cavus can be congenital or the consequence of neuromuscular disorders such as Charcot-Marie-Tooth disease.

■ FOREFOOT PAIN

METATARSALGIA

Metatarsalgia, or pain in the region of the metatarsal heads, can be generalized or localized to a single metatarsal head (Table 7–4).

METATARSOPHALANGEAL JOINT STRESS SYNDROME

ESSENTIALS OF DIAGNOSIS

- *"Central" metatarsalgia: pain over one or more of the central (second, third, or fourth) metatarsals.*
- *In the dislocation phase, palpable central metatarsal heads or positive luxation test for MTP joint instability.*

Clinical Findings

A. SYMPTOMS AND SIGNS

Predisposing conditions include synovitis of the MTP joints (such as occurs in rheumatoid arthritis and the spondyloarthropathies) and biomechanical flaws (such as hallux limitus/rigidus and Morton's foot [short first metatarsal]) that transfer stress from the weight-bearing first and fifth MTPs to the normally non-weight-bearing central MTP joints. The MTP joint stress syndrome consists of a predislocation and dislocation phase. In the predislocation phase, there is inflammation of the MTP joints; digital swelling and minimal digital splaying may be noted. The dislocation phase results from a rupture or attenuation of the plantar plate as it inserts into the base of the proximal phalanx. This rupture, together with loss of integrity of the stabilizing ligaments, leads to instability of the MTP joints and, ulti-

Table 7–4. Causes of central metatarsalgia.

Metatarsophalangeal joint stress syndrome
Intermetatarsal bursitis/neuritis
Morton neuroma
Stress fracture of the metatarsals
Freiberg disease (aseptic necrosis of the second metatarsal head)

mately, to dislocation. The second MTP joint is most often involved, but all of the central MTP joints can be affected. Digital deformities (hammertoe, claw toe, crossover toe) develop (Figure 7–8). Eventually, the digital deformities cause anterior dislocation of the fat pad cushion of the forefoot and prolapse of the unprotected metatarsal heads, producing painful plantar calluses.

The pain is generally described as a dull ache in the ball of the forefoot, but in the predislocation phase, the pain sometimes has a burning quality similar to the symptoms of a neuroma. Pain occurs with weight bearing and increases with activities that place stress on the forefoot (eg, wearing high-heeled shoes). The pain is usually worse when walking barefoot. On examination, there may be plantar calluses and digital deformities such as splaying, hammering, clawing, and dactylitis. The involved metatarsal heads are tender when compressed between the examiner's thumb and forefinger. When dislocation has occurred, one or more of the metatarsal heads are readily palpable on the plantar surface. In less severe cases, the MTP joint luxation test (Lachman or vertical load test) can assess stability and integrity of the flexor plate and restraining ligaments. One hand stabilizes the metatarsal while the other lifts

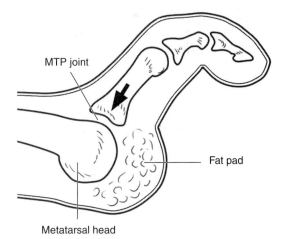

Figure 7–8. Diagram of a hammertoe deformity. There is dorsiflexion at the metatarsophalangeal joint and plantar flexion at the proximal interphalangeal joint. The protective fat pad normally beneath the metatarsal head displaces anteriorly. As the toe buckles, the retrograde digital force (arrow) places more stress upon the unprotected metatarsal head, creating metatarsalgia.

the proximal phalanx dorsally; findings of pain and ≥ 2 mm of dorsal displacement are pathognomonic for an unstable second MTP joint (Figure 7–9).

B. IMAGING STUDIES

Radiographs of the foot are not diagnostic but can rule out other conditions, such as a stress fracture.

Treatment

The involved digits should be splinted slightly plantar-flexed with tape. Patients should use supportive shoes with a rigid sole and should avoid higher-heeled shoes. In more severe cases, the patient should be referred for biomechanical evaluation for custom foot orthotics or rocker-soled shoes, or both. Periarticular or intra-artic-

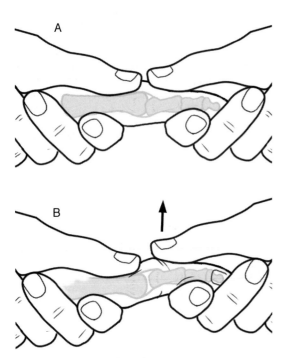

Figure 7–9. The metatarsophalangeal joint luxation test. The test is performed by stabilizing the metatarsal with one hand **(A)** while placing an upward force on the base of the proximal phalanx with the opposite hand. **(B)** When there is loss of integrity of the plantar plate (as seen in the metatarsophalangeal joint stress syndrome), this maneuver produces pain and dorsal dislocation of the base of the proximal phalanx.

ular injection of a glucocorticoid can be given if the digit is splinted in plantar flexion to prevent dislocation.

MORTON NEUROMA

ESSENTIALS OF DIAGNOSIS

- *Forefoot pain exacerbated by walking in shoes and often radiating to the third and fourth toes.*
- *Tenderness on palpation of the involved MTP interspace and Mulder click.*

Clinical Findings

Morton neuroma, a common cause of forefoot pain, is an entrapment neuropathy of an interdigital nerve, often associated with perineural fibrosis, that gives rise to a soft tissue mass. The third MTP interspace is the most common location, although Morton neuromas are also found in the second and, rarely, in the first or fourth interspaces. An intermetatarsal bursitis will create symptoms similar to a Morton neuroma as the bursa contacts the nerve distally. The patient describes burning, dull, or throbbing sensations that can radiate distally, transversely, or proximally, simulating a radiculopathy. The pain is intermittent and typically occurs while wearing shoes. Patients often remove their shoes and massage their feet in order to obtain relief. There is no pain with barefoot walking. There may be altered sensation on the sides or ends of the two toes adjacent to the involved interspace. Compressing the involved interspace with the thumb and forefinger of one hand while using the other hand to laterally compress the forefoot elicits pain. This maneuver also can cause the "neuromatous" mass to slip, producing a palpable click (Mulder click).

Treatment

Initial treatment consists of NSAIDs, contrast baths, and a lower-heeled, cushioned-soled shoe with a wide toe box. Using a dorsal approach, local anesthetic combined with a glucocorticoid can be injected into the involved interspace, making certain to deposit solution into the bursae as well as the area of nerve entrapment.

HALLUX LIMITUS/HALLUX RIGIDUS

 ESSENTIALS OF DIAGNOSIS

- *Limited or absent motion of the first MTP joint.*
- *Radiographic evidence of osteoarthritis of the first MTP joint.*

Clinical Findings

A. SYMPTOMS AND SIGNS

Hallux limitus and hallux rigidus are consequences of degenerative arthritis of the first MTP joint. Patients complain of a deep, dull ache at the base of the great toe with weight bearing. The pain increases with any activity that places stress upon the forefoot, such as walking barefoot, stooping, or wearing high-heeled shoes. Although a traumatic history (eg, ballet dancing) may be obtained, most often hallux limitus/rigidus is secondary to a biomechanical fault that leads to jamming of the first MTP joint. In hallux limitus, range of motion of the first MTP joint is decreased but not absent; pain is reproduced at the end points of motion. In hallux rigidus, joint motion is virtually absent, and what little there is creates pain and crepitation. Osteophytes may produce a prominence over the first MTP joint. Fragments of cartilage occasionally are sheared off and become lodged in the synovium, creating a detritic synovitis that is commonly mistaken for gout. The patient may also experience pain along the lateral column of the foot and lateral leg as he or she attempts to avoid bending the painful joint by adducting the foot and utilizing the oblique axis through the second through fifth MTP joints for propulsion.

B. IMAGING STUDIES

Radiographs reveal degenerative changes of the first MTP joint.

Treatment

Symptomatic treatment includes rest, contrast baths, and NSAIDs. Lower-heeled, rigid-soled shoes with soft uppers are advised. Injection of a local anesthetic and glucocorticoid into the first metatarsal interspace lateral to the joint will usually quiet the symptoms. More se-vere cases benefit from rigid custom foot orthotics. Surgical intervention may be indicated if the above measures fail.

HALLUX VALGUS

 ESSENTIALS OF DIAGNOSIS

- *Lateral deviation of the great toe.*
- *Medial bunion.*

Clinical Findings

Hallux valgus consists of medial deviation of the first metatarsal and a valgus deformity at the first MTP joint. It most likely results from the combination of a biomechanical fault, constrictive footgear, and walking on hard surfaces. Symptoms associated with the medial prominence of the first MTP joint usually are secondary to a pressure-induced bunion (an adventitious bursitis on the medial aspect of the joint), a nerve entrapment, or both. Sometimes the hallux valgus itself is asymptomatic but contributes to a painful forefoot deformity such as a hammer second toe or transfer metatarsalgia.

Treatment

Eliminating pressure from the bunion will minimize symptoms for patients with medial pain. Avoidance of high-fashion, constrictive footgear is imperative. Bunion splints that attempt to correct the deformity are of little use, but custom shoes can benefit patients with severe deformity. Patients with continual symptoms or progression of deformity should be referred for surgical consultation.

REFERENCES

Oloff LM, Schulhofer SD. Flexor hallucis longus dysfunction. *J Foot Ankle Surg.* 1998;37:101. [PMID: 9571456]

Relevant World Wide Web Sites

[ProLab Orthotics/USA]
www.prolaborthotics.com

Approach to the Painful Shoulder

Robin V. West, MD, & Mark W. Rodosky, MD

ESSENTIAL FEATURES

- *Pain is the most common symptom.*
- *An orthopedic consultation should be obtained early in the evaluation to rule out infection, tumor, or traumatic injury, which would require urgent treatment.*
- *Symptoms associated with shoulder pain may include numbness, weakness, instability, stiffness, redness, fevers, and weight loss.*

General Considerations

Because of the many sources of shoulder pain, diagnosis is often challenging. A thorough patient evaluation, including the interview, examination, and radiographic work-up, is mandatory. An orthopedic consultation should be obtained early in the evaluation if there is concern about an infection, tumor, or traumatic injury that may require urgent treatment. The injuries that may require early orthopedic intervention include a traumatic rotator cuff tear, displaced proximal humerus fracture, posterior sternoclavicular (SC) joint dislocation, septic joint, clavicle fracture that compromises the skin, or an irreducible shoulder dislocation.

Clinical Findings

A. HISTORY

The quality of the pain should be identified. Features of the pain that need to be addressed include the date of onset, history of trauma, character of the pain, associated symptoms, and all aggravating and relieving factors. Associated symptoms may include numbness, weakness, instability, stiffness, redness, fevers, and weight loss.

Pain is a subjective complaint but needs to be documented in an objective manner. Questions that should be answered include the presence of night pain (often indicates rotator cuff injury), analgesic requirements, degree of interference with work and activities of daily living, and an estimate of the amount of pain on a linear scale by the patient.

B. PHYSICAL EXAMINATION

The three basic steps of the physical examination include inspection, palpation, and range of motion.

1. Inspection—Scars provide information about trauma or previous surgery. Muscle wasting may be due to an underlying neurologic condition or to disuse atrophy. Paracervical spasm is common among patients with underlying cervical spine disease. Distal muscle wasting, such as in the interossei of the hand, may be found in cervical nerve root disorders. Deltoid wasting is best viewed over the anterior acromion and will produce a "squared-off" shoulder. Atrophy of the spinati will lead to a prominent scapular spine. Supraspinatus atrophy is more difficult to assess than infraspinatus atrophy since it is sheltered deep in the fossa under the trapezius.

Skin changes can aid in the diagnosis. Erythema, ecchymosis, or hair loss can indicate an infection, hemorrhage (seen with proximal biceps ruptures or fractures), or reflex sympathetic dystrophy. Deformities of the acromioclavicular (AC) joint may indicate previous trauma or underlying arthritis (Figure 8–1). Scapular winging is best assessed while the patient performs a push-up against a wall (Figure 8–2). Winging can be associated with thorax deformities, such as scoliosis, or with weakness of the major scapular stabilizers, including the trapezius, the serratus anterior, or the rhomboids. Severe scapular winging is most commonly due to dysfunction of the long thoracic nerve and secondary serratus anterior palsy.

2. Palpation—Sites that should be palpated during the physical examination include the AC and SC joints, the biceps tendon (in the bicipital groove), posterior joint line, and the rotator cuff at its insertion on the greater tuberosity. Deformities that may be tender along the course of the clavicle may be associated with an ununited fracture. Tenderness over the superior surface of the acromion may indicate an os acromiale with underlying impingement. The AC joint is best identified by following the clavicle and the spine of the scapula out laterally until they meet (Figure 8–3). Arthritis of the SC and AC joints is usually associated with tenderness. The greater tuberosity may be tender in patients with a fracture or rotator cuff tendinitis or tear. The bicipital groove is identified between the greater and lesser tuberosities. It can be palpated in thin

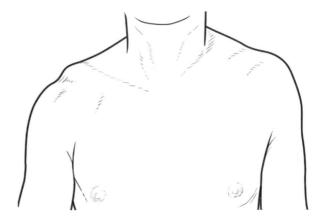

Figure 8–1. Acromioclavicular joint asymmetry.

patients as the arm is gently externally and internally rotated. The groove faces directly anterior when the arm is in about 10 degrees of internal rotation. Tenderness in the bicipital groove usually indicates biceps tendinitis. Biceps tendinitis is seldom an isolated diagnosis and is usually associated with underlying rotator cuff injury. Glenohumeral joint arthritis may elicit posterior joint line tenderness.

3. Range of motion—Range of motion of the shoulder can be assessed in the upright or supine positions. Active motion should always be compared with the contralateral side and documented. Passive motion only needs to be noted when active motion is incomplete. The motion of the opposite shoulder should also be documented. Because of the global nature of shoulder motion, a multitude of motions can be assessed. However, these various motions make documentation difficult. Therefore, the Society of the American Shoulder and Elbow Surgeons recommends recording the following four arcs of motion:

1. Total elevation
2. External rotation at side
3. External rotation in 90 degrees of abduction
4. Internal rotation

The Society has agreed that this list represents a standard protocol that is simple and reproducible. Total elevation represents a more functional measurement than forward flexion or abduction. With total elevation, the patient is allowed to find the most comfortable position in between the coronal and sagittal planes. Internal rotation is checked by having the patient scratch his or her back to the highest achievable point.

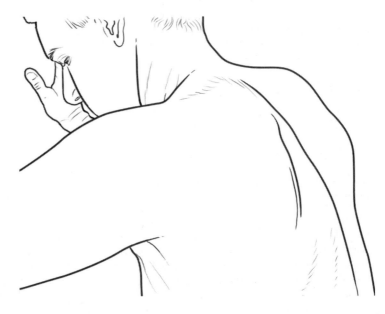

Figure 8–2. To evaluate a patient for scapular winging, have the patient perform a push-up against a wall.

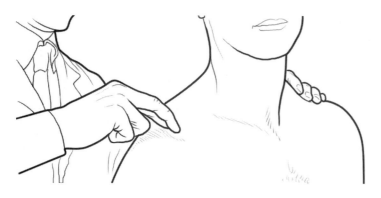

Figure 8–3. Acromioclavicular joint palpation.

The point where the patient's thumb touches is recorded (ie, the gluteus, L4, or T7).

Muscle strength should be assessed throughout all of the documented ranges of motion. Decreased strength may be found in a patient with a rotator cuff tear, brachial plexus lesion, or cervical disc disease. Sensory testing should also be performed, along with evaluation of reflexes, to assess for central or peripheral nerve involvement.

C. IMAGING STUDIES

1. Radiographs—Fractures, arthritis, calcific tendinitis, destructive bone lesions, and the bony morphology of the acromion can be seen on plain radiographs. There are multiple radiographic views that can be obtained to assess a painful shoulder.

The anteroposterior (AP) views in the plane of the scapula in neutral, internal, and external rotation are obtained to visualize the glenohumeral joint and the greater and lesser tuberosities. Cysts on the greater tuberosity may indicate rotator cuff disease. Calcium deposits in the supraspinatus can also be visualized on these views and indicate calcific tendinitis.

The axillary view can be used to assess for subtle joint space narrowing (early arthritis), an os acromiale, or a glenohumeral dislocation. The West Point axillary view is a slight variation of the standard axillary view. It provides a better evaluation of the anteroinferior glenoid rim, which is especially important when assessing for a bony Bankart lesion (capsulolabral avulsion) or glenoid rim fracture.

The supraspinatus outlet view shows the coracoacromial arch and is used to determine the acromial morphology. The acromion can be classified into three types, depending on the morphology. Type 1 acromions have a flat undersurface and have the lowest risk for impingement. Type 2 have a curved undersurface, and type 3 have a hooked undersurface. Type 3 acromions are associated with the highest percentage of rotator cuff tears.

The Stryker notch view demonstrates the posterolateral humeral head and is useful for identifying a Hill-Sachs deformity. A Hill-Sachs deformity is frequently found following an anterior shoulder dislocation and represents a compression fracture of the posterolateral humeral head.

2. Magnetic resonance imaging (MRI)—MRI can show rotator cuff abnormalities, labral disorders, and osseous integrity. The advantages of MRI include the lack of ionizing radiation and the ability to detect small changes in soft tissue composition without relying on an intravenous or an intra-articular injection of contrast material.

The accuracy in detecting full-thickness cuff tears has been reported to be between 93% and 100%. Partial-thickness tears are less accurately detected. The quality of the rotator cuff muscles, the size of the tear, and the involvement of the biceps tendon can be determined from the MRI. These MRI findings aid in the rehabilitation, surgical planning, and the postoperative planning following rotator cuff surgery.

3. Arthrography—An arthrogram can be used in addition to a plain radiograph or an MRI. The arthrogram, in association with a plain film, has been shown to have a 95–100% accuracy rate for detecting full-thickness rotator cuff tears. An MRI arthrogram can aid in detection of partial-thickness tears.

D. SPECIAL TESTS

Special tests are used to assess for instability, impingement, and AC and bicipital injuries. Examination of the elbow and cervical spine should also be included in this part of the evaluation.

1. Instability—Laxity is asymptomatic, passive translation of the humeral head on the glenoid as determined by clinical examination. Laxity is not associated with pain and is necessary for normal glenohumeral joint motion. Laxity changes with position of the arm as the static restraints tighten and decrease laxity at the extreme ranges of motion.

Instability is a pathologic condition that manifests as pain or discomfort in association with excessive translation of the humeral head during active shoulder motion. Clinical and experimental studies demonstrate a wide range of normal laxity in the glenohumeral joint; therefore, it is the association of pain that separates instability from excessive laxity.

General ligamentous laxity is commonly associated with shoulder instability and should be assessed by evaluating the range of motion of several other joints. The degree of thumb hyperabduction and elbow and knee hyperextension should be documented as part of the instability portion of the examination.

The specific instability tests include the sulcus sign test, the load and shift test, the apprehension test, and the relocation test. These tests should be initiated on the unaffected shoulder first to obtain baseline data. Two components should be addressed during this part of the examination: the amount of passive translation of the glenohumeral joint and the reproduction of symptoms of subluxation, dislocation, or apprehension by provocative testing.

The **sulcus sign test** establishes the presence of inferior laxity. This test is performed with the patient in the seated position. The arm is held at the side in neutral rotation. The examiner places a downward distraction force by grasping the distal humerus. The degree of the sulcus sign is determined by measuring the distance between the lateral acromion to the top of the humeral head. The contralateral shoulder is compared. An increased or symptomatic sulcus sign may indicate inferior instability and associated multidirectional instability.

The **shift and load test** is used to test for anterior and posterior translation. It is usually performed in the supine position but can also be performed in the upright position. To test for anterior translation of the patient's right shoulder, the examiner positions the patient's arm in the plane of the scapula, at about 45 degrees of abduction and neutral rotation. The examiner's right hand grasps the patient's arm and applies an axial load to the humeral head. This maneuver centers the humeral head in the glenoid. The examiner's right hand also controls the rotation of the patient's arm. The examiner uses his or her left hand, with the fingers placed anteriorly, to grasp the patient's upper arm. The examiner's left hand then shifts the humeral head anteriorly over the glenoid rim. The amount of translation can be determined by visual inspection and palpation. As the examiner maintains an axial load, the arm can be incrementally externally rotated. With progressive external rotation, the inferior glenohumeral ligament becomes taut, decreasing the anterior translation of the humeral head. The degree of translation can be graded. Grade 1 translation occurs when the diameter of the humeral head rides over the glenoid rim. Grade 2 occurs when the entire humeral head rides over the glenoid, but it reduces spontaneously. Grade 3 is de-

fined as a complete dislocation, which requires a reduction maneuver to relocate the humeral head.

Posterior translation is evaluated in the same position as described for testing anterior translation. The patient is supine, with the arm held in the plane of the scapula. However, the examination is initiated with the arm in 45 degrees of external rotation. The examiner's hands are positioned as described for testing anterior translation. An axial load is applied, and the humeral head is translated posteriorly. The patient's arm is then sequentially rotated internally, and the examination is repeated. The posterior-inferior capsule becomes increasingly taut during internal rotation, decreasing the posterior translation of the humeral head. The posterior translation is graded in the same way as for anterior translation.

The **apprehension test** places the shoulder in a provocative position of abduction and external rotation (Figure 8–4). This test should be performed in both the supine and seated positions. The examiner abducts the patient's arm to 90 degrees and gently begins to externally rotate the arm. With increasing external rotation and controlled gentle forward pressure on the humeral head, the patient may have an apprehensive feeling of impending instability. Isolated pain is poorly correlated with instability, and a subjective feeling of apprehension by the patient has been shown to be more specific to the diagnosis of instability.

The **relocation test** should be performed in conjunction with the apprehension test. During this test, the examiner applies a posteriorly directed force on the humeral head with the patient's arm in the position that produces apprehension. This test reduces the humeral head, and a positive result is recorded if the symptoms of apprehension are eliminated.

2. Impingement tests—Rotator cuff tendinitis has been termed shoulder impingement. The **impingement sign** and **impingement test** were described by Neer in 1977. The sign is considered positive when pain occurs with forcible elevation of the arm (Figure 8–5). This maneuver causes impingement of the inflamed supraspinatus tendon against the anterior inferior acromion. An alternative method for demonstrating impingement is to forward flex the arm to 90 degrees and then to forcibly internally rotate the shoulder (Figure 8–6).

The **impingement test** documents the patient's response to an injection of lidocaine into the subacromial space. After the injection is performed, the impingement maneuver is repeated. A significant reduction or abolition of the patient's pain constitutes a positive result and indicates a diagnosis of impingement.

3. Acromioclavicular disorders—AC pain can be caused by degenerative changes or trauma. Associated

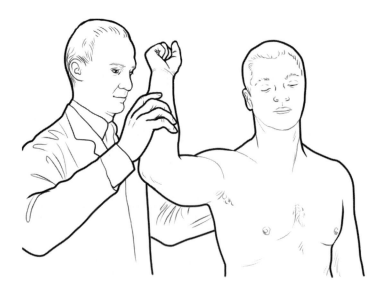

Figure 8–4. The apprehension test is useful in assessing anterior shoulder instability. Abduct and externally rotate the arm to elicit apprehension.

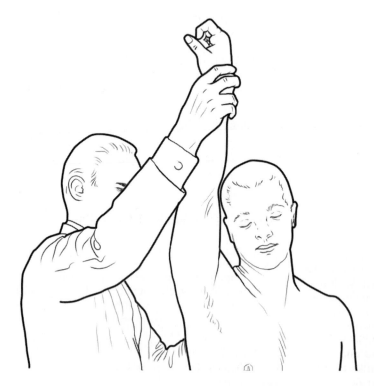

Figure 8–5. The Neer impingement sign involves forced forward elevation to 180 degrees with internal rotation of the arm.

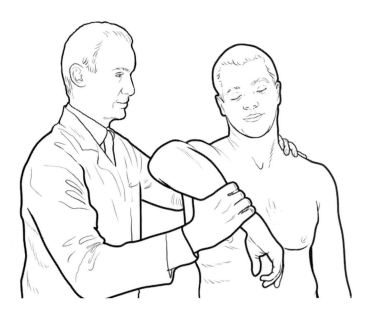

Figure 8–6. The Hawkins impingement sign involves forward elevation to 90 degrees and internal rotation.

tenderness and deformity are common after AC trauma or with arthritis. The cross-arm adduction test may also be used to diagnose AC joint disorders. This test is performed with forced crossed-arm adduction in the 90-degree forward-flexed position. Associated pain may indicate AC joint disease, usually degenerative arthritis.

4. Biceps evaluation—Biceps disorder is seldom an isolated entity. It is usually a secondary diagnosis to impingement. However, it can be a primary diagnosis. Although numerous tests that can evaluate the biceps have been described, their reliability is questionable. Palpating the bicipital groove, The Yergason test, and the Speed test are some of the tests used to assess biceps disease. Tenderness in the bicipital groove may indicate inflammation of the long head of the biceps tendon. The Yergason test is performed with the elbow flexed to 90 degrees and the forearm pronated. The patient is then asked to actively supinate the arm against resistance as the examiner holds the patient's wrist. The Speed test is performed with the elbow extended and the forearm supinated. Forward elevation of the arm to 60 degrees is resisted. A positive result with either of these tests may indicate biceps inflammation.

E. Special Examination

Vascular examination involves assessment of the entire upper limb. Skin texture, color, temperature, hair growth, pulses, and alterations in sensation should be documented and may relate to vascular problems. Vascular compression or thoracic outlet syndrome may cause shoulder pain. Thoracic outlet syndrome may cause a combination of neurologic and vascular signs. Several tests have been described to diagnose thoracic outlet syndrome. However, the reliability of these tests is not high.

1. Adson maneuver—The examiner palpates the radial pulse. The patient's head is then rotated toward the affected shoulder. The involved shoulder is then externally rotated and extended. The patient takes a deep breath and holds it. A positive test occurs when there is a decrease in the pulse with this maneuver.

2. Roos test (or provocative elevation test)—The arms are abducted to 90 degrees, the shoulders are externally rotated 100 degrees, and the elbows are flexed 90 degrees. The patient then opens and closes the hands slowly for 3 minutes. If the patient suffers from fatigue, cramping, or tingling before 3 minutes, the test is considered positive for thoracic outlet syndrome.

Differential Diagnosis & Treatment

Table 8–1 lists the major categories of disorders to be considered in the differential diagnosis of shoulder pain.

A. Cervical Disorders

Cervical spondylosis involves osteoarthritic changes of the joints of the cervical spine, including the facets and uncovertebral joints. Osteophytes may form and encroach upon the nerve root foramina. The cervical discs may also become desiccated and flattened.

Table 8–1. Differential diagnosis
of shoulder pain.

Cervical pathology
Neurologic disorder
    Serratus anterior nerve palsy
    Brachial plexus injury
    Suprascapular nerve compression
    Long thoracic nerve palsy
Congenital anomaly
Arthritis
Trauma
Instability
Rotator cuff pathology
Adhesive capsulitis
Tumor

Disc herniation consists of protrusion of the nucleus pulposus through a tear in the anulus fibrosus. The nerve root may become compressed within its foramen, producing cervical radiculopathy. Herniation can also occur in conjunction with cervical spondylosis.

Cervical radiculopathy and myelopathy may be caused by an acute, subacute, or insidious disc herniation. Subacute cervical radiculopathy is much more common than acute radiculopathy. Symptoms may include pain, paresthesias, and weakness. The dermatomal distribution of the pain, as well as weakness within certain muscles, may aid in differentiating the involved nerve root. The most commonly involved discs are C5–6 and C6–7.

The three main conservative treatments of cervical disorders include soft cervical collar immobilization, anti-inflammatory medications, and physical therapy. Cervical traction may be helpful in young patients with isolated disc herniations but less helpful in patients with spondylosis. Epidural steroids, root injections, and facet blocks can be used for the treatment of spondylosis. Experienced physicians should perform these blocks to minimize the risk of complications. Surgical intervention is usually required in patients who do not respond to nonsurgical management or in those patients who have significant neurologic deficits, particularly weakness.

B. Neurologic Disorders

There are multiple neurologic disorders that can present with pain around the shoulder. Some of the more common disorders include serratus anterior nerve palsy, brachial plexus injury, and suprascapular nerve compression. Patients with long thoracic nerve palsy present with weakness of the serratus anterior muscle, which results in periscapular pain, winging of the scapula, and difficulty elevating the arm above shoulder level. The long thoracic nerve arises from C5, C6, and C7 and provides motor innervation to the serratus anterior muscle. The serratus anterior muscle originates from the upper nine ribs, inserts onto the inferior angle of the scapula, and provides upward rotation and protraction of the scapula. There are many causes of long thoracic nerve palsy, including blunt trauma, stretching of the nerve, viral infection, or iatrogenic trauma (during a mastectomy with axillary dissection). The palsy results in a loss of normal scapular stability and rotation. Winging of the scapula occurs with elevation of the arm. Electromyography is used to confirm the diagnosis and to follow nerve recovery.

Most of the atraumatic palsies resolve over a 12- to 18-month period. Observation and periscapular muscle strengthening are appropriate therapies for patients who seem to be recovering. Surgical treatment may be considered for patients with symptomatic scapular winging for longer than 1 year and who demonstrate no electromyographic or clinical evidence of recovery. Multiple surgical procedures have been described, including scapulothoracic fusion and dynamic muscle transfers. The goal of these procedures is pain reduction and improvement of scapular function.

Brachial plexus injuries can also cause shoulder pain. The most common causes of plexus injuries are traction caused by extreme movements, such as when the head is forced laterally during a football game or motorcycle accident. Direct trauma, with an associated clavicle fracture, can also result in a plexus injury. A thorough history, complete neurologic examination, and electrodiagnostic studies are essential in diagnosing the location, extent, and completeness of the injury. Poor prognosis is associated with supraclavicular lesions, complete injuries, and root avulsions. Patients with less severe injuries who demonstrate neural recovery or mild signs and symptoms are treated conservatively. Nerve reconstruction or repair is considered in more severe postganglionic lesions or open injuries.

Patients with suprascapular nerve entrapment often present with posterior shoulder pain, which radiates to the neck or down the arm. The suprascapular nerve arises from the upper trunk of the brachial plexus at the Erb point. The nerve then courses posteriorly, deep to the trapezius, where it passes through the suprascapular notch. The notch is bounded by the transverse scapular ligament. After exiting the notch, the nerve innervates the suprascapular muscle and provides sensory branches to the AC joint, the rotator cuff, the glenohumeral joint, and the posterior capsule. The nerve then enters the spinoglenoid notch to finally reach the infraspinatus fossa, where it innervates the infraspinatus muscle.

Suprascapular nerve entrapment can occur from ganglion cysts arising from the glenohumeral joint, a hypertrophied spinoglenoid ligament, traction injuries, and microemboli that produce nerve ischemia. Ganglion cysts can cause entrapment at the suprascapular or spinoglenoid notch. Compression at the suprascapular notch causes weakness of both the supraspinatus and infraspinatus, while compression at the spinoglenoid notch causes isolated weakness of the infraspinatus. Physical examination may reveal atrophy of the spinati. Infraspinatus atrophy is more common and easier to identify than supraspinatus atrophy, since the supraspinatus muscle lies deep to the trapezius. Weakness in external rotation and forward elevation may also be noted. Routine shoulder radiographs rarely show abnormalities. Electromyographic and nerve conduction studies may localize the site of compression. An MRI of the shoulder can identify the ganglion cyst location and size. Initial treatment includes physical therapy and nonsteroidal anti-inflammatory drugs. Physical therapy should concentrate on the scapular stabilizers, deltoid, and rotator cuff. Surgical intervention is recommended if more than 6 months of conservative treatment is unsuccessful. Surgery focuses on the source of the compression. The ganglion cyst can be excised through an open incision or decompressed arthroscopically.

C. Congenital Anomalies

Congenital anomalies are rare and can be the most difficult and perplexing problems of the shoulder girdle. The anomalies can be classified into disorders of the bones, muscles, or neurovascular system. A thorough discussion of congenital anomalies is beyond the scope of this chapter.

D. Arthritis

Arthritis can involve the glenohumeral, SC, or AC joints. The arthritis can be degenerative, infectious, or inflammatory. Examination and radiographs can aid in the differentiation of the anatomic site and the type of arthritis. Examination findings may include decreased glenohumeral joint motion and tenderness to palpation over the posterior joint line in patients with glenohumeral arthritis. Tenderness over the AC joint and pain with cross-arm adduction may indicate AC joint arthritis. A long history of repetitive motion (manual labor, weight lifting) and chronic pain may lead to a diagnosis of degenerative arthritis. An insidious onset, with an associated family history, rashes, fevers, or involvement of multiple joints, may indicate an inflammatory arthritis. Infectious arthritis usually presents with an acute onset, occasional fevers, redness, and warmth. The involved joint can be aspirated, and the synovial fluid can be analyzed to confirm the diagnosis. White blood cell counts over 100,000 cells/μL strongly suggest an infection.

Radiographs may also help differentiate the type of arthritis. Degenerative arthritis usually shows sclerosis, asymmetric joint space narrowing, and osteophytes. Inflammatory arthritis usually shows osteopenia, symmetric joint space narrowing, and lack of osteophytes. In the later stages, infectious arthritis often shows joint destruction, with a mixed pattern of sclerosis and osteopenia.

Degenerative and inflammatory arthritis can be treated conservatively with anti-inflammatory drugs and physical therapy to maintain range of motion and strengthening. An intra-articular glenohumeral or AC cortisone injection may also be used to relieve some of the symptoms. Surgical intervention is recommended for patients who have not responded to a course of conservative management. A distal clavicle excision can be performed for AC joint arthritis. A medial clavicle excision can be performed for SC joint arthritis. Degenerative glenohumeral joint arthritis can be treated with either a hemiarthroplasty or a total shoulder arthroplasty. Infectious arthritis should be treated with surgical debridement and antibiotics.

E. Trauma

A traumatic event can result in a myotendinous injury, a fracture, or a dislocation. A thorough neurologic and vascular examination should be performed, and good radiographs are mandatory when evaluating a patient following an injury. Ecchymosis and deformity are common physical findings following a traumatic injury to the shoulder.

Most fractures can be treated in a sling initially, until further evaluation by an orthopedic surgeon. Open fractures, or ones that compromise the integrity of the skin, require emergency surgical intervention. Other injuries that should be treated urgently include posterior SC and glenohumeral dislocations. Anterior SC dislocations are much more common and less dangerous because posterior dislocations can compromise the underlying vessels and structures. These injuries are best assessed with a 40-degree cephalic tilt (serendipity) radiographic view or a paraxial computed tomography scan. An urgent reduction of the posteriorly dislocated SC joint is often required.

Myotendinous injuries, including an acute rotator cuff tear or a rupture of the pectoralis major or long head of the biceps, usually result in an acute onset of pain and weakness. Ecchymosis is a common finding. Initial treatment includes ice, rest, and nonsteroidal anti-inflammatory drugs. Surgical intervention is often required to perform a direct primary repair of the rotator cuff or pectoralis major acute ruptures.

F. Instability

The most common sequela of traumatic anterior shoulder dislocation is recurrence. Classic studies have documented a recurrence rate of 90% for patients under the age of 20. The recurrence rate is significantly lower among patients over the age of 40 years.

Pain and guarding of the affected arm are symptoms in patients with a traumatic dislocation. Motion will be limited, and the shoulder contour may be disrupted. A neurovascular examination is important to perform, since an associated axillary neuropraxia occurs in 5–35% of first-time anterior shoulder dislocations. Vascular injuries are rare but should be ruled out.

It is important to rule out a traumatic rotator cuff tear in older patients who sustain a shoulder dislocation. Associated cuff tears are common in older patients and can be confused with axillary neuropraxia during the clinical examination. Tears of the rotator cuff following dislocation have been reported to occur in 14–63% of patients. The incidence significantly increases among patients over the age of 50 years. Axillary neuropraxia will often present with weakness and numbness over the lateral aspect of the shoulder, while a rotator cuff tear presents only with weakness. An MRI can be performed to confirm the diagnosis of an associated rotator cuff tear.

Radiographic analysis should include a true AP in the plane of the scapula and an axillary view. The axillary view is mandatory to demonstrate an anterior or posterior glenohumeral dislocation. A West Point axillary view may better demonstrate an anterior-inferior glenoid rim fracture. Several recent studies correlating MRI arthrograms with surgical findings demonstrate an 88% sensitivity and 100% specificity in diagnosing inferior glenohumeral ligament tears.

Simple anterior dislocations without associated fractures can usually be reduced manually with sedation. Multiple reduction maneuvers have been described. The traction/countertraction technique is usually effective. From the contralateral side, an assistant holds a sheet that is wrapped around the patient's chest. The physician gently applies longitudinal traction to the injured side. A satisfying "cluck" sound is usually heard with the reduction. The reduction should be confirmed with a true AP and axillary radiograph.

Following the reduction, a brief period of immobilization and activity modification and a supervised rehabilitation program for rotator cuff and periscapular stabilizing exercises are prescribed. Conservative treatment is usually the first line of treatment, with acute surgical stabilization being considered in young athletes returning to contact sports. Once recurrent episodes of instability have occurred, conservative treatment has failed. Surgical intervention is then considered. Open and arthroscopic procedures that restore the normal glenohumeral anatomy are favored. The repair of the avulsed capsular-labral tissue (Bankart lesion) or reduction of the excessive capsular laxity is the goal of the reconstructive procedure.

Patients with multidirectional instability have symptomatic subluxation or dislocation in more than one direction: anterior, inferior, and posterior. The instability episodes are often atraumatic and painful. The primary cause is a loose redundant capsule. Swimmers, weight lifters, and gymnasts are particularly predisposed to multidirectional instability. The physical examination may demonstrate evidence of generalized ligamentous laxity, and a significant finding is usually the sulcus sign (see section, Special Tests). Once the diagnosis of multidirectional instability is established, a prolonged course of physical therapy is instituted. The therapy emphasizes deltoid, periscapular, and rotator cuff strengthening with the arm below the horizontal plane. Surgery is usually recommended after at least 6 months of supervised physical therapy. It is important to identify those persons who voluntarily dislocate their shoulder because they are poor candidates for surgical stabilization. Surgical intervention includes a capsular shift, which decreases the glenohumeral joint capsular volume.

G. ROTATOR CUFF

Rotator cuff disorders represent a spectrum of disease, including inflammation, partial- or full-thickness tears, and cuff tear arthropathy. Mechanical impingement and intrinsic degenerative processes have been cited as factors underlying rotator cuff disease.

Impingement syndrome is one of the most common causes of shoulder pain. It is a clinical diagnosis, which is made on the basis of a careful history and physical examination. Radiographs, especially the outlet view, are helpful in demonstrating the presence of subacromial spurs and acromion morphology. A subacromial lidocaine injection is useful in verifying the diagnosis. In some patients, especially overhead athletes, it may be difficult to differentiate between functional subacromial impingement, subtle instability, and "internal impingement" of the undersurface of the rotator cuff on the posterior glenoid rim. Treatment of subacromial impingement initially includes a subacromial cortisone injection and a physical therapy program for rotator cuff strengthening to improve humeral head centering and stretching to improve stiffness. Refractory cases are treated with an arthroscopic acromioplasty.

An MRI can be obtained to determine whether there is an associated rotator cuff tear. Patients with a rotator cuff tear will often demonstrate weakness, recalcitrant pain, and night pain. Many partial-thickness tears can be managed nonsurgically. If a patient with a partial-thickness rotator cuff tear continues to have symptoms, arthroscopic surgery is recommended. This procedure usually entails an arthroscopic acromioplasty, debridement, and possible repair of the rotator cuff.

Factors to consider in the choice of treatment for full-thickness rotator cuff tears include the severity and duration of symptoms, functional limitations, patient demands and expectations, as well as tear size and location. There is a high prevalence of cuff tears in the asymptomatic population, with a direct correlation between increasing age. In a prospective study of 411 asymptomatic volunteers, rotator cuff tears were identified by ultrasonography in 23% of patients. The incidence of tears was age-dependent. The prevalence increased to 31% and 51% in patients aged 70–79 years and over 80 years, respectively. These results provide evidence that patients with rotator cuff tears can exhibit relatively normal shoulder function. However, the natural history of rotator cuff tears remains unknown. A longitudinal analysis of asymptomatic cuff tears detected by ultrasonography was recently published. Fifty-eight patients with unilateral symptomatic rotator cuff tears and contralateral asymptomatic cuff tears were followed over a 5-year period. Twenty-three (51%) of the previously asymptomatic patients became symptomatic over a mean of 2.8 years. Twenty-three of the original patients returned for a repeat ultrasonography, and nine of these patients had tear progression. No patient had a decrease in the size of the tear. These ultrasonographic findings in asymptomatic patients may represent an early phase of the pathologic process of rotator cuff tears in which symptoms have not yet developed. The presence of a full-thickness rotator cuff tear is not necessarily an indication for surgery. Surgical intervention is usually recommended when there is an acute traumatic rotator cuff tear or when weakness is prominent or progressive.

H. Adhesive Capsulitis

Adhesive capsulitis or "frozen shoulder" is a poorly defined syndrome in which both active and passive motion is lost because of soft tissue contracture. The syndrome is characterized by thickening and contracture of the joint capsule, which results in decreased glenohumeral joint volume. It is believed to be a benign, self-limited disorder, which tends to resolve over 1–2 years, although patients are often left with residual loss of motion. A variety of causes have been implicated in the disorder, including, trauma, inflammation, and endocrine abnormalities. It is common among patients with diabetes and is more frequently bilateral and resistant to treatment in this subset of patients.

Most patients with frozen shoulder respond to nonsurgical treatment with stretching exercises in a supervised physical therapy program. If the therapy program is unsuccessful, manipulation under anesthesia can be done to regain motion. An arthroscopic capsular release can be used in addition to the manipulation in treating cases of resistant adhesive capsulitis. An indwelling interscalene or intra-articular catheter can also be used in addition to the surgical treatment to facilitate early postoperative therapy.

I. Tumor

Radiographic abnormalities and bone or soft tissue masses need to be evaluated in a well-organized and methodical fashion. The diagnostic work-up and treatment of bone and soft tissue tumors about the shoulder is based on the principles of oncologic surgery. The work-up should be performed promptly to improve patient survival and functional outcome. The goals of treatment are preservation of life followed by preservation of limb and function. Amputation was the primary treatment for primary bone tumors in the 1970s. However, successful limb salvage techniques have been developed for malignant and aggressive benign tumors.

The work-up of a tumor involves proceeding in a systematic fashion: clinical assessment, diagnostic studies, and biopsy in select cases. It is important to consult an orthopedic oncologist early in the work-up. Treatment should not be initiated until the oncologist has been consulted.

A thorough history should be documented. Patients often complain of associated symptoms including pain, fevers, and a mass. For example, an osteoid osteoma often causes night pain that is relieved by nonsteroidal anti-inflammatory medications. Patients with a Ewing sarcoma may have systemic signs and symptoms, such as fevers, sweats, and an elevated erythrocyte sedimentation rate.

Plain radiographs are the most useful and cost-effective study. Radiographs are relatively sensitive in detecting bony abnormalities, and they may show associated soft tissue masses. Specific findings on the radiographs, including the anatomic location and the bony reaction, can be helpful in the diagnosis.

Certain tumors have a predilection for the epiphysis (chondroblastoma), the diaphysis (Ewing sarcoma), or the metaphysis (conventional osteosarcoma). Well-circumscribed lesions are usually associated with benign lesions, and a permeative appearance on the radiographs suggests an aggressive lesion. Periosteal reaction is a useful measure of lesion aggressiveness. Slowly expanding lesions, either benign or malignant, may produce a lamellar periosteal reaction ("onion skinning"). More rapidly growing tumors can expand beyond the periosteal sleeve and give the appearance of a "sunburst" reaction.

In certain benign lesions, no further work-up is necessary after the radiographs. However, when treatment is indicated, other diagnostic studies are necessary. Technetium bone scans are helpful in determining polyostotic involvement or skip lesions. Computed tomography scans give excellent definition of bony structures, including cortical destruction, fractures, and soft tissue calcification. MRI is useful is determining the osseous and soft tissue extension. Occasionally, other studies are required, including angiography to assess vascular involvement, a biopsy to aid in the diagnosis, and a computed tomography scan of the chest to assess for metastatic disease.

Treatment is based on the diagnosis. Benign lesions (simple cysts) are usually treated nonoperatively. Aggressive-benign lesions (giant cell tumors) often require surgical intervention with curettage and bone grafting or cementation. Malignant lesions (Ewing sarcoma) usually require a combination of treatment modalities, including resection, chemotherapy, and radiation.

Techniques for Injection of the Shoulder

Prior to performing an injection, the patient should understand the risks and benefits of the procedure. The risks include an allergic reaction, infection, hypopigmentation of the skin, and poor blood glucose control in diabetics. The site should be thoroughly prepared with alcohol and povidone-iodine, and the injection should be performed under sterile conditions.

A. SUBACROMIAL SPACE

The subacromial space is the most common site for injection in patients with impingement. The cortisone can serve as treatment, and the lidocaine can aid in the diagnosis (the impingement test). The injection is performed from the posterior aspect of the shoulder. The posterolateral corner of the acromion is palpated. The injection is placed into the subacromial space with a 22-gauge needle about 1 cm distal and 1 cm medial to the posterior corner.

B. GLENOHUMERAL

This space is seldom the site for injection. It is more commonly aspirated to rule out an infection in patients who have a fever and a painful, warm shoulder. A cortisone injection can be performed for the treatment of glenohumeral arthritis. The posterolateral corner of the acromion is the landmark for the injection. A 22-gauge needle is usually used for injection, and an 18-gauge needle is used for aspiration. A spinal needle is sometimes needed in larger patients. The entry site is about 2 cm distal and 2 cm medial to the corner of the acromion. The needle is directed toward the coracoid.

C. ACROMIOCLAVICULAR

The AC joint can be injected with cortisone in patients with arthritis or distal clavicle osteolysis. The AC joint can be palpated by placing a finger in the corner formed by the transition of the scapular spine to the acromion. The AC joint is just anterior to this transition. The joint should be visualized radiographically prior to the injection, as the distal clavicle is often sloped about 15 degrees in the coronal plane. This slope should be documented to aid in a smooth, correct insertion of the needle into the AC joint. The injection is usually performed with a 22-gauge needle.

REFERENCES

Bottoni CR, et al. A prospective, randomized evaluation of arthroscopic stabilization versus nonoperative treatment in patients with acute, traumatic, first-time shoulder dislocations. *Am J Sports Med.* 2002;30:576. [PMID: 12130413] (This is a prospective, randomized clinical trial that was done to compare nonoperative treatment versus arthroscopic stabilization in acute, traumatic shoulder dislocations in young athletes.)

Chandnani VP, et al. Glenohumeral ligaments and shoulder capsular mechanism: evaluation with MR arthrography. *Radiology.* 1995;196:27. [PMID: 7784579] (This is a retrospective study that compared MRI arthrograms with surgical observations in patients with instability, impingement, or pain.)

Goldberg BA, et al. Outcome of nonoperative management of full-thickness rotator cuff tears. *Clin Orthop.* 2001;382:99. [PMID: 11154011] (This study documents the functional outcome of 46 patients with full-thickness rotator cuff tears who were treated nonoperatively.)

McConville OR, Iannotti JP. Partial-thickness tears of the rotator cuff: evaluation and management. *J Am Acad Orthop Surg.* 1999;7:32. [PMID: 9916188] (This is a review of the evaluation and management of partial-thickness rotator cuff tears.)

Morrison DS, et al. Nonoperative treatment of subacromial impingement syndrome. *J Bone Joint Surg.* 1997;79:732. [PMID: 9160946] (This is a retrospective analysis of 616 patients with subacromial impingement syndrome who were treated nonoperatively.)

Schenk TJ, Brems JJ. Multidirectional instability of the shoulder: pathophysiology, diagnosis, management. *J Am Acad Orthop Surg.* 1998;6:65. [PMID: 9692942] (This is a review of the pathophysiology, diagnosis, and treatment of multidirectional instability of the shoulder.)

Tempelhof S, et al. Age-related prevalence of rotator cuff tears in asymptomatic shoulders. *J Shoulder Elbow Surg.* 1999;8:296. [PMID: 10471998] (This is a prospective study to determine the prevalence of rotator cuff tears in asymptomatic shoulders and to determine an age-dependent relationship.)

Warner JP. Frozen shoulder: diagnosis and management. *J Am Acad Orthop Surg.* 1997;5:130. [PMID: 10797215] (This is a review of the diagnosis and management of adhesive capsulitis.)

Yamaguchi K, et al. Natural history of asymptomatic rotator cuff tears—a longitudinal analysis of asymptomatic tears detected sonographically. *J Shoulder Elbow Surg.* 2001;10:199. [PMID: 11408898] (This is a longitudinal study that evaluates the natural history of asymptomatic rotator cuff tears over a 5-year period to assess the risk for development of symptoms and tear progression.)

Relevant World Wide Web Sites

[American Academy of Orthopaedic Surgeons/American Association of Orthopaedic Surgeons]

http://www.aaos.org

[Arthroscopy Association of North America]

http://www.aana.org

[The American Orthopaedic Society for Sports Medicine]

http://www.sportsmed.org

Approach to the Patient with Neck Pain

David Borenstein, MD

9

Neck pain is a common musculoskeletal symptom that leads to approximately 1.9 million physician visits annually in the United States. Although neck pain has many possible causes (Table 9–1), 90% of cases are due to mechanical disorders. Mechanical neck pain may be defined as pain secondary to overuse of a normal anatomic structure or pain secondary to trauma or deformity of an anatomic structure (Figure 9–1). Mechanical disorders are characterized by exacerbation and alleviation of pain in direct correlation with particular physical activities. Neck pain due to mechanical disorders will decrease within 2–4 weeks in over 50% of patients; symptoms usually resolve within 2–3 months.

■ INITIAL EVALUATION

The goal of the initial evaluation is to differentiate patients with probable mechanical disorders from those with neck pain that requires more thorough immediate evaluation (Figure 9–2). A history should be taken and an examination should be performed in all patients with new-onset neck pain. The history should focus on symptoms suggestive of either associated neurologic deficits or an underlying systemic disease (Table 9–2). All patients should receive a neurologic examination to determine whether there are any signs of cervical nerve root compression (Table 9–3) or evidence of cord compression (ie, spastic weakness, hyperreflexia, clonus, and positive Babinski signs).

Diagnostic radiographic or laboratory tests are not necessary during the initial evaluation of patients with probable mechanical neck pain. These tests, however, are indicated for those patients whose history and physical findings suggest persistent compression of the spinal cord or nerve roots or raise the possibility of neck pain as a component of an underlying systemic disease.

Table 9–1. Causes of neck pain.

Biomechanical	Rheumatologic
Neck strain	Rheumatoid arthritis
Herniated disc	Spondyloarthropathies
Spondylosis	Polymyalgia rheumatica
Myelopathy	Fibromyalgia
Whiplash	Myofascial pain syndrome
Infectious	Diffuse idiopathic skeletal
Osteomyelitis	hyperostosis
Discitis	Microcrystalline disease
Meningitis	**Neoplastic**
Herpes zoster	Osteoblastoma
Lyme disease	Osteochondroma
Referred	Neurofibroma
Thoracic outlet syndrome	Gliomas
Pancoast tumor	Chordoma
Esophagitis	Chondrosarcoma
Angina	Metastasis
Vascular dissection	Giant cell tumor
Neurologic	Hemangioma
Brachial plexitis	**Miscellaneous**
Peripheral entrapment	Paget disease
Neuropathies	Sarcoidosis
Complex regional pain	Carotidynia
syndrome	
Syringomyelia	

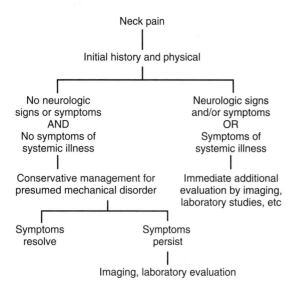

Neck pain

Initial history and physical

No neurologic
signs or symptoms
AND
No symptoms of
systemic illness

Neurologic signs
and/or symptoms
OR
Symptoms of
systemic illness

Conservative management for
presumed mechanical disorder

Immediate additional
evaluation by imaging,
laboratory studies, etc

Symptoms
resolve

Symptoms
persist

Imaging, laboratory evaluation

Figure 9–2. The initial evaluation of the patient with neck pain.

Table 9–3. Characteristics of radicular pain caused by cervical nerve root compression.

Nerve Root	Area of Pain	Sensory Loss	Motor Loss	Reflex Loss
C5	Neck to outer shoulder, arm	Shoulder	Deltoid	Biceps, supinator
C6	Outer arm to thumb, index finger	Index finger, thumb	Biceps	Biceps, supinator
C7	Outer arm to middle finger	Index, middle fingers	Triceps	Triceps
C8	Inner arm to ring and little fingers	Ring, little fingers	Hand muscles	None

■ DISORDERS REQUIRING URGENT EVALUATION

Suspected cervical myelopathy and neck pain in the setting of systemic disease require urgent evaluation in the form of imaging studies, laboratory investigation, and often, referral to the appropriate specialist.

Table 9–2. Symptoms that point to the need for urgent evaluation in a patient with neck pain.

- Constitutional symptoms such as fever, night sweats, weight loss
- Unusual quality of the neck pain
    Greatest at night; exacerbated by recumbency
    Well-localized within the neck
    Occurring in a regular pattern and extending to structures outside the neck
- Neurologic symptoms
    Lower extremity weakness; difficulty walking
    Combination of upper and lower extremity symptoms
    Rectal and/or urinary incontinence
- Associated medical conditions
    Cancer, diabetes, AIDS, and injection drug use, for example

CERVICAL MYELOPATHY

 ESSENTIAL FEATURES

- *Symptoms of weakness in upper and lower extremities; urinary or rectal incontinence.*
- *Upper motor neuron signs on examination of the lower extremities.*

Cervical myelopathy occurs secondary to compression of the neural elements (spinal cord or nerve roots) in the cervical spinal canal. Cervical spondylitic myelopathy is the most common cause of spinal cord dysfunction in persons older than 55 years. The cause of the compression is usually a combination of osteophytes and degenerative disc disease that leads to a decrease in the volume of the spinal canal. The distribution and severity of symptoms depend on the location, duration, and size of the lesion.

Clinical Findings

A. SYMPTOMS AND SIGNS

The most frequent presentation of myelopathy is a combination of arm and leg dysfunction. Patients with cervical myelopathy may have symptoms in four limbs, difficulty walking, and urinary or rectal incontinence. Only one-third of patients with cervical myelopathy

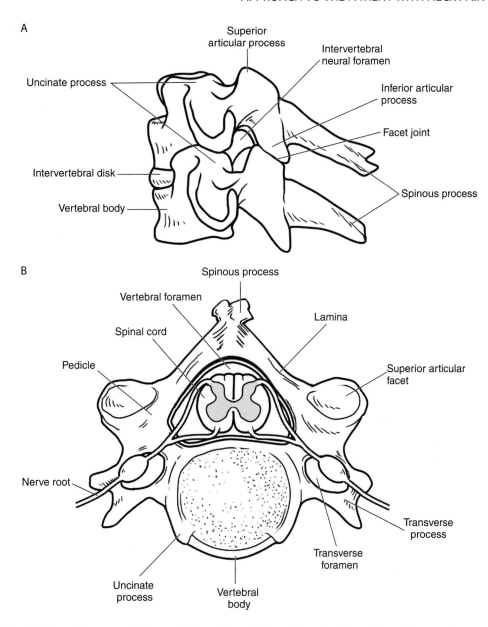

Figure 9–1. Schematic representations of a lateral view of the mid-cervical spine (**A**) and the superior aspect of C5 (**B**). The inferior articular processes form synovial-lined **facet joints** (also called **apophyseal joints**) with the superior articular processes of the vertebra below. The uncinate processes or posterolateral lips located on the superior aspect of the vertebral bodies interact with the inferolateral aspects of the vertebral body above, forming the small, non-synovial-lined **uncovertebral joints** (also referred to as the joints of Luschka). The spinal cord lies within the vertebral foramen formed by the vertebral body anteriorly, the pedicles laterally, and the laminae posteriorly. The cervical nerve roots course along "gutters" formed by the pedicles and exit through an intervertebral foramen. The vertebral artery passes through the transverse foramen. (From Polley HF, Hunder GS. *Rheumatologic Interviewing and Physical Examination of the Joints.* 2nd ed. WB Saunders, 1978, Figure 11–1A. With permission.)

mention neck pain. Older patients may describe leg stiffness, foot shuffling, and a fear of falling. Physical examination reveals weakness of the appendages in association with spasticity; hyperreflexia, clonus, and a positive Babinski sign are findings in the lower extremities.

B. IMAGING STUDIES

Magnetic resonance imaging detects the extent of spinal cord compression and is the imaging test of choice for most cases. Computed tomography myelograms help distinguish between osteophytes and protruding discs. Plain radiographs reveal advanced degenerative disease with narrowed disc spaces, facet joint sclerosis, and osteophytes.

Treatment

The natural history of cervical spondylitic myelopathy is gradual progression. Although some patients improve with conservative therapy, progressive myelopathy requires surgery to prevent further cord compression, vascular compromise, and myelomalacia. Outcomes are best when surgery is performed before severe neurologic deficits appear.

NECK PAIN ASSOCIATED WITH SYSTEMIC MEDICAL ILLNESS

 ESSENTIAL FEATURES

- *The history and examination help identify patients whose neck pain is not due to a mechanical disorder.*
- *The differential diagnosis and clinical context of each case determine the urgency and nature of the evaluation.*

Differential Diagnosis

Patients with neck pain require urgent evaluation if they have constitutional symptoms, symptoms that suggest either a focal process or referred pain, a history of cancer, or a condition that predisposes to infection (Table 9–2). If present, signs or symptoms of radiculopathy or spinal cord compression add to the urgency of the situation. The differential diagnosis, clinical setting, and findings of the individual case dictate the use of imaging, laboratory investigations, and need for consultations.

Neck pain in the presence of fever, night sweats, weight loss, or a predisposing condition such as injection drug use, AIDS, or diabetes raises the possibility of **infection.** Magnetic resonance imaging and computed tomography are indicated in cases of suspected vertebral osteomyelitis, discitis, and epidural abscess. In these conditions, radiographs of the cervical spine may demonstrate alterations of bone integrity but, especially early in the disease course, are often unrevealing.

Spinal cord infiltrative processes and vertebral column **tumors** tend to produce pain that is greatest at night or with recumbency. Patients with these symptoms and neurologic signs should undergo magnetic resonance imaging of the central nervous system. Patients with nocturnal pain and with normal neurologic examinations may have a bone tumor. Benign bone tumors affect the posterior elements of vertebral bodies, while malignant lesions affect the vertebral bodies. If plain radiographs are unable to detect alterations in bone architecture, bone scan is a sensitive means to detect lesions over the entire axial skeleton. Computed tomography can clarify the nature of abnormalities seen on bone scan.

Pain localized directly over the bony structures of the cervical spine is usually associated with either **fracture** or **expansion of bone.** Any condition that replaces bone with abnormal cells or increases mineral loss from trabeculae causes fractures that occur spontaneously or with minimal trauma. Fractures cause pain in the area of the lesion. Physical examination identifies the maximum point of tenderness. A bone scan may identify the area of fracture if the radiograph is normal. Magnetic resonance imaging can identify the presence of malignancies, such as **myeloma,** that do not stimulate osteoblast activity and thus are not detected by bone scan.

The **spondyloarthropathies** and **rheumatoid arthritis** can cause early morning stiffness of the cervical spine lasting for hours. Patients with neck symptoms due to these diseases usually have extensive disease of other joints, but women with ankylosing spondylitis may have neck disease without low back pain. Flexion-extension views of the cervical spine can reveal the presence of C1–C2 subluxation in either the spondyloarthropathies or rheumatoid arthritis.

Patients with **viscerogenic pain** (ie, neck pain secondary to cardiovascular, gastrointestinal, or neurologic disorders) have symptoms that recur in a regular pattern in structures that extend beyond the cervical spine. Pain with exertion raises the possibility of myocardial ischemia. Carotidynia is pain and tenderness over the carotid arteries. Esophageal disorders should be considered if neck pain occurs in association with eating. Posterior esophageal lesions, in particular, may affect the prevertebral space, causing neck pain. Disorders of the cranial nerves can cause cervical spine and facial pain.

Patients with **polymyalgia rheumatica** are over 50 years of age and have severe early morning muscle stiffness. Pain is localized to the proximal muscles of the shoulders and thighs. The erythrocyte sedimentation rate is elevated in most cases.

Treatment

Treatment of neck pain associated with systemic medical illnesses is chosen to remedy the specific disorder causing neck pain. For example, vertebral osteomyelitis requires sustained antibiotic therapy for eradication of the infection. Glucocorticoids are necessary for the treatment of polymyalgia rheumatica.

ACUTE NECK PAIN DUE TO A PROBABLE MECHANICAL DISORDER

ESSENTIAL FEATURES

- *There are no signs or symptoms of systemic disease, and the neurologic examination is normal.*
- *A trial of nonoperative therapy is indicated.*

Patients with neck pain but without symptoms or signs of myelopathy or an associated systemic disorder should be treated with nonoperative therapy for 3–6 weeks. In general, imaging studies and laboratory investigations are not necessary unless the neck pain persists.

Nonoperative Therapy

Nonselective nonsteroidal anti-inflammatory drugs (NSAIDs) and selective cyclooxygenase-2 inhibitors help decrease pain and inflammation that is associated with acute neck pain. Nonoperative management also includes muscle relaxants, nonnarcotic analgesics, temperature modalities, local injections, and range of motion and strengthening exercises.

Medications that have rapid onset of action and are effective analgesics are preferred. In addition, drugs with sustained relief properties may offer more constant pain relief with fewer tablets each day. Muscle relaxants do not produce peripheral muscle relaxation but do offer additional pain relief for persons with increased paracervical muscle contractions. Patients must be informed of the potential sedative effects of these medications. Patients may use ice massage on painful areas for

10 minutes for additional analgesia. Some patients may find the application of heat to the neck improves range of motion by decreasing muscle tightness. A local injection with 10 mg of triamcinolone and 2–4 mL of lidocaine into the area of maximum tenderness in the paravertebral musculature or trapezii may decrease pain.

Because of the pain, patients often have difficulty complying with the recommendation of returning to normal motion of the cervical spine. Patients will limit motion and prefer to wear a cervical collar. Short-term immobilization is useful, particularly at night when motion during sleep increases neck pain. A soft collar that does not extend the neck is appropriate in most cases. Patients should understand that the eventual goal of therapy is a return to normal neck motion. Therefore, the collar should be used less frequently as neck pain improves.

PERSISTENT NECK PAIN

Most patients, including those with cervical radiculopathy, will improve within 2 months. If initial nonoperative treatment fails after 6 weeks, symptomatic patients are separated into two groups: patients with neck pain as the predominant complaint and patients with arm pain as the predominant complaint.

NECK PAIN PREDOMINANT

ESSENTIAL FEATURES

- *Osteoarthritis is a frequent cause of local neck pain.*
- *Muscle tightness is a common exacerbating factor.*

Differential Diagnosis & Treatment

Cervical strain causes pain in the middle or lower portion of the posterior aspect of the neck. The pain may cover a diffuse area or both sides of the spine. Physical examination reveals local tenderness in the paracervical muscles, decreased range of motion, and loss of cervical lordosis. No abnormalities are found on neurologic or shoulder examination. Laboratory tests are normal. Cervical spine roentgenograms of patients with cervical strain may be normal or demonstrate a loss of cervical lordosis. Therapy for chronic cervical strain includes modification of the choice or dose of NSAID, muscle relaxant, local injections, and neck exercises, including strengthening and range of motion.

Cervical spondylosis is associated with disc degeneration and the approximation of articular structures. This instability results in osteoarthritis with osteophyte formation in the uncovertebral and apophyseal joints. Neck pain is diffuse and may radiate to the shoulders, occipital area, or the interscapular muscles. Physical examination may reveal midline tenderness and pain at the limit of motion with extension and lateral flexion. Factors that exacerbate and alleviate neck pain help differentiate among the various causes of mechanical neck pain. Plain roentgenograms of the cervical spine demonstrate intervertebral narrowing and facet joint sclerosis. Magnetic resonance imaging of the neck reveals degenerative disc disease in over 50% of persons 40 years of age or older, many of whom are asymptomatic. The radiographic findings are significant only if they correlate with the clinical symptoms of the patient. Therapy for osteoarthritis of the cervical spine requires a balance between stability and maintenance of motion. Patient education is essential to maximize neck flexibility with range of motion exercises while decreasing pain by restricting neck movement with a cervical collar. NSAIDs and local injections may also diminish neck and referred pain. Most patients with cervical spondylosis have a relapsing course with recurrent exacerbations of acute neck pain.

Cervical hyperextension injuries (whiplash) of the neck are most often associated with rear-impact motor vehicle accidents, but diving, falls, and other sports injuries also cause whiplash. Whiplash is an acceleration-deceleration injury to the soft tissue structures in the neck. Paracervical muscles are stretched or torn, and with severe injury, cervical intervertebral disc injuries occur. Severe whiplash also can damage the sympathetic ganglia, resulting in Horner syndrome, nausea, hoarseness, or dizziness. Symptoms of stiffness and pain on motion generally develop 12–24 hours after the accident. Patients may have difficulty swallowing or chewing. Physical examination reveals soreness of the neck with palpation, paracervical muscle contraction, and decreased range of motion. Neurologic examination is unrevealing, and radiographs demonstrate loss of cervical lordosis. Structural damage identified on radiographs occurs in patients with severe injuries that require immediate stabilizing therapy. Treatment of most whiplash injuries includes the use of a cervical collar for a minimal period of time. Longer use of collars may result in greater pain and decreased motion. Nonnarcotic analgesics, NSAIDs, and muscle relaxants decrease pain and facilitate motion of the neck. Patients with persistent symptoms have pain secondary to apophyseal joint injury. Patients with persistent symptoms for greater than 6 months rarely experience significant improvement.

If a patient with persistent neck pain does not have muscle tenderness and if the neurologic examination and imaging studies are unrevealing, the patient should have a complete psychosocial evaluation. Patients with neck pain who have psychiatric conditions may have conversion reactions or substance dependence as the cause of their symptoms.

ARM PAIN PREDOMINANT

 ESSENTIAL FEATURES

- Herniated intervertebral discs are a frequent cause of radicular pain.
- Cervical spinal stenosis is a cause of radicular pain in older persons.

Differential Diagnosis & Treatment

Patients with arm pain refractory to nonoperative management frequently have symptoms and signs owing to mechanical pressure from a herniated disc or hypertrophic bone and secondary inflammation of the involved nerve roots. Cervical disc herniation occurs with the sudden exertion of heavy lifting. A herniated cervical disc causes radicular pain that radiates from the shoulder to the forearm and hand. The pain may be so severe that the use of the arm is limited. Neck pain is minimal or absent. Physical examination reveals increased radicular pain with any maneuver that narrows the intervertebral foramen and places tension on the affected nerve. Compression, extension, and lateral flexion of the cervical spine (Spurling sign) cause radicular pain. Neurologic examination reveals sensory abnormalities, reflex asymmetry, or motor weakness corresponding to the damaged spinal nerve root and degree of impingement (see Table 9–3). Magnetic resonance imaging is the best technique to identify the location of disc herniation and nerve root impingement. Electromyography and nerve conduction tests document nerve dysfunction and are able to differentiate nerve root impingement from peripheral entrapment syndromes (eg, carpal tunnel syndrome).

If arm pain occurs during exertion, vascular evaluation is indicated. Patients who complain of neck and arm pain that occurs with exertion should be evaluated for coronary artery disease, particularly if chest pain occurs in conjunction with arm pain. If the exertional pain is limited to the arm alone, an evaluation for thoracic outlet syndrome, using the Adson test, is also appropriate. To perform the Adson test, the patient's radial pulse is examined at the wrist. While the pulse is continuously palpated, the arm is then abducted, extended, and externally rotated. The patient is then instructed to take a deep breath and turn the head toward the arm being tested. If there is compression of the subclavian artery, a marked diminution of the radial pulse is observed. Patients with thoracic outlet syndrome should be evaluated by appropriate imaging to rule out a Pancoast tumor (apical lung tumor). Patients with idiopathic thoracic outlet obstruction may benefit from isometric shoulder girdle exercises, improved posture, and limiting movements of the arm above the head. Surgery is helpful in a minority of patients.

REFERENCES

Dvorak J. Epidemiology, physical examination, and neurodiagnostics. *Spine*. 1998;23:2663. [PMID: 9879093] (A thorough review of the diagnostic evaluation of cervical spine disease.)

Kaiser JA, Holland BA. Imaging of the cervical spine. *Spine*. 1998;23:2701. [PMID: 9879096] (A discussion of the imaging methods for disorders affecting the cervical spine.)

Mochida K, et al. Regression of cervical disc herniation observed on magnetic resonance images. *Spine*. 1998;23:990. [PMID: 9589536] (Cervical disc herniations can resolve spontaneously.)

Relevant World Wide Web Sites

[The American College of Rheumatology]
http://www.rheumatology.org
[American Academy of Orthopaedic Surgeons]
http://www.aaos.org
[Hospital for Joint Diseases Orthopaedic Institute]
http://www.hjd.org
[Dr. David Borenstein America's Back Doctor]
http://www.drborenstein.com

Approach to the Patient with Low Back Pain

10

Rajiv K. Dixit, MD

ESSENTIAL FEATURES

- *Most patients with acute low back pain improve spontaneously within 4 weeks.*
- *Degenerative change in the lumbar spine is the most common cause of low back pain.*
- *Diagnostic testing is rarely indicated unless symptoms persist beyond 4 weeks.*
- *Presence of imaging abnormalities should be carefully interpreted since they are frequently seen in asymptomatic persons.*
- *Most patients respond to analgesia, education, and physical therapy. Surgery is rarely needed.*

General Considerations

Low back pain (LBP) is the most common musculoskeletal complaint and a leading cause of work disability; an estimated 80% of the population will experience it during their lifetime.

LBP affects the area between the lower rib cage and gluteal folds and frequently radiates into the thighs. Most LBP is benign and self-limited. Ninety percent of patients with acute LBP improve spontaneously within 4 weeks. Approximately half of these patients will experience one or more episodes of LBP over the next few years, but these too will generally be self-limited. Less than 1% of the patients with acute LBP have true **sciatica,** which is defined as pain in the distribution of a lumbar nerve root often accompanied by sensory and motor deficits.

Clinical Findings

A. HISTORY

Pain that is due to mechanical causes increases with activity and upright posture and is relieved by rest and recumbency. Nonmechanical LBP, especially when accompanied by nocturnal pain, suggests the possibility

of underlying infection or neoplasm. LBP in a patient under the age of 40 that is accompanied by marked early morning stiffness and improves with activity is characteristic of ankylosing spondylitis. On the other hand, acute LBP in a postmenopausal white woman suggests the possibility of a vertebral compression fracture secondary to osteoporosis.

Sciatica and pseudoclaudication suggest neurologic involvement. Sciatica results from nerve root compression, generally from a herniated disc, and produces lancinating pain in a radicular distribution. Sciatica should be differentiated from nonneurogenic **sclerotomal** pain, which arises from disease within the disc, facet joint, or lumbar paraspinal muscles and ligaments. Like sciatica, sclerotomal pain is often referred into the lower extremities but, unlike sciatica, sclerotomal pain usually does not radiate below the knee or have associated paresthesias, is nondermatomal in distribution, and is dull in quality.

Persistence of LBP may be associated with depression, job dissatisfaction, and pursuit of disability compensation or litigation.

B. PHYSICAL EXAMINATION

Examination of the back usually does not lead to a specific diagnosis. A general physical examination, including a neurologic examination, may help identify those few cases of LBP that are secondary to a systemic disease or those in which there is neurologic involvement.

Inspection may reveal the presence of **scoliosis.** Scoliosis can be either **structural** or **functional.** A structural scoliosis is associated with structural changes of the vertebral column and sometimes the rib cage as well. As the patient bends forward (flexing the spine), structural scoliosis persists whereas functional scoliosis usually disappears. Paravertebral muscle spasm and leg length discrepancy are leading causes of functional scoliosis.

Palpation can detect paravertebral muscle spasm that often leads to loss of the normal lumbar lordosis. Point tenderness over the spine has sensitivity but not specificity for vertebral osteomyelitis. A palpable step-off between adjacent spinous processes indicates spondylolisthesis.

Limited spinal motion (flexion, extension, lateral bending, and rotation) is not associated with any specific diagnosis since LBP due to any cause may limit motion. Range of motion measurements, however, can help in monitoring treatment.

The hip joints should be examined for any decrease in range of motion because hip arthritis, which normally causes groin pain, may occasionally present as LBP. Tenderness over the greater trochanter of the hip is seen in trochanteric bursitis, which can be confused with LBP. The presence of more widespread tender points, especially in a female patient, suggests the possibility that LBP may be secondary to fibromyalgia.

A **straight-leg raising test** should be performed on all patients with sciatica or pseudoclaudication. Straight-leg raising places tension on the sciatic nerve and thereby stretches the sciatic nerve roots (L4, L5, S1, S2, S3). If any of these nerve roots is already irritated, such as by impingement from a herniated disc, further tension on the nerve root by straight-leg raising will result in radicular pain that extends below the knee. The test is done by the examiner cupping the patient's heel in his or her hand and flexing the hip while keeping the knee extended. The test is positive if radicular pain (not merely back or hamstring pain) is produced when the leg is raised less than 60 degrees. The straight-leg raising test is very sensitive (95%) but not specific (40%) for clinically significant disc herniation at the L4–5 or L5–S1 level (the sites of 95% of disc herniations). False-negative tests are more frequently seen with herniation above the L4–5 level. The straight-leg raising test is usually negative in patients with spinal stenosis. The crossed straight-leg raising test (with sciatica reproduced when the opposite leg is raised) is insensitive (25%) but highly specific (90%) for disc herniation.

The neurologic examination (Table 10–1) should always include motor testing with focus on knee extension (L4), great toe dorsiflexion (L5), and foot plantar flexion (S1); determination of knee (L4) and ankle (S1) deep tendon reflexes; and tests for dermatomal sensory loss (Figure 10–1). The inability to toe walk (mostly S1) and heel walk (mostly L5) may indicate muscle weakness. Muscle atrophy can be detected by circumferential measurements of the calf and thigh at the same level bilaterally.

C. Laboratory Findings

Laboratory studies play a minor role in the investigation of LBP. They are used mostly in identifying patients with systemic causes of LBP. A patient with normal blood cell counts, erythrocyte sedimentation rate, and radiographs of the lumbar spine is unlikely to have an underlying systemic disease as the cause of LBP.

D. Imaging Studies

Diagnostic tests are not required unless symptoms persist for more than 4 weeks. However, diagnostic tests should be done early for patients who have evidence of a major or progressive neurologic deficit and in whom

Table 10–1. Neurologic features of lumbosacral radiculopathy.

Disc Herniation	Nerve Root	Motor	Sensory (light touch)	Reflex
L3–4	L4	Knee extension	Medial foot	Knee
L4–5	L5	Great-toe dorsiflexion	Dorsal foot	None
L5–S1	S1	Foot plantar-flexion	Lateral foot	Ankle

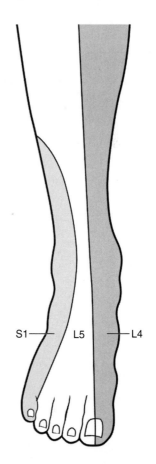

S1 — L5 — L4

Figure 10–1. Lower extremity dermatomes.

underlying infection or cancer is suspected (Table 10–2). Since 90% of patients with LBP recover spontaneously within 4 weeks, this approach avoids unnecessary early testing.

A major problem with imaging studies is that many of the anatomic abnormalities seen are common in asymptomatic persons. These abnormalities are often the result of age-related degenerative changes and are frequently present after the age of 30. Making causal inferences based on imaging abnormalities can be hazardous in the absence of corresponding clinical findings.

Plain radiographs of the spine do not usually help in determining the cause of LBP. Abnormalities such as single disc degeneration, facet joint degeneration, Schmorl's nodes, spondylolysis, mild spondylolisthesis, and mild scoliosis are equally prevalent in persons with and without LBP. Plain radiography should be limited to patients with clinical findings suggestive of infection, cancer, or trauma, or those who continue to have LBP after 4–6 weeks of conservative care. It is noteworthy that radiation exposure to the female gonads from standard views of the lumbar spine is equivalent to a daily chest radiograph for several years.

Computed tomography (CT) and magnetic resonance imaging (MRI) should be reserved for patients in whom there is a strong clinical indication of underlying infection or cancer, or for the evaluation of patients with significant or progressive neurologic deficits. MRI is the preferred modality for the detection of spinal infection and cancers, herniated discs, and spinal stenosis. When interpreting the results of MRI and CT, it is important to remember that most asymptomatic adults above age 30 will have evidence of either disc bulges (symmetric and diffuse extension of the disc) or disc protrusion (focal or asymmetric extension of the disc). When these findings are seen in a patient with LBP, therefore, they are not necessarily the cause. MRI with the intravenous contrast agent gadolinium is useful for the evaluation of patients with prior lumbar spine surgery (ideally with no hardware present) to help in the differentiation of scar tissue from recurrent disc herniation.

The significance of a focal high signal (high-intensity zone) in the posterior annulus on a T2-weighted image is controversial. It is thought to represent annular tears and to correlate with positive findings on discography (which in and of itself is a controversial procedure of questionable value). **Discogenic LBP** has been diagnosed in patients with these high-intensity zones, and spinal fusion surgery is often recommended. The high prevalence of high-intensity zones in asymptomatic individuals, however, calls this approach into question.

Bone scanning is used primarily to detect infection, bony metastases, and occult fractures. Bone scans have limited specificity due to poor spatial resolution, and thus abnormal findings often require confirmatory imaging, such as MRI.

E. SPECIAL TESTS

Nerve conduction studies and electromyography (EMG) are unnecessary when a patient has an obvious radiculopathy or isolated LBP. Electrodiagnosis, however, may be helpful in differentiating the limb pain of peroneal nerve palsy from that of L5 radiculopathy or in evaluating possible factitious weakness. EMG changes depend on the development of muscle denervation following nerve injury and cannot be detected until a few weeks after the injury.

Differential Diagnosis

LBP usually originates from the lumbar spine or associated muscles and ligaments (Table 10–3). Rarely, pain is referred to the back from visceral disease. Over 95% of LBP is mechanical (Table 10–4). **Mechanical LBP**

Table 10–2. Indications for early diagnostic testing.

Spinal fracture
    Trauma
    Glucocorticoid use
    Age > 50 years
Infection or cancer
    History of cancer
    Weight loss
    Fever or active infection
    Immunosuppression or injection drug use
    Nocturnal pain
    Age > 50 years
Cauda equina syndrome
    Urinary retention
    Bilateral or progressive motor deficit
    Saddle anesthesia
Spondyloarthropathy
    Morning stiffness in the low back
    Low back pain that improves with activity
    Age < 40 years

Table 10–3. Causes of low back pain.

Originating from spine
    Mechanical
    Neoplastic
    Infectious
    Inflammatory
    Metabolic
Originating from viscera

Table 10–4. Mechanical causes of low back pain.

Lumbar spondylosis[a]
Disc herniation[a]
Spondylolisthesis[a]
Spinal stenosis[a]
Diffuse idiopathic skeletal hyperostosis
Fractures
Idiopathic (sprain and strain, lumbago)

[a]Related to degenerative changes.

is due to an anatomic or functional abnormality without underlying inflammatory or neoplastic disease. Degenerative change (also referred to as lumbar spondylosis or lumbar osteoarthritis) is by far the most common disorder seen within the spine and the most important cause of mechanical LBP. Degenerative changes occur in both the intervertebral disc and facet joint (Figure 10–2).

A precise pathoanatomic diagnosis cannot be made in most patients with acute LBP. Because imaging abnormalities are often seen in asymptomatic persons, clinical disease cannot always be attributed to such abnormalities. The focus of the initial diagnostic evaluation, therefore, is to identify the small proportion of patients with systemic disease (infection, neoplasm, and

spondyloarthropathy together account for only 1% of patients with LBP) or with neurologic involvement that requires urgent intervention.

A. LUMBAR SPONDYLOSIS

Lumbar spondylosis, or osteoarthritis of the lumbar spine, is the most common cause of LBP. Symptomatic patients complain of mechanical LBP. Recurrent attacks of acute LBP may occur in some patients while chronic LBP may develop in others. In patients with facet joint osteoarthritis, the pain may radiate into the posterior thigh and be exacerbated by bending ipsilateral to the involved joint (**facet syndrome**).

Imaging evidence of degenerative changes (facet joint or disc space narrowing, osteophytosis, and subchondral sclerosis) increases with age and is common. However, the relationship between these changes and back pain is complex. Patients with severe LBP may have minimal radiographic changes and, conversely, patients with advanced changes may be asymptomatic.

Spinal instability (in the absence of fractures or spondylolisthesis) remains a controversial diagnosis. Spinal instability is identified by demonstrating abnormal vertebral motion (anteroposterior displacement or excessive angular change of adjacent vertebrae) on flexion-extension radiography. However, such spinal motion may be seen in asymptomatic persons, and its relationship to the causation of pain is unclear.

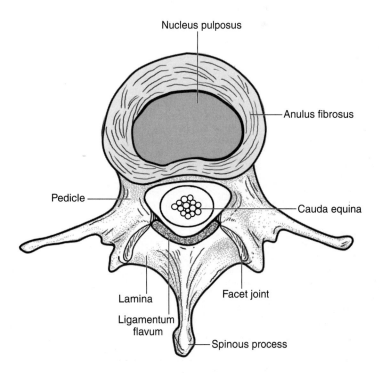

Figure 10–2. Schematic drawing showing a cross-sectional view through a normal lumbar vertebra. The facet joints are formed by the articulation between the superior facet of the vertebra below and the inferior facet of the vertebra above.

B. Disc Herniation

The nucleus pulposus in a degenerated disc may prolapse and push out the weakened annulus, usually posterolaterally. Imaging evidence of disc herniation (bulging or protrusion) is commonly seen, even in asymptomatic adults. Occasionally, however, disc herniation results in a nerve root impingement syndrome (Figure 10–3). This accounts for less than 1% of patients with LBP but is nevertheless important to identify. Such disc herniation may be precipitated by a wide range of activities from heavy lifting to trivial movement.

Ninety-five percent of lumbar disc herniations involve either the L4–5 or L5–S1 disc. In general, the more caudal nerve root is impinged, that is, the L5 nerve root with L4–5 herniation and the S1 nerve root with L5–S1 herniation. Nerve root impingement results in sciatica. Indeed, sciatica has such a high sensitivity (95%) that its absence makes clinically significant lumbar disc herniation unlikely.

The natural history of disc herniation is favorable. Studies using sequential MRI testing reveal that the herniated portion of the disc tends to regress with time. In most patients, the radicular pain resolves over a period of weeks, and less than 10% of patients with nerve root impingement will require surgical decompression.

Rarely, a massive midline disc herniation compresses the cauda equina, causing **cauda equina syndrome**—a surgical emergency. Patients usually present with bilateral sciatica and motor deficits. Sensory loss in a saddle distribution is common, and urinary retention with overflow incontinence is usually present.

Internal disc disruption is a controversial disorder diagnosed by provocative discography. Following contrast injection into the disc, the radiographic appearance and induced pain are assessed. Discographic anatomic abnormalities and induced pain are, however, frequently seen in asymptomatic persons, and more important the discogenic pain attributed to disc disruption frequently improves spontaneously.

C. Spondylolisthesis

Spondylolisthesis is the anterior displacement of a vertebra on the one beneath it. This displacement is usually the result of degenerative changes in the disc and facet joints (**degenerative spondylolisthesis**) but also can be due to a developmental defect in the pars interarticularis of the vertebral arch that produces **isthmic spondylolisthesis** (Figure 10–4).

Most patients with a minor degree of spondylolisthesis are asymptomatic, although some patients may have mechanical LBP. Greater degrees of spondylolisthesis occasionally cause nerve root impingement (usually L5) or spinal stenosis. Rarely, extreme slippage results in cauda equina syndrome.

D. Spinal Stenosis

Lumbar spinal stenosis is defined as a narrowing of the spinal canal, its lateral recesses, and neural foramina that may result in a compression of lumbosacral nerve roots.

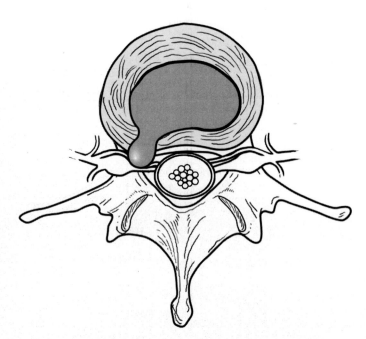

Figure 10–3. Schematic drawing showing posterolateral disc herniation resulting in nerve root impingement.

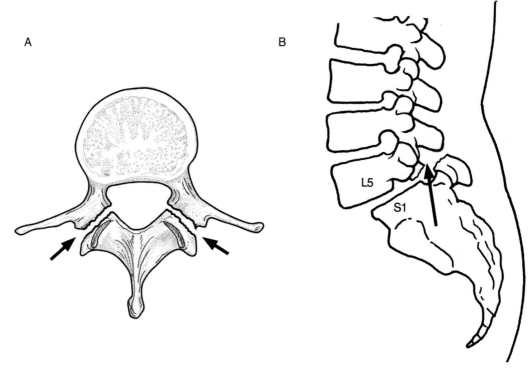

Figure 10–4. **A:** Spondylolysis with bilateral defects in the pars interarticularis (arrows). **B:** Spondylolysis of the L5 vertebra (arrow) resulting in isthmic spondylolisthesis at L5–S1.

Lumbar stenosis can be asymptomatic; up to 20% of asymptomatic adults over age 60 have evidence of spinal stenosis on imaging. Spinal stenosis can occur at one or more levels and the narrowing can be asymmetric.

Degenerative changes are the cause of spinal stenosis in an overwhelming majority of cases (Table 10–5). The intervertebral disc loses vertical height as it degenerates; this results in a bulging of the now redundant and often hypertrophied ligamentum flavum into the posterior part of the canal. Any herniation of the degenerated disc narrows the anterior part of the canal while hypertrophied facets and osteophytes may compress nerve roots in the lateral recess or intervertebral foramen (Figure 10–5).

The hallmark of spinal stenosis is **pseudoclaudication** (neurogenic claudication). The symptoms of pseudoclaudication are usually bilateral. The patient complains of pain and discomfort together with weakness ("spaghetti legs") or paresthesias in the buttocks, thighs, and legs. Unsteadiness of gait is a frequent complaint. The lumbar component of pain is frequently mild. Pseudoclaudication is induced by standing or walking and relieved by sitting or flexing forward. In fact, the most important finding may be a history of no

Table 10–5. Causes of lumbar spinal stenosis.

Congenital
  Idiopathic
  Achondroplastic
Acquired
  Degenerative
    Hypertrophy of facet joints
    Hypertrophy of ligamentum flavum
    Disc herniation
    Spondylolisthesis
    Scoliosis
  Iatrogenic
    Postlaminectomy
    Postsurgical fusion
  Miscellaneous
    Paget disease
    Fluorosis
    Diffuse idiopathic skeletal hyperostosis

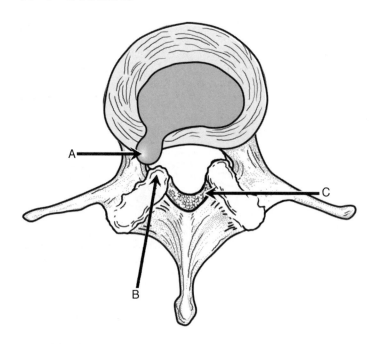

Figure 10–5. Spinal stenosis secondary to a combination of disc herniation (**A**), facet joint hypertrophy (**B**), and hypertrophy of ligamentum flavum (**C**).

pain when the patient is seated with the spine flexed. This forward flexion increases the canal diameter and may lead to the patient adopting a simian stance. It has been hypothesized that a diminished supply of arterial blood to the cauda equina is the cause of neurogenic claudication. Recent evidence, however, suggests that direct pressure on the nerve roots is the major mechanism. Factors that favor a diagnosis of pseudoclaudication over vascular claudication include the preservation of pedal pulses, provocation of symptoms by standing just as readily as by walking, and location of the maximal discomfort to the thighs rather than the calves.

The physical examination of a patient with lumbar spinal stenosis is often unimpressive. Severe neurologic deficits are rarely seen. Lumbar range of motion may be normal or reduced and the result of straight-leg raising is usually negative. Deep tendon reflexes and vibration sense may be reduced. Mild weakness is seen in some. The significance of these findings is often difficult to determine in elderly patients. The diagnosis of spinal stenosis is most often suspected when a history of pseudoclaudication is elicited and is best confirmed by MRI.

Spinal stenosis is an indolent condition, and the symptoms evolve gradually. Most patients remain stable, although some gradually worsen over a period of years.

E. DIFFUSE IDIOPATHIC SKELETAL HYPEROSTOSIS

Diffuse idiopathic skeletal hyperostosis (DISH) is characterized by florid hyperostosis of the spine. Marginal bony proliferation leads to the formation of anterior osseous ridges that fuse and give the appearance of "flowing wax" on the anterior bodies of the vertebrae. Ossification of paraspinous ligaments such as the anterior and posterior longitudinal ligaments may be seen. The thoracic spine is most commonly involved, although the cervical and lumbar regions may also be affected. Lesions are most prominent anteriorly and along the right lateral aspect of the spine. Involvement of the left lateral aspect in patients with situs inversus has led to speculation that the descending thoracic aorta plays a role in the location of calcification. Intervertebral disc spaces are preserved and sacroiliac and facet joints appear normal. This helps differentiate DISH from spondylosis and the spondyloarthropathies. Extraspinal manifestations include irregular new bone formation ("whiskering") and large bone spurs that are often seen at the olecranon process and calcaneus. Severe ligamentous calcification may be seen in the patellar, sacrotuberous, and iliolumbar ligaments.

DISH is usually seen in the middle-aged and the elderly. In spite of the extensive radiologic abnormalities, pain is often minimal or absent with only moderate limitation of spinal motion. Stiffness, which may be generalized, is a common complaint. Rarely, dysphagia or cervical myelopathy can occur secondary to extensive ossification of the anterior or posterior longitudinal ligaments, respectively. An association with diabetes mellitus has been noted.

F. IDIOPATHIC LBP

A definitive pathoanatomic diagnosis cannot be made in 80% of patients with LBP, largely because of the weak association between symptoms and the results of imaging. Thus, nonspecific terms, such as lumbago, strain, and sprain have come into use. Strain and sprain have never been anatomically or histologically characterized. Therefore, idiopathic LBP is a more accurate label for these patients who have a mostly self-limited syndrome of back pain.

G. NEOPLASTIC

Cancer is an unusual cause of LBP. Most cases result from involvement of the spine by metastatic carcinoma (prostate, lung, breast, thyroid, or kidney) or multiple myeloma.

Patients are usually older than 50 years and may give a history of weight loss or cancer in the past. Recumbency often does not improve the LBP and nocturnal pain is common. Missing the diagnosis can lead to irreversible neurologic compromise, ranging from cord compression to cauda equina syndrome.

Radiographs can reveal a compression fracture or lytic or blastic lesions that may be present in one or several vertebral bodies with sparing of the disc space. MRI is the test of choice to confirm bony metastases.

Patients with neurologic involvement may need urgent radiation therapy or surgical decompression.

H. INFECTIOUS

Vertebral osteomyelitis, epidural abscess, and septic discitis are infrequent but important causes of LBP. Osteomyelitis usually results from hematogenous spread from a distant source of infection and can lead to the formation of an epidural abscess. The most common organism is *Staphylococcus aureus,* followed by streptococci and gram-negative bacteria. Tuberculosis and nontubercular granulomatous infections (blastomycosis, cryptococcosis, actinomycosis, coccidioidomycosis, and brucellosis) of the spine are rare but should be considered in the appropriate clinical setting. Risk factors for osteomyelitis and epidural abscess include immunosuppression, diabetes, injection drug abuse, alcoholism, renal failure, and urinary tract infections. Septic discitis generally results from a procedure, such as disc excision, that inoculates the disc space.

Back pain that is not relieved by rest or recumbency, spine tenderness over the involved segment, and an elevated erythrocyte sedimentation rate are the most common findings. Fever may only be seen with abscess formation, and the white blood cell count is often normal. An untreated epidural abscess can result in spinal cord compression or cauda equina syndrome. Radiographs may show a narrowed disc space with erosion of adjacent vertebrae, but these changes often take weeks to appear. MRI is the most sensitive and specific imaging technique to detect spinal infections. A biopsy for culture is recommended, especially if blood cultures are negative. Treatment consists of intravenous antibiotics for 6 weeks and surgical decompression if an epidural abscess is present.

I. INFLAMMATORY

The spondyloarthropathies (see Chapter 18) cause inflammatory LBP characterized by prolonged early morning stiffness of the back that improves with activity and worsens with rest.

J. METABOLIC

The major consideration is the occurrence of acute LBP secondary to a vertebral compression fracture in a patient with osteoporosis (see Chapter 53). Most patients are postmenopausal women.

Paget disease of bone is often detected in an asymptomatic patient by the incidental finding of either an elevated alkaline phosphatase or characteristic radiographic abnormality. Back pain secondary to involvement of the spine is most common in the lumbar area. The pain may be due to the pagetic process itself, to secondary osteoarthritis in the facet joints or, rarely, to a pathologic fracture of a vertebra. Spinal cord and cauda equina compression secondary to Paget disease have been seen on rare occasions.

K. VISCERAL

Disease in organs that share segmental innervation with the spine can cause pain to be referred to the spine. In general, pelvic diseases refer pain to the sacral area, lower abdominal diseases to the lumbar area, and upper abdominal diseases to the lower thoracic spine area. Local signs of disease, such as tenderness to palpation, paravertebral muscle spasm, and increased pain on spinal motion, are absent.

A partial list of causes includes a contained rupture of an abdominal aortic aneurysm, pyelonephritis, ureteral obstruction due to renal stones, chronic prostatitis, endometriosis, ovarian cysts, inflammatory bowel disorders, colonic neoplasms, and retroperitoneal hemorrhage (usually in a patient taking anticoagulants).

Treatment

Specific treatment is available only for the small fraction of patients with LBP who either have major neural compression or have an underlying systemic disease. In the vast majority of patients with LBP, either the precise cause cannot be determined, or when the cause is determined, no specific treatment is available. These patients are then managed with a conservative program centered around analgesia, education, and physical therapy. Less than 1% of patients with LBP need surgery.

For management purposes, patients with LBP are considered under one of three clinical syndromes. They either have **acute LBP** (duration less than 3 months), **chronic LBP** (duration greater than 3 months), or a **nerve root compression syndrome.**

One should be wary of the proliferation of unproven medical, surgical, and alternative therapies. Most have not been rigorously tested in randomized controlled trials; uncontrolled studies can produce a misleading impression of efficacy due to the favorable natural history of LBP.

A. ACUTE LBP

In general, patients seek medical attention for sudden onset of severe mechanical LBP that can be associated with some physical activity. Examination usually reveals paravertebral muscle spasm and severe decrease in range of motion secondary to pain.

Patients with acute LBP are advised to stay active and continue ordinary daily activities within the limits permitted by pain. Bed rest of more than 1 or 2 days is discouraged.

Medications are used for symptomatic relief. Aspirin, acetaminophen, and nonsteroidal anti-inflammatory drugs (NSAIDs) are effective analgesics. Some patients, however, may need short-term narcotic analgesia. Muscle relaxants, used for a few days, may help some patients. Oral glucocorticoids are of no benefit in patients with acute LBP, including those with sciatica.

Back exercises are not helpful in the acute phase, and a physical therapy referral is usually unnecessary in the first month. A program of regular exercises, aerobic conditioning, and loss of excess weight are used later to prevent recurrences. The purpose of back exercises is to stabilize the spine by strengthening the trunk muscles. Flexion exercises strengthen the abdominal muscles and extension exercises strengthen the paraspinal muscles. Educational booklets that include back exercises and safe lifting techniques are helpful.

Spinal manipulation may be effective early on in some patients with acute LBP. However, there is no conclusive evidence about its effectiveness in LBP of greater than 1-month duration or in patients with radiculopathy.

There is limited evidence to support the use of epidural glucocorticoid injections for short-term relief of radicular pain. Epidural injections are not recommended for LBP without radiculopathy. Injections of trigger points, ligaments, sacroiliac joints, and facet joints with anesthetic agents or glucocorticoid are of unproven efficacy and are not recommended in the

management of LBP. Nerve root blocks are also not recommended for therapeutic or diagnostic purposes.

Self-application of heat or cold is an easy and inexpensive option. Shoe lifts are considered only when the leg length inequality is more than 1 inch.

Modalities such as ultrasound, cutaneous laser treatment, electrical stimulation, and transcutaneous electrical nerve stimulation are not effective in the treatment of LBP. Other physical treatments such as lumbar braces, traction, acupuncture, biofeedback, and massage are also ineffective and not recommended.

B. CHRONIC LBP

In most patients, the cause of chronic LBP is unclear. The clinical spectrum is wide. Some patients complain of severe unremitting pain, but most have a constant and nagging mechanical LBP that may radiate into the buttocks and is punctuated by periods of acute exacerbation. Treatment is centered around relief of pain and restoration of function. Results are often unsatisfactory, and complete relief of pain is unrealistic for most.

Acetaminophen and NSAIDs may provide some degree of analgesia. Long-term use of narcotic analgesics should be avoided. Antidepressants are useful in the one-third of patients who have associated depression. Low-dose tricyclic antidepressants (eg, amitriptyline 10–75 mg at bedtime) may help some patients without depression, but anticholinergic side effects are common.

Back exercises (see Acute LBP, above), aerobic conditioning, loss of excess weight, and patient education are effective in managing chronic LBP. Multidisciplinary pain centers offer a combination of drug therapy, behavioral therapy, physical therapy, and patient education. These therapies may be helpful in selected patients as long as the center is not procedure-oriented and avoids the use of unproven and expensive injections and physical treatments.

As a general principle, the results of back surgery are disappointing when the goal is relief of back pain rather than relief of radicular symptoms resulting from neurologic compression. It is therefore not surprising that the effectiveness of spinal fusion surgery for relief of chronic LBP remains unproven. Fusion surgery is generally performed when the pain is attributed to degenerative disc disease, spondylolisthesis, degenerative spinal instability, internal disc disruption, or facet syndrome.

Intradiscal electrothermal annuloplasty is an unproven new procedure that is gaining popularity for the relief of chronic LBP in patients with positive discography. A wire-containing catheter is inserted into the disc, positioned against the posterior annulus, and then heated. This presumably shrinks collagen fibrils and cauterizes granulation and nerve tissue.

Table 10–6. Indications for surgical referral.

Disc herniation
 Cauda equina syndrome (emergency)
 Severe neurologic deficit
 Progressive neurologic deficit
 Greater than 6 weeks of sciatica (elective)
 Persistence of significant neurologic deficit beyond
  6 weeks (elective)
Spinal stenosis
 Severe neurologic deficit
 Progressive neurologic deficit
 Persistent and disabling pseudoclaudication (elective)
Spondylolisthesis
 Significant or progressive neurologic deficit

C. NERVE ROOT COMPRESSION SYNDROMES

1. Disc herniation—Patients with radicular pain in whom a disc herniation with nerve root compression is suspected should be treated nonsurgically, as described under Acute LBP, for the first 6 weeks unless they have a severe or progressive neurologic deficit (Table 10–6). Most patients (approximately 90%) will respond. Elective surgery may be considered in the few patients who have a significant persistent neurologic deficit or severe sciatica after 6 weeks of conservative care.

Laminotomy with limited discectomy is generally the procedure of choice. A microdiscectomy is the same procedure but with the use of a microscope. Percutaneous techniques are less effective. Arthroscopic discectomy appears promising, but more studies are needed.

2. Spinal stenosis—The symptoms of spinal stenosis remain stable for years in most patients and may actually improve in a few. Even when symptoms progress, there is little likelihood of irreversible neurologic impairment. Therefore, nonoperative treatment is a rational choice for most patients. Analgesics, NSAIDs, loss of excess weight, physical conditioning, exercises (including those that reduce lumbar lordosis), and epidural glucocorticoid may provide symptomatic relief.

Patients with a progressive or severe neurologic deficit are surgical candidates (Table 10–6). Elective surgery may be considered in patients with severe and disabling pseudoclaudication. Surgical treatment is aimed at decompression of the neural elements. This is accomplished by laminectomy or laminotomy with excision of the ligamentum flavum and medial aspect of the hypertrophied facet joints and removal of any protruding disc material. If spinal instability is present (as with spondylolisthesis) or results from surgical decompression, fusion of vertebral segments may be required. Successful surgery is often followed by recurrence of symptoms a few years later.

3. Spondylolisthesis—The vast majority of patients are treated conservatively. Rarely, a patient may need decompression surgery with fusion if a significant or progressive neurologic deficit develops from nerve root impingement or as a result of spinal stenosis.

REFERENCES

Bigos S, et al. Acute low back problems in adults. Agency for Health Care Policy and Research, Public Health Service, US Department of Health and Human Services. Clinical Practice Guideline No. 14. Report No. 95-0642. December 1994. (A classic, comprehensive, and critical evaluation of the published literature with recommendations for managing acute LBP.)

Deyo RA, Weinstein JN. Low back pain. *N Engl J Med.* 2001; 344:363. [PMID: 2945917] (Concise overview of the clinical features, diagnostic evaluation, and treatment.)

Jarvik JG, Deyo RA. Diagnostic evaluation of low back pain with emphasis on imaging. *Ann Intern Med.* 2002;137:586. [PMID: 12353946] (A detailed review of the different imaging techniques.)

Relevant World Wide Web Sites

[American Academy of Orthopaedic Surgeons]
http://www.aaos.org
[Institute for Clinical Systems Improvement]
http://www.ICSI.org
[National Guideline Clearinghouse]
http://www.guideline.gov

The Patient with Hip Pain

Ilksen Gurkan, MD, James F. Wenz, MD†

General Considerations

Hip pain is a very common complaint of patients seeking medical care. However, since most patients have a broad definition of the hip, which often includes the thigh, low back, buttock, and groin areas, clinicians must determine whether the patient's pain originates from the hip joint itself or from other nearby structures such as the trochanteric bursa or lumbar spine. Therefore, accurate evaluation of patients with hip pain depends on a careful medical history and physical examination, a basic understanding of common radiographic findings, and a thorough appreciation of the differential diagnosis.

Clinical Findings

A. SYMPTOMS AND SIGNS

1. History—The location of the pain and activities associated with that pain are frequently the most reliable indicators of the cause: Pain located primarily in the groin associated with weight bearing or range of motion is the most reliable symptom of intra-articular hip disease.

The quality of the pain is also important. Severe hip pain that is generalized, unrelenting, constant, or worse at night may have an infectious or oncologic cause. Patients should be asked about the onset of symptoms to differentiate between chronic and acute hip pain. Pain that has been slowly progressive is common in noninfectious arthritic conditions. For example, a person with hip osteoarthritis experiences a gradual onset of slowly worsening hip pain and decreasing range of motion. It becomes progressively harder to walk normally, especially going up and down stairs. On the other hand, acute onset of pain in a previously nonsymptomatic patient suggests a systemic disease or joint infection. Systemic disease should be considered in all atypical and undiagnosed conditions. Lyme disease and other infections should always be considered early because the quality of the response to therapy may depend on the timing of intervention.

Radiation of pain down the leg or in conjunction with back pain may represent spine disease as a primary cause or trochanteric bursitis if the pain radiates from the lateral buttock to the knee. Also, factors that aggravate the pain need to be scrutinized carefully. For example, lateral thigh pain that is reproduced by palpation and worsens with lying on the affected hip is often soft tissue in nature. Questions regarding what type of activities exacerbate the pain can reveal important abnormal mechanics during running, such as the feet crossing the midline (increased adduction), wide pelvis and genu valgum, or running on tracks without banks. Such activities can exacerbate the discomfort of trochanteric bursitis.

Associated symptoms also help differentiate pain from the hip and from other sources. Extra-articular findings can help identify the type of associated arthritis (eg, tophi in gout, nodules in rheumatoid arthritis, pustular rash in gonococcemia). Coexisting periarticular disease also may facilitate the diagnosis. For example, tendinitis of the ankle or wrist commonly coexists with gonococcal arthritis, rheumatoid arthritis, and other systemic diseases; prominent tenderness of bones adjacent to joints and joint effusions occur in sickle cell disease and hypertrophic pulmonary osteoarthropathy; and enthesitis with tenderness and swelling at tendon insertions suggests reactive arthritis. Careful history taking may also uncover a traumatic event associated with the onset of pain, which strongly suggests fracture or injury to the soft tissues about the hip. Landing on the knee and jarring the hip may result in a subluxation or labral tear or both. However, a fall on the lateral aspect of the hip can indicate a fracture or, in less severe cases, trochanteric bursitis.

Patients who report snapping in and around the hip may have one of the "snapping hip syndromes." Mechanical abnormalities that can result in snapping occur at approximately 45 degrees of flexion, when the hip is moving from flexion to extension. An internal snapping sensation can be caused by the iliopsoas tendon slipping over the osseous ridge of the lesser trochanter or the anterior acetabulum or by the iliofemoral ligament riding over the femoral head. In contrast, external snapping sensations are produced by a tight iliotibial band or gluteus maximus tendon riding over the greater tuberosity of the femur. This condition can be exacerbated by trochanteric bursitis. In addition, acetabular labral tears or loose bodies can cause intra-articular snapping; snapping in these conditions is always associated with sharp pain in the groin and anterior thigh.

2. Physical examination—A basic understanding of the hip anatomy and biomechanics is the cornerstone

†Deceased

of an accurate physical examination of the patient with hip pain. The hip is formed by the proximal femur and the articulation with the pelvis. The bony anatomy of the proximal femur includes the femoral head, the femoral neck, and the greater and lesser trochanters. The acetabulum, the mating socket for the femoral head, is coated with articular cartilage. A rim of fibro-cartilage at the outer edge of the acetabulum helps stabilize the hip joint. The abductor muscles, which attach to the greater trochanter, are the main abductor of the hip. The iliopsoas tendon, which inserts on the lesser trochanter, is the primary hip flexor. These tendinous insertions have an associated bursa where the tendon traverses over the bony margins. The iliotibial band originates along the brim of the iliac wing (along the anterior and posterior margins), consolidates over the greater trochanter, travels laterally along the thigh, and inserts in the proximal leg.

The femoral triangle is formed by the inguinal liga-ment (the top border), the sartorious muscle (the lateral border), and the adductor longus muscle (the medial border). This triangle includes the femoral nerve,

artery, and vein that run through it (lateral to medial) (Figure 11–1). Any muscle of the pelvis can cause rota-tion of the pelvis. Muscles around hip can be summa-rized in groups (Figure 11–2).

The trochanteric bursa decreases friction between the gluteus maximus and the greater trochanter; the gluteofemoral bursa, between the gluteus maximus and the vastus lateralis origin; and the ischial bursa, between the ischial tuberosity and gluteus maximus.

a. Inspection of the hip—Inspection of the hip be-gins with careful observation of the patient's gait. Two phases of gait need to be observed: stance phase (when the foot is on the ground and bears weight) and swing phase (when the foot moves forward and does not bear weight). Most problems appear during the stance phase.

The width of the gait, the shift of the pelvis, and flexion of the knee should be observed as well as the lumbar portion of the spine. With the patient in the supine position, the lumbar spine reflects a slight lordo-sis. Loss of lordosis may reflect vertebral muscle spasm,

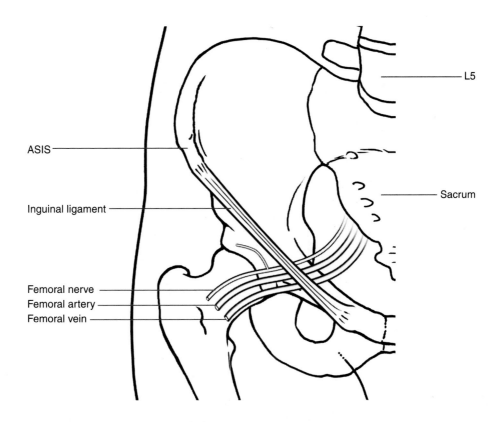

Figure 11–1. The mnemonic **NAVEL** may be a helpful reminder of the lateral-to-medial sequence of **N**erve-**A**rtery-**V**ein-**E**mpty Space-**L**ymph node. ASIS, anterior superior iliac spine.

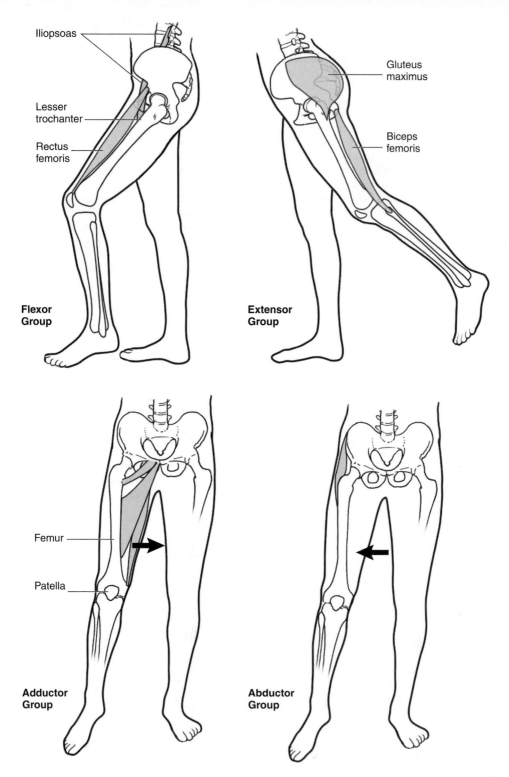

Figure 11–2. Four powerful muscle groups that move the hip are shown with their attachments to the femur and pelvis.

Flexor Group

Iliopsoas

Lesser trochanter

Rectus femoris

Extensor Group

Gluteus maximus

Biceps femoris

Adductor Group

Femur

Patella

Abductor Group

and excess lordosis may suggest a flexion deformity of the hip. Therefore, this observation should always be followed by assessment of leg length symmetry. Leg shortening and external rotation with pain suggest hip fracture. Inspect the anterior and posterior surfaces of the hip for any areas of muscle atrophy or bruising caused by trauma or neuromuscular diseases (eg, polymyositis and dermatomyositis).

It is important to detect and characterize any limp. An antalgic limp is characterized by a shortened stance phase on the affected side. An antalgic gait usually reflects substantial hip arthritis or disease in other joints of the lower extremity. A Trendelenburg limp or gait occurs when the trunk lurches laterally to one side during the stance phase, producing a "waddling" effect. Trendelenburg gait results from weakness of the hip abductors, which in turn may result from primary muscle disease or from muscle weakness caused by chronic hip disease. A limp may also result from shortening of the leg, flexion contracture, or muscle weakness in the pelvic girdle muscles or in other parts of the lower limb, such as in paralyzed quadriceps gait pattern, triceps surae gait pattern, and dorsiflexor gait pattern. Therefore, a thorough evaluation of the lower extremity muscle strength is essential for diagnosing the cause of the limp. Manual muscle testing is useful for evaluating flexors (iliopsoas and rectus femoris), extensors (gluteus maximus and hamstrings), abductors (gluteus medius and minimus), and adductors (adductor longus, magnus, and brevis, pectineus, and gracilis).

b. Palpation—With the patient supine, the clinician should ask the patient to place the heel of the leg being examined on the opposite knee. This position fa-cilitates palpation along the inguinal ligament. Bulges along the ligament can be inguinal hernias or aneurysms, which can be secondary causes of hip pain outside the hip joint (eg, ischemia secondary to a vascular disease or compression of an aneurysm). From lateral to medial, a sequence of nerve, artery, vein, and lymph nodes can be palpated. Enlarged nodes suggest infection. With the patient on one side and the hip flexed and internally rotated, the trochanteric bursa over the greater trochanter can be palpated (Figure 11–3). Tenderness over the femoral greater trochanter indicates local bursitis rather than hip arthritis. The ischiogluteal bursa cannot be palpated unless it is inflamed (Figure 11–4). When the ischiogluteal bursa is inflamed, it can mimic sciatica. Bursitis is one of the major causes of tenderness around the hip joint. Crepitus, or a grating sensation in the joint, felt by the patient or detected by the examiner is a late manifestation of arthritic condition and is neither a sensitive nor specific indicator.

c. Range of motion—Motions of the hip include flexion, extension, abduction, adduction, and rotation. The hip can flex further when the knee is also flexed. In the case of a hip with a flexion deformity, flexion of the unaffected hip prevents full leg extension of the affected hip, which appears flexed (Figure 11–5). By placing one hand on the patient's iliac crest, the clinician can detect pelvic movement that might be mistaken for hip movement. Flexion deformity may be masked by an increase in lumbar lordosis and an anterior pelvic tilt. Assessment of hip extension can be aided by positioning the patient face down and extending the thigh toward the clinician in a posterior direction. Stabilizing the pelvis by pressing down on the opposite anterior supe-

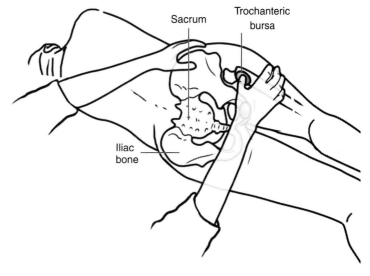

Figure 11–3. With the patient lying on the unaffected side and the affected hip flexed and internally rotated, the trochanteric bursa over the greater trochanter can be palpated. Swelling with tenderness suggests trochanteric bursitis. Tenderness without swelling along the posterolateral aspect suggests localized tendinitis.

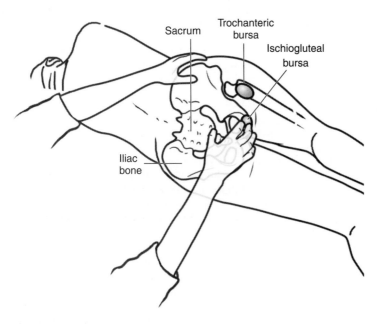

Sacrum

Trochanteric bursa

Ischiogluteal bursa

Iliac bone

Figure 11–4. The ischiogluteal bursa, unless inflamed, cannot be palpated. Shown are the location of (directly over the ischial tuberosity) and the palpation technique for the ischiogluteal bursa.

rior iliac spine with one hand, grasping the ankle with the other, and abducting the extended leg marks the limit of hip abduction (Figure 11–6). Restricted abduction (normal range, 45–50 degrees) is common in hip osteoarthritis. In the same manner, moving the leg medially across the body and over the opposite extremity marks the adduction limit. Flexing the leg to 90 degrees at hip and knee, stabilizing the thigh with one hand, grasping the ankle with the other, and rotating the lower extremity externally (normal, 45 degrees) and internally (normal, 35 degrees) identifies the hip's rota-

tion limits (Figure 11–7). The earliest motion affected, and therefore the most sensitive indicator of true hip disease, is loss of internal rotation. As the disease progresses, prolonged joint stiffness and limitations of movements become more evident. Limitation of joint movement may be secondary to flexion contractures or mechanical obstructions.

d. Symmetry and other joint involvement—Involvement of other joints may provide clues about the primary disease affecting the hip. For example,

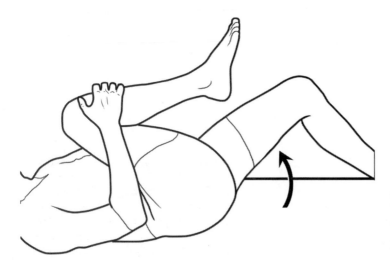

Figure 11–5. In flexion deformity of the hip, the affected hip does not allow full leg extension when the opposite hip is flexed. Therefore, the affected hip appears flexed.

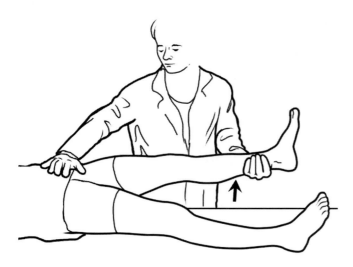

Figure 11–6. The limit of hip abduction is determined by stabilizing the pelvis with one hand pressing down on the opposite anterior superior iliac spine and with the other hand grasping the ankle and abducting the extended leg.

metacarpophalangeal and proximal interphalangeal deformity and involvement indicate rheumatoid arthritis, whereas distal interphalangeal involvement can indicate osteoarthritis.

B. LABORATORY FINDINGS

Additional evaluation is indicated when the diagnosis remains uncertain after the history and physical examination, response to therapy is not as expected, or substantial clinical changes occur. Certain problems require immediate attention and prompt treatment.

Acute monarthritis is one example; joint fluid examination is essential for this condition. Hemorrhagic joint fluid suggests fracture, bleeding diathesis, or malignancy. Intensely inflammatory effusions suggest pyogenic infection, requiring immediate antibiotic therapy and aspiration or other drainage procedures to establish the diagnosis and prevent joint destruction.

When systemic rheumatic diseases are suspected, clinically indicated laboratory work may include tests for erythrocyte sedimentation rate and rheumatoid factor. Blood tests are useful in diagnosing some specific

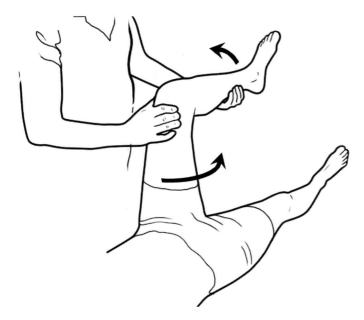

Figure 11–7. Establishing the rotation limits of the hip is done by flexing the leg to 90 degrees at the hip and knee, stabilizing the thigh with one hand, and with the other hand grasping the ankle and rotating the lower extremity externally (normal, 45 degrees) and internally (normal, 35 degrees).

types of arthritis (for specific tests, see the chapters for each disease).

Synovial fluid analysis, especially the synovial fluid white blood cell count, allows effusions to be classified as normal, noninflammatory, inflammatory, or septic (see Chapter 2, Aspiration & Joint Injection). Effusions can also be hemorrhagic. Thus, each type of effusion suggests certain joint diseases, and differential diagnosis can be based on the joint fluid findings (see Chapter 2). If infection is suspected, a portion of the synovial fluid sample should be sent to the laboratory for Gram stain and culture. Synovial fluid analysis provides a definitive diagnosis for infections and crystal arthropathies (which rarely affect hip joints) (Table 11–1).

C. IMAGING STUDIES

1. Plain radiographs—Routine radiographs for a patient with hip pain include anteroposterior and lateral views of the pelvis and hip. Plain radiographs can delineate the alignment, bone mineralization, articular cartilage, and soft tissue. Alignment abnormality may indicate a fracture, a dislocation, or secondary causes of osteoarthritis such as congenital dislocation of the hip or slipped capital-femoral epiphysis. Articular cartilage changes, such as joint space narrowing or the presence of osteophytes, subchondral sclerosis, cysts, or subluxation, can occur early or late in the course of rheumatoid or systemic diseases or both. Each finding provides clues about the extent of the cartilage damage in the hip joint as well as the stages of certain diseases such as avascular necrosis (AVN) of the hip. Specialized views can provide clearer images of certain aspects of the joint. For example, the frog-leg lateral view provides a better view of the anterolateral femoral head and is useful in evaluating for AVN. This view can also show breaks in the cortex and a "rim sign" (a subcortical black lucent line) characteristic of AVN as well as femoral head collapse in later stages of AVN. A 40-degree cephalad

anteroposterior view is useful for elucidating subtle femoral neck and pubic fractures.

Radiographic findings of osteoarthritis include joint space narrowing, subchondral sclerosis, subchondral cyst formation, irregularity of the femoral head, osteophyte formation, and increased subchondral bone density. Since some patients with radiographic evidence of hip osteoarthritis are asymptomatic, radiographic changes in the absence of characteristic symptoms should not lead to the diagnosis of osteoarthritis as the cause of the patient's pain. The radiographic signs for joint effusion are lateral displacement of the femoral head (especially common in juvenile rheumatoid arthritis), a vacuum effect (defined as the lack of the normal radiolucent crescent between the joint surfaces when manual traction is applied to the hip during the radiograph), and demineralization of subchondral bone and apparent joint space widening. Radiographic evidence of calcification within soft tissue also indicates abnormality in the hip joint. This finding is fairly nonspecific but is most frequently associated with rheumatoid arthritis, systemic lupus erythematosus, heterotopic ossification or post-traumatic soft tissue calcification.

The anteroposterior pelvic view can help evaluate sacroiliac joint changes as a source of referred hip pain (Table 11–2).

2. Other imaging methods—Frequently used imaging tools other than the plain radiographs include computed tomography (CT), magnetic resonance imaging (MRI), and bone scans. Bone scans are useful for detecting metastatic disease (when suspected), AVN, and Paget disease of bone. They delineate the regions of increased metabolic activity ("hot spots") by increased uptake of a radioactive tracer. Pelvic/acetabular fractures, osseous sequelae of hip dislocation, and intra-articular osseous fragments are better visualized by CT than by plain radiographs. CT is also useful in characterizing calcifications secondary to tumor matrix within bone

Table 11–1. Analysis of synovial fluid in hip.

Parameter	Normal	Noninflammatory	Inflammatory	Infectious	Hemorrhagic
Color	Clear	Clear	Opaque	Opaque	Sanguinous
Viscosity	High	High	Low	Variable	Variable
White blood cell count/μL	< 200	< 2000	> 2000	> 50,000	Variable
% Polymorphonuclear neutrophils	< 25	< 25	> 25	> 50	Variable
Examples		Traumatic, osteoarthritis, neuropathic, hypertrophic arthropathy	Rheumatoid arthritis, gout	Septic arthritis	Trauma, hemophilia

Table 11–2. Expected radiographic changes on anteroposterior radiograph of patient with hip pain.

Decreased bone density
  Rheumatoid arthritis
  Late ankylosing spondylitis
Bony erosions
  Erosive osteoarthritis in postmenopausal women
  Rheumatoid arthritis
  Psoriatic arthritis
  Ankylosing spondylitis
  Pigmented villonodular synovitis
Cyst formation
  Osteoarthritis (subchondral cysts)
  Rheumatoid arthritis (synovial cysts)
  Calcium pyrophosphate deposition disease
Joint space narrowing
  Osteoarthritis (nonuniform narrowing)
  Rheumatoid arthritis (uniform)
  Calcium pyrophosphate deposition disease (uniform)
  Psoriatic arthritis
  Ankylosing spondylitis
Bone production
  Osteophytes
    Osteoarthritis
    Calcium pyrophosphate deposition disease
    Diffuse idiopathic skeletal hyperostosis
  Subchondral sclerosis
    Osteoarthritis
    Calcium pyrophosphate deposition disease
  Tendon and ligament ossification
    Diffuse idiopathic skeletal hyperostosis
    Myositis ossificans
  Chondrocalcinosis
    Calcium pyrophosphate deposition disease
Distortion of normal skeletal structure
  Fracture
  Tumor invasion
  Infections (especially tuberculosis)
  Rapidly progressive osteoarthropathy

---

or soft tissue or to ossification, and is best for imaging cortical bone.

MRI is the most specific and sensitive imaging modality for AVN. MRI is also useful in detecting soft tissue lesions (tumors), transient osteoporosis, synovial pitting, bone cysts, and stress fractures. Compared with CT, MRI provides better visualization of medullary bone and soft tissues.

Depending on the patient history and physical examination results, other useful studies may include needle or surgical synovial biopsy, ultrasonography, arthroscopy, arthrography (especially to evaluate labral tears), electromyography, nerve conduction times (for the differential diagnosis of lumbar causes or lower extremity muscle weakness as the source of limp), thermography, and muscle or bone biopsy (Table 11–3).

D. SPECIAL TESTS

The Stinchfield resisted hip flexion test helps distinguish between intra-articular and extra-articular hip causes of groin, thigh, buttock, and even pretibial leg pain. With the patient supine, the test is performed by asking the patient to elevate the leg while the examiner applies gentle manual resistance to the ankle with the knee extended. Reproduction of pain in a typical pattern related to the sensory innervation of the hip (groin, thigh, buttock, or knee) makes the test positive for hip disease.

In the Patrick test, the patient lies supine and the clinician holds the affected leg and rotates it externally. Pain so elicited suggests sacroiliitis, hip disease, or an L4 nerve root lesion.

For the Gaenslen test, the patient lies supine on a treatment table, hangs one leg over the side of the table in hyperextension, and draws the other knee to the chest (Figure 11–8). The clinician may aid the patient in moving the hip into hyperextension. Pain in the ipsilateral sacroiliac joint makes this reliable test positive and indicates ipsilateral joint lesion, hip disease, or an L4 nerve root lesion.

Differential Diagnosis

Table 11–4 lists the possible causes of hip pain (and conditions that mimic hip disease) most commonly seen in different age groups and populations. The differential diagnosis of hip pain includes referred pain. Pain reproduced by the patient sitting in a forward position suggests referred pain from the lumbar spine, discs, or nerve roots. Coughing and the Valsalva maneuver raise the intratechal pressure, and stretching nerve roots worsen discal pain. An abnormal neurologic examination of the lower extremity can also suggest radiculopathy. Pain can also be referred to the hip from the bladder and reproductive organs (Table 11–4).

The location of hip pain plays an extremely important role in shaping the differential diagnosis. Anterior hip pain may be caused by hip fracture, septic arthritis, AVN osteoarthritis, rheumatoid arthritis, or iliopectineal bursitis. Lateral or trochanteric hip pain can result from bursitis, bone tumor, fracture, or referred hip pain from lumbar disc herniation. Lumbar disc disease without herniation or facet disease rarely causes lateral hip pain. On the other hand, posterior hip pain necessitates ruling out sciatic nerve irritation and sacroiliitis secondary to spondyloarthropathy, lumbar disc disease, or facet disease.

In athletes, rapid sartorius contraction in a jumping sport can result in an anterosuperior iliac spine avulsion

Table 11–3. Conditions and diagnostic tools for hip pain.

Test	Fracture	Trauma	Avascular Necrosis	Degen-erative Arthritis	Soft Tissue Pathology	Tumors	Pigmented Villo-nodular Synovitis	Osteo-porosis	Infection	Labral Tear
Ultrasonography	N/O	N/O	N/O	N/O	U	N/O	N/O	N/O	N/O	U
Radiography	U	U	U	U	U	U	U	U	U	N/O
Bone scan	U	N/O	U	N/O	N/O	U	S	U	N/O	N/O
Tomography	U	N/O	N/O	N/O	N/O	N/O	N/O	N/O	N/O	N/O
Magnetic resonance imaging	U	U	U	N/O	U	U	U	U	S	U
Computed tomography	U	U	U	N/O	U	U	U	N/O	N/O	N/O
Arteriography/venography	N/O	S	U	N/O	N/O	U	N/O	N/O	N/O	N/O
Arthrography	S	S	N/O	N/O	N/O	N/O	N/O	N/O	N/O	U

N/O, not often used; U, used; S, sometimes used (but not as the first diagnostic tool).

fracture. Strong rectus femoris contraction in a kicking sport can cause an anteroinferior iliac spine avulsion fracture, and rapid hamstring contraction in sprinting and hurdling can cause an ischial tuberosity avulsion fracture. Such fractures are displaced less than 1 cm and usually respond to nonoperative therapy. Larger injuries may require surgical fixation. Therefore, a high-risk patient with a recent sports injury should be assessed with anteroposterior pelvic views to determine the method of treatment.

Patients with upper lateral hip pain and without groin pain can have trochanteric bursitis, a common cause of hip discomfort. Trochanteric bursitis is often exacerbated by direct pressure (eg, rolling onto the affected side in bed) and may refer the pain to the knee. Pain below the inguinal ligament and lateral to vessels indicates iliopectineal bursitis. Other soft tissue conditions causing hip pain include strains (an acute injury to a muscle or tendon) and tendinitis (inflammatory changes secondary to overuse). Acute direct trauma can

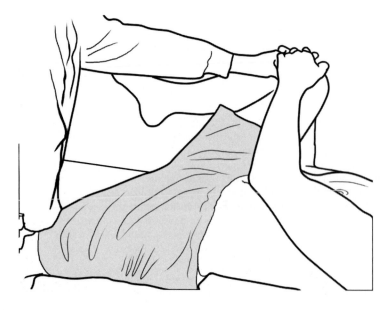

Figure 11–8. Gaenslen test. (Available at: http://www.hughston.com/hha/a_15_1_1a.htm)

Table 11–4. Causes of groin or hip pain.

I. Nonmusculoskeletal causes
- A. General
  1. Inguinal hernia
  2. Inguinal lymphadenopathy or lymphadenitis
  3. Lumbar disc disease with L1–2 radiculopathy
  4. Nephrolithiasis
  5. Abdominal aortic aneurysm
  6. Appendicitis
  7. Diverticulitis
  8. Inflammatory bowel disease
  9. Malignancy
- B. In women
  1. Ovarian cyst
  2. Urinary tract infection
  3. Pelvic inflammatory disease
- C. In men
  1. Epididymitis
  2. Hydrocele
  3. Varicocele
  4. Prostatitis
  5. Testicular cancer

II. Hip joint disorders
- A. In pediatric patients (> 10 years old)
  1. Malignancies (uncommon)
  2. Legg-Calvé-Perthes disease
  3. Septic joint
  4. Toxic synovitis
- B. In adolescent patients
  1. Slipped capital-femoral epiphysis
  2. Hip avulsion fracture
  3. Juvenile rheumatoid arthritis
- C. In adults
  1. Osteoarthritis or rheumatoid arthritis
  2. Avascular necrosis
  3. Stress fractures
     a. Pubic rami
     b. Supra-acetabular region
     c. Femoral neck
     d. Acetabular labral tear
     e. Rheumatic manifestations of systemic disease: sarcoidosis, malignancy, amyloidosis, etc (rare)
     f. Connective tissue disease with hip involvement
     g. Paget disease
     h. Pigmented villonodular synovitis
     i. Hip fractures
- D. In Athletes
  1. Idiopathic in 30% of cases
  2. Adductor strain or adductor tendinitis (groin pull)
  3. Pubic instability
  4. Osteitis pubis
  5. Myositis ossificans
  6. Sports hernia
  7. Groin disruption
  8. Iliopsoas strain or iliopsoas bursitis
  9. Snapping hip syndrome
  10. Femoral neck stress fracture
  11. Pubic ramus stress fracture
  12. Avulsion fracture (adolescent athletes)
     a. Anterosuperior iliac spine avulsion fracture
     b. Anteroinferior iliac spine avulsion fracture
     c. Ischial tuberosity avulsion fracture
- E. Nerve entrapment
  1. Genitofemoral nerve entrapment
  2. Lateral femoral cutaneous nerve entrapment
  3. Ilioinguinal nerve entrapment
  4. Obturator nerve entrapment

III. Other common hip conditions
- A. Trochanteric bursitis: iliopectineal bursitis

cause contusion or contusion with hematoma, which can progress to myositis ossificans in 2–4 weeks.

Hip tumors can be characterized by the extent of bone destruction. Large, aggressive lesions with irregular margins or soft tissue extensions are often associated with malignant tumors. Benign lesions have sclerotic or nonsclerotic well-defined borders. The periosteal reaction also provides clues about the aggressiveness of the tumor and the rate of growth. Slow-growing lesions may leave the periosteal sleeve intact as new bone formation continues, but a rapidly growing tumor mass can exceed new bone formation capacity and produce the characteristic "sunburst" appearance. Alleviating factors may also help identify certain hip tumors: The pain from osteoid osteoma typically responds to nonsteroidal anti-inflammatory medications (Table 11–5).

Nerve entrapment can cause hip pain (see Table 11–4). Nerves can be compressed as they pass under ligaments and between muscles. The sciatic and lateral femoral cutaneous nerves are most frequently affected.

Neuromuscular hip conditions can cause isolated hip pain and can be classified as intrinsic or extrinsic. Intrinsic disorders include spasticity (such as cerebral palsy), cerebrovascular accidents, spinal cord injuries in the young, and flaccid paralysis (such as myelomeningocele, poliomyelitis, and Charcot-Marie-Tooth disease). Extrinsic causes involving the hip joint can include upper motor neuron injury or multiple sclerosis.

When to Refer to a Specialist

Patients in whom a hip infection is suspected should be referred urgently to a specialist (eg, orthopedist, radiologist, or rheumatologist) for joint aspiration and synovial fluid analysis. Patients with fractures or bone tumor should be referred to an orthopedist. Patients in

Table 11–5. Common hip disorders: clinical findings and management.

Characteristic	Osteoarthritis	Inflammatory Arthritis	Septic Joint	Trochanteric Bursitis	Trauma	Tumor	Avascular Necrosis
Onset	Insidious	Insidious	Acute, severe	Insidious, can be acute	Acute, severe	Acute or chronic	Sudden
Progression and duration	Slow, temporary exacerbations after periods of overuse	Chronic with remissions and exacerbations	Acute, unrelenting	Acute, or acute exacerbation of of chronic condition	Acute, accompanied by history of falling	Acute exacerbations in chronic setting, night pain in osteoid osteoma	Sudden severe pain becomes rapidly worse, worse at night
Location	Groin, anterior	Groin, anterior	Groin, inner thigh, radiates to knee	Lateral, radiates from lateral hip to knee	Anywhere, depending on the fracture	Anywhere, depending on the invasion	Groin or thigh pain
Aggravating factors	Activity	Exacerbation of systemic disease	Hip movements	Lying on affected side	Weight bearing	Weight bearing	Weight bearing
Alleviating factors	Rest	None	Hip in flexion and rest	Lying on unaffected side, NSAIDs	External rotation and rest	NSAIDs in osteoid osteoma, or strong pain medications	Early in the course NSAIDs, rest
Associated symptoms	Bony enlargement, possibly tender, seldom warm, morning stiffness < 1 hour	Swelling, tender, warm, seldom red, stiffness lasts > 1 hour, symmetric and polyarthritis	Localized and generalized fever, tenderness, warmth	Swelling, tenderness, w/wo warmth, snapping	Tenderness, warmth	Swelling, may be tender, warm	Tender
Range of motion	Limited	Limited	Extremely limited	Slightly limited	Extremely limited	Restricted	Limited
Generalized symptoms	Usually none	Weakness, fatigue, weight loss, low fever	Fever, weakness, fatigue, weight loss	Usually absent	Symptoms of osteoporosis in other joints	W/wo weakness, fatigue, weight loss, low fever	Symptoms related to secondary causes of avascular necrosis
Physical findings	Periarticular muscle atrophy, loss of internal rotation first	Effusion, tenosynovitis, nodules, bone-on-bone creptitus	Hip in flexion, slight abduction or adduction, and external rotation	Pain on palpation of bursa with patient lying on unaffected side	Shortened limb, externally rotated, antalgic gait, trauma signs	Pain on palpation, restricted range of motion	Antalgic gait, decreased flexion, internal rotation, and abduction
Management	Weight loss, physiotherapy, NSAIDs, glucocorticoid injections, surgery	NSAIDs, glucocorticoid, synovectomy, hip replacement	Surgical drainage, intravenous antibiotic, Gram stain guides subsequent treatment, physiotherapy	NSAIDs, ice, injection, physiotherapy, bursectomy	Surgery	Surgical resection w/wo reconstruction, w/wo chemotherapy and/or radiation	Early, nonoperative; Late, hip replacement

NSAIDs, nonsteroidal anti-inflammatory drugs; w/wo, with or without.

whom AVN of bone or a systemic rheumatic disease such as rheumatoid arthritis is suspected should usually be referred to a rheumatologist for treatment. Referral to a specialist is also warranted if the cause of hip pain eludes diagnosis or fails to respond appropriately.

REFERENCES

Bird PA, et al. Prospective evaluation of magnetic resonance imaging and physical examination findings in patients with greater trochanteric pain syndrome. *Arthritis Rheum.* 2001;44:2138. [PMID: 11592379] (Bird et al evaluated patients with greater trochanteric pain syndrome via magnetic resonance imaging for the prevalence of gluteus medius pathology.)

Gonzalez della Valle A, et al. Pigmented villonodular synovitis of the hip: 2- to 23-year followup study. *Clin Orthop.* 2001;388:187. [PMID: 11451119] (Gonzalez della Valle et al compiled a comprehensive review of the condition in the hip, a rare occurrence.)

Hamilton J, et al. The hip or not. *J Rheumatol.* 2001;28:1398. [PMID: 11409137] (Hamilton et al compiled several excellent case presentations to show the importance of CT in differentiating between soft tissue etiology and other causes arising from the hip joint itself. The diagnostic capability of CT for soft tissue pathologies is emphasized.)

Hedger S, et al. Unexplained hip pain: look beyond the obvious abnormality. *Ann Rheum Dis.* 1998;57:131. [PMID: 9640126] (Hedger et al present a case and emphasize the underestimation of bursitis incidence as a cause of hip pain.)

Rossi F, Dragoni S. Acute avulsion fractures of the pelvis in adolescent competitive athletes: prevalence, location and sports distribution of 203 cases collected. *Skeletal Radiol.* 2001;30:127. [PMID: 11357449] (Rossi and Dragoni reviewed the distribution of this common injury among athletes according to the sports activities in which they participated.)

van der Wurff P, et al. Clinical tests of the sacroiliac joint. A systemic methodological review. Part 1: reliability. *Man Ther.* 2000;5:30. [PMID: 10688957] (van der Wurff et al reviewed numerous studies examining specific tests used to detect joint mobility or pain provocation and analyzed the reliability of these tests.)

Relevant World Wide Web Sites

[Johns Hopkins Arthritis Center]
http://www.hopkins-arthritis.som.jhmi.edu
[Partners against Pain]
http://www.partnersagainstpain.com
[The Five Minute Orthopaedic Consultant]
http://www.jhbmc.jhu.edu/ortho/consultant/index.html

Approach to the Patient with Knee Pain

Carl A. Johnson, MD

GENERAL CONSIDERATIONS

Knee pain may result from trauma, overuse, internal derangement, osteoarthritis, or inflammatory arthritis. In addition, pain about the knee may be due to vascular or neurologic conditions. Hip disease may also refer pain to the knee, distal thigh, or both. The initial evaluation of a patient with knee pain should provide sufficient information to determine whether the pain is the result of intra-articular or periarticular knee pathology, or whether it may be produced by or referred from another source. In addition, the initial history and physical examination must identify specific conditions, such as septic arthritis or arterial occlusion, that may require urgent surgical intervention, other conditions that are amenable to nonoperative treatment, and those that may require further specialized evaluation or treatment (Table 12–1). The initial evaluation should provide clues to enable the examiner to formulate a provisional differential diagnosis, which may then be confirmed or refined through use of imaging studies or laboratory findings.

INITIAL CLINICAL ASSESSMENT

 ESSENTIAL FEATURES

- Conditions such as septic arthritis or vascular occlusion may require acute intervention.
- Knee pain may be referred from ipsilateral hip disease or may be due to a neurologic condition resulting from degenerative arthritis of the lumbosacral spine, lumbar disc herniation, or spinal stenosis.

History

The significant features of the history should include the onset and history of the pain as well as any prior history of similar problems in the knee or other joints. A history of trauma, whether recent or remote, should be noted. The nature of the onset of pain, including the location of the pain, whether the pain began suddenly, or whether symptoms began gradually and insidiously should be determined. The examiner should seek information about the response of pain to activity; whether the pain is constant or intermittent; and whether it is present only with weight bearing, at rest, or both. The history should elicit information about whether activities such as negotiating stairs or inclines, weather changes, rest, or position exacerbate the symptoms and whether rest, moving about, stretching, or other factors may relieve them. Specific questions to determine whether the onset of symptoms may have been associated with any specific activity or change in activity, such as recreational exercise, physically demanding work, or hobbies, may be helpful.

A history of swelling as well as its location should be sought. A history of stiffness, locking, catching, snapping, grinding, and crepitus should be obtained (Table 12–2). Locking symptoms must be further characterized as either true mechanical locking or nonmechanical locking due to apprehension or reluctance to move the knee because of pain or anticipation of pain. Similarly, symptoms of giving way should also be further investigated to determine whether they are the result of mechanical instability, weakness, or possible neurologic problems. A history of change in sensation, low back pain, radicular symptoms, feelings of leg weakness or heaviness, muscle cramps, and claudication may alert the examiner to the possibility of neurologic or vascular problems. Fevers, chills, or a history of infection elsewhere should also be noted.

A more comprehensive past medical history may be required in selected cases. A history of prior glucocorticoid use or alcohol abuse should alert the examiner to the possibility of avascular necrosis of the hip, which may initially present with thigh pain, knee pain, or both. Diabetes, systemic glucocorticoid use, HIV, and other conditions that may compromise immune function should similarly raise the clinician's index of suspicion to the possibility of septic arthritis.

Table 12–1. Diagnoses to be excluded as a cause of knee pain.

- Critical exclusionary diagnoses
    - Septic arthritis
    - Arterial occlusion
- Mimics of knee pain
    - Ipsilateral hip disease (osteoarthritis, osteonecrosis, fracture)
    - Neuropathic conditions (lumbar disc disease, spinal stenosis, saphenous nerve entrapment)

Physical Examination

The physical examination should include observation and characterization of the patient's gait, when possible, specifically seeking abnormal gait features such as antalgic limp, Trendelenburg gait, and ataxic gait (Table 12–3). An antalgic gait is characterized by shortened stance phase of gait on the affected side, as the patient avoids weight bearing on the painful limb. An unsteady walk, generally wide-based, with the feet thrown outward due to impaired coordination, is a feature of an ataxic gait. A Trendelenburg gait is characterized by listing of the trunk toward the affected side with each step. Overall limb alignment should be assessed for varus or valgus deformity. Extensor mechanism alignment is measured by the Q-angle (normally 15 degrees valgus ± 5 degrees), determined by the angle between the orientation of the quadriceps tendon and the patellar ligament (Figure 12–1). Excessive Q-angle valgus correlates with increased likelihood of patellar subluxation. Muscle atrophy, abnormal joint contours, and patellar tracking should be assessed. Abnormalities of the skin, including old scars, color, or temperature changes, should be noted. Swelling should be character-

Table 12–2. History for evaluation of knee pain.

Onset and history
History of trauma, prior problems, or similar problems with other joints
Response to activity and rest
Factors that exacerbate symptoms
Factors that improve symptoms
History and nature of swelling
Stiffness, locking, catching, grinding, or crepitus
Symptoms of giving way or instability
Changes in sensation or muscle strength
Muscle cramps, claudication
Fevers or chills
Hip, groin, or thigh pain
Pertinent general medical conditions

Table 12–3. Physical examination for evaluation of knee pain.

Observation of gait, alignment, deformities
Presence and location of warmth
Presence and location of swelling
Active and passive range of motion
Patellar tracking, mobility, apprehension
Collateral and cruciate stability
Meniscal tests
Tenderness to palpation and localization
Hip pain or stiffness
Vascular examination (pedal pulses, skin, hair distribution)
Neurologic examination (sensation, muscle strength, straight leg raise)

---

ized as diffuse or localized and by whether it represents an intra-articular effusion or soft tissue swelling. Localized swelling may also be specifically described as medial, lateral, popliteal, or prepatellar.

Active and passive range of motion should be measured and compared with the contralateral knee, noting flexion contractures, hyperextension, and any extension lag. Crepitus should be noted and localized, and patellar tracking should be observed. A sudden lateral deviation of the patella occurring as the knee approaches full extension, described as a positive "J-sign," may indicate patellar subluxation. The patellar apprehension sign, in which the examiner attempts to subluxate the patella laterally with the knee slightly flexed, often provokes the quadriceps to contract in response to the sensation of impending pain or patellar dislocation in patients with patellar tracking problems.

Medial and lateral stability should be examined at full extension and 30 degrees of knee flexion. Anterior cruciate ligament stability is determined by the Lachman test (Figure 12–2), anterior drawer sign (Figure 12–3), and flexion rotation drawer test or pivot shift. The posterior drawer test is used to assess posterior cruciate ligament integrity. Ligament stability findings should be compared with those of the contralateral knee to evaluate whether any perceived laxity is pathologic. In persons with apparent generalized laxity conditions, it may be helpful to examine the elbow and wrist joints for hyperextensibility and ability to touch the thumb to the ipsilateral forearm. McMurray and Appley meniscal compression tests may detect meniscal tears, although the sensitivity and specificity of these tests are not sufficient to rely entirely on those findings alone. Palpation about the knee can provide substantial information by localizing tenderness to a specific area or anatomic structure, such as the medial or lateral joint lines, patellar facets, pes anserine bursa, tibial tubercle, tendons, ligaments, or bony structures.

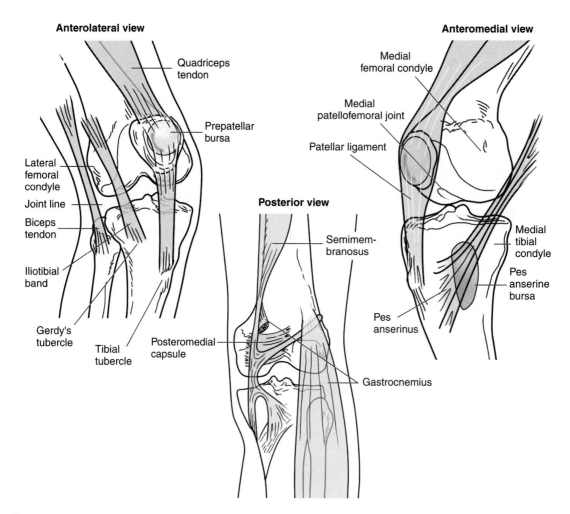

Figure 12–1. Functional anatomy of the knee.

The hip joint must be examined to exclude the possibility that knee pain may be referred from ipsilateral hip disease. If pain is produced in the groin or thigh by active straight leg raising against resistance or if significant limitation of hip range of motion is detected, further evaluation, including radiographic imaging of the hip, may be indicated. Pedal pulses, skin quality and pigmentation, and hair distribution on the feet and legs provide information about vascular status. When indicated, motor and sensory testing, examination of reflexes, and straight leg raise testing may help identify pain from lumbosacral spine pathology.

Oberlander MA, et al. The accuracy of the clinical knee examination documented by arthroscopy. A prospective study. *Am J Sports Med.* 1993;21:773. [PMID: 8291625] (Discusses the accuracy of clinical examination findings in diagnosing intra-articular knee pathology.)

Shybut GT, McGinty JB. The office evaluation of the knee. *Orthop Clin North Am.* 1982;3:497. [PMID: 7099586] (Describes a systematic approach to the clinical examination of the knee.)

SEPTIC ARTHRITIS

 ESSENTIAL FEATURES

- *Early recognition and treatment of septic arthritis is essential to minimize articular cartilage destruction and potentially life-threatening infection.*

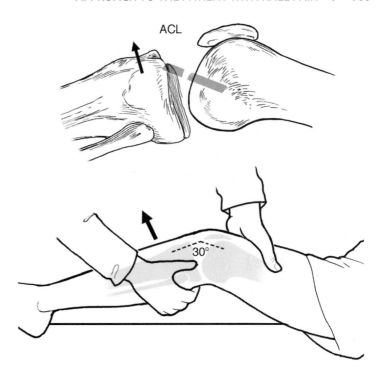

Figure 12–2. Lachman test for anterior cruciate ligament tear is at 30 degrees flexion. The extremity does not have to be lifted or foot stabilized.

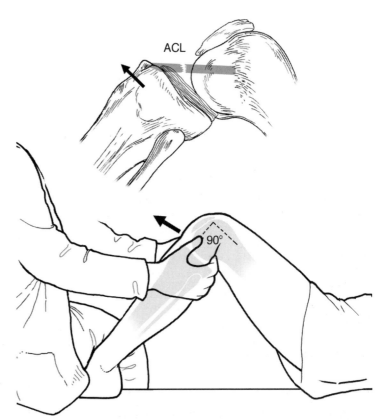

Figure 12–3. Anterior drawer test determines anterior cruciate instability. Flex knee to 90 degrees and stabilize foot. Note forward shift of tibia.

• *Joint aspiration and synovial fluid analysis are the most helpful diagnostic tests.*

Clinical Findings

A. SYMPTOMS AND SIGNS

Septic arthritis of the knee is generally associated with a history of severe, unremitting pain of recent onset exacerbated by motion and weight bearing and with swelling, fevers, chills, or infection elsewhere. Pain is improved at rest. Physical findings include limited range of motion, associated with pain. Erythema, warmth, and diffuse tenderness are present about the knee. Swelling and an effusion are also present. Septic arthritis is unlikely when pain is intermittent, when range of motion is normal, and in the absence of warmth or effusions.

B. LABORATORY FINDINGS

Joint aspiration and synovial fluid analysis should be performed in all cases of suspected septic arthritis of the knee. Analysis of the synovial fluid for cell count with differential, Gram stain, and polarized light microscopy analysis for crystals should be performed. Cultures should be evaluated for bacteria, mycobacteria, and fungus. A complete review of the results of synovial fluid analysis can be found in Chapter 2. Routine peripheral blood tests including a complete blood cell count with differential, erythrocyte sedimentation rate, C-reactive protein, and blood cultures should also be obtained, both to help establish the diagnosis of septic arthritis and to assist in monitoring the effectiveness of subsequent treatment.

C. IMAGING STUDIES

Radiographs generally provide little information to establish the diagnosis of septic arthritis of the knee. However, radiographs may confirm the presence of pre-existing osteoarthritis, which may predispose patients to the development of septic arthritis. Baseline radiographs may also be useful as a reference to assess possible future joint destruction and osteomyelitis, which may result from septic arthritis.

Differential Diagnosis

The clinical presentation of septic arthritis may be virtually indistinguishable from that of a crystal-induced arthritis, yet the diagnosis must be made without delay in order to minimize the likelihood of articular cartilage destruction and potentially life-threatening sepsis. Synovial fluid analysis is essential to differentiate between the diagnoses of gout, pseudogout, or septic arthritis. Other entities that may present as an inflammatory monoarthritis are outlined in Chapter 4.

ARTERIAL OCCLUSION

 ESSENTIAL FEATURES

• *Prompt recognition of acute arterial occlusion is essential to prevent gangrene and possible loss of limb.*
• *Absent pulses with loss of sensation and strength should alert the examiner to the possibility of arterial occlusion.*

Clinical Findings

A history of acute and constant pain, unrelieved by any means, and associated with altered sensation and strength should suggest the possibility of arterial occlusion. Acute arterial occlusion generally produces diffuse leg pain, not localized to the knee alone. Physical findings including absent pedal pulses, objective motor weakness, cyanosis, and decreased skin temperature may also be evident. The knee examination is often normal. The consequences of delayed recognition and treatment of acute vascular occlusion include paralysis, compartment syndrome, contractures, gangrene, and amputation. When suspected on the basis of the physical findings above, vascular consultation should be obtained without delay.

ANTERIOR KNEE PAIN

 ESSENTIAL FEATURES

• *Pain provoked or exacerbated by climbing stairs, squatting, and arising from a chair associated with peripatellar tenderness are common features of the syndrome of anterior knee pain.*
• *Laboratory and imaging studies are not generally indicated in the initial evaluation.*

Clinical Findings

The syndrome of anterior knee pain refers to a constellation of symptoms and physical findings that generally localizes to the patellofemoral articulation and the surrounding structures. Patellofemoral arthralgia, historically known as "chondromalacia patellae," usually begins insidiously without a specific provocative injury or incident.

A. SYMPTOMS AND SIGNS

Climbing or descending stairs or inclines generally exacerbates the pain. Symptoms are also provoked by squatting, kneeling, or arising from chairs. On closer questioning, there is frequently an identifiable activity in which the patient participates, or may have participated, that may have contributed to precipitating the symptoms. Exercise programs that include leg presses, full arc knee extensions, squatting, or high-impact loading (such as running or jogging) may generate extremely high patellofemoral joint reaction forces and can often precipitate the syndrome. Other activities such as housework, gardening, and hiking can provoke patellofemoral pain. Although the pain is usually most apparent with activity, patients with patellofemoral arthralgia often experience pain when sitting for prolonged periods with the knee flexed. This symptom, commonly noted when driving a car or sitting in a movie theatre, is referred to as a positive "movie sign" or a positive "theatre sign." Crepitus, nonmechanical locking, and sensations of giving way are common. True mechanical locking is rare.

On palpation, there is often tenderness over the articular surface of the patella. The medial and lateral aspects of the patellar articular surfaces, referred to as the medial and lateral facets, respectively, may be examined by manually subluxing the patella medially or laterally and palpating under the edges of the patellar facets. The knee must be fully extended and the quadriceps must be fully relaxed in order to allow the patella to be subluxed sufficiently to palpate its articular aspect. Tenderness associated with patellofemoral arthralgia is frequently noted over the medial patellar facet and often in the soft tissues adjacent to the patella. In patients with patellar tracking problems, the patellar apprehension sign, in which the examiner attempts to subluxate the patella laterally with the knee slightly flexed, often provokes the quadriceps to contract in response to a sensation of impending pain or patellar dislocation. Patients with increased generalized laxity, joint hypermobility, and relative dysplasia of the vastus medialis portion of the quadriceps musculature may be at increased risk for patellofemoral arthralgia, although these are not essential findings for the diagnosis. Similarly, abnormalities of lower extremity alignment including genu valgus, internal femoral torsion, and external tibial torsion may increase the likelihood of developing the syndrome, although these findings are not universal. Excessive tightness or contracture of the peripatellar retinaculum is noted in some cases, determined by measuring the amount of mediolateral patellar excursion possible in the fully extended knee with the quadriceps muscles relaxed. Normally, there should be at least 2 cm of side-to-side passive patellar movement. Excessive retinacular tightness may produce pain in the peripatellar tissues and potentially further increase patellofemoral pain by increasing joint pressures. The anterior knee pain syndrome is generally not associated with swelling, fevers or chills, erythema, instability, loss of motion, sensory changes, or muscle weakness.

B. LABORATORY FINDINGS

No laboratory studies are generally indicated for the syndrome of anterior knee pain. In cases presenting with an effusion, or if there is significant prepatellar bursal swelling, aspiration may be considered. Fluid obtained at aspiration should be examined for crystals if gout or pseudogout is suspected. Blood tests are rarely helpful in this setting.

C. IMAGING STUDIES

When the history and physical findings strongly support the diagnosis of anterior knee pain, radiographic assessment may be deferred. In such cases, a therapeutic trial of activity modification, avoidance of patellar loading activities (stairs, squatting, running), a home exercise program, analgesics, and nonsteroidal anti-inflammatory medications (unless contraindicated) may be initiated. The response of symptoms to such a trial may be useful from a diagnostic perspective. If symptoms continue, formal physical therapy may be prescribed for isometric quadriceps sets; straight leg raising; short arc extensions; and stretching of the hamstrings, quadriceps, and calf muscles. Retinacular stretching and passive patellar mobilization should be prescribed when retinacular tightness has been noted.

Radiographs should be obtained when symptoms have persisted for 6 weeks despite the above measures. In addition to routine anteroposterior and lateral radiographs of the knee, patellar sunrise or Merchant views, which specifically demonstrate the axial representation of the patellofemoral articulation, should be obtained. The sunrise or Merchant views often demonstrate degenerative arthritic changes involving the patellofemoral articulation better than anteroposterior and lateral views, and may also demonstrate patellar subluxation or tilt with respect to the femoral trochlea. The length of the patellar ligament, as measured from the distal pole of the patella to its insertion on the tibial tubercle, and the length of the patella should be approximately equal (± 20%). If the length of the patellar ligament exceeds the patellar length by more than 20%, patella alta is present, a condition that is also frequently seen in association with patellar tracking abnormalities. Patella baja, defined as the condition when the length of the patellar ligament is less than 80% of the length of the patella, may indicate fibrosis and contracture of the infrapatellar tissues following injury or surgery and may be associated with anterior knee pain. Magnetic resonance imaging (MRI) is rarely indicated in the initial evaluation of anterior knee pain.

Differential Diagnosis

The differential diagnosis of anterior knee pain includes patellofemoral arthralgia, osteoarthritis, patellar tendinitis, quadriceps tendinitis, prepatellar bursitis, synovial plica, Osgood-Schlatter disease, Sinding-Larsen-Johansson disease, internal derangement of the knee, and saphenous nerve entrapment (Table 12–4). Radiographs, particularly the patellar sunrise view, provide the best means of differentiating between osteoarthritis and anterior knee pain without arthritis. Precise anatomic localization of the pain and tenderness usually enables the examiner to differentiate patellofemoral arthralgia from tendinitis of the quadriceps or patellar ligaments. The tenderness in patellofemoral arthralgia is usually most pronounced in the area of the medial patellar facet, whereas the most common site of tenderness due to quadriceps or patellar tendinitis is at the tendon-bone insertion. Osgood-Schlatter disease also presents with pain and tenderness, usually accompanied by swelling at the tibial tubercle in an adolescent. Prominence of the tibial tubercle and bony ossicles adjacent to the tubercle are frequently seen on radiographs in Osgood-Schlatter disease. In Sinding-Larsen-Johansson disease, similar pain, tenderness, and radiographic changes are localized to the distal pole of the patella. Prepatellar swelling, present in cases of

Table 12–4. Differential diagnosis of anterior knee pain.

Patellofemoral arthralgia
Osteoarthritis
Patellar tendinitis
Quadriceps tendinitis
Prepatellar bursitis
Synovial plica
Osgood-Schlatter disease
Sinding-Larsen-Johansson disease
Internal derangement of the knee
Saphenous nerve entrapment (Hunter's canal syndrome)

---

prepatellar bursitis, is absent in patellofemoral arthralgia. Plica syndrome, often associated with a history of repetitive overuse or minor direct trauma to the anteromedial aspect of the knee, is characterized by pain and tenderness localized specifically to a palpable fold or thickening of the synovium over the edge of the medial femoral condyle, adjacent to the patella. The patient may also note a snapping sensation in this area. Internal derangement of the knee may mimic anterior knee pain and should be considered in cases refractory to initial treatment. The clinical assessment of internal derangement of the knee is discussed later in this chapter.

Another uncommon condition, which may also present with pain localized to the anteromedial aspect of the knee, results from compression or irritation of the saphenous nerve in the region of Hunter's adductor canal in the medial aspect of the distal thigh. The symptoms may mimic the pain of patellofemoral arthralgia, although the tenderness in this condition usually extends well proximal to the knee joint to the area of Hunter's canal in the thigh and often extends distally along the course of the saphenous nerve medially in the calf.

Fulkerson JP, Shea KP. Disorders of patellofemoral alignment. *J Bone Joint Surg Am.* 1990;72:1424. [PMID: 2229126] (Comprehensive discussion of chondromalacia patellae, anterior knee pain, and patellar alignment.)

Jacobson KE, Flandry FC. Diagnosis of anterior knee pain. *Clin Sports Med.* 1989;8:179. [PMID: 2665950] (Presents a systematic approach to the clinical evaluation and differential diagnosis of anterior knee pain.)

Patel D. Plica as a cause of anterior knee pain. *Orthop Clin North Am.* 1986;17:273. [PMID: 3714211] (Review of the anatomy and clinical presentation of symptomatic synovial plicae.)

BURSITIS OR TENDINITIS

 ESSENTIAL FEATURES

- *The most helpful diagnostic information is the precise localization of the pain and tenderness.*
- *Laboratory and imaging studies are generally not indicated in the initial evaluation.*

Clinical Findings

A. SYMPTOMS AND SIGNS

Pain due to bursitis or tendinitis about the knee is usually related to activity, although the onset is generally spontaneous and atraumatic. Symptoms improve with rest. Physical findings include localized extra-articular swelling and point tenderness, directly related to the anatomic location of a bursa or tendon. Common sites for bursitis are the bursa of the pes anserine, located between the anteromedial tibial metaphysis and the tendons of the pes anserine near their insertion, and the prepatellar bursa, located subcutaneously directly anterior to the patella. Frequent sites for tendinitis include the quadriceps tendon at or near its insertion on the proximal patellar pole, the patellar ligament at its origin on the distal pole of the patella, and the iliotibial band in the area of the lateral femoral epicondyle. Since these structures are extra-articular, there is no joint effusion and swelling is localized to the involved bursa or tendon. Range of motion is not restricted except for guarding due to the pain itself. Instability, locking, and other mechanical symptoms are not present.

Infection may occasionally present in the setting of bursitis. A history of fevers, extreme pain and tenderness localized to the bursa, and local erythema should alert the examiner to the possibility of septic bursitis.

B. Laboratory Findings

Routine laboratory studies are not indicated except in the rare setting in which septic bursitis may be suspected. In such cases, the bursa should be aspirated and the fluid analyzed using Gram stain and cultures. The fluid should be tested for crystals and cell count.

C. Imaging Studies

Radiographs are of little value in the evaluation of a patient with bursitis or tendinitis. However, since the pain and tenderness are extra-articular and often overlying the bony structures, anteroposterior, lateral, and sunrise view radiographs may be indicated in selected cases to exclude the possibility of stress fracture, tumor, or other osseous conditions that may produce pain in the same area.

Differential Diagnosis

The differential diagnosis of bursitis or tendinitis about the knee includes the syndrome of anterior knee pain or patellofemoral arthralgia, meniscal disease, and osteoarthritis (Table 12–5). Precise clinical localization of

Table 12–5. Differential diagnosis of bursitis or tendinitis.

Anterior knee pain syndrome
Meniscal pathology
Osteoarthritis
Occult bony pathology (stress fracture, osteonecrosis, tumor)
Soft tissue lesions (cysts, ganglions)

the pain and tenderness is usually sufficient to determine the most likely diagnosis, and radiographs may help exclude such possibilities as fractures or other bony abnormalities. In refractory cases with normal radiographs, bone scans may help exclude other occult bony pathology such as stress fractures, osteonecrosis, or neoplasms. Similarly, MRI may identify soft tissue lesions such as cysts, ganglions, and tumors. Bursitis may also be confirmed by a diagnostic injection of local anesthetic into the bursa.

INTERNAL DERANGEMENT OF THE KNEE

 ESSENTIAL FEATURES

- *Symptoms and physical findings of internal derangement of the knee are primarily mechanical.*
- *Radiographs and MRI are the most helpful diagnostic tools.*

Clinical Findings

A. Symptoms and Signs

Internal derangement of the knee refers to a group of disorders involving the intra-articular structures of the knee joint. Symptoms of locking, snapping, or popping suggest an internal derangement of the knee. The onset of symptoms is often sudden and may be associated with a specific provocative event or injury. The symptoms are generally intermittent, mechanical in nature, and associated with and exacerbated by activity. They improve with rest. Crepitus is frequently present but may be intermittent. The patient should be asked specifically about a history of prior knee injuries or episodes. Prior injuries, often temporally remote and sometimes seemingly trivial or even forgotten by the patient, may provide clues to the diagnosis.

On physical examination, there is often an effusion, which may fluctuate in size, swelling localized to the joint line, mechanical restriction of motion, and joint line tenderness. Palpation about the knee, including the suprapatellar, medial, and lateral synovial recesses, may reveal evidence of an intra-articular loose body, a fragment of bone or cartilage (also commonly referred to as a "joint mouse") that may move freely about the knee resulting in intermittent pain, popping, and locking. When extension is restricted by an apparent mechanical obstruction, gentle passive pressure may be applied to attempt to obtain further extension. If such pressure produces pain and the knee returns to its previously flexed position, this represents a positive "Spring sign," usually indicative of a displaced meniscal tear. Meniscal compression tests may be positive, although the sensitivity and specificity of these tests are limited and the findings must be considered in the context of the remainder of the history and examination.

Collateral and cruciate ligament testing should be performed. Medial and lateral stability should be assessed by varus and valgus stress of the knee at full extension and with the knee flexed 30 degrees. Instability resulting from an injury of the anterior cruciate ligament may be detected by the anterior drawer test, Lachman test, or flexion rotation drawer test. The posterior drawer test is used to assess the integrity of the posterior cruciate ligament. Stability findings should be compared with those of the contralateral knee to assess their significance and to identify those persons in whom generalized laxity conditions may exist. The patellofemoral joint should also be examined for tenderness and possible tracking abnormalities. A positive apprehension test or other abnormal evidence of patellar subluxation may be indicative of patellar instability, which may mimic other disorders of internal knee derangement.

B. Laboratory Findings

Laboratory testing is rarely indicated in the evaluation of suspected internal knee derangement. Aspiration of the knee may be considered in the setting of an acutely painful knee with a significant effusion. Although it is not always necessary to obtain a laboratory analysis of the fluid, the nature of the fluid may be helpful diagnostically. An acute hemarthrosis may suggest a tear of the anterior cruciate ligament, patellar dislocation, or synovial impingement. Hemarthrosis may also occur in patients taking anticoagulation medications or in the setting of other coagulation disorders. A hemarthrosis with associated fat globules may indicate the presence of an intra-articular fracture. Dark brown serosanguinous synovial fluid may suggest the possibility of pigmented villonodular synovitis, a disorder characterized by proliferation of synovium with formation of brown villous and nodular projections. Although uncommon, this disorder may also present as a chronic inflammatory arthritis, most frequently involving the knee joint. A clear or amber effusion with high viscosity, a white blood cell count < 2000/µL, and no crystals suggests a noninflammatory etiology. An inflammatory etiology may be suspected when the fluid is yellow to cloudy, turbid, and of low viscosity, and the white blood cell count exceeds 3000/µL. Crystals, when present, also denote an inflammatory process.

C. Imaging Studies

Radiographs including anteroposterior, lateral, and patellar sunrise or Merchant views (axial views of the patellofemoral articulation) should be obtained when internal derangement of the knee is suspected. Plain films may reveal fractures, arthritic changes, bony loose bodies, and chondrocalcinosis. Additional views such as femoral notch or tunnel views may be necessary to reveal loose bodies, osteochondritis dissecans, or spontaneous osteonecrosis of the femoral condyles. An anteroposterior radiograph angled 15 degrees caudally may reveal an occult fracture of the tibial plateau, and occult fractures of the femoral condyles or tibial plateau may be demonstrated on oblique radiographs obtained in 45-degree internal and 45-degree external rotation. Weight-bearing views may be necessary to demonstrate joint space narrowing due to osteoarthritis. Standing anteroposterior views may be sufficient in many cases, although posteroanterior standing views obtained with the knees flexed 45 degrees may be necessary in those instances in which arthritis is suspected but not demonstrated on routine standing views (Figures 12–4 and 12–5).

Bone scans may reveal occult fractures not seen on plain radiographs, particularly stress fractures or insufficiency fractures associated with osteoporosis. Avascular necrosis and spontaneous osteonecrosis may also present with normal radiographs, yet may be evident on bone scan and MRI. A bone bruise or bone marrow edema, also seen on MRI, may be seen following trauma or in association with osteoarthritis, even in the absence of plain radiographic abnormalities. MRI is also sensitive in detecting meniscal tears and may reveal useful information about the condition of the articular cartilage, ligaments, and other periarticular soft tissue structures. The presence of a Baker cyst on MRI in an adult knee is indicative of intra-articular disease that results in increased production of synovial fluid, which accumulates in the medial aspect of the popliteal fossa, distending the synovium posteriorly through the interval between the medial head of the gastrocnemius and the semimembranosus tendon. Seen frequently in association with degenerative arthritis and posterior medial meniscal tears, the finding of a Baker cyst in an adult should prompt further evaluation for intra-articular disease, if none has previously been apparent.

Differential Diagnosis

Conditions that result in symptoms and physical findings characteristic of internal knee derangement include meniscal pathology, loose bodies, osteochondritis dissecans, ligamentous instability, synovial impingement, arthritis, and bony abnormalities ranging from fracture

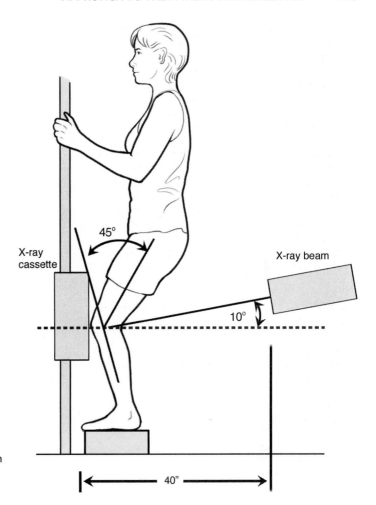

Figure 12–4. Technique for positioning the patient and X-ray equipment to obtain the 45-degree posteroanterior weight-bearing radiograph of the knee.

to osteonecrosis (Table 12–6). Symptomatic meniscal tears may be suspected when there is a history of locking, crepitus, and positive McMurray or Appley meniscal compression tests. The most reliable finding on examination is tenderness localized specifically to the joint line, particularly in the absence of significant radiographic evidence of degenerative arthritis. Although MRI is quite sensitive in the detection of meniscal tears, it should be noted that approximately one-third of asymptomatic individuals over 50 years of age would be found to have a torn meniscus on MRI. Thus, the mere presence of a torn meniscus on MRI in an older person does not necessarily indicate that the symptoms are attributable to the tear, and further clinical correlation is indicated. Congenital or developmental meniscal abnormalities, such as discoid lateral meniscus, may present in a fashion similar to a torn meniscus, although radiographic findings of abnormal widening

and squaring of the lateral compartment joint space should lead to suspicion of a discoid meniscus. MRI is also helpful in firmly establishing the diagnosis.

Loose bodies are often suspected on the basis of the patient's perception of something moving about within the knee, with episodes of mechanical locking, and often a palpable fragment of bone or cartilage on examination. Radiographs may reveal the presence and location of bony loose bodies, although cartilaginous loose bodies will not be evident on radiographs and are often not seen on MRI. Osteochondritis dissecans, which most often occurs during adolescence, may also present in adulthood with mechanical symptoms of pain, crepitus, popping, and locking. The radiographic appearance usually reveals fragmentation, irregularity, or a lucent defect of the articular surface of one of the femoral condyles, most often involving the lateral aspect of the medial femoral condyle. The fragment may partially or

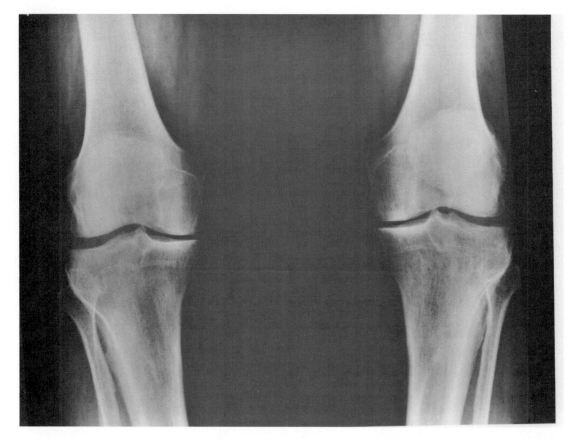

Figure 12–5. **A:** Weight-bearing anteroposterior radiograph reveals sclerosis of the medial compartments of both knees, although the joint space appears to be only mildly narrowed.

completely separate from the condyle, causing symptoms of a loose body. Loose bodies and the condylar lesion seen in osteochondritis dissecans are often better seen radiographically on a tunnel view or femoral notch view than on routine anteroposterior and lateral radiographs.

Ligamentous instability is generally suspected or diagnosed on the basis of the history and physical findings. Laxity on one or more of the tests previously described for the collateral and cruciate ligaments is often sufficient to make the diagnosis. Increased side-to-side motion of the knee may also be seen when performing the collateral ligament examination in patients with osteoarthritis of the medial and/or lateral compartments. This "pseudolaxity" is the result of thinning or absence of articular and meniscal cartilage associated with the arthritic process, in contrast to true laxity resulting from incompetence of the ligament itself. The age of the patient as well as other information from the history and examination, especially a varus or valgus defor-

mity, may help differentiate between laxity or instability due to ligamentous injury and pseudolaxity associated with arthritis. Radiographs will generally reveal the presence of joint space narrowing if pseudolaxity is the result of medial or lateral compartment arthritis. If significant arthritis is suspected and not evident on standing anteroposterior and lateral radiographs, 45-degree flexed standing posteroanterior radiographs (see Figures 12–1 and 12–2) should be obtained to look further for joint space narrowing. MRI may be helpful in documenting the diagnosis of a ligament injury when in doubt and may also reveal associated pathology such as meniscal or osteochondral injuries.

Synovial plicae, intra-articular folds of synovium, and portions of the infrapatellar fat pad may occasionally become pinched or entrapped between the articular surfaces of the patella and femur or between the femur and tibia. Such impingement may cause sharp localized pain, swelling, and popping. In some cases, locking or loss of motion may also be seen. Localization of the area

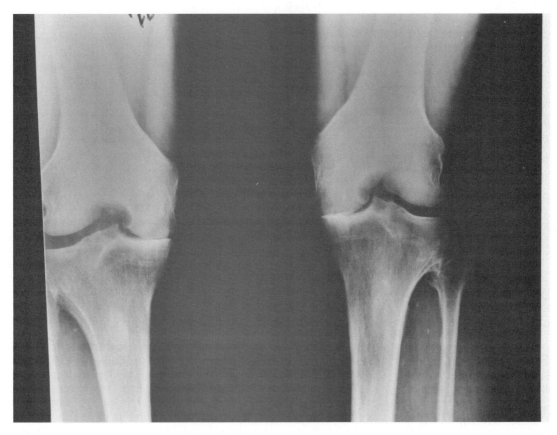

Figure 12–5. (***Continued***) **B:** The 45-degree posteroanterior radiograph of the same patient reveals complete loss of joint space in the medial compartments of both knees. Osteophytes of the tibial spines and intercondylar notch of the femur are also more apparent on the 45-degree flexion posteroanterior view.

of tenderness can help distinguish this entity from meniscal pathology, and in some cases, the plica or fold of tender synovium may be palpable. Synovial nodules associated with pigmented villonodular synovitis may also produce similar mechanical symptoms. Aspiration of the characteristically dark brown serosanguinous fluid associated with pigmented villonodular synovitis

Table 12–6. Differential diagnosis of internal derangement of the knee.

Meniscal pathology
Loose bodies
Osteochondritis dissecans
Ligamentous instability
Synovial conditions (plica, impingement, pigmented
 villonodular synovitis)
Arthritis
Bony abnormalities (fracture, osteonecrosis)

---

is helpful in the diagnosis. Radiographic studies, although not usually helpful with other disorders of synovial plicae or impingement, may reveal juxta-articular subchondral erosions involving both sides of the joint in pigmented villonodular synovitis, with preservation of the articular cartilage. MRI may also reveal hemosiderin deposition, with low signal intensity, in the synovium of pigmented villonodular synovitis.

Arthritis may be associated with several other intra-articular abnormalities such as meniscal tears, loose bodies, synovial impingement, and ligamentous laxity or pseudolaxity that may produce symptoms of internal derangement of the knee. In some cases, the arthritis may otherwise be relatively asymptomatic, although its presence may greatly influence the choice of treatment. The possibility that arthritis may be presenting with symptoms of internal knee derangement should be considered in older persons, patients with a past history of meniscectomy or long-standing instability, patients with significant obesity, and patients with a family history of arthritis. (See the following sections on osteoarthritis and inflammatory arthritis for discussion of clinical features.)

Fowler PJ, Lubliner JA. The predictive value of five clinical signs in the evaluation of meniscal pathology. *Arthroscopy.* 1989;5: 184. [PMID: 2775390] (Compares the relative accuracy of various clinical examination findings in diagnosing a torn meniscus.)

Hughston JC, et al. Osteochondritis dissecans of the femoral condyles. *J Bone Joint Surg Am.* 1984;66:1340. [PMID: 6501330] (Review of the etiology, clinical findings, and management of osteochondritis dissecans.)

OSTEOARTHRITIS OF THE KNEE

 ESSENTIAL FEATURES

- *Pain due to osteoarthritis of the knee is generally increased with activity and improved with rest.*
- *Weight-bearing radiographs are the most useful diagnostic study.*

Clinical Findings

A. SYMPTOMS AND SIGNS

Patients who seek medical attention for pain due to osteoarthritis of the knee often describe long-standing pain that began insidiously and worsened gradually. Symptoms are generally chronic, as opposed to episodic, and are exacerbated by activity and weight bearing, particularly during stair climbing and when arising from a seated position. Although pain is usually improved at rest, it may sometimes persist after activity and may also be influenced by weather changes. Mechanical symptoms such as locking and popping may occur due to coexistent meniscal pathology or loose bodies, although such symptoms are otherwise not commonly associated with the arthritis alone. Physical findings frequently include crepitus, deformity, fixed contractures, and decreased range of motion. When present, tenderness is usually greatest over the joint lines but may also be noted over osteophytes and occasionally over the juxta-articular aspect of the tibial metaphysis and/or the femoral condyles. Periarticular osteophytes may be palpable. An effusion and slight increase in warmth about the knee may also be seen intermittently in osteoarthritis due to the inflammatory response of the synovium to the products of cartilage degradation. Localized swelling, erythema, fevers, and chills are not characteristic of osteoarthritis, however.

B. LABORATORY FINDINGS

Routine laboratory studies are rarely necessary in the initial evaluation of suspected osteoarthritis. However, if inflammatory arthritis is suspected, arthrocentesis should be performed and the synovial fluid analyzed for cell count and crystals. See Chapter 4 for a discussion of laboratory studies in osteoarthritis.

C. IMAGING STUDIES

The most useful imaging studies in the evaluation of a patient with suspected osteoarthritis of the knee are plain radiographs, specifically anteroposterior weight-bearing, lateral, and patellar sunrise views of the knee. Early radiographic features of osteoarthritis include spurring of the tibial spines and squaring of the edges of the femorotibial compartments. Irregularity of the articular surfaces, marginal osteophytes, and subchondral cyst formation may be seen later. Joint space narrowing reflects the loss of articular cartilage, which may be underestimated on non-weight-bearing films. Standing anteroposterior films may also fail to demonstrate joint space narrowing in some cases, and the lateral view should be closely scrutinized to assess the distance between the medial and lateral femoral condyles and their respective tibial articulations. In addition, weight-bearing posteroanterior radiographs taken with the patient standing with both knees flexed 45 degrees (see Figures 12–4, 12–5, and 12–6) may reveal significant narrowing of the femorotibial compartments not seen on the previous views. In addition, as this view also resembles a femoral tunnel or notch view, the 45-degree flexed standing view may also reveal loose bodies, osteochondritis dissecans lesions of the femoral condyle, and femoral notch osteophytes better than routine anteroposterior and lateral views. Patellofemoral arthritis may be evident on the lateral radiograph, although the severity of joint space narrowing and presence of subluxation are usually better visualized on patellar sunrise views.

MRI is rarely necessary in the initial assessment of suspected osteoarthritis of the knee, particularly in advanced disease. In early arthritis, MRI may demonstrate coexistent meniscal pathology, which may sometimes produce symptoms of internal derangement. It must be remembered, however, that asymptomatic meniscus tears are frequently seen on an MRI of persons over age 50. The finding of a torn or degenerative meniscus on MRI in an older individual must be correlated with the history and physical findings before attributing the symptoms to the meniscal pathology. Similarly, effusions and cruciate ligament abnormalities are often seen on MRI in older individuals in the absence of symptoms. The presence of a Baker cyst on MRI in an adult is highly suggestive of intra-articular disease, usually degenerative arthritis, meniscal pathology, or synovitis.

Table 12–7. Differential diagnosis of osteoarthritis of the knee.

Inflammatory arthritis
Osteonecrosis
Internal derangement
Anterior knee pain syndrome

Bone marrow edema seen on MRI may correlate with the pain of arthritis, although the pathophysiology of this process is not yet known.

Differential Diagnosis

The differential diagnosis of osteoarthritis of the knee includes inflammatory arthritis, osteonecrosis, and internal derangement of the knee (Table 12–7). The syndrome of anterior knee pain may also mimic the clinical presentation of patellofemoral arthritis. Clinically, the pain in osteoarthritis is exacerbated by activity and relieved at rest, whereas inflammatory arthritis is associated with stiffness after rest, which improves with activity. Synovial fluid analysis and the distinguishing radiographic features of both conditions are discussed elsewhere in this chapter and in Chapter 4. Anterior knee pain from other sources may be distinguished from patellofemoral arthritis on the basis of the presence or absence of patellar osteophytes, sclerosis, articular irregularity, subchondral cysts, and joint space narrowing, usually seen best on patellar sunrise views.

Rosenberg TD, et al. The forty-five degree posteroanterior weight-bearing radiograph of the knee. *J Bone Joint Surg Am.* 1988; 70:1479. [PMID: 3198672] (Describes a supplementary radiographic technique that is more sensitive in detecting osteoarthritic changes in some patients.)

Lotke PA, Ecker ML. Osteonecrosis of the knee. *J Bone Joint Surg Am.* 1988;70:470. [PMID: 3279040] (Discusses the presentation, evaluation, etiology, and treatment of osteonecrosis of the knee.)

INFLAMMATORY ARTHRITIS OF THE KNEE

 ESSENTIAL FEATURES

- *Prompt recognition and treatment of septic arthritis are essential.*
- *Synovial fluid analysis is the most helpful test.*

Clinical Findings

A. SYMPTOMS AND SIGNS

The pain due to inflammatory arthritis of the knee is frequently associated with stiffness after rest and improvement after activity. Patients may also experience similar problems in other joints as well as fevers, chills, or other systemic symptoms. Mechanical symptoms such as locking or popping are uncommon. Physical findings include presence of an effusion, synovial thickening, warmth, and decreased range of motion. Tenderness is diffuse rather than localized.

B. LABORATORY FINDINGS

Joint aspiration and synovial fluid analysis provide the most helpful diagnostic information in the assessment of suspected inflammatory arthritis of the knee. Synovial fluid that is yellow or cloudy, turbid, with low viscosity, and in which the white blood cell count is > 3000/μL is consistent with inflammatory arthritis. Crystals may also be present in association with gout or pseudogout. Gram stain and cultures of the synovial fluid should be obtained in the setting of presumed inflammatory arthritis to exclude the possibility of septic arthritis. Blood studies including complete blood cell count, erythrocyte sedimentation rate, and serum uric acid level may also be helpful. Further information outlining the laboratory findings associated with inflammatory arthritis can be found in Chapter 4.

C. IMAGING STUDIES

Radiographic findings in early inflammatory arthritis are usually normal. Diffuse, symmetric joint space narrowing, juxta-articular osteopenia, and periarticular erosions may be seen within weeks of the onset of acute inflammatory arthritis. Radiographs may also be helpful in distinguishing inflammatory arthritis from osteoarthritis, osteonecrosis, and neuropathic arthritis. Although no radiographic abnormalities may be evident in early osteonecrosis, a radiolucent lesion and flattening of the femoral condyle may be seen later. In addition, bone scans reveal intense uptake in the femoral condyle in osteonecrosis. MRI in osteonecrosis may be extremely helpful, with T2-weighted images demonstrating a low-signal area in the central portion of the lesion in the femoral condyle, surrounded by high-intensity signal around the periphery, most likely due to edema. MRI may also help determine the size of the lesion, which determines treatment and prognosis. However, MRI changes may not be seen early in the course of osteonecrosis and may persist long after clinical symptoms have resolved.

Differential Diagnosis

The differential diagnosis of inflammatory arthritis includes septic arthritis, crystal-induced arthritis, osteoarthritis, osteonecrosis, neuropathic arthropathy, and pigmented villonodular synovitis (Table 12–8). Analysis of the synovial fluid is key to establishing the diagnosis. The clinical presentation of fever and elevated peripheral white blood cell count is suggestive of infection but may also occur in crystalline arthropathy. Conversely, some cases of septic arthritis may present without fever and with a normal peripheral white blood cell count. See Chapter 4 for additional information about synovial fluid analysis and peripheral blood studies in inflammatory arthritis.

Osteonecrosis involving the distal femur may present suddenly and is often associated with an effusion. This condition may be distinguished from an acute inflammatory arthritis by tenderness localizing to the bone rather than diffuse synovial tenderness. Radiographs, nuclear bone scans, and MRI may also confirm the diagnosis of osteonecrosis.

The presentation of neuropathic arthropathy or Charcot joint may resemble that of an inflammatory arthritis, with a severe effusion, diffuse tenderness, and warmth. Once again, however, the synovial fluid in this process is characteristically noninflammatory and the radiographic features of neuropathic arthropathy are quite diagnostic, with severe joint destruction and shards of fragmented bone.

Pigmented villonodular synovitis may also present as an inflammatory arthritis. Although this disorder is relatively uncommon, the knee is more frequently involved than other joints. Aspiration of dark brown serosanguinous synovial fluid should raise suspicion of this disease. Juxta-articular subchondral erosions involving both sides of the joint may be seen on radiographs. Articular cartilage is preserved, despite extensive marginal erosions. MRI may also be helpful, revealing hemosiderin deposition in the synovium with characteristic low signal.

Lee YU, Sartoris DJ. Imaging of the knee. *Curr Opin Orthop.* 1995;6:56. (Thorough review of the applications of imaging modalities including conventional radiography, arthrography, radionuclide imaging, computed tomography, ultrasound, and MRI to the knee.)

WHEN TO REFER TO A SPECIALIST

Patients with a septic knee should be referred urgently to an orthopedist to evaluate the need for surgical drainage. Patients with fractures or bone tumor should also be referred to an orthopedist.

Patients in whom avascular necrosis of bone or a systemic rheumatic disease such as rheumatoid arthritis is suspected should be referred to a rheumatologist for treatment.

Referral to a specialist is also warranted if the cause of knee pain eludes diagnosis or fails to respond appropriately to initial therapy.

Table 12–8. Differential diagnosis of inflammatory arthritis of the knee.

Septic arthritis
Crystal-induced arthritis
Osteoarthritis
Osteonecrosis
Neuropathic arthropathy
Pigmented villonodular synovitis

The Patient with Diffuse Pain

13

John B. Winfield, MD

ESSENTIALS OF DIAGNOSIS

- *Consider fibromyalgia when a patient complains of the following:*
  - *Widespread pain for longer than 3 months*
  - *Fatigue associated with usual daily activities*
  - *Sleep disturbances*
  - *Changes in personality and mood*
  - *Multiple symptoms that cannot be easily explained*
- *Consider alternative explanations to a diagnosis of fibromyalgia. Conversely, if an alternate diagnosis is present, ask: "Which symptoms are due to concomitant fibromyalgia?" Specifically, assess the following:*
  - *Onset, location, and nature of pain, together with ameliorating and exacerbating factors*
  - *Sleep quality*
  - *Current and past stressors*
  - *Adverse experiences during childhood, such as physical, emotional, or sexual abuse*
  - *How the patient deals with the usual stresses of daily life, feelings of anxiety, and feelings of depression*
  - *Presence of regional pain syndromes, such as temporomandibular joint pain, irritable bowel syndrome, and chronic pelvic pain. These disorders overlap with fibromyalgia and very frequently coexist in the same patient.*
- *Physical and neurologic examinations will be normal unless there are coexisting diagnoses.*

General Considerations

Chronic pain and fatigue are extremely prevalent in the general population, especially among women and persons of lower socioeconomic status: regional pain, 20%; widespread pain, 11%; fibromyalgia by American College of Rheumatology (ACR) criteria, 3–5% in females

and 0.5–1.6% in males; and chronic fatigue, ~ 20%. Fibromyalgia may develop in both children and older persons. Although there is debate about whether fibromyalgia is a discrete illness or simply the extreme end of a spectrum of pain and distress in the general population, abnormal central nociceptive processing appears to be the basis for a generalized decrease in thresholds for pain perception and pain tolerance.

The 1990 ACR classification criteria for fibromyalgia specify that widespread pain be present for longer than 3 months and that pain can be elicited by manual pressure at 11 or more defined tender points (Figure 13–1). Not all patients have tenderness at all 11 points. Fibromyalgia frequently coexists with systemic lupus erythematosus, rheumatoid arthritis, and other systemic disorders. In addition, fibromyalgia overlaps with chronic fatigue syndrome, irritable bowel syndrome, and multiple other regional pain syndromes. Associated psychiatric conditions, especially depression, anxiety, and personality disorders, are prevalent.

In assessing patients with fibromyalgia, a detailed social and behavioral history, identification of current and past stressors, and recognition of depression are essential. The physician should validate the patient's complaints. Therapy combines pharmacologic treatment of pain, depression, and sleep disturbances with nonpharmacologic approaches, including education, graded aerobic exercise, and promotion of self-efficacy for control of pain through self-management, rather than health care–seeking behavior. The therapeutic goal is *care* not *cure*.

Pathogenesis

The precise etiology and pathogenesis of pain in fibromyalgia is currently unknown. Nevertheless, a clinically useful conceptual basis for understanding the nature of pain is provided by the International Association for the Study of Pain definition: Pain is "an unpleasant sensory and emotional experience associated with actual or potential tissue damage, or described in terms of such damage." The pain *experience* involves simultaneous parallel processing of sensory-discriminative elements of nociception (twisting your ankle), afferent input from somatic reflexes (sweating, heart rate acceleration), and major contributions from pathways and regions of the brain concerned with cognitive (Is

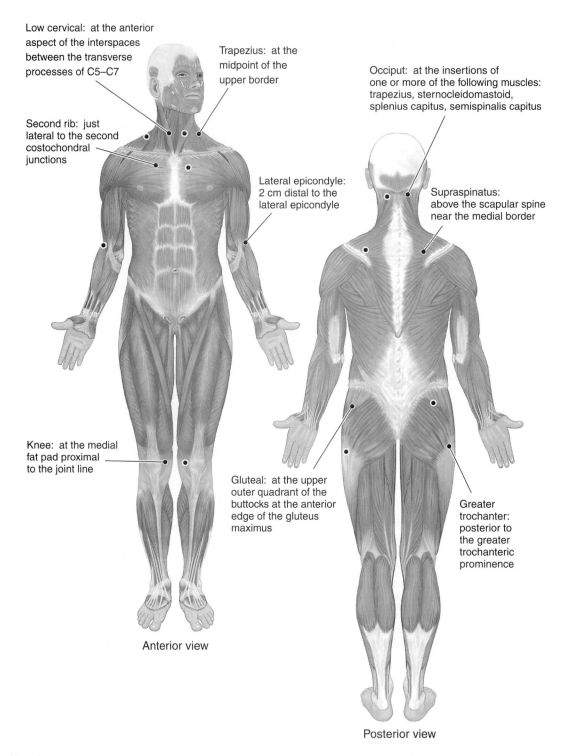

Low cervical: at the anterior aspect of the interspaces between the transverse processes of C5–C7

Trapezius: at the midpoint of the upper border

Occiput: at the insertions of one or more of the following muscles: trapezius, sternocleidomastoid, splenius capitus, semispinalis capitus

Second rib: just lateral to the second costochondral junctions

Lateral epicondyle: 2 cm distal to the lateral epicondyle

Supraspinatus: above the scapular spine near the medial border

Knee: at the medial fat pad proximal to the joint line

Gluteal: at the upper outer quadrant of the buttocks at the anterior edge of the gluteus maximus

Greater trochanter: posterior to the greater trochanteric prominence

Anterior view

Posterior view

Figure 13–1. Eighteen tender points used in the American College of Rheumatology classification criteria for fibromyalgia.

my ankle broken?) and emotional aspects of pain. Collectively, these determine the subjective intensity of pain. Negative psychological factors (depression and anxiety, loss of control, unpredictability in one's environment) and certain cognitive aspects (negative beliefs and attributions, catastrophizing) amplify perceived pain. The principal effectors of the stress response system (hypothalamic-pituitary-adrenocortical axis and the sympathetic nervous system) become activated in pain states, as well. Normally adaptive, the stress response may become maladaptive in chronic pain syndromes, thereby contributing to diffuse aching pain, fatigue, poor sleep, low mood and anxiety, and "flu-like" illness.

Psychological variables clearly operative in fibromyalgia include pain beliefs and attributions; hypervigilance (expectancy); active and passive coping strategies; perceived self-efficacy for pain control; mood, depression, and anxiety; personality traits and disorders; and pain behaviors. Certain environmental and sociocultural variables also contribute to chronic diffuse pain, such as a history of poor health in parents; parental pain history; poor family environment; and childhood abuse, particularly sexual abuse. Other environmental and sociocultural variables that can serve to perpetuate symptoms in fibromyalgia include lack of spousal and family support, poor work environment and job dissatisfaction, focus on definable causes, media hype, primary and secondary gain, diagnostic "waffling" and inappropriate diagnostic testing, and prescription of long courses of physical therapy by well-meaning physicians.

Clinical Findings

A. SYMPTOMS AND SIGNS

The hallmark of fibromyalgia is widespread pain (above and below the waist, both sides of the body) for longer than 3 months. Pain is described as "exhausting," "miserable," or "unbearable" and diffusely radiates from the axial skeleton over large areas of the body, primarily in muscles. Arthralgias may be present together with a subjective sense of joint swelling, which is not confirmed by physical examination unless another coexisting rheumatic disease is present. Morning stiffness may be prominent. The patient may complain that a light touch by the spouse or even a breeze is unpleasant (allodynia, defined as pain with stimulation that should not be painful). The skin may "burn." Nondermatomal paresthesiaes are common.

Regional pain syndromes, such as headache, temporomandibular joint pain, irritable bowel syndrome, and chronic pelvic pain overlap with fibromyalgia and very frequently coexist in the same patient. Indeed, the diagnostic label applied often is determined by which specialist the patient sees first.

Marked fatigue with usual activities is almost universal and may dominate the clinical picture. As with diffuse pain, physical and laboratory examinations fail to define abnormal findings other than deconditioning. Associated symptoms are subjective muscle weakness not confirmed by loss of muscle power or elevated creatinine kinase levels, hypersomnolence during the day, and exhaustion after mild exercise. Pain and fatigue may be intermittent, with "good days and bad days." On good days, the patient may overexert herself or himself, for example, with an exercise routine, with consequent flare in pain and fatigue. Exercise often is feared and avoided.

Poor sleep almost always is present, and the patient awakens unrefreshed. Specific sleep abnormalities may be demonstrable, particularly α-wave intrusion into slow δ-wave non-REM sleep, restless legs syndrome, and sleep apnea. Formal sleep testing should be sought in patients whose sleep does not improve with hypnotics and proper sleep hygiene.

Current and past stressors and adverse experiences should be explored. Persons with fibromyalgia often carry a huge psychological burden of stress and distress that may precede chronic pain.

Patients often report difficulty dealing with the usual stresses of daily life, feelings of anxiety, and feelings of depression. A majority of patients have current or lifetime depression. Recognition of mood disorders, anxiety, and insomnia is the essential first step in developing approaches for improving chronic pain and fatigue.

Reporting of multiple symptoms that cannot be explained ("diffusely positive" review of systems) is very common. Many patients meet the criteria established in the fourth edition of the *Diagnostic and Statistical Manual for Mental Disorders* for somatoform disorder (Figure 13–2). When physical and neurologic examinations are normal, it is important that the physician not pursue unnecessary diagnostic laboratory or imaging evaluations for each symptom. Conversely, it should be recognized that fibromyalgia and somatiform disorders are extremely common in primary care, and therefore frequently coexist with other significant illnesses. Optimum care requires recognition and treatment of both fibromyalgia and any comorbid illnesses present.

Cognitive impairment ("fibro-fog") manifests as difficulty finding the right word, decreased short-term memory, forgetting names, or difficulty concentrating and is extremely common. In some cases, this is exacerbated by central effects of psychotropic medications.

Many patients exhibit functional impairment in multiple activities of daily living, such as performing household chores, shopping, or working an 8-hour day.

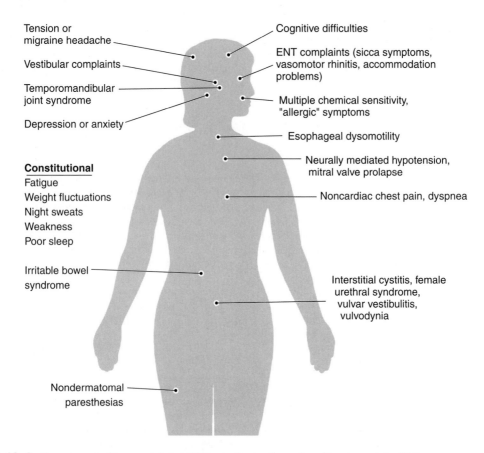

Tension or migraine headache

Vestibular complaints

Temporomandibular joint syndrome

Depression or anxiety

Cognitive difficulties

ENT complaints (sicca symptoms, vasomotor rhinitis, accommodation problems)

Multiple chemical sensitivity, "allergic" symptoms

Esophageal dysomotility

Neurally mediated hypotension, mitral valve prolapse

Noncardiac chest pain, dyspnea

Constitutional
Fatigue
Weight fluctuations
Night sweats
Weakness
Poor sleep

Irritable bowel syndrome

Interstitial cystitis, female urethral syndrome, vulvar vestibulitis, vulvodynia

Nondermatomal paresthesias

Figure 13–2. Symptoms in fibromyalgia in addition to "pain all over" and tender points. ENT, ear, nose, and throat.

Patients with fibromyalgia suffer frustration with respect to their perceived poor states of health and the apparent inability of the medical profession to help them.

Patients with fibromyalgia often have fixed beliefs that minor traumatic events, viruses (Epstein-Barr), chemical sensitivities ("sick building syndrome"), or other physical agents (silicone breast implants, "black mold") caused their illness. Such false beliefs not infrequently lead to litigation and can be a barrier to recovery.

The physician should be aware of pending litigation regarding causation of fibromyalgia, disability determination, or worker's compensation claims because therapy will be fruitless until such issues are resolved.

B. LABORATORY FINDINGS

There are no characteristic laboratory findings in fibromyalgia. The results of routine testing are normal unless a coexisting or alternative diagnosis is present. Additional laboratory tests are unnecessary unless there is a specific indication from the history and physical examination. Antinuclear antibodies, complete blood cell count, erythrocyte sedimentation rate, C-reactive protein levels, urine dipstick, thyroid-stimulating hormone levels, creatine kinase, aspartate aminotransferase, and alanine aminotransferase are useful screening tests for autoimmune diseases, hematologic problems, systemic inflammatory states, hypothyroidism, myopathies, and occult liver disease. Illnesses in these categories can present with chronic pain and fatigue.

C. IMAGING STUDIES

Radiographs of the spine or other joints may be indicated to confirm the presence of conditions that serve as "pain generators," such as osteoarthritis or degenerative spondylosis.

D. SPECIAL EXAMINATIONS

A tender point examination should be performed. Manual pressure of ~ 4 kg at the characteristic tender points shown in Figure 13–1 elicits pain, often accompanied by pain behaviors, such as withdrawal, grimacing, or groaning.

Differential Diagnosis

The diagnoses listed in Table 13–1 should be considered. Objective signs on physical or neurologic examinations should be present before the clinician embarks on extensive diagnostic evaluations.

Treatment

Much of the current treatment of fibromyalgia is empiric, based on proposed rather than on established models of pathophysiology. Pain, poor sleep, low mood and depression, anxiety, and fatigue usually are amenable to pharmacologic therapy, but the treatment plan should be multifaceted, incorporating pharmacologic, physical, psychological, and behavioral approaches. The goal is palliation of symptoms, not cure.

Table 13–1. Differential diagnosis of fibromyalgia.

Rheumatologic disorder	SLE,[a] rheumatoid arthritis, Sjögren syndrome[a]
	Polyarticular osteoarthritis, degenerative spondylosis
	Polymyalgia rheumatica[a]
	Polymyositis, statin myopathy
	Regional pain syndromes[a]
	Osteomalacia
	Hypermobiltiy syndromes
Neurologic disorder	Carpal tunnel syndrome[a]
	Cervical radiculopathy[a]
	Metabolic myopathies
	Multiple sclerosis[a]
	Cervical cord compression
Chronic infection	SBE, brucellosis, hepatitis C, HIV, for example
Endocrine disorder	Hypothyroidism[a]
	Non-IDDM
	Hyperparathyroidism
Neoplastic disorder	Myeloma; metastatic breast, lung, and prostate cancer
Psychiatric disorder	

[a]Diagnoses commonly encountered.
SLE, systemic lupus erythematosus; SBE, subacute bacterial endocarditis; Non-IDDM, non-insulin-dependent diabetes mellitus.

Special approaches are required for treatment of diffuse pain in older persons and in children. Most common in preadolescent to adolescent girls, unexplained diffuse or localized pain is associated with incongruent affect disproportional dysfunction. Psychological distress in the child or the family is common. Elements of therapy include discontinuation of all medications, a psychological evaluation and psychotherapy if necessary, and a program of intense exercise. Most children do well.

A. PHARMACOLOGIC

"Peripheral pain generators," such as osteoarthritis, inflammatory arthritis, neuropathic pain, herniated discs, and spinal stenosis, should be identified and treated using nonsteroidal anti-inflammatory drugs (NSAIDs) and analgesics. Such medications are effective in peripheral nociceptive pain but are less useful in the central pain of complex etiology in fibromyalgia. Their use should be based on a stepwise approach using nonopioid and opioid analgesics either singly or in combination, as determined by pain intensity: acetaminophen, 325–650 mg every 4–6 hours or 1000 mg 3 or 4 times daily, not to exceed 4 g/d; NSAIDs (newer cyclooxygenase-2 [COX-2] inhibitors in older patients and in those with risk factors for peptic ulcer disease); tramadol, 50–100 mg every 4 hours; or opioids. Depending on the specific musculoskeletal disorder, various combinations of glucocorticoid injections, activity modification, splints, counterforce bracing, local heat or cold, and in some cases surgical procedures may also be indicated for "pain generators."

For treatment of the chronic pain of complex etiology in fibromyalgia, use a multifaceted therapeutic approach incorporating various adjuvant medicines, graded aerobic exercise, and psychological and behavioral approaches to reduce distress and promote self-efficacy and self-management. First-line agents are a tricyclic antidepressant (eg, 10–50 mg of amitriptyline at bedtime) in combination with a selective serotonin reuptake inhibitor (eg, 10–40 of fluoxetine every morning) and a centrally acting muscle relaxant (eg, 20–40 mg/d of oral cyclobenzaprine divided 2 to 4 times daily not to exceed 60 mg/d).

If there is marked allodynia and hyperalgesia, addition of an antiepileptic drug is indicated, both for the pain sensitivity and as adjunctive medications for disturbed sleep and depression: gabapentin, escalating from 300 mg at bedtime to 600 mg 3 times daily over several weeks; topiramate, escalating at weekly intervals from 25–50 mg at bedtime to 200 mg twice daily; tiagabine, escalating from 2–4 mg at bedtime to 16–32 mg/d in divided doses; or pregabalin (not yet available in US markets).

Centrally acting skeletal muscle relaxants, including cyclobenzaprine, are not effective as single agents but may provide some benefit in combination with other agents, at least over the short term. Multiple choices are available: baclofen (activates GABA beta-receptors), start 5 mg 3 times daily, increasing by 5 mg/dose every 3 days until reaching 20 mg 3 times daily; tizanidine (α_2-adrenergic agonist), 4–8 mg every 6–8 hours, maximum 36 mg/d; and others. Topical capsaicin can be very useful when applied twice daily to painful areas with gentle massage; the patient should be informed that the beneficial effects may require 3–4 weeks of therapy). Anxiolytics of different durations of action frequently are useful adjuncts: clonazepam (long half-life), escalate after 3 days from 0.25 mg twice daily to a maximum of 4 mg/d; lorazepam (medium half-life), 2–3 mg/d given 2 or 3 times daily; temazepam (medium half-life), 7.5–30 mg at bedtime; alprazolam (short half-life), 0.25–0.5 mg 2 or 3 times daily; or buspirone, start 7.5 mg twice daily (usual dose is 15 mg twice daily). Other drugs that have effects on the abnormal central nociceptive processing in fibromyalgia include mexilitine (sodium channel blocker), clonidine (centrally acting antiadrenergic), and tropisetron (highly selective, competitive antagonist of 5-HT_3, not currently available in the United States).

Sleep disturbances should be treated aggressively. If good sleep hygiene and sleep medications are ineffective, request a formal sleep study to identify sleep apnea and restless legs syndrome, which are particularly common in fibromyalgia. Useful drugs to improve sleep are a single bedtime dose of a tricyclic antidepressant, alprazolam, trazodone, cyclobenzaprine, or temazepam; zolpidem, 5–10 mg at bedtime; or triazolam, 0.125–0.5 mg at bedtime. Clonazepam, 0.5–1.5 mg at bedtime, or L-Dopa/carbidopa, 1–2 tablets at bedtime, may be effective for restless legs syndrome.

Depression should be treated aggressively. Encourage formal or informal counseling and treat pharmacologically with one of the following: a tricyclic antidepressant; a bicyclic antidepressant (venlafaxine, start 37.5–75 mg/d divided twice daily, maximum 375 mg/d); a selective serotonin reuptake inhibitor (fluoxetine, 10–40 mg every morning, maximum 80 mg/d; citalopram, start 20 mg/d, maximum 60 mg/d; fluvoxamine, start 50 mg at bedtime, maximum 150 mg twice daily; paroxetine, start 20 mg every morning, maximum 50 mg/d; or sertraline, start 50 mg every morning, maximum 200 mg/d); a serotonin antagonist (mirtazapine, start 15 mg at bedtime, usual effective dose 15–45 mg/d); bupropion, start 100 mg twice daily, increase to 100 mg 3 times daily after 1 week; nefazodone, start 100 mg twice daily, maximum 600 mg/d; or trazodone, start at 50 mg twice daily, usual effective dose 200–300 mg twice daily.

Fatigue generally improves with effective treatment of pain, depression, and sleep disturbances in combination with a graded aerobic exercise program. Modafinil (approved by the US Food and Drug Administration for narcolepsy), 100–200 mg/d, or tropisetron (5-HT_3 receptor antagonist, not currently available in the United States) may benefit those patients in whom overwhelming fatigue is a persistent complaint.

Clonidine, 0.1 mg orally 3 times daily, is useful in neuropathic pain and to decrease withdrawal symptoms when tapering opioids.

B. NONPHARMACOLOGIC

When nonpharmacologic treatments have been compared with pharmacologic treatments alone, nonpharmacologic treatments generally have been of greater benefit. A meta-analysis of 49 fibromyalgia outcome treatment studies concluded that "the optimal intervention for fibromyalgia would include nonpharmacologic treatments, specifically exercise and cognitive-behavioral therapy (CBT), in addition to appropriate medication management as needed for sleep and pain symptoms." Various forms of exercise, strengthening and stretching, biofeedback and relaxation, acupuncture and electroacupuncture, CBT, hypnotherapy, or combinations of such treatments have all been shown to be of benefit.

Biofeedback alone or combined with relaxation therapy, CBT, and various forms of exercise significantly improves physical status and self-reported fibromyalgia symptoms but not daily functioning. Whether biofeedback/relaxation training plus exercise training maintains improvement over the long term is less certain, however.

Graded aerobic exercise, especially aquatherapy, is effective in fibromyalgia with respect to overall well-being, tender point count, self-reported pain, depression, state-trait anxiety, and self-efficacy, at least over the short term. The degree of response is significantly determined by the patient's capacity to effectively cope with her or his illness. High-intensity fitness programs should be avoided because they are associated with increased pain and fatigue, with consequent poor compliance.

Not all experts agree that CBT in fibromyalgia syndrome is cost-effective and provides additional benefit over other interventions. Other psychological interventions, such as guided imagery, may improve self-reported pain over the short term.

Many widely used nonpharmacologic treatments are of uncertain benefit. Although trigger point injections are commonly used by some health care practitioners for treatment of myofascial pain, the definition and reliability of "trigger points," "taut bands," and "muscle twitch" responses upon which myofascial pain syndromes are based are open to question. Randomized, controlled clinical trials examining dry needling, saline injections, anaesthetic injections, botulinum toxin, acupuncture, and sham acupuncture as therapies have not shown significant benefit beyond nonspecific, placebo-related effects. Ultrasound treatment of myofascial "trigger points" is no more effective in reducing pain than sham ultrasound. Similarly, low-level laser therapy and sphenopalatine blocks have no place in the treatment of fibromyalgia.

Almost all patients with fibromyalgia use complementary and alternative medicine (CAM), at least in part because of distrust of physicians and frustration with the limited efficacy of much traditional care. Acupuncture, hypnotherapy, relaxation techniques (yoga, Tai Chi, and meditation), and osteopathic manipulation appear to have efficacy. In other cases, such as vegetarian diets and exposure to static magnetic fields, efficacy has not been demonstrable. Properly designed controlled trials have not been reported for most other CAMs. The physician should inquire about self-administered herbs and other substances because many are potent pharmacologic agents with potential for interaction with conventional medicines.

C. Education and Lifestyle Measures

Although time consuming, educational efforts validate symptoms, inform regarding the nature of fibromyalgia and the role of stress, lessen fear regarding outcome, promote self-efficacy, and provide a rationale for the treatment program. Begin education at the first visit, emphasizing that an *active* role for the patient in the treatment plan is essential, particularly with respect to compliance with a regular *graded* (go slow and not overdo) aerobic exercise program. Advise the patient regarding the effects of stress and counsel regarding approaches to reduce current stressors. Encourage self-efficacy (the belief that the patient can control pain and fatigue through self-management).

Complications

The adverse impact of fibromyalgia on the patient, on family, and on society is high. Scores on the Rand 36-item Health Survey (SF-36), a self-report questionnaire measuring functional impairment and well-being, usually are in the severely impaired range in all areas (physical functioning, pain, role limitations, emotional well-being, social functioning, energy/fatigue, general health perception). More than 25% of patients receive some type of disability or other compensation payment.

When treating patients with fibromyalgia, two other potential complications should be kept in mind. First, be alert for dependence on opioids, benzodiazepines, and muscle relaxants, recognizing that drug-seeking behavior ("pseudoaddiction") often means that chronic pain is not being controlled adequately. Abrupt cessation of such medications may be associated with withdrawal symptoms. Second, use of the term "post-traumatic" fibromyalgia by physicians may unwittingly contribute to the development of chronic pain in patients with acute pain following minor injury. The current consensus of experts in this area is that this term not be used.

When to Refer to a Specialist

Referral to a rheumatologist familiar with fibromyalgia is appropriate when diagnosis is unclear, when response to therapy is inadequate, and when comorbid musculoskeletal or autoimmune conditions are present. Psychiatric referral is indicated when significant psychiatric comorbidity is present and is essential for severe depression with suicidal ideation and for comorbid psychosis. Psychotherapeutic counseling is helpful for many patients.

Prognosis

Most patients will improve with respect to self-reported pain, disturbed sleep, and fatigue, but daily functioning often remains impaired. The goal of therapy is care, not cure. Distinct subsets of patients vary in their prognosis: "Adaptive copers" do well clinically, whereas "dysfunctional" patients with high levels of pain, anxiety, and opioid dependence and those with pending litigation do poorly. While it is not possible to reverse entirely the allodynia and hyperalgesia in fibromyalgia, quality of life can be improved for many patients in response to therapy if ongoing stressors are relieved and if self-efficacy for control of pain can be achieved.

REFERENCES

American Geriatrics Society Panel on Chronic Pain in Older Persons, 1998.

Arnold LM, et al. Antidepressant treatment of fibromyalgia. A meta-analysis and review. *Psychosomatics.* 2000;41:104. [PMID: 10749947]

Barkhuizen A. Rationale and targeted pharmacologic treatment of fibromyalgia. *Rheum Dis Clinics North Am.* 2002;28:261. [PMID: 12122917]

Clauw D, Chrousos GP. Chronic pain and fatigue syndromes: overlapping clinical and neuroendocrine features and potential pathogenic mechanisms. *Neuroimmunomodulation.* 1997;4:134. [PMID: 9500148]

Merskey H. Classification of chronic pain: description of chronic pain syndromes and definition of pain terms. *Pain.* 1986; Suppl 3:S1.

Rossy LA, et al. A meta-analysis of fibromyalgia treatment interventions. *Ann Behav Med.* 1999;21:180. [PMID: 10499139]

Turk DC, et al. Differential responses by psychological subgroups of fibromyalgia syndrome patients to an interdisciplinary treatment. *Arthritis Care Res.* 1998;11:397. [PMID: 9830884]

Winfield JB. Psychological determinants of fibromyalgia and related syndromes. *Curr Rev Pain.* 2000;4:276. [PMID: 10953275]

Wolfe F, et al. The American College of Rheumatology 1990 Criteria for the Classification of Fibromyalgia. Report of the Multicenter Criteria Committee. *Arthritis Rheum.* 1990;33: 160. [PMID: 2306288]

Relevant World Wide Web Sites

[Arthritis Foundation]

http://www.arthritis.org/conditions/DiseaseCenter/Fibromyalgia/fibromyalgia.asp

[Medlineplus Health Information: A service of the U.S. National Library of Medicine and the National Institutes of Health]

http://www.nlm.nih.gov/medlineplus/fibromyalgia.html

[American College of Rheumatology]

http://www.rheumatology.org/patients/factsheets/fibromya.html

[Missouri Arthritis Rehabilitation Research and Training Center]

http://www.muhealth.org/fibro

[A Physician's Guide to Fibromyalgia Syndrome]

http://www.hsc.missouri.edu/~fibro/fm-md.html

[Fibromyalgia.com]

http://www.fibromyalgia.com

[The American Fibromyalgia Syndrome Association]

http://www.afsafund.org/

[Chronic Fatigue Syndrome and Fibromyalgia]

http://www.co-cure.org/

Health information for the whole family from the American Academy of Family Physicians]

Familydoctor.org

Complex Regional Pain Syndromes: Reflex Sympathetic Dystrophy & Causalgia

14

Ralf Baron, MD, & Jon D. Levine, MD, PhD

ESSENTIALS OF DIAGNOSIS

- *Spontaneous pain, hyperalgesia, swelling, autonomic abnormalities, and impairment of motor function are symptoms of complex regional pain syndrome (CRPS).*
- *Abnormalities, regardless of the site of the precipitating event, have a distal distribution with a spreading tendency that is not confined to innervation territories of peripheral nerves or roots.*
- *No overt nerve lesion is detectable in CRPS type 1 (also called reflex sympathetic dystrophy), which typically develops after minor tissue trauma or bone fracture.*
- *Diagnosis of CRPS 2 is confirmed by the identification of a partial peripheral nerve lesion.*

General Considerations

Complex regional pain syndromes (CRPS) are painful disorders that may develop as a disproportionate consequence of trauma affecting the limbs. The pathophysiology of CRPS is not well understood. Localized neurogenic inflammation may be involved in the edema, vasodilation, and increased sweating observed in the acute phase of CRPS. The spontaneous pain and various forms of stimulus-evoked pain (induced by touch, heat, or cold) that characterize CRPS are thought to be generated by peripheral and central sensitization of the nociceptive system.

Altered somatosensory perceptions are probably the result of changes in the central representation of somatosensory maps in the thalamus and cortex. CRPS 1 is associated with alterations in sympathetic reflex patterns that cause unilateral abnormalities in skin blood flow, temperature, and sweating. Pathologic interactions of sympathetic and afferent neurons may stimulate nociceptors after physiologic activation of sympathetic neurons (eg, by thermoregulatory stress). About half of patients with CRPS 1 show evidence of motor abnormalities, possibly as a result of abnormal central programming and processing of motor tasks.

Clinical Findings

A. SYMPTOMS AND SIGNS

1. CRPS type 1 (reflex sympathetic dystrophy)— Bone fracture, surgeries (eg, for carpal tunnel syndrome), minor soft tissue trauma and, rarely, stroke or myocardial infarction may precipitate CRPS type 1. Characteristically, asymmetric pain and swelling of a distal extremity develops after trauma; no overt nerve lesion is produced. The swelling and pain often develop at a site that is remote from the inciting injury, and obvious local tissue-damaging processes may be absent at the site of pain and swelling. Patients with CRPS 1 often report a **burning spontaneous pain** in the distal part of the affected extremity. The intensity of the pain is disproportionate to the inciting event and usually increases when the extremity is in a dependent position. Pain evoked by mechanical and thermal stimuli is a striking clinical feature.

These sensory abnormalities often appear early, are most pronounced distally, and have no consistent spatial relationship to individual nerve territories or to the site of the inciting lesion. Typically, pain is elicited by movement and pressure at the joints (deep somatic pain), despite the fact that these joints are not directly affected by the inciting lesion. In many cases, associated deep somatic symptoms are also present in more proximal joints (eg, the shoulder).

Autonomic abnormalities include swelling and changes in sweating and blood flow in the skin (Table 14–1). In the acute stages of CRPS 1, the affected limb is often warmer than the contralateral limb. Sweating abnormalities (hypohidrosis or, more frequently, hyperhidrosis) are present in nearly all CRPS 1 patients. The acute distal swelling of the affected limb depends on aggravating stimuli. **Trophic changes,** such as abnormal

Table 14–1. Symptoms of complex regional pain syndromes (CRPS).

Sensory system
   Spontaneous pain, hyperalgesia, allodynia, Deep somatic
      hyperalgesia
   Sensory deficits
   Sensory hemisyndrome
   Sensory "neglect-like" symptoms
Autonomic system
   Temperature side differences
   Vascular abnormalities
   Sudomotor dysfunction
   Edema
   Trophic changes
Motor system
   Weakness
   Tremor
   Deficits in coordination
   Dystonia
   Motor "neglect-like" symptoms
Increase of the periarticular bone metabolism
   "Active" osteoporosis
   Stiffness of joints
   Ankylosis

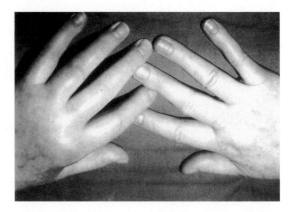

Figure 14–1. Complex regional pain syndrome developed in this patient after a radial fracture in the left hand. The marked swelling seen in the left hand started 2 weeks after the initial trauma. (Reproduced with permission from Baron R, et al. Causalgia and reflex sympathetic dystrophy: does the sympathetic nervous system contribute to the generation of pain? *Muscle Nerve.* 1999;22:678.)

nail growth, increased or decreased hair growth, fibrosis, thin glossy skin, and osteoporosis, may be present, particularly in chronic stages. Restrictions of passive movement are often seen in long-standing cases and may be related to both functional motor disturbances and trophic changes of joints and tendons. Weakness of all muscles of the affected distal extremity is often present. Small accurate movements are characteristically impaired. Nerve conduction and electromyography studies are within normal ranges, except among patients in whom CRPS 1 is chronic or advanced. About half of patients have postural or action tremors that represent exaggerated physiologic tremors. In about 10% of cases, dystonia of the affected hand or foot develops.

Identifying who is at risk for CRPS following a potential precipitating event (such as a radial fracture; Figure 14–1) is not possible. During the normal course of fracture healing, pain is felt predominantly within the traumatized area. If CRPS develops, the pain changes in quality (often described as burning), becomes more intense, spreads to the entire affected distal extremity, and is located deep within the bone or joints. Movement of all distal joints elicits discomfort, and the patient experiences disproportionate muscle weakness.

2. CRPS type 2 (causalgia)—Causalgia is described as a burning pain that develops in the distal extremity after a traumatic partial injury of a peripheral nerve. In addition to spontaneous pain, patients report hypersensitivity of the skin to light mechanical stimulation. Movement, loud noise, or strong emotion can trigger the pain. Distal extremity swelling, smoothness and mottling of the skin, and in some cases, acute arthritis are present. In most cases, the affected limb is cold and sweaty. Sensory and trophic abnormalities spread beyond the innervation territory of the injured peripheral nerve and often occur at a site remote from the original injury. Because of the many similarities to the symptoms of CRPS 1, this syndrome is called CRPS 2. It occurs in approximately 1–5% of partial nerve lesions. As with CRPS 1, no predictors for the development of CRPS 2 have been identified.

3. Sympathetically maintained pain—Patients with CRPS 1 and 2 who have similar clinical signs and symptoms can be divided into two groups: responders and nonresponders to selective sympathetic blockade or antagonism of α adrenoceptors. The pain component that is relieved by sympatholytic procedures is considered sympathetically maintained pain and is defined as a symptom of the underlying mechanism in a subset of patients with neuropathic disorders and not a clinical entity.

B. Imaging and Special Tests

Several tests and procedures can help confirm the diagnosis of CRPS. Bone scintigraphy can provide information about vascular bone changes but only shows significant changes during the subacute period (up to 1 year). Plain radiographs can be used to evaluate the status of mineralization but are abnormal only in chronic stages. Quantitative sensory testing can provide information about the sensory symptom profile (function of unmyelinated and myelinated afferent fibers), but no sensory profile is diagnostic for CRPS. Autonomic testing with the quantitative sudomotor axon reflex test can provide information about the function of sudomotor reflex loops. Swelling can be quantified by measuring water displacement. Autonomic vascular function can be tested by laser Doppler flowmeter and infrared thermography.

Skin temperature measurements (using infrared thermometry) assess vascular function and are particularly helpful in the diagnosis of CRPS. Under resting conditions, only minor skin temperature asymmetries are present between both limbs. Asymmetries are most prominent, however, at a high to medium level of sympathetic activity and distinguish CRPS from other extremity pain syndromes with high sensitivity and specificity.

Differential Diagnosis

A. OTHER DISORDERS WITH UNILATERAL VASCULAR DISTURBANCES

Inflammatory arthritis and soft tissue infections can cause unilateral skin warming as well as produce a vascular regulation pattern that mimics CRPS. Arterial or venous occlusive diseases can present with marked temperature differences between the affected and healthy limbs. Repetitive artificial occlusion of the blood supply to a limb (as in the psychiatric factitious syndrome) can induce secondary structural changes of the blood vessels with consecutive abnormalities in perfusion.

B. POST-TRAUMATIC NEURALGIA AND TERRITORIAL NEUROPATHIC PAIN SYNDROMES

Neuralgia (eg, trigeminal neuralgia) is a type of neuropathic pain located within the innervation territory of the affected nerve (Table 14–2). Some patients with focal painful neuropathies are more complex than neuralgia patients but do not have the full clinical picture of CRPS 2. Patients with territorial neuropathic pain syndromes, which can follow traumatic or postherpetic nerve damage, have spontaneous burning pain and pain that can be evoked by mechanical or cold stimuli. In contrast to CRPS 2, these sensory symptoms are confined to the territory of the affected peripheral nerve, although the mechanically evoked pain may extend somewhat beyond the border of nerve territories. Patients with territorial neuropathic pain syndromes do

Table 14–2. Diagnostic criteria for different focal neuropathic pain syndromes.

Neuralgia
Pain is located within the innervation territory of a lesioned nerve

Territorial neuropathic pain syndromes
Sensory symptoms (mechanical allodynia, cold allodynia, hyperalgesia) extend beyond the innervation territory of a lesioned nerve for several centimeters.
No distal generalization of symptoms
No joint pain
No changes of bone metabolism

Complex regional pain syndrome
Distal generalization of all symptoms (deep pain, allodynia, and hyperalgesia), swelling

not have marked swelling and do not exhibit a progressive spread of symptoms.

C. METABOLIC AND TOXIC NEUROPATHIES

Polyneuropathies induced by metabolic (eg, diabetes mellitus) or toxic (eg, alcohol-related) disorders characteristically demonstrate a diffuse symmetric distribution of symptoms and therefore can be distinguished clearly from CRPS, which in most cases is confined to one extremity.

Treatment of CRPS

Only a few evidence-based treatment regimens for CRPS are available, and the clinician must rely on studies of other neuropathic pain syndromes or on treatments based on hypothetical mechanisms.

The general principles of pharmacologic treatment are the individualization of therapy and the titration of a specific pharmacologic agent to maximize effect and minimize negative side effects. "No response" should not be accepted as a result until enough time (2–4 weeks) has passed to accurately judge the efficacy of the drug. Destructive surgery on the peripheral or central afferent nervous system in patients with CRPS always generates further deafferentation and provides an increased risk for the persistent pain associated with destruction of afferent pathways.

In rare cases, treatment of an underlying disorder is associated with complete resolution of CRPS. In patients with carpal tunnel syndrome, for example, continuous nociceptive input from the nerve compression site can initiate and maintain CRPS 2. Adequate decompression of the nerve will rapidly relieve CRPS symptoms in these patients.

A. Pharmacologic Therapy

Nonsteroidal anti-inflammatory drugs can be used for relief of mild to moderate pain. Opioids have been shown in short-term studies to be efficacious in other neuropathic pain syndromes but have not been rigorously studied in CRPS; however, the use of opioids in a comprehensive pain treatment program is supported by expert pain clinicians. Tricyclic antidepressants have analgesic effects in several neuropathic pain states and should be tested as part of the treatment regimen. Lidocaine, mexiletine, tocainide, and the anticonvulsant carbamazepine relieve neuropathic pain. Intravenous lidocaine is effective in CRPS. The mechanism of action of gabapentin is not completely understood but probably includes an inhibition of central calcium channels. In one study, gabapentin had a promising effect on CRPS. Oral glucocorticoids have demonstrated efficacy in controlled trials. There is clinical evidence of efficacy for radical scavengers. Transdermal application of the α_2-adrenoceptor agonist clonidine, which is thought to prevent the release of catecholamines by a presynaptic action, may be helpful when small areas of hyperalgesia are present. The administration of intravenous bisphosphonates (alendronate, clodronate) has been shown to provide significant relief from pain and swelling and improve movement.

B. Interventional Therapy in the Sympathetic Nervous System

Sympatholytic therapy can result in substantial or even complete pain relief in some patients and can improve other symptoms of CRPS. Approximately 85% of patients report a positive short-term effect, but far fewer experience long-term relief. Two therapeutic techniques to block sympathetic nerves are used currently: (1) injections of a local anesthetic around sympathetic paravertebral ganglia that project to the affected body part (sympathetic ganglion blocks), and (2) regional intravenous application of guanethidine, bretylium, or reserpine (which deplete noradrenaline in the postganglionic axon) to an isolated extremity blocked with a tourniquet (intravenous regional sympatholysis).

C. Stimulation Techniques and Spinal Drug Application

Transcutaneous electrical nerve stimulation may be effective in some cases and produces minimal side effects. Epidural spinal cord stimulation was effective in one randomized study in selected patients with chronic CRPS and may be a promising treatment for such individuals. Other stimulation techniques, such as peripheral nerve stimulation with implanted electrodes and deep brain stimulation (sensory thalamus and medial lemniscus), have been reported to be effective in selected cases of CRPS.

In selected patients with severe refractory CRPS, epidural administration of the N-methyl-D-aspartate antagonist ketamine or the adrenoceptor agonist clonidine induced analgesia associated with marked side effects such as sedation and hypotension. Intrathecal baclofen resulted in positive outcomes for CRPS patients with severe dystonia (Figure 14–2).

D. Physical Therapy

Aggressive physical therapy is not feasible and may be harmful in the acute stage of CRPS, when patients still suffer from severe pain. Immobilization and careful contralateral physical therapy should be the treatment of choice in the acute stages. Later, when pain subsides, passive physical therapy followed by active isometric and later active isotonic training should be combined with sensory desensitization programs. Clinical experience strongly suggests that physiotherapy and occupational therapy are of utmost importance in achieving recovery of function and in rehabilitation.

When to Refer to a Specialist

In mild cases of CRPS (defined by pain present only under load and with only mild symptoms at the joints), conventional pain therapy and carefully increasing physiotherapy may be associated with resolution within weeks. If symptoms are severe, however, pain therapy should be immediate, aggressive, and most importantly, directed toward restoration of full function of the extremity. This objective is best attained in a comprehensive multidisciplinary setting with emphasis on conventional and interventional pain management and functional restoration. Pain specialists should include neurologists, anesthesiologists, orthopedists, physiotherapists, and psychologists.

Prognosis

In patients with mild CRPS who experience pain only under physical load and have few articular symptoms, conventional pain therapy and carefully increased physiotherapy may relieve the disorder within weeks. In patients with moderate CRPS, a multidisciplinary approach with interventional treatment options and frequent occupational and physiotherapy often leads to successful relief of symptoms within 1 year. In most patients with severe CRPS, however, the prognosis is poor despite aggressive therapy. Improvement followed by relapse of symptoms is common. More than 60% of patients with severe CRPS 2 continue to suffer from many of the primary symptoms for years after the initiating trauma. Spontaneous remissions of associated

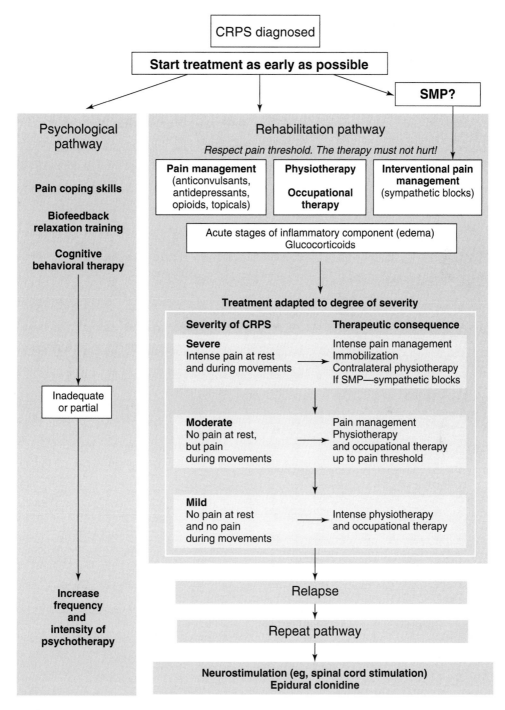

Figure 14–2. Treatment algorithm. CRPS, complex regional pain syndrome; SMP, sympathetically maintained pain. (Modified from Stanton-Hicks M, et al. An updated interdisciplinary clinical pathway for CRPS: report of an expert panel. *Pain Practice.* 2002;2:1. Modified from Baron R, et al. Complex regional pain syndrome. Reflex sympathetic dystrophy and causalgia. *Nervenarzt.* 2002;73:305.) (Reproduced with permission from *Wall & Melzack`s Textbook of Pain,* 5th edition. Churchill Livingstone, in press.)

shoulder symptoms occur more often than remissions of hand symptoms, which often progress to severe dystonia. Complete loss of function is the final stage in severe CRPS 2 cases.

REFERENCES

Jänig W, Baron R. Complex regional pain syndrome: mystery explained? *Lancet Neurology.* 2003; Nov, 2(11):687–697. [PMID: 14572737].

Jänig W, Stanton-Hicks M, eds. *Reflex Sympathetic Dystrophy: A Reappraisal.* IASP Press, 1995.

Perez RS, et al. Treatment of reflex sympathetic dystrophy (CRPS type 1): a research synthesis of 21 randomized clinical trials. *J Pain Symptom Manage.* 2001;21:511. [PMID: 11397610]

Stanton-Hicks M, et al. Complex regional pain syndromes: guidelines for therapy. *Clin J Pain.* 1998;14:155. [PMID: 9647459]

Relevant World Wide Web Sites

[International Research Foundation for RSF/CRPS]
www.rsdfoundation.org

Approach to the Patient with a Painful Prosthetic Joint

15

Steven A. Lietman, MD

ESSENTIALS OF DIAGNOSIS

- *Revision arthroplasty is indicated for a painful prosthetic joint in three major circumstances: prosthetic failure, loosening, and infection.*
- *Prosthetic joints that are infected are generally not as painful as native septic joints with range of motion.*
- *Infection is always in the differential diagnosis.*
- *Wound drainage beyond the third postoperative week is usually related to infection.*
- *Prosthetic loosening usually occurs more than 10 years after the procedure.*
- *Radiographs are insensitive for early osteolysis.*
- *The spine is the most common cause of referred pain when the prosthetic joint itself is not the cause of the pain.*

Total joint arthroplasty represents one of the most successful operations performed in the United States, with excellent results for greater than 90% of patients. There is a small subset of patients, however, who have chronic pain after total joint replacement.

Prevention

The life of a prosthetic joint can be extended by the following preventive measures:

- *Prophylaxis against infection.* The risk of infection after joint replacement can be decreased with antibiotic prophylaxis with amoxicillin for dental visits or a cephalosporin for surgical procedures.
- *Avoidance of high-impact exercise.* Patients with prosthetic joints should avoid high-impact activities such as running, aerobics, and playing tennis on hard courts.
- *Body positioning.* In order to decrease the risk of dislocation, patients should avoid crossing their legs and sitting in low chairs for at least 6 weeks after surgery.

- *Moderation in physical therapy.* Overly aggressive physical therapy may lead to periarticular muscle damage in tissues already compromised by the operation. Gentle passive and active assisted range of motion exercises are preferred to extreme range of motion maneuvers, particularly in the hip and shoulder.

Clinical Findings

A. HISTORY

There are several critical questions to ask in taking the history of a patient with prosthetic joint pain:

- Is pain present at the time of the visit?

  If the patient has no pain that can be elicited with use of the extremity at the time of the visit, major problems with the prosthesis are unlikely unless the patient is immunosuppressed (in which case infection remains a possibility).

- Where is the pain?

  Many patients say they have hip pain, but when they are asked to show the clinician the specific location, they point to the sacrum or lumbar spine, indicating a possible disc herniation or spinal stenosis, or to the trochanteric bursa, indicating the possibility of trochanteric bursitis.

- When did the pain start?

  If the patient's pain is unchanged from before the initial prosthetic implantation, then the pain for which the joint replacement was performed may not have been related to the joint at all. With the exception of Charcot joints, pain relief obtained from a joint replacement correlates well with the severity of joint disease before surgery.

- What triggers the pain?

  Except in infection and fracture, pain without use of the extremity is rarely related to a prosthetic problem.

- Could the pain be referred and due to other medical problems?

  Spinal stenosis, disc herniation, and arthritis of the lumbar and cervical spine are the most common causes of referred extremity pain.

B. PHYSICAL EXAMINATION

A general physical examination can delineate other potentially relevant issues, such as hernias or spinal disease. The area around the prosthetic joint must be examined systematically by inspection, palpation, evaluation of range of motion, and special tests.

For patients with lower extremity joint prostheses, observation of their gait is extremely important and can help define the cause of the pain. Patients with pain from their prostheses generally walk with limps, and frequently have worse pain with the use of the extremity. Specific tenderness in the area of the prosthesis is generally present. Range of motion is generally decreased.

C. RADIOGRAPHS

A set of radiographs should always be taken of at least the entire painful prosthesis. The standard radiographic approach to painful prosthetic joints according to the joint involved is shown in Table 15–1.

Aspiration of the joint should be performed if infection is suspected. Aspiration is urgent if the problem is acute (present for less than 2–3 weeks), because irrigation and debridement may salvage the prosthesis.

Differential Diagnosis

The differential diagnosis for the patient with a painful prosthetic joint is listed in Table 15–2.

A. INFECTION

Infection is always in the differential diagnosis of the painful prosthetic joint. Prosthetic joint infections can cause myriad symptoms and signs, including constitutional symptoms such as fever, chills, night sweats, and pain at rest. An infected prosthesis generally is less painful with range of motion exercises than a native septic joint. A history of difficulty with healing of the

Table 15–1. Radiographic evaluation of the painful prosthetic joint.

Joint	Radiographic Studies
Hip	AP pelvis and AP and lateral of the entire femur
Knee	AP weight-bearing, sunrise view, and lateral knee (consider hip films if the patient also has groin pain or decreased hip ROM)
Shoulder	Axillary view (Y view can be substituted if the patient cannot raise arm high enough for the cassette to be placed properly) and AP and lateral of the entire humerus
Elbow	AP and lateral of the elbow

AP, anteroposterior; ROM, range of motion.

Table 15–2. Differential diagnosis in the patient with a painful prosthesis.

- Infection
- Prosthetic loosening
- Osteolysis
- Fracture of the bone around the prosthesis
- Component fracture or failure
- Prosthetic dislocation or subluxation
- Bursitis
- Scar neuromata
- Reflex sympathetic dystrophy
- Referred pain
- Prosthetic stem pain

wound postoperatively and or what was termed a "superficial infection" should be noted. In addition, a history of infections in other areas and particularly a history of recent dental procedures should be obtained.

On physical examination, the wound and area around the involved joint should always be examined for evidence of drainage. Wound drainage beyond the third postoperative week is usually related to infection. Laboratory tests such as white blood cell count, C-reactive protein, and erythrocyte sedimentation rate are frequently, but not always, elevated.

Aspiration of the joint (under fluoroscopy in the case of the hip and sometimes shoulder) is the gold standard and should be performed at least 2 weeks after the patient has discontinued antibiotic therapy. At the time of all revision surgery for hip pain or loosening, Gram stains and cultures for aerobic and anaerobic organisms as well as acid-fast bacilli and fungal organisms are essential.

B. PROSTHETIC LOOSENING

The patient with prosthetic loosening generally has pain of the involved joint, which is present with the use of the extremity. The pain is particularly severe with weight bearing in the lower extremity and with lifting objects or simply lifting the involved extremity. This pain can be present even immediately after the surgery (if the implant was improperly fixed) but more commonly occurs more than 10 years after implantation. The average longevity of a prosthetic implant is variable depending on many factors including patient age, but is generally 10–20 years.

Patients with prosthetic loosening in a lower extremity joint nearly always have an antalgic gait or limp, and the pain is generally demonstrable with lifting or use of that extremity. They may have pain with palpation or range of motion of the involved joint. Some patients have more pain in the area of loosening with an active straight leg raise (raising the leg off the examination table with the knee straight) than with a passive straight leg raise. This pain is presumably due to the increased joint reaction force created by the contraction of the hip flexor muscles.

Radiographs nearly always demonstrate at least a 2-mm lucency around the entire prosthesis. Radiographic techniques should be standardized so that accurate serial radiographs can reveal progressive loosening. Standardization of radiographic technique is particularly important in the evaluation of the knee arthroplasty where lucency may not be seen if the x-ray beam is not tangential to the interface between the cement and bone.

C. Osteolysis

Osteolysis manifests itself as a lucent area around the prosthesis and is the most common cause for eventual prosthetic loosening. It is generally the result of polyethylene wear debris that stimulates a foreign-body inflammatory response, resulting in bone resorption and manifested as radiographic lucency. Osteolysis can, but does not always, cause pain in the absence of loosening; it is a progressive process in which there is probably a release of polyethylene particles with every motion of prosthetic joint. However, the rate of bone resorption can be variable and can be quite slow. Osteolysis may cause pain with the provocative maneuvers described above for prosthetic loosening, and the patient may limp. Radiographs frequently do not demonstrate osteolysis until the bone mass in the area of lucency has been decreased by 30–50%.

D. Periprosthetic Fracture

Fracture around the prosthesis is relatively uncommon, but it is usually related to at least osteolysis and frequently implant loosening. The history may relate relatively minor trauma, particularly in areas of significant osteolysis. Physical examination should be limited based on the significant discomfort generally present with motion of the involved extremity. Standard radiographs will nearly always reveal the fracture.

E. Component Fracture or Failure

The metal of modern prostheses rarely fractures, but the polyethylene, particularly as it wears in a joint arthroplasty, can suddenly break. This will usually—but not always—present with a change in pain and instability, and the use of the extremity will be less effective. Radiographs demonstrate joint asymmetry.

F. Prosthetic Dislocation or Subluxation

Prosthetic dislocation is most common in the hip, less common in the shoulder, and rare in the knee and elbow. In general, the patient describes an unusual or extreme motion of the joint and pain afterwards. The dislocated joint is not functional and can be seen by standard radiographs; however, it can be missed if only one radiographic view is used.

G. Referred Pain

Pain at a site remote from the joint is particularly important to try to identify. The most common cause of referred pain is a spinal disorder, although abdominal and pelvic abnormalities can cause pain in the hip and thoracic tumors can cause shoulder pain. Nerve root impingement in the neck can cause pain very similar to that of a loose shoulder implant, and impingement in the lumbar spine can cause pain similar to that of a loose hip or knee. In general, the symptoms and signs of nerve root impingement from either spinal stenosis or a herniated disc are numbness and weakness. Also, the pain will not generally increase with an active straight leg raise compared with a passive straight leg raise. The classic presentation of nerve root impingement at the neck is reproducible pain with neck range of motion or rotation. The classic manifestation of spinal stenosis is a stooped posture; leaning forward (as when pushing a grocery cart) relieves the pain. Radiographs, computed tomography scans, and magnetic resonance imaging all may be helpful if a spinal disorder is suspected.

H. Bursitis

Bursae around prosthetic joints are potential sites of inflammation and sources of pain after joint arthroplasty. Patients with subacromial, olecranon, trochanteric, pes, patellar, or anserine bursitis describe pain in the bursal region and tenderness to touch.

I. Scar Neuromata

Theoretically, any adjacent cutaneous nerve can be cut and cause pain after the incision for joint arthroplasty, in particular the infrapatellar branch of the saphenous nerve after knee replacement. Patients with painful neuromata generally have pain out of proportion to physical examination and cutaneous hypersensitivity.

J. Reflex Sympathetic Dystrophy

Patients with reflex sympathetic dystrophy generally have less focal pain than those with scar neuromata. They generally will have joint stiffness, which may be increasing, and they may have increased sweating or discoloration over the involved area. They may also demonstrate local osteopenia on radiograph.

K. Prosthetic Stem Pain

Pain in the area of long uncemented stems can be present even with well-fixed implants and is primarily believed to be due to a mismatch in the modulus between a stiff implant and the less stiff bone. In most cases, this condition is believed to improve within 2 years of implantation and is not common with newer uncemented prostheses with lower moduli of elasticity.

Treatment

A. INFECTION

The treatment of the infected total joint involves careful irrigation and debridement and change of the polyethylene liner if it is started within 3 weeks of the onset of the infection. In most cases, however, the infection is not detected within 3 weeks of onset and all foreign bodies in the joint (prosthetic components, methylmethacrylate, cement restrictors, cables and plate and screws) should be removed. At this point, multiple culture specimens should be obtained and at least a 6-week course of antibiotics should be given. Following this initial treatment, antibiotic therapy should be discontinued for at least 2 weeks and an aspiration of the joint should be performed. If there is no evidence of infection at this point, a revision arthroplasty can be performed. If infection persists, then another course of antibiotics for at least 3 months is given before reimplantation. Reimplantation is not recommended if the aspirate or a Gram stain at the time of surgery reveals evidence of continued infection.

B. OSTEOLYSIS

The treatment of osteolysis in the patient with minimal symptoms and bone loss is somewhat controversial. Antiresorptive agents, such as alendronate, may be considered. In the patient with severe pain or dysfunction, joint revision—or rarely, bone grafting of the defect without implant revision in the patient with easily accessible lesions, significant comorbidities, and well-fixed components—may be recommended.

C. PERIPROSTHETIC FRACTURE

Usually, fracture of the bone around the prosthesis does not heal with immobilization and requires surgery, except in the severely debilitated or ill patient. Often, there is component loosening with these fractures, and at the time of fixation, the components should be examined for signs of loosening. The revision surgery in these situations generally requires implant change to a long stem model, which will in essence bypass the fracture or defect.

D. COMPONENT FRACTURE OR FAILURE

The failure of a component requires exchange of at least that component, except in the most severely ill or debilitated patients.

E. PROSTHETIC DISLOCATION OR SUBLUXATION

Prosthetic subluxation can generally be treated with avoidance of the activity that causes the subluxation. Progressively increasing prosthetic subluxation, however, can be a harbinger of polyethylene wear and failure.

F. BURSITIS

The approach to the patient with bursitis following joint arthroplasty is different than that in the patient with bursitis around a native joint. Postsurgical joints are less likely to have capsules or boundaries between the bursae and the joint space. Contamination of the bursa is associated with a greater risk of joint infection. Consequently, bursal injections are discouraged.

G. SCAR NEUROMATA AND REFLEX SYMPATHETIC DYSTROPHY

Cutaneous nerve resection may be useful in patients who have pain for at least 6 months after a joint replacement in the absence of other causes. Sympathetic nerve block has relieved pain in selected patients with reflex sympathetic dystrophy.

H. PROSTHETIC STEM PAIN

This condition is usually self-limited, resolving within 2 years. Revision of uncemented to cemented components in this situation has not yielded consistently favorable results.

REFERENCES

Gusenoff JA, et al. Outcome and management of infected wounds after total hip arthroplasty. *Ann Plast Surg.* 2002;49:587. [PMID: 12461440] (Salvage of the infected hip prosthesis is accomplished best via early recognition, irrigation, and debridement. In the setting of complex wounds, plastic surgery consultation may be important for muscle flap coverage.)

Tsukayama DT, et al. Diagnosis and management of infection after total knee arthroplasty. *J Bone Joint Surg Am.* 2003;Suppl 1:S75. [PMID: 12540674]

Relevant World Wide Web Sites

[The Cleveland Clinic]
http://www.clevelandclinic.org/quality/leaders/orthopaedics.htm

Common Injuries from Running

Calvin R. Brown Jr., MD

GENERAL CONSIDERATIONS

Approximately 11 million people in the United States run more than 100 days per year. Recreational exercise is attractive because it improves the quality of life and increases longevity. Runners note a range of salutary effects, from improved cardiopulmonary capacity to enhanced mental health, less depression and anxiety, and a greater sense of tranquility.

Regular exercise enhances sleep patterns; promotes a stronger and more stable musculoskeletal system; and results in decreases in disability, hypertension, diabetes, cancer, stroke, and osteoporosis. Runners report increased appetite and healthier weight, a desirable combination. Except for walking, running may be the most easily accessible and least expensive form of regular exercise.

However, there are important health concerns occurring as a consequence of running as well. These include the risk of sudden death, musculoskeletal injuries, and potential effects on joints. Approximately 45–70% of runners will experience musculoskeletal injuries each year.

RISK FACTORS

Repetitive use, rather than a single traumatic event, causes the majority of running injuries. Table 16–1 lists the 10 most common injuries seen in one clinic and is representative of reports from other large series. Risk factors for running injuries include history of a previous injury, competitive running, high weekly mileage (> 25 miles per week), and abrupt increases in the intensity or duration of training. Injuries are more likely to occur when the runner's shoes are worn down, leading to the recommendation that shoes be replaced every 6 months.

Stretching is of particular interest because runners frequently report performing better and feeling better after stretching. However, a large controlled trial of stretching as taught by an Olympic marathon coach showed no difference in injury type or frequency between the intervention and control groups. Thus, the well-entrenched lore of stretching and running does not have evidence-based support. Similarly, there is little or no evidence to support proposed links between running injuries and age, gender, body mass, hill running, running on hard surfaces, time of year, and time of day.

CLINICAL FINDINGS

Physical Examination

The physical examination of an injured runner should not only focus on the area of pain but should also include an examination of adjacent joints, alignment, and flexibility. Approximately 20–40% of running injuries can be related to structural abnormalities. The foot must dissipate 110 tons of force for every mile run, and alignment abnormalities of the foot are associated with increased frequency of injury. A high-arched (cavus) foot is rigid and tends to transmit impact up the leg. A flat (pes planus) foot leads to excessive pronation of the foot during running, which in turn increases stress on the medial structures of the ankle, shin, and knee. Orthotics may be helpful for either type of structural abnormality.

Hamstring and calf flexibility can be assessed with the runner in the supine position on the examining table, the femur at 90 degrees to the table, and the foot at 90 degrees to the tibia. The physician should be able to passively extend the knee to within 15 degrees of full extension. Although there is little evidence that stretching prevents running injuries, stretching may be of therapeutic value for the injured runner with limited flexibility.

Shoe Evaluation

Current thinking is that runners with excessive pronation need a shoe that has more rearfoot control but can have a bit less shock absorption. People with a high-arched (cavus) foot need more cushioning because of the rigid nature of their foot. An examination of well-worn running shoes can often reveal biomechanical abnormalities. This would include abnormal wear patterns on the soles and deformation of upper shoe indicating motion abnormalities.

PATELLOFEMORAL PAIN SYNDROME

Far and away the most common injury in runners, and probably the most common cause of knee pain in all active individuals, is the patellofemoral or anterior knee pain syndrome. Persons seek medical attention complaining of the insidious onset of poorly localized pain on the anterior surface of the knee. Pain is worse when arising from a seated position, particularly after sitting

Table 16–1. The top 10 most common running injuries.[a]

Medical Diagnosis	%	n
Patellar pain syndrome	25.8	468
Stress fractures	13.2	239
Achilles tendinitis	6.0	109
Plantar fasciitis	4.7	85
Patellar tendinitis	4.5	81
Iliotibial band syndrome	4.3	78
Metatarsalgia	3.2	58
Tibial stress syndrome	2.6	47
Tibialis posterior tendintis	2.5	45
Peroneas tendinitis	1.9	34
Total	68.7	1224

[a]Note 20–30% of running injuries do not involve the lower extremity; other musculoskeletal injuries (spine, upper extremity), dog bites, amenorrhea, hyperthermia, and frostbite.

for several minutes (the "theater sign") and when walking up or, more commonly, down stairs.

On physical examination, the Q angle between the femur and tibia should be measured (see Chapter 12). An angle greater than 16 degrees is associated with a higher incidence of patellofemoral pain syndrome. Compression of the patella will cause pain, particularly when the quadriceps muscle is contracted simultaneously. The patient may be reluctant to do so because of apprehension of pain (the "patellar inhibition" sign).

STRESS FRACTURES

A stress fracture is an incomplete fracture that results from repetitive strain on the bone rather than a single traumatic episode. Stress fractures occur in all sports that require repetitive running and jumping but are far more common in long-distance runners than in any other athletes. The vast majority occurs in people who are running more than 20 miles per week. Continued, repetitive stress on the bone leads to a normal remodeling response that is gradually overcome, and trabecular microfractures occur. The tibia and fibula are most commonly involved (Figure 16–1). Displacement of stress fractures is rare except for femoral neck fractures, which also carry the risk of avascular necrosis.

In most patients, the diagnosis of a stress fracture should be made on the clinical history. Any running athlete who complains of pain localized to a bone in the lower extremity should be considered to have a stress fracture. If local tenderness over the bone is found, further work-up should include radiographs or bone scan. Magnetic resonance imaging (MRI) is expensive but can be used in rare instances when the lesion on bone scan is indistinct (Figure 16–2).

Some general rules can be applied to treatment of stress fractures regardless of their location. Pain can usually be controlled with nonsteroidal anti-inflammatory drugs. The patient must significantly decrease or stop running to reduce the excess strain that is causing the stress fracture. During this rest phase of treatment, alternative exercise possibilities include swimming, biking, and the use of a stair-climber or elliptical trainer. This hiatus offers an excellent chance to increase muscle mass and strength and thereby avoid further stress fractures. When local tenderness has disappeared, a final radiograph can be obtained, and running activities can be gradually reintroduced. At this point one has to know the previous running history and must be certain that the return to running is gradual.

MEDIAL TIBIAL STRESS SYNDROME (SHIN SPLINTS)

Persons with medial tibial stress syndrome complain of diffuse, nagging pain over the tibia that worsens with running. If the pain persists after running and is noted with routine ambulation, the diagnosis of a tibial stress fracture should be suspected. Medial tibial stress syndrome is common in beginning runners. The pathophysiology is thought to be inflammation of the anterior and posterior calf musculature and periostitis of the tibia. Treatment consists of a break from full or vigorous training, correction of any misalignment, and substituted aerobic activities to prevent deconditioning.

ACHILLES TENDINITIS

Runners and jumping athletes may complain of pain in the substance of the Achilles tendon, which connects the soleus and the gastrocnemius muscles to the calcaneus. A relatively avascular or "watershed" area in the Achilles tendon approximately 4–5 cm proximal to its insertion is a factor in its vulnerability to injury and rupture. Diverse factors are thought to incite overuse injuries of the Achilles tendon, including running on hard surfaces, abrupt increases in mileage or training intensity, and shoe design. Fortunately, the latter has been addressed in contemporary running shoes. A person with a high-arched foot may also be at increased risk for Achilles tendinitis and rupture.

Clinically, fusiform swelling with or without warmth may be evident along the Achilles tendon. Crepitation

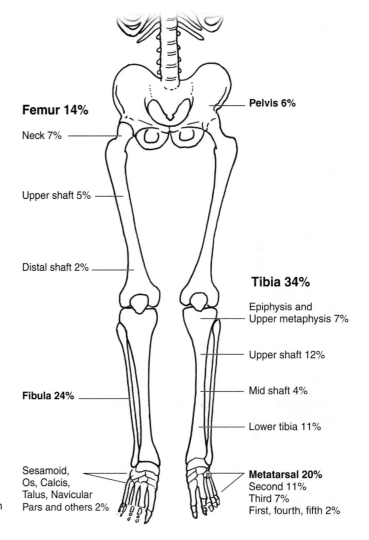

Femur 14%

Neck 7%

Upper shaft 5%

Distal shaft 2%

Pelvis 6%

Tibia 34%

Epiphysis and
Upper metaphysis 7%

Upper shaft 12%

Mid shaft 4%

Lower tibia 11%

Fibula 24%

Sesamoid,
Os, Calcis,
Talus, Navicular
Pars and others 2%

Metatarsal 20%
Second 11%
Third 7%
First, fourth, fifth 2%

Figure 16–1. Stress fracture resulting from failure of bone remodeling.

may be present with motion. Palpation along the tendon will elicit pain. The calf should be squeezed with the foot held in dorsiflexion; this should result in a modest amount of plantar flexion if the Achilles tendon is intact (the Thompson squeeze test).

Treatment of Achilles tendinitis consists of reduction of activities, anti-inflammatory medication, heel lifts or orthotics, and gentle stretching. Once the Achilles tendon is no longer tender to palpation and the athlete has restored his or her flexibility, slow progressive return to activity is permitted. There have been reports of iatrogenic Achilles tendon rupture secondary to inadvertent intratendinous glucocorticoid injection, and thus injection should be avoided.

PLANTAR FASCIITIS

Plantar fascitis typically occurs over the midportion of the plantar fascia and is usually exacerbated by dorsiflexion of the toes and direct pressure over the fascia. Lateral squeeze of the heel also precipitates pain. Individuals with chronic plantar fascial pain have microtears and partial rupture of the plantar fascia near its origin. In the case of rupture, a gap in the tendon is often palpable.

Treatment consists of ice, anti-inflammatory drugs, and physical therapy to increase heel and Achilles flexibility in order to relieve stress and tension on the plantar fascia. Orthotics may be useful.

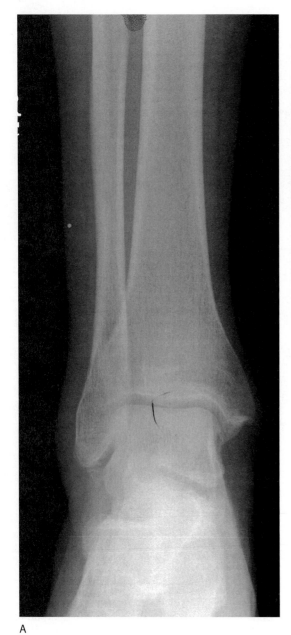

A

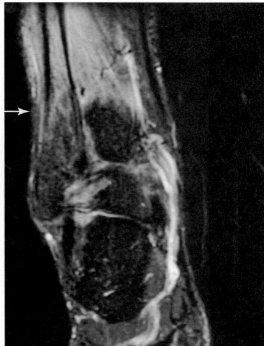

B

Figure 16–2. **A:** The initial radiograph shows no abnormality. **B:** The fat suppression magnetic resonance image shows increased signal in the fibula at the area indicated by arrow, indicative of bone injury.

PATELLAR TENDINITIS

Patellar tendinitis is often referred to as "jumper's knee" because of its common association with jumping sports such as basketball. However, it can occur in any running sport, which can be thought of as a series of one-legged-jumps. Abnormal foot biomechanics and running up hills are cited as aggravating factors.

Pain is localized to the inferior pole of the patella, and swelling is generally not present. Knee range of motion is within normal limits. Affected persons feel a sensation of the knee giving way with hard jumping. On examination, tenderness is felt directly on the lower tip of the patella. Radiographs are normal, but bone scans may be positive at the inferior pole of the patella, and MRI may show chronic tendinopathy.

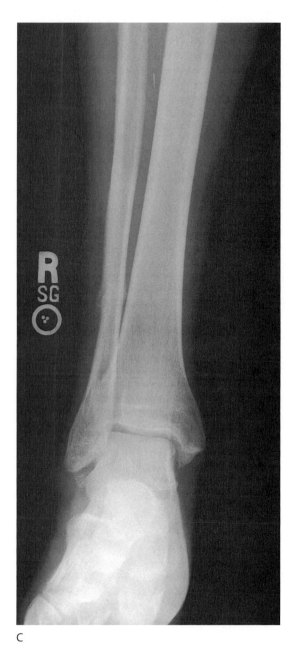

C

Figure 16–2. **(Continued) C:** The follow-up radiograph 1 month later confirms periosteal bone reaction indicative of stress fracture.

Unfortunately, patellar tendinitis is often chronic, taking many months to a year for complete healing. Nonsteroidal anti-inflammatory drugs are helpful, as are exercises to stretch and strengthen leg muscles. In some cases, surgery is needed to remove scarred portions of the ten-

don. Long-term restriction of jumping may be required for 1 or 2 years. Patellar tendinitis can affect the long-term playing ability of jumping athletes, such as volleyball or basketball players and long-distance runners.

ILIOTIBIAL BAND SYNDROME

Iliotibial band (ITB) syndrome is an overuse condition that is common in runners and cyclists and is characterized by an ache or burning sensation of the lateral aspect of the knee during or after activity. ITB syndrome is thought to be due to local friction of the tendon band as it rubs over the lateral femoral condyle. Clinically, pain symptoms are localized to the lateral aspect of the femoral condyle and may radiate up the side of the thigh to the hip. Motion of the knee is normal, but tightness and snapping may be perceived. Apart from well-localized tenderness, the knee examination is normal. Radiographs generally are normal, and MRI is not indicated.

Progressive healing is the rule with ITB syndrome. The athlete can continue moderate activities during this condition. Treatment consists of local icing both before and after activities, and frequent regular stretching of the lateral hip muscles and ITB.

METATARSALGIA

Metatarsalgia, which is more a description than a diagnosis, refers to a syndrome of pain in one or more metatarsophalangeal (MTP) joints due to a variety of causes, including capsulitis and synovitis, degenerative arthritis, neuroma, synovial cyst, and stress fracture. Synovitis and capsulitis are probably the most common causes. Although any of the MTP joints can be affected, the second MTP joint is the most commonly involved.

Biomechanical factors such as a hypermobile first MTP joint accompanied by a long second metatarsal can result in second MTP synovitis. Anterior ankle impingement may cause diffuse forefoot pain. Plantar fat pad atrophy and plantar flexion of the metatarsal may also cause MTP joint synovitis.

Physical findings associated with MTP joint synovitis include swelling and pain with manipulation of the joint. Vertical subluxation of the toe places pressure on the plantar capsule, eliciting pain.

Treatment is almost always conservative and is generally successful. Ice massage and anti-inflammatory medications reduce swelling and pain. Orthotics with metatarsal relief padding reduce stress on the joint and can be of great help. In resistant cases, an intra-articular injection is indicated. This should be done judiciously because repeated injections may be destructive to the ligamentous capsular support of the joint. Surgery, in the form of synovectomy and metatarsal osteotomy, is rarely necessary.

SECTION II

Rheumatoid Arthritis & Spondyloarthropathies

Rheumatoid Arthritis

17

James R. O'Dell, MD

ESSENTIALS OF DIAGNOSIS

- *Symptoms generally start in proximal interphalangeal (PIP), metacarpophalangeal (MCP), and metatarsophalangeal (MTP) joints.*
- *Symptoms must be present for 6 weeks.*
- *Diagnostic criteria include morning stiffness, arthritis in three joint areas, arthritis in hands, symmetric arthritis, rheumatoid nodules, serum rheumatoid factor, and radiographic changes.*

General Considerations

Rheumatoid arthritis (RA) is the second most common form of chronic arthritis and affects approximately 1% of the adult population worldwide. This potentially crippling disease shortens survival and, most importantly, significantly compromises quality of life in most affected patients. RA is an inflammatory disease of unknown etiology, and most patients have systemic features such as fatigue, low-grade fevers (≤ 38 °C), anemia, and elevations of acute phase reactants (erythrocyte sedimentation rates [ESR] and C-reactive protein [CRP] levels). Despite these systemic features, the primary target of this disease is the synovium. Some clinicians have likened RA to a cancer of the synovial tissues; these tissues proliferate in an uncontrolled fashion, resulting in excess fluid production and erosion of surrounding bone as well as tendon and ligament damage.

The good news is that over the last decade there has been a dramatic change in how clinicians think about and treat RA. Current therapeutic strategies, particularly if the disease is diagnosed and treated early, will result in substantial clinical benefit for the majority of patients.

Clinical Findings

A. SYMPTOMS AND SIGNS

RA may present at any age in any patient. However, it is more common in women (3:1) (Table 17–1). The typical age of onset in women is the late childbearing years, while men are often in their sixth to eighth decade. Although RA has a significant genetic component, most patients will have no significant family history. The onset may be fulminant, coming on almost overnight, but is more commonly insidious, building up over several weeks to months.

The distribution of involved joints is a critical clue to the underlying diagnosis (Figure 17–1). Most patients report involvement of small joints first, classically the PIP, MCP, and MTP joints, with involvement of large joints occurring later. Symptoms include pain, swelling, and stiffness, with stiffness often dominating, particular in the mornings. Rings that no longer fit are a common complaint.

1. Articular manifestations—RA can affect any of the synovial joints (Figure 17–1). Most commonly, the disease starts in the MCP, PIP, and MTP joints followed by the wrists, knees, elbows, ankles, hips, and shoulders in roughly that order. Early treatment helps limit the number of joints involved. Of particular importance, RA almost always spares the distal interphalangeal

Table 17–1. Classic manifestations.

- Gender: Female (3:1 ratio)
- Age: Late childbearing years in women (sixth to eighth decade in men)
- Onset: Insidious (builds up over several weeks to months)
- Distribution: Symmetric small joints—MCP, PIP, and MTP (spares DIP) joints
- Systemic: Fatigue, possible weight loss, occasional low-grade fevers
- Symptoms: Joint stiffness (worse in morning), pain, swelling
- Laboratory: Anemia, elevated ESR or CRP or both, thrombocytosis, positive rheumatoid factor in 60–80%

MCP, metacarpophalangeal; PIP, proximal interphalangeal; MTP, metatarsophalangeal; DIP, distal interphalangeal; ESR, erythrocyte sedimentation rate; CRP, C-reactive protein.

(DIP) joints (these joints are, however, often involved in osteoarthritis [OA] and psoriatic arthritis). RA may involve the temporomandibular, cricoarytenoid and sternoclavicular joints, but less commonly and usually in more advanced cases. RA may involve the upper part of the cervical spine, particularly the C1–C2 articulation, but, unlike the spondyloarthropathies rarely, if ever, involves the rest of the spine. Patients with RA are, however, at an increased risk for osteoporosis, and this risk should be considered and dealt with early.

The hands are a major site of involvement in almost all patients with RA; hand involvement is responsible for a significant portion of the disabilities caused by RA. Typical early disease is shown in Figure 17–2A with the swelling of the PIP joints easily seen. The DIP joints, are almost always spared unless the patient also has OA; both diseases are common and can coexist,

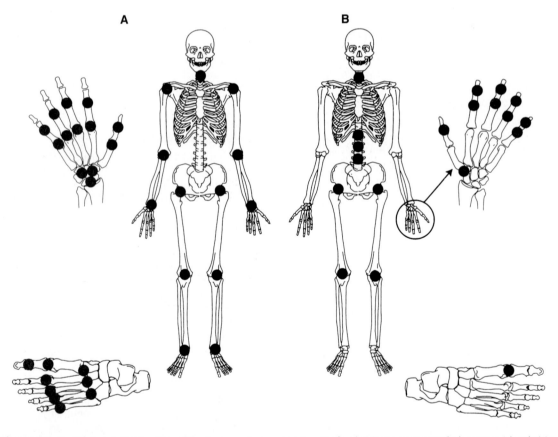

Figure 17–1. The joint distribution of the two most common types of arthritis are compared: rheumatoid arthritis (**A**) and osteoarthritis (**B**). Rheumatoid arthritis involves almost all synovial joints in the body. Osteoarthritis has a much more limited distribution. Importantly, rheumatoid arthritis rarely, if ever, involves the distal interphalangeal joints, but osteoarthritis commonly does.

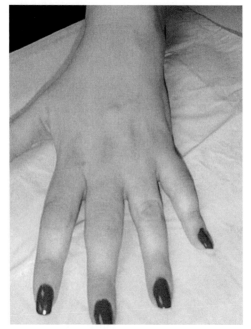

A

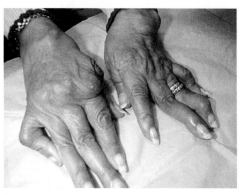

B

Figure 17–2. **A:** A patient with early rheumatoid arthritis. There are no joint deformities, but the soft tissue synovial swelling around the third and fifth proximal interphalangeal (PIP) joints is easily seen. **B:** A patient with advanced rheumatoid arthritis with severe joint deformities including subluxation at the metacarpophalangeal joints and swan neck deformities (hyperextension at the PIP joints.)

particularly in elderly patients. Figure 17–2B illustrates the classic ulnar deviation and swan neck deformities (hyperextension of the PIP joints) that are all too commonly seen in late, more established disease. Boutonnière (or buttonhole) deformities result from hyperextension of the MCP joints. If the clinical disease remains active, hand function will slowly deteriorate. Sudden loss of function of individual fingers may result from tendon ruptures, which will require the expertise of a carefully selected hand surgeon to repair.

Wrists are involved in most patients with RA; radial deviation is the rule, and patients with severe involvement may progress to volar subluxation. Even early in the course of the disease, synovial proliferation in and around the wrists may compress the median nerve, causing carpal tunnel syndrome. Later, this synovial proliferation may invade tendons and lead to rupture.

The feet, particularly the MTP joints, are involved early in almost all cases of RA and are second only to hand involvement in terms of the problems they cause. Radiographic erosions occur at least as early in the feet as in the hands. Subluxation of the toes, at the MTP joint, is common and leads to the dual problem of skin ulceration on the top of the toes and painful ambulation because of loss of the cushioning pads that protect the heads of the MTP joints.

Involvement of **large joints** (knees, ankles, elbows, hips, and shoulders) is common but generally occurs somewhat later than small joint involvement. Characteristically, the whole joint surface is involved in a symmetric fashion. Therefore, RA is not only symmetric from one side of the body to the other, but symmetric within the individual joint with the entire joint surface area involved. In the case of the knee (Figure 17–3A), the medial and lateral compartments are both severely narrowed in RA, whereas OA usually involves only one compartment (Figure 17–3B).

Fluctuant masses may occur around any of the joints (large or small) and represent synovial cysts. **Synovial cysts** from the knee are perhaps the best examples of this phenomenon. The knee produces excess synovial fluid that may accumulate in the popliteal space (popliteal or Baker cyst). These cysts may cause problems by pressing on the popliteal nerve, artery, or veins; they may dissect into the tissues of the calf (usually posteriorly); or they may rupture. Dissections may produce only minor symptoms such as a feeling of fullness; ruptures of the cyst with extravasation of the inflammatory content produce significant pain and swelling and may be confused with thrombophlebitis, the so-called pseudothrombophlebitis syndrome. Ultrasonography of the popliteal fossa and calf is useful to confirm the diagnosis and to rule out thrombophlebitis, which may be precipitated by popliteal cysts. Short-term treatment

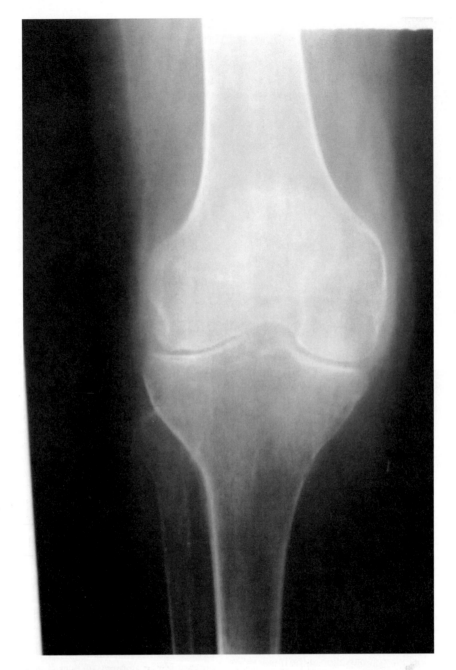

Figure 17-3. The radiographic features of rheumatoid arthritis and osteoarthritis are compared with regard to large joint involvement. **A:** Symmetric loss of cartilage space that is typical of inflammatory arthritis such as rheumatoid arthritis. Note that both the medial and lateral compartments are severely narrowed. Despite this severe narrowing, there is very little in the way of subchondral sclerosis or osteophyte formation since these repair mechanisms are generally shut off in active rheumatoid arthritis.

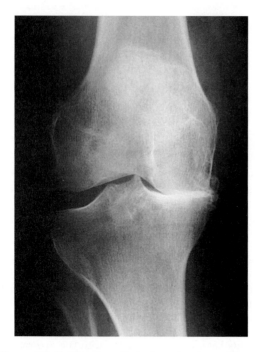

***Figure 17–3.* (Continued) B:** Complete loss of the cartilage in the medial joint compartment with significant subchondral sclerosis and osteophyte formation. The lateral compartment in this patient is not involved. These features are typical of osteoarthritis.

of popliteal cysts usually involves injecting the knee with glucocorticoids to interrupt the inflammatory process.

Most of the spine is spared in RA; however, the cervical spine (especially the C1–C2 articulation) is not. As with RA elsewhere, bony erosions and ligament damage can occur in this area and may lead to subluxation. Most often, subluxation is minor, and patients and caregivers need only be cautious and avoid forcing the neck into positions of flexion. Occasionally, it may be severe and require complex surgical intervention in an attempt to prevent compromise of the cervical cord and, in some cases, death.

Wherever synovial tissue exists, RA may cause problems; the temporomandibular, cricoarytenoid, and sternoclavicular joints are examples. The cricoarytenoid joint is responsible for abduction and adduction of the vocal cords. Involvement of this joint may lead to a feeling of fullness in the throat, to hoarseness, or rarely to a syndrome of acute respiratory distress with or without stridor when the cords are essentially fused in a closed position. In this latter situation, emergent tracheotomy may be lifesaving.

2. Extra-articular manifestations—RA is a systemic disease and features such as fatigue, weight loss, and low-grade fevers (≤ 38 °C) occur frequently, and like all the other extra-articular features, tend to be more common in those patients with rheumatoid factor (seropositive).

Subcutaneous nodules are seen in approximately one-quarter of patients with RA, almost exclusively in patients who are seropositive for rheumatoid factor. Patients with nodules but without rheumatoid factor should be carefully evaluated for an alternative diagnosis, such as chronic tophaceous gout. Nodules may occur almost anywhere (lungs, heart, and eye, for example), but most commonly occur subcutaneously on extensor surfaces (particularly forearms [Figure 17–4]), over joints or pressure points. They are firm on examination, are usually nontender (unless traumatized), have a characteristic histologic picture, and are thought to be triggered by small vessel vasculitis. A syndrome of increased nodulosis (despite good control of the disease) has been described with methotrexate therapy.

Digital infarcts and leukocytoclastic vasculitis are other features of RA-associated **small vessel vasculitis** and should prompt more aggressive treatment with disease-modifying antirheumatic drugs (DMARDs). A vasculitis of small and medium arteries, which is indistinguishable from **polyarteritis nodosa,** can be seen and requires aggressive systemic therapy. Finally, **pyoderma gangrenosum** occurs with increased frequency in patients with RA.

Clinical manifestations of **cardiac involvement** directly related to RA are uncommon; however, patients with RA have significantly increased morbidity and mortality from **coronary artery disease.** The reasons for this have not been completely elucidated, but chronic inflammation, some of the medications used, and sedentary lifestyle may be significant risk factors. **Pericardial effusions** are common (detected in up to 50% of patients by echocardiography) but are usually asymptomatic. Rarely, long-standing pericardial disease may result in a fibrinous pericarditis, and **constrictive pericarditis** may present clinically in these patients. Uncommonly, rheumatoid nodules may occur in the conduction system and cause heart block.

Pulmonary manifestations of RA include pleural effusions, rheumatoid nodules, and parenchymal lung disease. **Pleural effusions** occur more commonly in men and are usually small and asymptomatic. Of interest, pleural fluid in RA is characterized by low glucose and pH and, therefore, may at times be confused with empyema. **Rheumatoid nodules** may occur in the lung, especially in men; they are usually solid but may calcify, cavitate, or become infected. An aggressive diagnostic work-up should be performed when rheumatoid

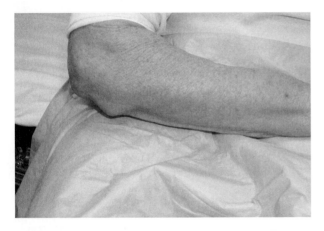

Figure 17–4. A rheumatoid nodule in a typical location on the extensor surface of the forearm is apparent in this patient with seropositive, erosive rheumatoid arthritis.

nodules are detected. Differentiating rheumatoid nodules from lung cancer may be difficult, particularly if they are solitary.

Diffuse interstitial fibrosis causes dyspnea and may progress to a honeycomb appearance on radiographs. Rarely, bronchiolitis obliterans can be seen with or without organizing pneumonia. Bronchiolitis obliterans carries a poor prognosis and may occur more often in association with D-penicillamine or gold therapy.

Keratoconjunctivitis sicca (dry eyes) from secondary **Sjögren syndrome** is the most common **ophthalmologic** manifestation of RA. Patients may have associated xerostomia (dry mouth), parotid gland swelling and occasionally, lymphadenopathy.

Scleritis, which also occurs in RA, is usually painful and can progress to thinning of the sclera (seen as a bluish discoloration as the deep pigment shows through) and even to perforation of the orbit (scleromalacia perforans).

Neurologic manifestations include peripheral nerve entrapment syndromes, such as carpal tunnel syndrome (entrapment of the median nerve at the wrist) and tarsal tunnel syndrome (entrapment of the anterior tibial nerve at the ankle). Vasculitis can lead to **mononeuritis multiplex** and a host of neurologic problems. Subluxations at C1–C2 can produce myelopathy. Rheumatoid nodules in the central nervous system have been described but are rare and usually asymptomatic.

Felty syndrome is the triad of RA, splenomegaly, and neutropenia. Felty syndrome is seen in patients with severe, seropositive disease and may be accompanied by hepatomegaly, thrombocytopenia, lymphadenopathy, and fevers. Most patients with Felty syndrome do not require specific therapy; instead, treatment should be focused on severe RA. Splenectomy may be indicated if severe neutropenia exists (< 500 cells/µL) accompanied by recurrent bacterial infections or chronic nonhealing leg ulcers. A few RA patients, who were previously thought to have Felty syndrome, have white blood cell counts dominated by large granular lymphocytes and have almost complete absence of neutrophils. This condition is known as the "large granular lymphocyte (LGL) syndrome" and is thought to be a variant of T-cell leukemia. When seen in the setting of RA, these patients have a good prognosis, with the neutropenia often responding dramatically to methotrexate therapy.

B. Laboratory Findings and Imaging

Anemia (of chronic disease) is seen in the majority of patients with RA, and the degree of anemia is proportional to the activity of the disease. Therapy that controls the disease will result in normalization of the hemoglobin. Rarely, erythropoietin administration may be indicated. Thrombocytosis is common, with platelet counts returning to normal as the inflammation is controlled. Acute phase reactants, **ESR** and **CRP** levels, also parallel the activity of the disease, and their persistent elevation portends a poor prognosis, both in terms of joint destruction and mortality. White blood cell counts may be elevated, normal, or in the case of Felty syndrome, profoundly depressed.

The most characteristic laboratory abnormality in RA is the presence of **rheumatoid factor.** Rheumatoid factor will be positive in about 50% of cases at presentation and 20–35% of cases will become positive in the first 6 months after diagnosis. Rheumatoid factor is an antibody that recognizes IgG as its antigen. Rheumatoid factor has an unfortunate name since it is not unique to RA and is seen in association with many other diseases, particularly in processes that provide chronic stimulation of the immune system (Table 17–2). In patients with RA, the presence of rheumatoid factor is strongly associated with more severe articular disease, as well as essentially all of the extra-articular features. RA is associated with multiple other autoantibodies, including **antinuclear antibodies** (ANA ~ 30%

Table 17–2. Differential of a positive rheumatoid factor.

- Rheumatic diseases
  — RA, Sjögren syndrome, SLE, others
- Infections
  — Viral: Hepatitis C, EBV, parvovirus, influenza, others
  — Bacterial: Endocarditis, osteomyelitis, others
- Chronic inflammatory conditions
  — Liver disease, inflammatory bowel, others
- Aging

RA, rheumatoid arthritis; SLE, systemic lupus erythematosus; EBV, Epstein-Barr virus.

of patients); anticyclic citrullinated peptide (CCP) antibodies (~80% of patients); and antineutrophil cytoplasmic antibodies (ANCA), particularly of the perinuclear type (~30% of patients).

Synovial fluid in RA is characterized by white blood cell counts in the 5000- to 50,000-per-microliter range with approximately two-thirds of the cells being neutrophils. Unfortunately, there are no synovial fluid findings that are pathognomonic of RA.

Making the Diagnosis

Unfortunately, there is no one single finding on physical examination or laboratory testing that is pathognomonic of RA. Instead, the diagnosis of RA is a clinical one, requiring a collection of historical and physical features, as well as an alert and informed clinician. Early consultation with a rheumatologist should occur to help solidify the diagnosis. Table 17–3 lists the classification criteria for RA, and although not designed specifically for the purpose of diagnosis, these criteria are ubiquitously used as a diagnostic aid. The first five criteria are all clinical; in other words, they are met by physical examination or talking to the patient. Only the last two criteria require

laboratory tests or radiographs. It is critical to note that the first four criteria need to be present for at least 6 weeks before a diagnosis of RA can be made. This is true because a host of conditions, including many viral-related syndromes, often cause self-limited polyarthritis syndromes that look identical to RA (Table 17–4), including, at times, the presence of rheumatoid factor. These syndromes, which usually last 2–3 weeks, have caused many clinicians to be overly cautious and delay the diagnosis of RA for months and sometimes years, resulting in delays in therapy. The goal for the majority of RA patients should be to establish a diagnosis and to start DMARD therapy by 3 months of disease.

Although most patients with RA present with the onset of pain, stiffness, and swelling in multiple joints over the course of weeks to months, some may have a fulminant presentation and other may have an onset so insidious that the patient hardly notices. Alternatively, patients may have persistent monoarthritis or oligoarthritis for prolonged periods before manifesting the more typical pattern of polyarticular involvement. Rarely, patients may present with extra-articular features of RA before the joint problems occur.

The distribution of involved joints is a critical clue to the underlying diagnosis (Figure 17–1). The joints that are involved in patients with RA at presentation are also variable; the typical presentation has been described above. While the patient's history of joint symptoms (arthralgia) is important, the diagnosis of RA requires the presence of inflammation (swelling or warmth or both) on examination of the joints.

Morning stiffness is a hallmark of inflammatory arthritis and is a prominent feature of RA. Patients with RA are characteristically at their worst first thing in the morning or after prolonged periods of rest. This stiffness in and around joints will often last for hours and quantifying it is one way to measure improvement. Stiffness is relieved by warmth and activity, and reducing or eliminating it is a clear goal of therapy.

Table 17–3. American College of Rheumatology criteria for rheumatoid arthritis.

- Morning stiffness[a]
- Arthritis of three joint areas[a]
- Arthritis of the hands[a]
- Symmetric arthritis[a]
- Rheumatoid nodules
- Serum rheumatoid factor
- Radiographic changes

---

[a]These criteria must be present for more than 6 weeks.

Table 17–4. Differential diagnosis.

- Viral syndromes, especially hepatitis B and C, Epstein-Barr virus, parvovirus, rubella
- Psoriatic arthritis
- Reactive arthritis
- Tophaceous gout
- Systemic lupus erythematosus
- Calcium pyrophosphate disease
- Polymyalgia rheumatica
- Osteoarthritis, especially hereditary osteoarthritis of the hand
- Sarcoidosis, Lyme disease, rheumatic fever, etc

Differential Diagnosis

While the early and accurate diagnosis of RA may at times be challenging, it is now more critical than ever if patients are to benefit maximally from the many effective therapeutic interventions that are available. Once disease has been present and active for a number of years and the characteristic deformities on physical examination (Figure 17–2B) and radiographs (Figure 17–3A) have occurred, the diagnosis in most cases is all too obvious. Unfortunately, once deformities are present, they will not respond to medical therapy.

Since many diseases can mimic RA (particularly early in its course), it is critical to rule out these processes (Table 17–4). **Viral syndromes,** especially hepatitis B and C, parvovirus, rubella (infection or vaccination), and Epstein-Barr virus need to be considered since they may produce a self-limited syndrome that can mimic RA for their duration (usually 2 to 4 weeks). Obviously, the key here is the duration of symptoms. **Systemic lupus erythematosus, psoriatic arthritis,** and **reactive arthritis** may present diagnostic challenges. With these three mimics, a targeted history and examination to elucidate their associated clinical features (such as rashes, oral ulcers, nail changes, dactylitis, and urethritis) and renal, pulmonary, gastrointestinal or ophthalmologic problems is critical. Hypothyroidism, which causes a collection of rheumatic manifestations and also occurs commonly in conjunction with RA, should be kept in mind. In the elderly with fulminant-onset RA, remitting seronegative symmetric synovitis with pitting edema (RS3PE) or paraneoplastic syndromes should be considered. Chronic tophaceous gout may mimic severe nodular RA. Finally, OA with severe deformities of the hands from bony proliferation of the DIP and PIP joints (Heberden and Bouchard nodes) may confuse some inexperienced clinicians; the keys here are DIP joint involvement and the bony, instead of soft tissue, involvement.

Treatment

There is no cure for RA; it is a lifelong disease process that requires lifelong therapies. These factors magnify the importance of the patient-physician interaction, and since many treatment options exist, a premium is often placed on the art rather than the science of medicine. The optimal care for patients with RA always requires effective interactions between primary care physicians and rheumatologists; often physical therapists, occupational therapists, and orthopedic surgeons will need to be part of the team as well. Because of the serious nature of the disease, the rapid introduction of new treatments, and the need for expertise in monitoring these therapies, the importance of all patients with RA being monitored by a rheumatologist needs to be emphasized. Often, once the diagnosis is established and therapeutic programs are in place, follow-up may be primarily with primary care physicians, with rheumatologists involved two to four times per year.

The goal of therapy for RA is to put the disease in remission and to maintain this remission by continuing therapy. If RA is treated early using currently available therapies (Figure 17–5), remission is possible in 20–40% of patients. Unfortunately, remissions require the ongoing use of medications and even then are not always long-lasting. Some combination of nonsteroidal anti-inflammatory drugs (NSAIDs), glucocorticoids, and DMARDs will be necessary in almost all patients. In many and perhaps most patients, combinations of different DMARDs or DMARDs plus biologics will be necessary for optimal control. It is of critical importance that therapy be escalated rapidly to assure maximal suppression of disease with minimal toxicity and expense. In addition, all patients with RA should be educated about their disease and the therapies that will be used. In most cases, patients should have an opportunity to spend time with physical and occupational therapists to learn about range of motion exercises, joint protection, and assistive devices. When treating RA, four types of medical therapies are used: NSAIDs, glucocorticoids, DMARDs, and biologics (Figure 17–5).

NSAIDs are important for symptomatic relief; however, they play only a minor role, if any, in altering the underlying disease process. Therefore, NSAIDs should rarely, if ever, be used to treat RA without the concomitant use of DMARDs. Many clinicians waste valuable time switching from one NSAID to another before starting DMARD therapy.

Much has been written about the gastrointestinal toxicity of NSAIDs, and many of these concerns are particularly relevant to RA patients who have a significant number of risk factors that are associated with toxicities. Therefore, selective cyclooxygenase-2 (COX-2) agents have been particularly popular in this group of patients. Several caveats should be kept in mind. RA patients have a significantly increased risk of cardiovascular problems, and since COX-2 drugs provide little antiplatelet activity, many of these patients will need to take low-dose aspirin therapy in addition to the selective COX-2 drug. The effect the addition of aspirin has on gastrointestinal toxicity is unclear. In addition, the COX-2 drugs appear to differ little from the nonselective COX agents in terms of their effects on the kidney and on blood pressure.

Glucocorticoids have had a significant role in the treatment of RA for over half a century. RA was chosen as the first disease to test this new therapy in 1948, partly because it was believed that RA was a disease of glucocorticoid deficiency (an issue that remains unresolved). As was the case with the first patient treated in

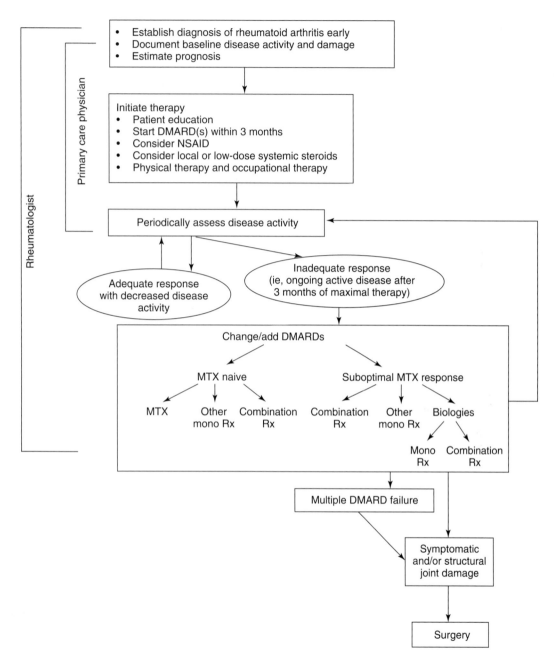

Figure 17–5. Guidelines for the management of rheumatoid arthritis. (Adapted from the American College of Rheumatology 2002 Guidelines for the Management of Rheumatoid Arthritis.)

1948, glucocorticoid therapy can be dramatically and rapidly effective in patients with RA. Glucocorticoids are not only useful for symptomatic improvement, but significantly decrease the radiographic progression of RA. Unfortunately, the toxicities of long-term glucocorticoid therapy are legend. Therefore, the optimal use of these drugs requires an understanding of the principles of glucocorticoid use in RA (Table 17–5).

Glucocorticoids remain among the most potent anti-inflammatory treatments available; because of this and their rapid onset of action, they are ideally suited to help control the inflammation in RA while the much slower acting DMARDs are starting to work. Prednisone, the most commonly used glucocorticoid, should rarely be used in doses higher than 10 mg/d to treat the articular manifestations of RA. This dose should be slowly tapered to the lowest effective dose and the concomitant DMARD therapy adjusted to make this possible. Glucocorticoids should rarely, if ever, be used to treat RA without concomitant DMARD therapy. The paradigm is to shut off inflammation rapidly with glucocorticoids, and then to taper them as the DMARD is kicking in ("bridge therapy"). In all patients receiving glucocorticoids, strong consideration should be given to the prevention of osteoporosis, and bisphosphonates have been shown to be particularly effective in this regard. Higher doses of glucocorticoids may be necessary for extra-articular manifestations, especially for vasculitis and scleritis.

DMARDs are a group of medications that have the ability to modify or change the course of RA. Drugs included in this class have, in most cases, met the "gold standard" of halting or slowing the radiographic progression of RA. Included in this group of medications are methotrexate, sulfasalazine, gold, antimalarials, leflunomide, azathioprine, penicillamine, and minocycline. It is critically important that clinicians and patients alike understand that these medications take 2–6 months to reach maximal effect. Therefore, other measures, such as glucocorticoid therapy, may be needed to control the disease while these medications are starting to work.

Table 17–5. Glucocorticoid treatment guidelines.

- Prednisone > 10 mg/d rarely indicated for articular disease
- Avoid using glucocorticoids without DMARDs
- Use glucocorticoids as a "bridge" to effective DMARD therapy
- Minimized duration and dose: Taper to the lowest dose that controls arthritis
- Always consider prophylaxis to avoid osteoporosis

DMARDs, disease-modifying antirheumatic drugs.

All of the above-mentioned DMARDs have been shown to be effective in treating both early and more advanced RA. The choice of which DMARD to start with depends on patient and physician concerns about toxicity and monitoring issues as well as the activity of disease and comorbid conditions. Until additional research elucidates factors that allow clinicians to select the best initial therapy for each patient, there are many reasonable choices for initial therapy. The critical factor is not which DMARD to start first, but the fact that DMARD therapy is started early in the disease process.

Methotrexate is the preferred DMARD of most rheumatologists, in part because patients have a more durable response, and when monitored correctly, serious toxicities are rare. Methotrexate is dramatically effective in slowing the radiographic progression of RA and is usually given orally in doses ranging from 5 to 25 mg as a single dose once a week. **This once a week administration is worthy of emphasis;** prior experience with daily therapy in psoriasis has taught us the importance of allowing the liver time to recover between doses. Oral absorption of methotrexate is variable; therefore, subcutaneous methotrexate may be effective when oral is not. Side effects include oral ulcers, nausea, hepatotoxicity, bone marrow suppression, and pneumonitis. With the exception of pneumonitis, these toxicities respond to dose adjustments. Monitoring of blood cell counts and liver blood tests (albumin and alanine transaminase or aspartate transaminase) should be done every 4–8 weeks for the duration of methotrexate therapy, with dosage adjustments as needed. Renal function is critical for clearance of methotrexate; previously stable patients may experience severe toxicities when renal function deteriorates. Pneumonitis, while rare, is less predictable and may be fatal, particularly if the methotrexate is not stopped or is restarted. Importantly, folic acid in the dose of 1–4 mg/d can significantly decrease most methotrexate toxicities without apparent loss of efficacy against RA. Methotrexate in combination with sulfasalazine and hydroxychloroquine has been shown to be more effective than methotrexate alone.

Hydroxychloroquine or chloroquine is frequently used for the treatment of RA. They have the least toxicity of any of the DMARDs and do not require monitoring of blood tests. Yearly monitoring by an ophthalmologist is recommended to pick up any signs of retinal toxicity (rare). Hydroxychloroquine is the most commonly used preparation and is given orally 200–400 mg/d. These drugs are frequently used in combination with other DMARDs, particularly methotrexate.

Sulfasalazine is the most commonly used DMARD in Europe. It is an effective treatment when given in doses of 1–3 g/d. Monitoring blood cell counts, particularly white blood cell counts, in the first 6 months is recommended. **Minocycline,** 100 mg twice daily, has been shown to be an effective treatment for RA, particularly when used in early seropositive disease. Long-term therapy (more than 2 years) with minocycline may lead to cutaneous hyperpigmentation.

Leflunomide, a pyrimidine antagonist, is the newest DMARD approved for use in RA. It has a very long half-life and is given daily in a dose of 10–20 mg. Previously, because of the long half-life, a loading dose of 100 mg/d for 3 days was given but is no longer recommended by most experts (due to increased diarrhea, etc). The most common toxicity is diarrhea, which may respond to dose reduction. Also, because of its long half-life and its teratogenic potential, women wishing to become pregnant who have previously received leflunomide (even if therapy was years ago) should have blood levels drawn. If toxicity occurs or if pregnancy is being considered, leflunomide can be rapidly eliminated from the body with cholestyramine.

Gold, the oldest DMARD, when given intramuscularly, remains an extremely effective therapy for a small percentage of patients. It is less commonly used because of its slow onset of action, need for intramuscular administration, frequent monitoring required (complete blood cell count and urinalysis), and frequent toxicities. Toxicities include skin rashes, bone marrow suppression, and proteinuria.

Biological therapies have had a significant impact on the treatment of patients with RA. Recent research has continued to elucidate the central role that cytokines, most notably tumor necrosis factor-α (TNF-α) and interleukin-1 (IL)-1, play in the pathophysiology of RA. This has lead directly to the development and clinical use of biological agents directed against TNF-α (**etanercept** and **infliximab**) and IL-1 (**anakinra**). Etanercept is a recombinant TNF receptor fusion protein and is administered subcutaneously 25 mg twice weekly. Infliximab is a mouse/human chimeric monoclonal antibody against TNF-α that is given intravenously (3–10 mg/kg) every 4–8 weeks. Both have been shown to be highly effective against both clinical symptoms and radiographic progression of RA. A rapid onset of action (days to weeks) is apparent with both of these agents and is a significant advantage that these treatments have over conventional DMARDs. Current disadvantages include cost and concern about long-term toxicities, in particular infections (especially tuberculosis) and demyelinating syndromes. Unfortunately, there is a paucity of data comparing biologics with conventional DMARD therapy.

Anakinra, a recombinant human IL-1 receptor antagonist, is given subcutaneously 100 mg/d. It has been shown to be effective against signs and symptoms of RA, as well as radiographic progression. Its onset of action is somewhat slower and less dramatic than the TNF inhibitors. Toxicities include injection site reactions and pneumonia (especially in patients with asthma).

Optimal care of patients with RA requires a recognition of the **comorbid conditions** that are associated with RA, including an increased risk of cardiovascular death, osteoporosis, infections (especially pneumonia) and certain cancers. Increasingly, cardiovascular disease is being recognized as the cause of much of the excess mortality in RA. A number of factors probably contribute to this, including sedentary lifestyle, glucocorticoid therapy, and treatments that increase homocysteine levels such as methotrexate and sulfasalazine. However, with the recent identification of the strong association between chronic inflammation and cardiovascular disease, it is likely that this may be the most significant factor. Therapies that control RA earlier and better can be expected to decrease cardiovascular morbidity and mortality. A recent study indicates that methotrexate decreases cardiovascular mortality by 70% in patients with RA. Clinicians should consider RA a risk factor for cardiovascular disease and should aggressively address other cardiovascular risk factors in these patients.

Osteoporosis is ubiquitous in patients with RA, and early therapy directed at this problem will result in long-term benefits. Patients with RA are at an increased risk for infections, and this risk is further increased by some therapies. Patients should be cautioned to seek medical attention early for even minor symptoms suggestive of infection, especially if receiving anti-TNF therapy. All patients with RA should receive pneumococcal and yearly influenza vaccinations. Finally, patients with RA have an increased risk of lymphomas. Occasionally, B-cell lymphomas may be associated with immunosuppression and regress after immunosuppression is discontinued. Interestingly, RA patients have significantly decreased risk (odds ratio = 0.2) of developing colon cancer. This is thought to be secondary to chronic inhibition of COX by NSAIDs in this group of patients.

Complications

Historically, RA has been described as an indolent and relatively benign disease. Unfortunately, it is now clear that once established, RA is a lifelong, progressive disease that produces significant morbidity in most and premature mortality in many. Long-term studies have found that 50% of RA patients have had to stop working after 10 years (approximately 10 times the average rate). Patients who are rheumatoid factor positive and those who have HLA-DR alleles expressing the shared epitope have a worse prognosis with more erosions and more extra-articular disease. Once deformities are found on examination or erosions on radiography, the damage is largely irreversible. It has been clearly shown that erosions occur in the majority of patients in the first 1 or 2 years and that the rate of radiographic damage can be affected by early therapy. Therefore, early DMARD therapy is critical. Although, long-term data are not yet available, short-term data strongly suggest that current patients have the opportunity to benefit greatly if the newer principles of therapy are practiced (Table 17–6).

When to Refer to a Specialist

Consultation with a rheumatologist should be the rule for all patients with RA. This is important to establish a definitive diagnosis early and to initiate appropriate therapy. Once the diagnosis has been established, patients should be seen by a rheumatologist two to four times per year with primary care physicians closely involved for management of associated comorbid conditions, as well as to address other health care problems.

Additional situations that should precipitate prompt referral should include persistent active disease (swollen and tender joints) or declining functional capacity; toxicities or concern for possible toxicities; red swollen joints, particularly if out of proportion to other joints; and extra-articular disease (eg, vasculitis, pulmonary involvement, eye involvement).

Prognosis

The duration of disease prior to DMARD therapy may be one of the strongest predictors of outcome; therefore, making the correct diagnosis quickly is of critical importance. All current treatment paradigms for RA stress the early aggressive use of DMARDs.

Table 17–6. Keys to optimize outcome.

- Early diagnosis
- DMARD therapy as early as possible
- Strive for remissions in all patients
- Recognize and treat comorbid conditions
- Cooperation and communication between primary care physician and rheumatologist

DMARD, disease-modifying antirheumatic drug.

REFERENCES

American College of Rheumatology Subcommittee on Rheumatoid Arthritis Guidelines. 2002 Update: guidelines for the management of rheumatoid arthritis. *Arthritis Rheum.* 2002;46: 328. [PMID: 11840435]. (State of the art guidelines for the treatment of rheumatoid arthritis as formulated by the American College of Rheumatology in 2002.)

Bathon JM, et al. A comparison of etanercept and methotrexate in patients with early rheumatoid arthritis. *N Engl J Med.* 2000; 343:1586. [PMID: 11096165] (An important article focusing on the use of biologics in the treatment of early rheumatoid arthritis.)

Gabriel SE. The epidemiology of rheumatoid arthritis. *Rheum Dis Clin North Am.* 2001;27:269. [PMID: 11396092] (This is an excellent article on the epidemiology of rheumatoid arthritis.)

Goldbach-Mansky R, et al. Rheumatoid arthritis associated autoantibodies in patients with synovitis of recent onset. *Arthritis Res.* 2000;2:236. [PMID: 11056669] (This study of patients with early rheumatoid arthritis is a terrific summary of what is known about early antibody markers of rheumatoid arthritis.)

Lipsky PE, et al. Infliximab and methotrexate in the treatment of rheumatoid arthritis. *N Engl J Med.* 2000;343:1594. [PMID: 11096166] (An important article that focuses on the use of biologics in the treatment of advanced rheumatoid arthritis.)

Mikuls TR, Saag KG. Comorbidity in rheumatoid arthritis. *Rheum Dis Clin North Am.* 2001;27:283. [PMID: 11396093] (This article summarizes the importance of comorbidity in rheumatoid arthritis and discusses strategies to address these comorbid conditions.)

Moreland LW, O'Dell JR. Glucocorticoids and rheumatoid arthritis: back to the future? *Arthritis Rheum.* 2002;46:2553. [PMID: 12384910] (This article reviews the use of glucocorticoids in the treatment of rheumatoid arthritis from their initial use in 1949 to the current use. It also reviews toxicities and measures to help prevent these toxicities.)

O'Dell JR. Treating rheumatoid arthritis early: a window of opportunity? *Arthritis Rheum.* 2002;46:283. [PMID: 11840429] (This editorial summarizes the rationale for treating patients with rheumatoid arthritis early in their course of disease and discusses different approaches.)

O'Dell JR, et al. Treatment of rheumatoid arthritis with methotrexate alone, sulfasalazine, and hydroxychloroquine, or a combination of all three medications. *N Engl J Med.* 1996;334: 1287. [PMID: 8609945] (This is the classic initial paper that showed that combinations of DMARDs are superior to what had previously been the gold standard, methotrexate, in the treatment of patients with rheumatoid arthritis.)

Relevant World Wide Web Sites

[American College of Rheumatology]
http://www.rheumatology.org

Spondyloarthropathies

Jennifer D. Gorman, MD, MPH

The spondyloarthropathies are a group of inflammatory diseases characterized by enthesitis (inflammation at sites where tendons, ligaments, and joint capsule insert onto bone), arthritis of the axial skeleton (sacroiliac joints and spine), and an oligoarticular arthritis of peripheral joints. Inheritance of HLA-B27 increases the relative risk of developing spondyloarthropathy, particularly when there is involvement of the axial skeleton. These diseases are not associated with rheumatoid factor and thus are often referred to as the "seronegative" spondyloarthropathies.

The spondyloarthropathies are ankylosing spondylitis, reactive arthritis, psoriatic arthritis, and enteropathic arthritis (arthritis associated with inflammatory bowel disease). Although these conditions share a number of features, each one has distinct epidemiologic and clinical features that distinguish it from the others (Table 18–1). Some patients, particularly those early in the disease course, cannot be clearly placed in one of these disease categories and are referred to as having "undifferentiated spondyloarthropathy."

Enthesitis is a characteristic feature of spondyloarthropathy and is observed in only a few other inflammatory arthropathies (primarily gout, disseminated gonococcal infection, and sarcoidosis). Enthesitis is the hallmark of spondyloarthropathy in children (juvenile spondyloarthropathy; Chapter 5), and in many cases, the disease is limited to this manifestation. Dactylitis, the distinctive sausage-like swelling of a finger or toe, has increased specificity for psoriatic arthritis and reactive arthritis. The characteristic clinical appearance is caused by inflammation of the tendons and, in some cases, the adjacent synovium.

On average, 9 years elapse between the onset of symptoms and the eventual diagnosis of a spondyloarthropathy. Because primary care physicians are typically the first to evaluate these patients, they can play a major role by identifying affected individuals earlier in the course of the disease.

ANKYLOSING SPONDYLITIS

 ESSENTIALS OF DIAGNOSIS

- *Inflammatory back pain in young adults.*
- *Radiographic demonstration of sacroiliitis.*
- *Reductions in spinal mobility, particularly lumbar flexion.*
- *Association with anterior uveitis.*
- *Increased relative risk conferred by inheritance of HLA-B27.*
- *Positive family history.*

General Considerations

Ankylosing spondylitis is regarded as the prototype of the spondyloarthropathies. Axial skeletal involvement predominates in ankylosing spondylitis, which invariably involves the sacroiliac joints and typically presents with the insidious onset of inflammatory low back pain during late adolescence or early adulthood. Onset of symptoms after the age of 40 is uncommon.

Although environmental factors are important in the development of ankylosing spondylitis, the environmental triggers appear to be ubiquitous, and genetic background is the major determinant of susceptibility to ankylosing spondylitis. The only known susceptibility gene, HLA-B27, confers a relative risk of close to 100 but probably accounts for only 10–50% of the overall genetic risk for ankylosing spondylitis.

The disease course varies considerably, ranging from mild disease with little impact on functional status to severe disease that produces substantial disability. The

Table 18–1. Clinical and epidemiological features of the spondyloarthropathies.

	Ankylosing Spondylitis	Psoriatic Arthritis	Reactive Arthritis	Enteropathic Arthritis
Prevalence[a]	0.1%	0.1%	> 0.05%	> 0.05%
Male: female ratio	3:1	1:1	9:1	1:1
Axial arthritis				
Frequency	100%	20%	20%	15%
Radiographic features				
Sacroiliitis	Bilateral	Unilateral	Unilateral	Bilateral
Syndesmophytes	Symmetric Marginal	Asymmetric Bulky	Asymmetric Bulky	Symmetric Marginal
Peripheral arthritis				
Frequency	25%	60–95%	90%	20%
Typical distribution	Monoarticular, oligoarticular	Oligoarticular, polyarticular	Monoarticular, oligoarticular	Monoarticular, oligoarticular
Typical affected joints	Hip, knee, ankle	Knee, ankle, DIPs	Knee, ankle	Knee, ankle
Uveitis frequency	30%	15%	15–20%	~5%
Dactylitis frequency	Uncommon	~25%	~30–50%	Uncommon
Cutaneous findings	None specific	Psoriasis Onycholysis Nail pitting	Oral ulcerations Keratoderma blennorrhagica	Erythema nodosum Pyoderma gangrenosa
HLA-B27 positivity[a]				
All cases	90%	40%	50–80%	30%
With axial disease	90%	50%	90%	50%

[a]Disease prevalence and HLA-B27 positivity greatly vary according to geographic and race/ethnicity.
DIPs, distal interphalangeal joints.

extent of spinal involvement is a major determinant of the impact of the disease on functional status. Unfortunately, there are no reliable predictors of long-term functional outcome early in the disease course.

Clinical Findings

A. SYMPTOMS AND SIGNS

1. Axial spine—The typical presenting symptom in ankylosing spondylitis is the insidious onset of inflammatory low back pain due to sacroiliitis. The pain is dull and located in the lower lumbar regions, although some describe a deep alternating buttock pain. The characteristic inflammatory nature of the pain differentiates it from mechanical back pain; most notably, the pain worsens with rest, improves with activity, and is accompanied by morning stiffness that lasts 30 minutes or longer. Patients often describe awakening from sleep and pacing in order to relieve nocturnal pain—a rare complaint in patients with mechanical back pain.

There may be few objective findings in patients with early disease, making diagnosis a challenge. Palpation and specific maneuvers can elicit pain in the sacroiliac joints, but these tests are relatively insensitive and non-

specific due to the number of other anatomic structures that overlap within the same area.

Involvement of the spine (spondylitis) is the major source of morbidity. Unlike rheumatoid arthritis, which only affects the cervical spine, ankylosing spondylitis can involve the lumbar, thoracic, and cervical spine. Over time the accumulation of pathologic changes can lead to loss of spinal mobility, particularly of the lumbar spine. The **Schober test** is the standard examination to assess impaired lumbar flexion. Two marks are made on the patient's back: one at the level of the sacral dimples (approximately at the fifth lumbar spinous process) and the other 10 cm above. The patient then bends forward as far as possible (ie, attempts to touch toes with knees extended), and the distance between the two marks is again measured. In normal individuals, the overlying skin will stretch to 15 cm; values less than this can be indicative of reduced lumbar mobility. Some clinicians prefer the **modified Schober test** in which marks are made 5 cm below and 10 cm above the sacral dimples; the distance between these marks increases from 15 cm to at least 20 cm with lumbar flexion. Reductions in lumbar lateral bending and rotation are also commonly observed. Spinal fusion results in irreversible impairments, but reductions in mobility also can be induced by pain or muscle spasm and, therefore, vary somewhat with time and treatment. With advancing disease, a characteristic posture often develops as the spine fuses in flexion, leading to loss of lumbar lordosis, exaggeration of thoracic kyphosis, an inability to extend the neck, and compensatory hip flexion deformities (Figure 18–1). The extent of spondylitis varies greatly, from minimal to complete fusion of the cervical, thoracic, and lumbar spine.

Involvement of the costovertebral and costochondral joints commonly leads to impaired chest expansion (< 5 cm difference between full inspiration and full expiration when measured at the fourth intercostal space) and occasionally produces pain with deep breathing, coughing, or sneezing.

2. Peripheral joint manifestations—Peripheral arthritis, typically monarticular or asymmetric oligoarticular, develops in approximately one-third of patients with ankylosing spondylitis and most often affects large joints of the lower extremities. Hip disease is a major source of morbidity.

3. Enthesitis—Involvement of insertion sites around the pelvis (the ischial tuberosities, iliac crests, and greater trochanters) is common and appears on radiographs as bony "whiskering" at these sites of attachment. Achilles tendinitis and enthesitis at the site of the insertion of the plantar fascia onto the calcaneus can cause unilateral or bilateral heel pain, although not as often as in reactive arthritis.

4. Ocular—The most common extra-articular manifestation of ankylosing spondylitis is acute anterior uveitis, and one-third of patients experience at least one episode. It is heralded by the acute onset of unilateral eye pain, photophobia, blurred vision, and increased lacrimation. Ciliary flush (an increased conjunctival injection at the rim of the iris) is a characteristic finding (Figure 18–2). The presence of cells and flare in the anterior uveal chamber detected by slit-lamp examination establishes the diagnosis. The need for specialized equipment and expertise necessitates prompt ophthalmologic consultation when this diagnosis is suspected. Anterior uveitis can precede the onset of ankylosing spondylitis by several years, and a history of anterior uveitis is a helpful diagnostic clue in a patient with inflammatory back pain or other symptoms of ankylosing spondylitis. Anterior uveitis is strongly associated with HLA-B27.

5. Other organs—The majority of patients with ankylosing spondylitis have histologic evidence of inflammation on biopsy specimens of the small or large bowel. These changes are asymptomatic but may be of pathogenetic importance in view of the link between clini-

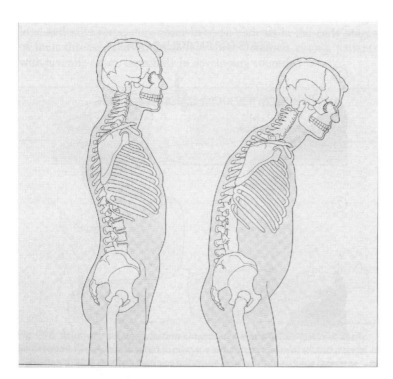

Figure 18–1. Characteristic posture in ankylosing spondylitis with advanced spinal disease. There is a loss of the lumbar lordosis, exaggeration of thoracic kyphosis, and compensatory hip flexion deformities. Severe deformity can interfere with the ability to look straight ahead. (Reprinted from Khan MA. Ankylosing spondylitis: clinical features. In: Klippel JH, Dieppe PA, eds. *Rheumatology*. Elsevier, © 1994, p 3.25.4. With permission from Elsevier Science.)

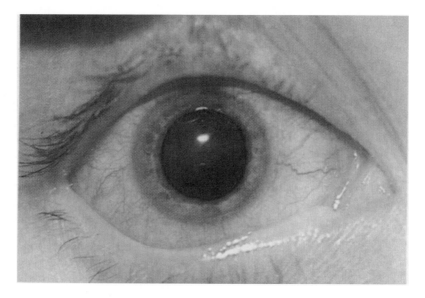

Figure 18–2. Acute anterior uveitis. Pinkish to purple conjunctival injection appearing around the iris is the result of uveal inflammation. The pupil is dilated in this picture to prevent damage to the edges of the pupil. (Reprinted from Shipley M. *A Colour Atlas of Rheumatology.* Elsevier, © 1993, p 82. With permission from Elsevier Science.)

cally overt inflammatory bowel disease and spondyloarthropathy and the apparent importance of colitis in the transgenic rat model of HLA-B27-associated disease.

Cardiac involvement in the form of ascending aortitis, aortic regurgitation, conduction abnormalities, and myocardial disease occurs in approximately 10% of patients with ankylosing spondylitis, and, like uveitis and axial disease, is strongly associated with HLA-B27. The prevalence of aortic regurgitation, which is the most common cardiac problem, increases with the duration of disease but remains < 10% even after 30 years of disease.

Restriction in chest wall motion from enthesitis or bony fusion commonly produces mild impairment of pulmonary function; characteristic spirometry findings include a slight reduction of vital and total lung capacity and normal diffusion capacity. Most patients, however, are asymptomatic, and clinically significant pulmonary disease is uncommon. A rare pulmonary finding in ankylosing spondylitis is the development of apical fibrobullous disease that radiographically resembles reactivation of tuberculosis and that can become a site for bacterial or fungal infections.

Of the neurologic consequences of spondyloarthritis, the most important is spinal fracture, which often goes unrecognized and leads to neurologic compromise in about one-third of cases (see the following section, Complications). Cauda equina syndrome can develop in long-standing ankylosing spondylitis and is associated with large subarachnoid diverticula on magnetic resonance imaging.

Rare manifestations of the spondyloarthropathies include the late development of secondary amyloidosis. An association of ankylosing spondylitis with retroperitoneal fibrosis has been suggested.

B. Laboratory Findings

Routine laboratory investigations often reveal a mild, normocytic, normochromic anemia, reflective of chronic disease. Only about half of patients with active disease will have elevations of the erythrocyte sedimentation rate or C-reactive protein. These inflammatory markers appear to correlate more with peripheral arthritis than the activity of axial skeleton disease. There is no association with rheumatoid factor or antinuclear antibodies.

No laboratory test is diagnostic of ankylosing spondylitis or the other spondyloarthropathies. Inheritance of HLA-B27 is strongly associated with these diseases, but **testing for HLA-B27** has limited usefulness in clinical practice. Several key facts should inform the use and the interpretation of this test. First, inheritance of HLA-B27 is not sufficient to produce spondyloarthropathy. The great majority of HLA-B27-positive persons (95% in some studies) do not have a spondyloarthropathy, and indiscriminate testing for HLA-B27 will produce many more false-positive tests for spondyloarthropathy than true positives. Second, inheritance of HLA-B27 is not absolutely essential for the development of a spondyloarthropathy (Table 18–1). Third, the strength of the association between HLA-B27 and disease varies according to the presence of axial involvement and the specific spondyloarthropathy (Table 18–1). Fourth, there are important ethnic differences in the prevalence of HLA-B27 in normal populations. Finally, although HLA-B27 confers an increased relative risk of spondyloarthropathy in most ethnic groups studied, ethnicity influences the prevalence of HLA-B27 in disease populations. For example, HLA-B27 is present in 8% of the general white population, and 90% of whites with ankylosing spondylitis are HLA-B27 positive. In contrast, HLA-B27 is present in 2% of the African American population and in 50% of African Americans with ankylosing spondylitis. Therefore, in a patient with symptoms suggestive of ankylosing spondylitis, the absence of HLA-B27 substantially decreases the probability of disease if the patient is white but not if the patient is African American.

In general, HLA-B27 testing should only be ordered in patients with inflammatory back pain when the diagnosis is uncertain after appropriate clinical evaluation and radiographs. Even when used in these circumstances, however, the test results only increase or reduce the probability of disease and do not establish or exclude the diagnosis. Because the presence of HLA-B27 does not have important therapeutic or prognostic implications, there is no need to order the test in patients with known disease.

C. IMAGING STUDIES

The inflammatory disease of the axial spine results in characteristic pathologic changes; however, it may take years before these become evident by plain radiographic techniques.

1. Sacroiliac joints—The most distinctive finding is inflammation of both sacroiliac joints. A standard anteroposterior radiograph of the pelvis is commonly used to evaluate these S-shaped joints, although some believe a superior image is achieved with the Ferguson view, in which the radiograph is taken at a 15-degree angle to the prone pelvis.

The first radiographic finding is the appearance of iliac erosions, described as resembling postage stamp serrations, in the lower one-third of the sacroiliac joint (Figure 18–3). With time, the erosions become more prominent and produce "pseudowidening" of the sacroiliac joint. Progressive inflammation leads to fusion, and the end result can be complete obliteration of the sacroiliac joint by bone and fibrous tissue (Figure 18–4). The pattern of sacroiliac joint involvement is bilaterally

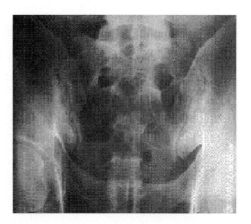

Figure 18–3. Early sacroiliitis of ankylosing spondylitis. Bilateral, symmetric erosions of the sacroiliac joint, with characteristic appearance of postage stamp serrations. (Reprinted from Bevens DL. Roentgen features of ankylosing spondylitis. In: *Clinical Orthopaedics and Related Research*. Vol. 74. Lippincott Williams & Wilkens, © 1974, p 23.)

symmetric in ankylosing spondylitis and enteropathic arthritis, in contrast to the unilateral changes observed in early psoriatic and reactive arthritis. However, in the latter two diseases, the progressive joint changes can become bilateral with time.

Scintigraphy has been used for evaluation of inflammatory back pain but has very limited usefulness. Increased uptake in the sacroiliac joints is highly sensitive for sacroiliitis but is nonspecific due to the normally high bone turnover of these joints, which leads to increased uptake without associated disease. Moreover, positive scintigraphic findings can result from a variety of other inflammatory or infectious causes, such as septic sacroiliitis. A diagnosis of spondyloarthropathy should not be based solely on scintigraphic results.

The superior technique for diagnosing early axial inflammation is by magnetic resonance imaging with gadolinium-DPTA or fat suppression. This method is the most sensitive and specific for the diagnosis of sacroiliitis and also avoids exposure to radiation, making it particularly advantageous in the assessment of women of childbearing age and children. Magnetic resonance imaging allows for visualization of acute sacroiliitis, spondylitis, and spondylodiscitis and can also detect acute inflammation of the entheses, bone, and synovium. The ability to detect early inflammation and accurately visualize cartilaginous and enthesal lesions makes magnetic resonance imaging a useful assessment tool in the spondyloarthropathies.

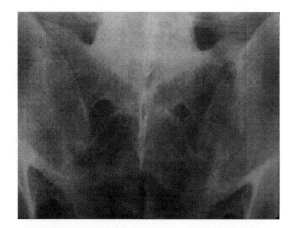

Figure 18–4. Sacroiliac joint fusion. The sacroiliac joints are completely obliterated by bony and fibrous fusion in advanced disease. (Reprinted from Bevens DL. Roentgen features of ankylosing spondylitis. In: *Clinical Orthopaedics and Related Research.* Vol. 74. Lippincott Williams & Wilkens, © 1974, p 23.)

In clinical practice, a reasonable initial evaluation of patients with symptoms of inflammatory back pain is to obtain a plain radiograph of the pelvis. If this study fails to demonstrate sacroiliitis, then dynamic magnetic resonance imaging should be considered.

2. Spine—A subtle radiographic change observed relatively early in the course of spondylitis is the appearance of vertebral "shiny corners." Also referred to as Romanus lesions, these are a reaction to inflammation at the site where the annulus fibrosus of the disks inserts onto the vertebral bodies. With progressive erosions and formation of new periosteal bone, the lumbar vertebral bodies become "squared off" in the lateral view (Figure 18–5).

The most characteristic finding is the formation of syndesmophytes—bony bridges between vertebral bodies due to gradual ossification of the edges of the annulus fibrosus (Figure 18–6). The vertical orientation of syndesmophytes and preservation of the disk space distinguish these from osteophytes associated with degenerative disease of the spine. The morphology and symmetry of syndesmophytes can help distinguish among the spondyloarthropathies. Ankylosing spondylitis and enteropathic arthritis exhibit symmetric delicate-appearing syndesmophytes that are marginal, meaning that they are almost completely vertical in their alignment and arise from the margins of the vertebral body. In contrast, psoriatic arthritis and reactive arthritis typically have more bulky, asymmetric bony growths that tend to initially protrude laterally before progressing vertically (nonmarginal syndesmophytes; Figure 18–6).

3. Peripheral joints—Radiographic changes in the peripheral joints mainly result from disease of the synovium or entheses. Hip involvement can produce symmetric narrowing of the joint space. Enthesitis can result in a faint periosteal reaction at bony prominences, such as the greater trochanters, calcaneus, and malleoli.

D. Special Tests

Spinal immobility and persistent inflammation are believed to contribute to the increased prevalence of osteoporosis in ankylosing spondylitis and other spondyloarthropathies. However, the formation of syndesmophytes in these diseases creates a unique problem in evaluation of bone mineral density. For example, in an ankylosed spine with paravertebral calcification, anterior-posterior measurement of bone density by dual energy x-ray absorptiometry can lead to spuriously increased values. Greater diagnostic specificity may be achieved by densitometry of the lateral spine or proximal femur or evaluation of density with quantitative computed tomography.

Differential Diagnosis

The diagnosis of ankylosing spondylitis usually rests on the combination of inflammatory back pain and radiographic evidence of bilateral sacroiliitis. The bilateral nature of the sacroiliitis, the prominence of axial skeleton involvement, and the absence of mucocutaneous disease help distinguish ankylosing spondylitis from reactive arthritis and psoriatic arthritis. The presence of bowel symptoms in a patient with "ankylosing spondylitis" should prompt a search for inflammatory bowel disease. The sacroiliitis and spondylitis of inflammatory bowel disease are radiographically indistinguishable from ankylosing spondylitis.

Inflammatory sacroiliac joint disease is not limited to the spondyloarthropathies, and a number of disease processes can cause radiographic sacroiliac changes (Table 18–2). Degenerative disease of the sacroiliac joints does occur, although its radiographic appearance is distinct from the inflammatory changes of the spondyloarthropathies. Osteitis condensans ilii is a condition seen in young, multiparous women and radiographically manifests as a characteristic triangle of ilial sclerosis adjacent to the sacroiliac joint. The sacroiliac joint itself is normal, and patients are usually asymptomatic.

Sacroiliitis from prolonged hyperparathyroidism, such as that induced by hemodialysis, can closely resemble the changes of ankylosing spondylitis. Other causes of sacroiliac erosions include familial Mediterranean fever, Whipple and Paget disease, and rarely, paraplegia. Whether Behçet disease is associated with

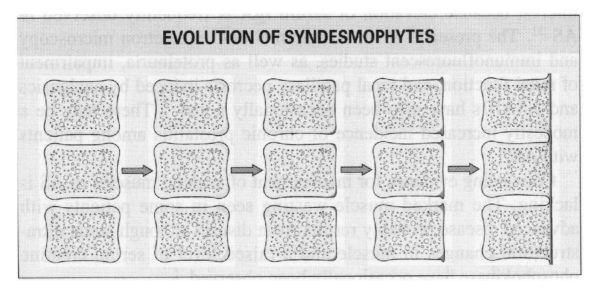

Figure 18–5. Lateral view of the progression of spinal pathology in ankylosing spondylitis. The appearance of "shiny corners" from erosions of the vertebral body edges is one of the first subtle changes. The vertebral bodies then become square from the lateral view due to deposition of new periosteal bone. Eventually, syndesmophytes form bony bridges between the anterior vertebral bodies. (Reprinted from Khan MA. Ankylosing spondylitis: clinical features. In: Klippel JH, Dieppe PA, eds. *Rheumatology*. Elsevier, © 1994, p 3.25.6. With permission from Elsevier Science.)

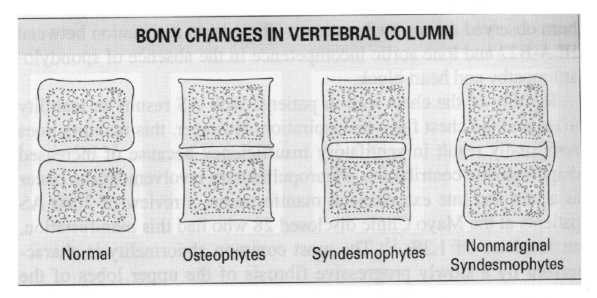

Figure 18–6. Bony changes of the vertebrae. A schematic of the bony growths of degenerative disease (osteophytes), ankylosing spondylitis, and enteropathic arthritis (marginal symmetric syndesmophytes), and psoriatic and reactive arthritis (bulky, nonmarginal syndesmophytes). The nonmarginal syndesmophytes of the latter two diseases are typically asymmetric. On occasion, the osteophytes of diffuse idiopathic hyperostosis can appear similar to those of psoriatic and reactive arthritis. (Reprinted from Khan MA. Ankylosing spondylitis: clinical features. In: Klippel JH, Dieppe PA, eds. *Rheumatology*. Elsevier, © 1994, p 3.25.6. With permission from Elsevier Science.)

Table 18–2. Differential diagnosis
of the spondyloarthropathies.

Sacroiliac abnormalities	
Sacroiliitis	Hyperparathyroidism
	Familial Mediterranean fever
	Whipple disease
	Paget disease
	Paraplegia
	Beçhet disease
	Tuberculosis
	Brucellosis
	Pyogenic sacroiliitis
	Malignancy
	Retinoid treatment
	SAPHO syndrome
Other changes	Degenerative joint disease
	Osteitis condensans ilii
	Chondrocalcinosis
	Gout
Vertebral hyperostosis	DISH
	Ochronosis
	SAPHO syndrome
	Retinoid treatment
Enthesopathy	Gout
	Disseminated gonococcal
	infection
	SAPHO syndrome
	Retinoid treatment
	BCG-induced

SAPHO, synovitis-acne-pustulosis-hyperostosis-osteitis; DISH, diffuse idiopathic skeletal hyperostosis; BCG, bacillus Calmette-Guérin.

sacroiliitis is still debated. Infections that seem to have a particular tropism to the sacroiliac joints include tuberculosis and brucellosis. However, infection with more typical organisms is also described, such as *Staphylococcus aureus,* particularly in injecting drug users. In rare instances, the sacroiliac joint and surrounding structures are the sites for primary malignancies or metastatic lesions.

The prominent osteophytes of diffuse idiopathic skeletal hyperostosis (DISH) may mimic syndesmophytes, particularly the nonmarginal syndesmophytes characteristic of psoriatic or reactive arthritis. In DISH, however, the sacroiliac joints should appear normal. Symptomatically, the diseases are easily differentiated since DISH patients lack inflammatory back pain. Moreover, approximately half of patients with DISH also exhibit prominent osteoarthritic changes in other joints.

Ochronosis can cause calcification of vertebral disk spaces and bony bridging that can mimic marginal syndesmophytes. In some cases, sacroiliac involvement is also observed, complicating diagnosis. The SAPHO (synovitis-acne-pustulosis-hyperostosis-osteitis) syndrome has sometimes been considered a spondyloarthropathy due to the frequency of sacroiliitis, enthesopathies, and oligoarticular peripheral arthritis. In addition, bony hyperostosis can be induced by retinoid treatment.

Treatment

The goals of therapy are to reduce inflammation and pain and to improve function, mobility, and strength. Best results are achieved by a multidisciplinary treatment approach, with physical therapy being an essential adjunct to pharmacologic methods. In general, patients should be advised to be aware of their posture and to avoid maintaining a flexed spine. For example, the height of work surfaces should be adjusted to avoid prolonged leaning over or slouching.

A. NONSTEROIDAL ANTI-INFLAMMATORY DRUGS

Almost all patients are prescribed at least one nonsteroidal anti-inflammatory drug (NSAID) during the course of the disease. These agents can provide significant reductions in pain, although many patients require additional pharmacologic agents. Of the NSAIDs currently available, indomethacin is commonly mentioned as the most effective, although this is mainly based on anecdotal clinical experience. As in other rheumatic diseases, there can be a wide individual variation in response to a given agent, and it is reasonable to prescribe what is most effective with the least amount of toxicity for each individual patient.

B. DISEASE-MODIFYING ANTIRHEUMATIC DRUGS (DMARDs)

NSAIDs alone do not control the symptoms of many patients. Sulfasalazine has established efficacy in treating the peripheral arthritis of ankylosing spondylitis but does not appear to be of benefit for disease of the axial skeleton. The typical therapeutic dose is 2–3 g/d in divided doses. Methotrexate is sometimes used; the rationale for this is based mainly on its efficacy in rheumatoid arthritis, as controlled studies are lacking.

Intravenous bisphosphonates have recently been demonstrated to effectively treat the pain and inflammation of both the peripheral and axial disease of spondyloarthropathy. Pamidronate is typically given as a 30–60-mg intravenous dose monthly for 6 months. Acute arthralgia, myalgia, and fever after the first infusion are not uncommon, but reactions are generally mild and usually decrease with continued treatment.

Etanercept and infliximab, both anti-tumor necrosis factor (TNF) therapies, have dramatic and rapid efficacy in the therapy of the ankylosing spondylitis and the other spondyloarthropathies. The main toxicities include injection site or infusion reactions and a slight increase in minor uncomplicated infections. Serious toxicities, although uncommon, include reactivation of tuberculosis, the induction of demyelinating disease, and possibly an increase in lymphoproliferative diseases. Since the long-term safety of these agents is still relatively unknown, treatment should not be undertaken lightly and patients should be properly advised of potential risks.

C. OTHER PHARMACOLOGIC THERAPIES

Systemic glucocorticoids are not commonly used and can worsen osteopenia. In certain cases, intra-articular glucocorticoid injection into the sacroiliac joint can provide short-term symptomatic relief. However, the anatomy of the joint is extremely complicated, and radiographic guidance for this procedure is required.

D. SURGICAL THERAPY

The deformities that result from extensive disease of the spine can lead to disabling decreases in the field of vision and ambulation. Corrective surgeries of spinal alignment, however, are major procedures and have limited indications. Typically, osteotomy with fixation is performed, with corrections of the lumbar spine being most common. Neurologic complications and perioperative mortality are not insignificant with these procedures.

Hip involvement requires artificial replacement in approximately 5% of patients with ankylosing spondylitis. The outcome of total hip arthroplasty is good, with long-term joint survival of 60% at 20 years. The occurrence of postoperative heterotopic bone formation is increased in those undergoing repeat hip surgery and those with more spinal ankylosis.

Complications

The fused, osteopenic spine of ankylosing spondylitis is at great risk for fracture, which can be precipitated by such minor trauma as insignificant falls, sneezing, or manual manipulation of the spine. The most common sites of fracture are the thoracolumbar and cervicothoracic junctions. Although cervical fractures may result immediately in quadriplegia or death, the symptoms of spinal fracture are often subtle and include new, localized back or neck pain and, in some cases, the description of recently increased spinal mobility. Plain radiographs are relatively insensitive and fail to identify many spinal fractures, especially in the acute setting. Magnetic resonance imaging is the preferred technique when plain radiographs are unrevealing. Depending on the fracture site, the degree of instability, and the neurologic status, treatment may require early surgical stabilization.

Because of the ability to manually fracture the ankylosed spine, particularly in patients with altered mental status, preoperative assessment for patients with significant axial disease is essential before surgical procedures requiring general anesthesia. Specifically, since damage to the spine and spinal cord can result from endotracheal intubation, the need for awake fiberoptic intubation should be considered in appropriate situations.

Patients previously treated with spinal radiation for spondylitis have an increased risk of cancer, specifically myeloid leukemias and other hematologic malignancies. This highly effective therapy was widely performed from the early 1920s until the last few decades but is no longer used because of the unacceptable long-term morbidity and mortality. Questions regarding previous therapeutic radiation should be included in a complete past medical history of patients with long-standing ankylosing spondylitis.

When to Refer to a Specialist

Vertebral fracture of the ankylosed spine can lead to serious neurologic complications, and prompt identification and early treatment are essential. Many fractures are not acutely identified, in part because of the absence of preceding significant trauma and the failure to recognize a change in the characteristics of the back pain. In a case of suspected vertebral fracture, care should be taken to immobilize the patient and obtain urgent imaging.

Most uveitis associated with the spondyloarthropathies can be effectively treated with topical glucocorticoids, NSAIDs, and mydriatics. However, the diagnosis requires specialized evaluation, and prompt referral to an ophthalmologist is required. In addition, some cases require more aggressive therapy, such as direct injection of glucocorticoid agents to the affected area, requiring professional expertise.

REACTIVE ARTHRITIS

 ESSENTIALS OF DIAGNOSIS

- *Asymmetric, oligoarticular inflammatory arthritis of the lower extremities.*
- *Enthesitis and dactylitis.*
- *Axial skeleton involvement characterized by unilateral sacroiliitis.*
- *Associations with antecedent genitourinary and gastrointestinal infections.*

• Extra-articular manifestations, including conjunctivitis, anterior uveitis, urethritis, oral ulcers, circinate balanitis, and keratoderma blennorrhagicum.

General Considerations

The typical patient is a male in his 20s, but reactive arthritis also occurs in women and can affect individuals over a wide age span. Peripheral arthritis, usually in the form of an oligoarthritis of the lower extremities and acute in onset, characterizes reactive arthritis. Enthesitis and dactylitis are often prominent, and approximately 50% of patients have mucocutaneous manifestations. Reiter syndrome refers to the triad of reactive arthritis, conjunctivitis, and urethritis, but this term has fallen out of favor, particularly following recent revelations of Reiter's involvement in war crimes during World War II.

Genitourinary infections with *Chlamydia trachomatis* or gastrointestinal infections with *Shigella, Salmonella, Yersinia,* or *Campylobacter* species can trigger reactive arthritis, generally after a lag of 1–4 weeks. Cultures of synovial fluid and synovium, however, are sterile (hence the term "reactive"). Often, however, there is no history of antecedent infection, suggesting that reactive arthritis can follow subclinical infections or that there are other environmental triggers. The prevalence and severity of reactive arthritis may be increased in persons infected with HIV (see Chapter 49).

The majority of cases of reactive arthritis spontaneously resolve over months, but a substantial minority will have either a relapsing course or persistent arthritis.

Clinical Findings

A. Symptoms and Signs

The onset of the joint disease is usually acute with the appearance of an additive, asymmetric oligoarthritis most commonly affecting the knees and ankles. Involvement of upper extremity joints occurs but is uncommon. Urethritis and mild conjunctivitis may precede articular symptoms. In contrast to rheumatoid arthritis, fever > 38 °C is not uncommon at the outset of reactive arthritis, and weight loss can be striking.

Heel pain, due either to Achilles tendinitis or enthesitis where the plantar fascia inserts onto the inferior aspect of the calcaneus, is common. Dactylitis, usually in the form of "sausage toes," occurs in approximately half of cases.

Approximately 50% of patients have low back pain, but radiographic evidence of involvement of the axial skeleton occurs in only 20%. Sacroiliitis and spondylitis, however, become more prevalent with disease duration, and up to 70% with persistent disease have disease of the axial skeleton. Sacroiliitis is usually unilateral but may become bilateral with time. In a small minority of cases, spondylitis leads to extensive fusion of the spine as can be seen in ankylosing spondylitis.

Mucocutaneous disease is common and can provide important clues to the diagnosis. Although urogenital infections with *C trachomatis* can induce reactive arthritis, urethritis and cervicitis also can be manifestations of the mucosal inflammation that is part of the disease process and can occur with the postenteric forms of reactive arthritis, particularly early in the disease course. Other early mucocutaneous manifestations include shallow, painless ulcers of the palate, tongue, and the glans penis (circinate balanitis). Approximately 25% of patients with reactive arthritis have keratoderma blennorrhagicum, a papulosquamous rash of the soles and palms (Figure 18–7) that clinically and histologically resembles pustular psoriasis. Subungual deposits of keratotic material can produce nail changes similar to those of psoriasis.

Up to one-third of cases have conjunctivitis that is usually mild and present early in the disease course. Conjunctivitis is not associated with HLA-B27 and is the least specific extra-articular manifestation of reactive arthritis. Anterior uveitis and aortitis also occur although the prevalence of these in reactive arthritis is less than in ankylosing spondylitis (Table 18–1).

B. Laboratory Findings

Patients with active disease often have mild anemia, modest leukocytosis, and moderate to marked thrombocytosis. The erythrocyte sedimentation rate and levels of C-reactive protein are usually elevated. Tests for rheumatoid factor and antinuclear antibodies are negative.

Synovial fluid is inflammatory with white blood cell counts usually ranging from 5000 to 50,000/μL. Synovial fluid cultures are negative. Patients with genitourinary symptoms should be tested for infection with *C trachomatis*.

Testing for HLA-B27 can aid diagnosis in selected cases. The association with HLA-B27 is strongest in the subset of patients with persistent disease and involvement of the axial skeleton.

C. Imaging Studies

Enthesopathy at the insertion of the plantar fascia produces periostitis and "inflammatory heel spurs." These can be differentiated from degenerative spurs of the calcaneus by the degree of cortication, as the inflammatory lesions tend to be fluffy in appearance, in contrast to well-corticated degenerative spurs. Patients with disease

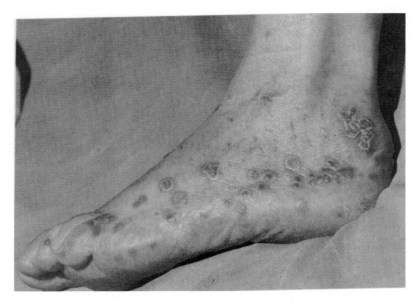

Figure 18–7. Keratoderma blennorrhagica. Lesions typically consist of confluent papules, vesicles, and/or pustules ranging from red to brown in appearance. (Reprinted from Fitzpatrick TD, Johnson RA, Polamo MK, Summon D, Wolff K. *Color Atlas and Synopsis of Clinical Dermatology.* McGraw-Hill, © 1994, p 529. With permission from McGraw-Hill.)

of the axial skeleton have sacroiliitis that is usually unilateral and spondylitis characterized by nonmarginal syndesmophytes (Figure 18–6).

Differential Diagnosis

The diagnosis of reactive arthritis is based on the clinical presentation and the exclusion of alternative explanations for an inflammatory oligoarthritis.

In the early stages it is critical to exclude infectious causes of arthritis. Disseminated gonococcal infection (DGI) can be particularly difficult to distinguish from acute-onset reactive arthritis because oligoarthritis, tenosynovitis, and fever occur in both diseases. Urethral, pharyngeal, cervical, and rectal swabs for gonococci have, in combination, a sensitivity of 70–90% in DGI. Synovial fluid cultures, in contrast, are positive in < 50% of cases of DGI, and therefore, sterile synovial fluid cultures do not distinguish reactive arthritis from DGI. Occasionally, a therapeutic trial of antibiotics is necessary to make this diagnostic distinction; a prompt response to appropriate antibiotic therapy points to a diagnosis of DGI.

Nongonococcal septic arthritis can be oligoarticular and occasionally mimics reactive arthritis; synovial fluid cultures are usually positive, underscoring the importance of diagnostic arthrocentesis in cases of unexplained acute oligoarthritis. Bacterial endocarditis can produce an oligoarthritis due to either direct infection

(with positive synovial fluid cultures) or immune complexes (with sterile synovial cultures); back pain is common, especially with acute endocarditis. Acute viral infections, such as parvovirus B19, usually cause an acute polyarthritis, but occasionally the arthritis involves only a few joints. An antecedent sore throat suggests post-streptococcal arthritis which, in adults, usually is additive and is not associated with the extra-articular manifestations of acute rheumatic fever.

Occasionally, rheumatoid arthritis begins as an oligoarthritis and causes some diagnostic confusion with reactive arthritis. Inflammatory low back pain and dactylitis are not features of rheumatoid arthritis, and their presence should point to reactive arthritis or another spondyloarthropathy. Dactylitis can a helpful clue to the presence of a spondyloarthropathy (particularly reactive arthritis or psoriatic arthritis) but also can be seen in gout and sarcoidosis.

Treatment

The treatment of reactive arthritis mirrors the therapeutic approach to ankylosing spondylitis discussed earlier. NSAIDs are widely used. Sulfasalazine appears to be efficacious for peripheral arthritis but of little or no efficacy for disease of the axial skeleton. Methotrexate has been widely used and is likely beneficial, although its efficacy in this disease has not been established in rigorously performed clinical trials. The anti-TNF therapies, infliximab and etanercept, produce prompt and sub-stantial responses. These are currently the treatment of choice for severe disease.

The use of antibiotics in the treatment of reactive arthritis is still somewhat contentious. Genitourinary infections with *Chlamydia* should be treated. Prolonged (months) treatment with tetracyclines has been reported to be beneficial for patients with post-chlamydial reactive arthritis, but there is not general agreement on this issue. Antibiotics do not appear to be effective in the treatment of postenteric and idiopathic forms of reactive arthritis.

Complications

Disability due to destructive peripheral arthritis or extensive disease of the spine develops in a minority of patients. Amyloidosis and aortic regurgitation are rare complications of long-standing disease.

PSORIATIC ARTHRITIS

Arthritis occurs in about 10% of patients with psoriasis. Psoriatic arthritis typically develops after, or coincident with, the onset of psoriasis, but the arthritis precedes the skin disease by as much as 2 years in a minority of cases (~15%). A range of joint manifestations occurs in association with psoriasis: monarticular or oligoarticular arthritis, polyarthritis, arthritis mutilans, and arthritis of the axial skeleton.

Two-thirds of patients with psoriatic arthritis have an asymmetric oligoarthritis or a monoarthritis, but others have polyarticular disease that mimics osteoarthritis or rheumatoid arthritis in its distribution. Involvement of the distal interphalangeal joints, which are spared by rheumatoid arthritis, can help distinguish psoriatic arthritis from rheumatoid arthritis. Psoriatic arthritis of the distal interphalangeal joints is associated with abnormalities of the nail bed and dystrophic changes of the nail, such as pitting, onycholysis, ridging, and brown-yellow discoloration (oil-drop sign).

The skin disease can be subtle. When psoriatic arthritis is suspected based on the distribution of affected joints or suspicious radiographic findings, skin examination should include evaluation of the gluteal fold, umbilical region, and scalp because cutaneous findings can be limited to these sites. Of significance, the explosive development of psoriatic skin disease, with or without articular involvement, can be a sign of HIV infection and should prompt appropriate testing (see Chapter 49).

Psoriatic arthritis has a distinctive radiographic appearance, specifically the concurrence of both bony destruction and proliferation at an affected site (Figure 18–8). In addition, psoriatic arthritis can be highly destructive, with development of a pencil-in-cup appear-

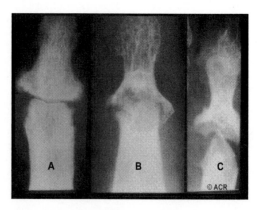

Figure 18–8. Radiographic changes from psoriatic arthritis of the distal interphalangeal joint. **A:** Subtle periosteal erosions at the margins of the joint space are an initial appearance. **B:** Progressive erosive and proliferative changes occur over time and can be greatly destructive. **C:** Distinctive "pencil-in-cup" appearance with severe disease. (© 1972–1999, American College of Rheumatology Clinical Slide Collection. Used with permission.)

ance of the finger bones, and in some cases, arthritis mutilans. Involvement of the axial skeleton resembles that of reactive arthritis. Sacroiliitis is usually unilateral, and nonmarginal syndesmophytes characterize the spondylitis.

NSAIDs are used for mild disease. Once-weekly methotrexate is effective for treatment of both the cutaneous and peripheral articular disease. Sulfasalazine is superior to placebo in the treatment of joint disease, but the effect, although statistically significant, is small. Anti-TNF therapies show considerable promise and improve both the articular and cutaneous manifestations of psoriatic arthritis. Cyclosporine A has been used with severe, refractory disease.

Oral glucocorticoids should be avoided, but intra-articular injections of glucocorticoids can be useful adjunctive therapy. Care should be taken to make certain that the needle does not pass through psoriatic plaques, which are heavily contaminated with bacteria. Psoriatic skin lesions overlying a joint are a contraindication to arthrocentesis because of the added risk of procedure-induced septic arthritis.

ENTEROPATHIC ARTHRITIS

Enteropathic arthritis, which develops in approximately 20% of patients with either Crohn disease or ulcerative colitis, has two forms: (1) a peripheral arthritis whose activity can correlate with the activity of the inflammatory bowel disease, and (2) arthritis of the axial skeleton whose activity is independent of the bowel disease. The peripheral arthritis can take the form of either migratory arthralgias or an asymmetric oligoarthritis of the lower extremities. Erythema nodosum and pyoderma gangrenosa sometimes occur coincident with peripheral arthritis. Involvement of the axial skeleton is clinically and radiographically indistinguishable from that of ankylosing spondylitis.

Treatment of the underlying inflammatory bowel disease can ameliorate peripheral arthritis. Sulfasalazine appears to be effective for peripheral arthritis. There is some evidence that NSAIDs can induce gastrointestinal flares of inflammatory bowel disease; therefore, their use in treating enteropathic arthritis should be considered on a case-to-case basis. Small, uncontrolled studies report that infliximab, which is approved for use in the treatment of Crohn disease, is beneficial for both peripheral arthritis and arthritis of the axial skeleton.

REFERENCES

Sieper J, Braun J. New treatment strategies in ankylosing spondylitis: proceedings of the Ankylosing Spondylitis Workshop, Berlin, Germany, 18-19 January 2002. *Ann Rheum Dis.* 2002;61:iii1-2. [PMID: 12381504] (Comprehensive summary of current knowledge regarding the pathogenesis, genetics, natural progression, and treatment of ankylosing spondylitis.)

Bellamy N, et al. What do we know about the sacroiliac joint? *Semin Arthritis Rheum.* 1983;12:282. [PMID: 6867741] (Although 2 decades old, the most complete review on the anatomy, function, and diseases of the sacroiliac joint.)

Relevant World Wide Web Sites

[The Spondylitis Association of America]
http://www.spondylitis.org
[National Ankylosing Spondylitis Society]
http://www.nass.co.uk

SECTION III

Lupus & Related Autoimmune Disorders

Systemic Lupus Erythematosus

19

Michelle Petri, MD, MPH

ESSENTIALS OF DIAGNOSIS

- *Onset after puberty in young women.*
- *More common in African Americans.*
- *Common presentations are photosensitive rashes, polyarthritis, or nephritis.*
- *Characterized by autoantibody formation (specific autoantibodies include anti-dsDNA and anti-Sm) and often low complement levels (C3, C4, CH50).*

General Considerations

Systemic lupus erythematosus (SLE) is usually a multi-organ, multisystem autoimmune disease. It must be distinguished from chronic cutaneous lupus (in which only discoid lupus occurs and progression to a systemic disease occurs in only 5%) and from drug-induced lupus erythematosus (associated with isoniazid, procainamide, hydralazine, and some other drugs, presenting as arthritis and serositis especially, but resolving after cessation of the culprit drug).

Mixed connective tissue disease is a term proposed for patients with high-titer anti-RNP antibodies and a syndrome of Raynaud phenomenon, polyarthritis, and myositis. Long-term follow-up has suggested that the diagnosis is often not appropriate because true systemic lupus erythematosus or scleroderma develops in many patients. In addition, the term is often misused to designate patients with an undefined autoimmune disease. A better diagnostic code for such patients is undifferentiated connective tissue disease.

SLE predominantly occurs in women, with a gender ratio of 9:1. Onset is usually after puberty, typically in the 20s and 30s. It is more common in African Americans than in whites. The incidence in white females is 3.9 per 100,000 and in white males is 0.4 per 100,000. The prevalence in white females is 130 per 100,000. The incidence of SLE may have tripled since the 1970s.

Multiple predisposing factors have been identified. The genetic predisposition is complex, likely involving more than 100 genes. HLA-DR and DQ alleles are associated not just with the risk of developing lupus, but with the kinds of autoantibodies produced. Genes that control programmed cell death (apoptosis) are important in murine lupus models and in human lupus as well. The proteins to which the lupus patient mounts an autoantibody response are exposed on nuclear blebs during programmed cell death. Genes involved in immune complex clearance (Fc gamma receptor alleles) may predispose patients to lupus nephritis. However, the genetic predisposition is not overwhelming. Only 10% of patients have a first-degree relative with SLE, and SLE develops in only 2% of children who have an afflicted parent.

Environmental factors play a role not only in the onset of SLE but also in triggering the "flares" (relapses). The most recognized environmental trigger is UV light exposure. UV light, both UV-B and UV-A, can trigger photosensitive rashes and, more rarely, systemic flares. SLE patients are more likely than controls to have drug allergies, especially to sulfonamide antibiotics. The common cold remedy echinacea has precipitated SLE flares in several patients. In several case-control studies, smoking has been found to be a risk factor for SLE. Once SLE is diagnosed, patients who continue to smoke are at greater risk for discoid lupus. Infection with Epstein-Barr virus has been strongly associated with SLE in a multicase family registry.

Hormonal factors are obviously important, given the female predominance of SLE and the usual onset of SLE after puberty. In the Nurses' Cohort study, use of oral contraceptives or estrogen replacement therapy was a risk factor for later SLE. However, several case-control studies have suggested that hormone replacement therapy is not associated with flare in patients with established SLE. Pregnancy is associated with SLE flares in some, but not all, studies. Elevation of prolactin may be associated with activity of SLE.

The activity of SLE follows several patterns. The classic pattern, the "flare" pattern, is characterized by a relapsing-remitting pattern. However, an equal number of SLE patients have a pattern of continuously active disease. Only a minority of patients are lucky enough to have long periods of disease quiescence. The antimalarial drug hydroxychloroquine, which is widely used for cutaneous lupus and lupus arthritis, reduces future flares if patients continue to take it. Dehydroepiandrosterone, DHEA, which is not approved by the US Food and Drug Administration (FDA), has also been shown to reduce flares.

Over half of SLE patients have acquired permanent damage in one or more organ systems. Although damage, such as renal failure and interstitial pulmonary fibrosis, can occur from SLE itself, glucocorticoid therapy accounts for a large proportion as well. For example, long-term prednisone therapy may cause osteoporotic fractures and osteonecrosis of bone.

Survival of SLE patients plateaued at about 80% at 10 years after diagnosis in the 1980s. The Centers for Disease Control and Prevention reported in 2002 that mortality in young women had actually increased. The major cause of death in SLE is accelerated atherosclerosis. Although SLE itself can damage the endothelial surface of the coronary arteries, part of the atherosclerotic process resulted from elevated levels of traditional cardiovascular risk factors, including hypertension, hyperlipidemia, obesity, and homocysteine levels. Prednisone increases the patient's weight, blood pressure, and glucose and lipid levels. SLE nephritis can lead to hypertension and hyperlipidemia. Renal insufficiency can increase homocysteine levels.

Clinical Findings

A. Symptoms and Signs

The American College of Rheumatology has established criteria for the classification (not diagnosis) of SLE. Four of the 11 criteria must be present for the classification of SLE (Table 19–1). The criteria are heavily weighted toward mucocutaneous findings but do serve to emphasize the multisystem nature of the disease. However, a patient with a classic finding, such as lupus nephritis, has SLE even if she or he does not have 4 of the 11 classification criteria.

Early signs and symptoms of SLE may not be specific—a delay in diagnosis is commonplace. Early signs

Table 19–1. Systemic lupus erythematosus classification criteria.

Systemic lupus erythematosus may be classified if 4 or more of the following 11 disorders are present:
Malar rash
Discoid rash
Photosensitivity
Oral ulcers
Arthritis
Serositis
Renal disorder
a. > 0.5 g/d proteinuria, or—
b. ≥ 3+ dipstick proteinuria, or—
c. Cellular casts
Neurologic disorder
a. Seizures, or—
b. Psychosis (without other cause)
Hematologic disorder
a. Hemolytic anemia, or—
b. Leukopenia (< 4000/µL), or
c. Lymphopenia (< 1500/µL), or
d. Thrombocytopenia (< 100,000 µL)
Immunologic disorder
a. Positive LE cell preparation, or—
b. Antibody to native DNA, or—
c. Antibody to Sm, or—
d. False-positive serologic test for syphilis
Positive antinuclear antibodies

and symptoms include fatigue, mild hair loss, anemia, arthralgias, nausea, and weight loss.

1. Head, ears, eyes, nose, and throat—Alopecia can occur as a diffuse alopecia or as an alopecia especially marked around the face (Table 19–2). Discoid lupus can cause a scarring alopecia. Ear involvement is sometimes seen in discoid lupus. Rarely, polychondritis may develop in a patient with lupus. Secondary Sjögren syndrome occurs in some patients with SLE, leading to keratoconjunctivitis sicca (dry eyes, dry mouth). Additional ocular involvement includes episcleritis, scleritis, uveitis, retinitis, and optic neuropathy. Both the nose and mouth (palate and buccal mucosa) may have aphthous ulcers (both painful and painless). Discoid lupus can occur in the mouth.

2. Cutaneous—SLE rashes are most often, but not always, photosensitive. The malar rash occurs in sun-exposed areas, such as nose and cheeks, and spares the nasolabial folds and below the nares. Maculopapular lupus eruptions can occur on the face, V- of the neck, forearms, and elsewhere. Discoid lupus lesions occur in these areas and also the ears and scalp. Discoid lesions often heal with hypopigmentation or hyperpigmentation. Subacute cutaneous lupus, which may be mis-

Table 19–2. Organ involvement in systemic lupus erythematosus.

Involved Organ or System	Typical	Unusual
Head, ears, eyes, nose, and throat	Alopecia Discoid lupus of scalp, ears Oral/nasal ulcers Keratoconjunctivitis sicca Dry mouth Episcleritis, scleritis Uveitis	Angioedema Polychondritis Retinitis Optic neuritis
Cutaneous	Malar rash Discoid rash Maculopapular rash Subacute cutaneous lupus Cutaneous vasculitis Nailfold capillary changes Livedo reticularis	Bullous lupus
Cardiopulmonary	Pleurisy/pleural effusion Pericarditis/pericardial effusion Interstitial pneumonitis (acute or chronic) Pulmonary hypertension	Myocarditis Libman-Sacks endocarditis Pulmonary hemorrhage Coronary arteritis/aneurysm
Gastrointestinal	Esophageal dysmotility Hepatomegaly Splenomegaly Elevated liver function tests	Mesenteric vasculitis (with or without infarcts) Colitis Protein-losing enteropathy Primary biliary cirrhosis Budd-Chiari syndrome Ascites
Neurologic	Cognitive impairment Seizures Psychosis Stroke (or transient ischemic attack) Transverse myelitis Mononeuritis multiplex Peripheral neuropathy Encephalopathy/coma	Cranial neuropathy Chorea Pseudotumor cerebi
Constitutional	Fever Weight loss Fatigue Lymphadenopathy	
Musculoskeletal	Polyarthralgias/arthritis Myalgias Myositis	

taken for a fungal rash, occurs as a psoriaform type or an annular type. It may develop idiopathically or in a response to a drug, often hydrochlorthiazide. Livedo reticularis occurs with or without antiphospholipid antibodies. Nailfold capillary changes can be seen. A rare lupus rash, bullous lupus, presents as blistering lesions.

3. Cardiopulmonary—Pleuritic pain (sometimes with pleural effusions) and pericardial pain (with or without effusion) occur in SLE. Rare cardiac manifestations include Libman-Sacks endocarditis with valvular vegetations, myocarditis, and coronary arteritis. Pulmonary hypertension can occur. Interstitial pneumonitis, both acute and chronic, may occur. Life-threatening pulmonary hemorrhage is an unusual finding.

4. Gastrointestinal—Esophageal dysmotility occurs in SLE, but is usually mild. Hepatomegaly and splenomegaly may occur, especially in children. Pancreatitis is a rare manifestation. Mesenteric vasculitis can lead to postprandial pain, abdominal pain, infarcts, and bowel perforation. Colitis and protein-losing enteropathy are extremely rare. A few SLE patients will have overlap with primary biliary cirrhosis or autoimmune hepatitis.

5. Neurologic—SLE can present with or include psychosis, seizures, encephalopathy (organic brain syndrome), coma, pseudotumor cerebri, meningitis, transverse myelitis, mononeuritis multiplex, and peripheral neuropathy.

6. Constitutional—Many SLE patients have low-grade fever (a few with temperatures higher than 39 °C), fatigue, and weight loss. Lymphadenopathy is common in active disease.

7. Musculoskeletal—Polyarthralgias and polyarthritis eventually occur in 90% of SLE patients. The arthritis is usually nonerosive, involving the small joints of the hands and wrists initially. Myositis, or an overlap with dermatomyositis, can also occur. As many as 30% of SLE patients have coexisting fibromyalgia.

B. LABORATORY FINDINGS

1. Hematologic—Anemia is very common in SLE but is multifactorial. The classic anemia, a hemolytic anemia with increased reticulocyte count, direct Coombs test, and low haptoglobin, is not the most common. Anemia of chronic disease is the most common finding (Table 19–3). Anemia may also be due to iron deficiency, renal insufficiency or failure, or to sickle cell (or trait) and thalassemia.

Leukopenia is common but usually mild. It is rare for the white blood count to be below 1000/μL. Lymphopenia is frequent (glucocorticoids also cause lymphopenia). Neutropenia can occur but is rare.

Mild or profound thrombocytopenia can occur. Antiphospholipid antibodies are associated with thrombocytopenia.

The partial thromboplastin time may be prolonged due to a lupus anticoagulant.

The erythrocyte sedimentation rate (ESR) or C-reactive protein (CRP) level may be elevated.

2. Chemistries—The blood urea nitrogen (BUN) and creatinine may be elevated due to renal insufficiency or failure. Cholesterol may be elevated secondary to nephrotic syndrome.

The transaminases may be elevated (usually mildly) due to SLE. An elevated alkaline phosphatase may indicate renal osteodystrophy or primary biliary cirrhosis.

The creatine kinase may be elevated secondary to myositis. Homocysteine, a risk factor for atherosclerosis

Table 19–3. Laboratory findings in systemic lupus erythematosus.

Test	Typical	Unusual
Hematologic	Anemia of chronic disease Hemolytic anemia, with elevated reticulocyte count Leukopenia Thrombocytopenia Elevated erythrocyte sedimentation rate or C-reactive protein Prolonged partial thromboplastin time, dRVVT, or other test for lupus anticoagulant	Neutropenia
Comprehensive metabolic panel	Elevated blood urea nitrogen and creatinine Elevated liver function tests	
Other chemistry tests	Elevated creatine kinase or aldolase Elevated homocysteine Elevated cholesterol	
Urinalysis	Proteinuria Red blood cells or red blood cell casts	

RVVT, dilute Russel viper venom time.

and thrombosis, is elevated in up to 30%, especially if there is renal insufficiency.

3. Urinalysis—Lupus nephritis may present as proteinuria alone or proteinuria with an active urine sediment (red blood cells, red blood cell casts).

C. IMAGING STUDIES

Magnetic resonance imaging (MRI) of the brain is preferred over computed tomography (CT) in the evaluation of central nervous system lupus. The most common finding is small white matter lesions, which may represent immune complex deposition. A true vasculitis is almost never seen on cerebral arteriogram.

MRI of the hip is the best way to find osteonecrosis at an early stage, when it may be ameliorated by core decompression. Bone scan can detect subclinical involvement of other sites.

D. SPECIAL TESTS

1. Autoantibodies—Most (96% or more) SLE patients have a positive antinuclear antibody (ANA) test result. Because 20% of healthy young women also have a positive ANA, the presence of an ANA alone is not given much weight. Titers of 1:640 or higher are more indicative of a connective tissue disease of some sort.

Some autoantibodies are very specific for lupus, such as anti-dsDNA (which occurs in about 30%) or anti-Sm (this is an abbreviation for Smith, not smooth muscle). Other autoantibodies, such as anti-Ro/SS-A, anti-La/SS-B, and anti-RNP, occur in SLE but also in rheumatoid arthritis and in Sjögren syndrome.

Antiphospholipid antibodies, lupus anticoagulant, anticardiolipin, anti-β_2 glycoprotein I, and the false-positive test for syphilis are found in about 50% of SLE patients during the course of disease.

A recent autoantibody, anti-SR, has received FDA approval for testing in SLE.

2. Complement—Reduction in the complement components C3 and C4 or in total hemolytic complement occurs but is not specific for lupus.

E. SPECIAL EXAMINATION

A skin biopsy, with immunofluorescence, is helpful in the diagnosis of SLE cutaneous lesions.

In patients with nephritis, a renal biopsy can determine the World Health Organization subtype (mesangial, focal proliferative, diffuse proliferative, or membranous) and give information on both activity and chronicity (damage).

In patients with neuropathy, a nerve conduction study and biopsy may be necessary to document vasculitis. An electromyelogram and muscle biopsy may be needed in the evaluation of myositis.

Differential Diagnosis

SLE is diagnosed in some patients based on a positive ANA, which is inappropriate. Patients with a positive ANA and fatigue or chronic pain are likely to have fibromyalgia rather than lupus.

SLE may be confused with other connective tissue diseases, especially rheumatoid arthritis. SLE patients may have positive rheumatoid factor. The usual presentation of lupus arthritis is identical to that of rheumatoid arthritis, but SLE arthritis is rarely erosive. SLE and dermatomyositis may be hard to differentiate, or they may overlap.

Drug-induced lupus must be excluded. In young women, minocycline can cause a drug-induced lupus, often with autoimmune hepatitis and P-antineutrophil cytoplasmic antibodies (P-ANCA).

Some viral infections may mimic lupus. Parvovirus can cause a polyarthritis and positive ANA. HIV can cause thrombocytopenia and direct Coombs test. Hepatitis B can cause vasculitis, and hepatitis C can cause cryoglobulinemia (with renal and neurologic manifestations) that can be confused with lupus.

A malignancy can cause anemia, elevated ESR, positive ANA, vasculitis, and other autoimmune phenomena. Anemia and an elevated ESR should also bring to mind multiple myeloma.

Treatment

A. GENERAL MEASURES

SLE patients who are stable should be seen quarterly for routine physical examination and laboratory monitoring (at a minimum, complete blood cell count, comprehensive metabolic panel, and urinalysis).

The patient with SLE should receive preventive care, including yearly influenza vaccine and a pneumococcal vaccine every 5 years.

SLE patients on glucocorticoids should have a screening bone density scan.

Because of the risk of accelerated atherosclerosis, patients should have cardiovascular risk factors checked and appropriate teaching on lifestyle modification. Compliance with antihypertensive therapy should be monitored.

Patients with SLE should avoid sulfonamide antibiotics, which can be associated with disease flares (dapsone 100 mg, 3 times weekly, can be substituted in those patients who require *Pneumocystis carinii* pneumonia [PCP] prophylaxis). Echinacea, an alternative cold remedy, is an immune stimulant associated with lupus flares. Oral contraceptives and estrogen replacement therapy are contraindicated in patients with SLE who have antiphospholipid antibodies.

B. CUTANEOUS LUPUS

Avoidance of sun exposure and use of sunblocks (that block both UV-A and UV-B) form the baseline approach to cutaneous lupus. The antimalarial hydroxychloroquine is used to treat photosensitive rashes. Its onset is slow, with some improvement seen at 1 month and maximal effect at 3 months. Bridging therapy with glucocorticoids may be necessary while waiting for the hydroxychloroquine effect, especially in patients with discoid lupus, given its propensity to scar.

If there is an incomplete response to hydroxychloroquine, quinacrine may be added. Quinacrine is only available through compounding pharmacists. Several immunosuppressive drugs are beneficial for cutaneous lupus and are used both to control disease and to "steroid spare." These include methotrexate and mycophenolate mofetil.

Cyclophosphamide is used for severe cutaneous vasculitis or disfiguring lupus rashes unresponsive to other immunosuppressant therapy. Thalidomide can be considered in a postmenopausal patient or a premenopausal patient with hysterectomy or tubal ligation.

Thalidomide has been associated with peripheral neuropathy and rarely with thrombosis or ovarian failure.

C. ARTHRITIS

Nonsteroidal anti-inflammatory drugs (NSAIDs) are the mainstay of treatment. Specific cyclooxygenase-2 (COX-2) NSAIDs have not yet been studied for safety in SLE. Hydroxychloroquine is frequently added to NSAIDs for control of arthralgias or arthritis. Because of its slow onset, bridging therapy with glucocorticoids may be necessary.

To control severe arthritis and to "steroid spare," two medications approved for rheumatoid arthritis, methotrexate or leflunomide, can be added. Folic acid must be given with methotrexate. However, the biologics that block tumor necrosis factor (etanercept, infliximab, adalimumab) are not recommended for SLE arthritis because they can induce antiphospholipid antibodies and anti-dsDNA.

D. SEROSITIS

Mild pleurisy and pericarditis may be controlled with NSAIDs and low-dose prednisone (10 mg/d or less). More severe presentations may require pulse intravenous methylprednisolone, 1000 mg daily for 3 days, followed by moderate-dose prednisone (up to 40 mg/d) and later taper. Patients who have frequent recurrences may benefit from the addition of hydroxychloroquine. If there is a high glucocorticoid requirement, azathioprine or mycophenolate mofetil can be added. Pericardial tamponade may require pericardiocentesis; recurrent large effusions may require a pericardial window.

E. RENAL LUPUS

Treatment of acute lupus nephritis requires knowledge of the World Health Organization classes. Mesangial and mild focal proliferative nephritis will respond well to glucocorticoids and sometimes require the addition of azathioprine or mycophenolate mofetil. Diffuse proliferative glomerulonephritis that is not rapidly progressive may be treated with mycophenolate mofetil, but the severe form requires the addition of cyclophosphamide, usually following the National Institutes of Health regimen of induction (monthly for 6 months) followed by maintenance (quarterly for 2 more years). Toxicity of intravenous cyclophosphamide includes cytopenias, infections, nausea, alopecia, hemorrhagic cystitis (which can be prevented by giving mesna to bind the metabolite acrolein), premature gonadal failure (the risk of ovarian failure can be lessened by giving leuprolide 2 weeks before each infusion), and malignancy. Treatment of membranous nephritis varies, but may include an initial trial of glucocorticoids followed by mycophenolate mofetil, cyclosporine, or cyclophosphamide.

Patients who do not have a complete response may require a second renal biopsy to determine whether there is still a component of active nephritis. If the activity index is low, efforts to reduce the progression of sclerosis should be instituted. Strict control of hypertension, using angiotensin-converting enzyme (ACE)-inhibitors (or angiotensin receptor blockers if there is ACE-inhibitor cough), is recommended.

Patients with SLE in whom renal failure develops are candidates for renal transplantation. The risk of recurrence of lupus nephritis in the graft is low. In general, when the patient is undergoing dialysis, disease activity is more likely to be low with hemodialysis than with peritoneal dialysis.

F. NEUROLOGIC LUPUS

The most common neurologic complaint of SLE patients is cognitive dysfunction. On formal testing, this is usually mild and not rapidly progressive. Therefore, it is not clear that it represents active lupus, nor is it reversible by immunosuppression. The goal is careful follow-up. Progression should lead to a repeat MRI of the brain with gadolinium, lumbar puncture, and consideration of a cerebral arteriogram. Antiphospholipid antibodies should be checked and low-dose aspirin instituted if they are present, even if no brain infarct has been detected.

Major presentations of central nervous system lupus, such as psychosis and seizures, are treated in the usual fashion (antipsychotics for psychosis, antiepileptics for seizures) with an evaluation to determine whether there is an active lupus component. If active central nervous system SLE is present, treatment with glucocorticoids and usually other immunosuppressive drugs is instituted. Psychosis can also be caused by high-dose glucocorticoids. Seizures can be due to past infarcts (such as those due to antiphospholipid antibody syndrome, hypertension, or atherosclerosis), eclampsia, infection, or hypertensive encephalopathy.

Encephalopathy (organic brain syndrome) caused by lupus is treated with 1000 mg/d of intravenous methylprednisolone for 3 days, followed by high-dose glucocorticoids (such as prednisone, 0.5–1 mg/kg/d). If there is lack of response, the National Institutes of Health regimen of intravenous cyclophosphamide can be instituted (see above Renal Lupus section). If a patient is unresponsive to high-dose glucocorticoids and to intravenous cyclophosphamide, plasmapheresis can be considered.

G. HEMATOLOGIC LUPUS

Most hematologic lupus is mild and does not require treatment. Treatment can sometimes be harmful. For example, if the white blood cell count drops to less than 1000/μL from intravenous cyclophosphamide, granulocyte colony-stimulating factor (G-CSF) is not initially indicated, because G-CSF can precipitate lupus flare. Any infection should be treated, and the next monthly cyclophosphamide dose reduced appropriately.

Platelet counts less than 30,000/μL can be associated with bleeding (although most patients do not bleed unless the platelet count is below 10,000/μL). Acute profound thrombocytopenia is treated with 1000 mg/d of intravenous methylprednisolone for 3 days, followed by high-dose oral prednisone (0.5–1.0 mg/kg). If there is no response, intravenous gammoglobulin is added at 400 mg/kg/d; immunoglobulin (Ig) A deficiency is a contraindication. If there is no response after 5 days, the dose is increased to 1000 mg/kg/d. Patients who respond to intravenous gammaglobulin but frequently relapse may be candidates for laparoscopic splenectomy. Splenectomy should not be considered curative. Patients who respond but have a high prednisone maintenance dose are candidates for a steroid-sparing approach with immunosuppressive drugs such as azathioprine.

Acute profound hemolytic anemia is treated with pulse methylprednisolone (1000 mg/d for 3 days) followed by high-dose glucocorticoids (such as 0.5–1.0 mg/kg/d of prednisone). Folic acid is given daily. Lack of response may lead to the use of intravenous gammaglobulin, as described above for thrombocytopenia. For patients with chronic hemolytic anemia, steroid-sparing approaches can be tried, including danazol and azathioprine.

H. CONSTITUTIONAL SYMPTOMS

Acute fatigue from a lupus flare will improve with treatment of the flare. Chronic fatigue is rarely responsive to any lupus treatment and is highly correlated with the presence of fibromyalgia. Depression, if present, should be treated. Any comorbid conditions, such as hypothyroidism, should be recognized and treated. In individual cases, consideration can be given to stimulants such as methylphenidate or drugs not yet formally studied in lupus, such as modafinil.

Complications

A. SLE COMPLICATIONS

The major cause of death in patients with SLE is accelerated atherosclerosis. This is a multifactorial process, with lupus playing a role along with traditional cardiovascular risk factors (many of which are aggravated by glucocorticoid therapy). Attention to weight, hypertension, hyperlipidemia, smoking, diabetes, and homocysteinemia is crucial.

Renal failure occurs in lupus nephritis in spite of aggressive treatment with intravenous cyclophosphamide. Hypertension is a major comorbidity and should be aggressively managed with ACE inhibitors, which may have a renal protective effect.

Strokes can occur from active central nervous system lupus, but also from antiphospholipid antibody syndrome, hypertension, atherosclerosis, and infection. Antiphospholipid antibody syndrome (see Chapter 20) is a major source of morbidity in SLE and contributes to mortality.

B. GLUCOCORTICOID COMPLICATIONS

Glucocorticoid use contributes to cataracts; osteoporotic fractures; osteonecrosis; diabetes mellitus; multiple cardiovascular risk factors; infections; and quality-of-life issues with Cushingoid habitus, weight gain, acne, and emotional lability or frank depression.

Recognition of glucocorticoid toxicity has led to a steroid-sparing approach, with prednisone taper; if taper is unsuccessful, then other immunosuppressive drugs are added to control disease activity.

C. OPPORTUNISTIC INFECTIONS

Until proved otherwise, consider infection in a patient with SLE who is febrile. Opportunistic infections are often missed until a postmortem examination. Prophylaxis against *Pneumocystis carinii* pneumonia can be given to neutropenic SLE patients using 100 mg of dapsone 3 times a week to avoid giving sulfonamide antibiotics, which can sometimes precipitate lupus flares.

D. MALIGNANCY

Recent cohort studies have suggested an increased risk of malignancy in SLE. Certainly, this is true in SLE patients who received oral cyclophosphamide at the National Institutes of Health. Women with SLE are more likely to have cervical dysplasia and carcinoma. Papanicolaou smears should be done yearly.

E. ASSOCIATED AUTOIMMUNE DISEASES

Hypothyroidism develops in about 10% of SLE patients. Secondary Sjögren syndrome can occur in SLE patients, with or without the Sjögren antibodies anti-Ro and anti-La.

If anti-Ro (especially with anti-La) is present, there is a risk of neonatal lupus in the fetus, presenting as congenital heart block or neonatal lupus rash (the latter being transient).

When to Refer to a Specialist

A rheumatologist is usually needed to make a firm diagnosis of SLE. Often, the need for procedures, such as skin, nerve/muscle, or renal biopsy, will lead to the involvement of dermatologists, neurologists, and nephrologists, as appropriate.

SLE patients receiving glucocorticoids or other immunosuppressive drugs require follow-up by a rheumatologist. Often, comorbid conditions, such as depression or fibromyalgia, lead to complaints that appear to mimic lupus. Recognition, before the patient is unnecessarily exposed to glucocorticoids, is essential.

Communication between the patient, primary care provider, and rheumatologist is crucial in laboratory monitoring and identifying which new events or complications are lupus-related.

Prognosis

The 10-year survival of lupus patients plateaued at 80% in the 1980s. The improvement up to the 1980s reflected not just rheumatologic care but successful treatment of infections and supportive care for renal failure.

Early deaths in lupus tend to reflect disease activity and infections, whereas late deaths are largely due to cardiovascular complications.

REFERENCES

American College of Rheumatology Ad Hoc Committee on Systemic Lupus Erythematosus Guidelines. Guidelines for referral and management of systemic lupus erythematosus in adults. *Arthritis Rheum.* 1999;42:1785. [PMID: 10513791] (The committee report reviews general guidelines in the care of SLE.)

Austin HA, et al. Therapy of lupus nephritis: controlled trial of prednisone and cytotoxic drugs. *N Engl J Med.* 1986;314:614. [PMID: 3511372] (This is one of the classic NIH papers reviewing the better outcome of lupus nephritis with immunosuppressive drugs [specifically cyclophosphamide] than with glucocorticoids alone.)

Barr S, et al. Patterns of disease activity in systemic lupus erythematosus. *Arthritis Rheum.* 1999;42:2682. [PMID: 10616018] (Two patterns of activity characterize SLE: a relapsing-remitting pattern (flare) and a chronically active pattern. Long periods of disease quiescence are rare.)

Chan TM, et al. Efficacy of mycophenolate mofetil in patients with diffuse proliferative lupus nephritis. Hong Kong-Guangzhou Nephrology Study Group. *N Engl J Med.* 2000;343:1156. [PMID: 11036121] (Mycophenolate mofetil may be useful in some patients with diffuse proliferative glomerulonephritis.)

Esdaile JM, et al. Traditional Framingham risk factors fail to fully account for accelerated atherosclerosis in systemic lupus erythematosus. *Arthritis Rheum.* 2001;44:2331. [PMID: 11665973] (Atherosclerosis in SLE cannot be explained by traditional risk factors alone.)

Manzi S, et al. Age-specific incidence rates of myocardial infarction and angina in women with systemic lupus erythematosus: comparison with the Framingham Study. *Am J Epidemiol.* 1997;145:408. [PMID: 9048514] (Atherosclerosis in SLE is much more frequent than in Framingham controls.)

Tan EM, et al. The 1982 revised criteria for the classification of systemic lupus erythematosus. *Arthritis Rheum.* 1982;25:1271. [PMID: 7138600]

Uramoto KM, et al. Trends in the incidence and mortality of systemic lupus erythematosus, 1950-1992. *Arthritis Rheum.* 1999;42:46. [PMID: 9920013] (This population-based study in Rochester, Minnesota, shows an apparent tripling in the incidence of SLE.)

Urowitz MB, Gladman DD. Late mortality in SLE—"the price we pay for control." *J Rheumatol.* 1980;7:412. [PMID: 7401073] (Mortality in SLE is bimodal, with later deaths largely due to atherosclerosis.)

Zonana-Nacach A, et al. Damage in systemic lupus erythematosus and its association with corticosteroids. *Arthritis Rheum.* 2000;43:1801. [PMID: 10943870] (In this prospective study, both chronic use of prednisone and exposure to high doses led to later morbidity.)

Relevant World Wide Web Sites

[Lupus Foundation of America]

http://www.lupus.org

[The National Institute of Arthritis and Musculoskeletal and Skin Diseases (NIAMS)]

http://www.nih.gov/niams

[Arthritis Foundation]

http://www.arthritis.org

Antiphospholipid Antibody Syndrome

20

Michelle Petri, MD, MPH

ESSENTIALS OF DIAGNOSIS

- *An acquired hypercoagulable state.*
- *Presentation with arterial or venous thrombosis, pregnancy loss, or thrombocytopenia.*
- *About 50% have systemic lupus erythematosus.*
- *Antiphospholipid antibodies include the lupus anticoagulant, anticardiolipin antibody, and anti-β_2 glycoprotein I.*

General Considerations

About 5% of the general population, but 50% of patients with systemic lupus erythematosus, have an antiphospholipid antibody, such as the lupus anticoagulant, anticardiolipin antibody, or anti-β_2 glycoprotein I. Because phospholipids are integral parts of the control of coagulation, these antibodies can lead to a hypercoagulable state, antiphospholipid antibody syndrome (APS). If no connective tissue disease is present, the term "primary" is used.

Classification criteria for APS are listed in Table 20–1. The two clinical criteria are (1) arterial or venous thrombosis or vasculopathy or (2) pregnancy loss (three first-trimester losses; one or more late fetal deaths) or morbidity from placental insufficiency in the setting of a lupus anticoagulant or moderate to high immunoglobulin (Ig) G or IgM anticardiolipin (confirmed twice over at least 6 weeks).

Venous thrombosis, usually a deep venous thrombosis with or without pulmonary emboli, is the most common thrombotic presentation. Arterial thrombosis is most commonly a transient ischemic attack or stroke. Some strokes in APS patients are embolic, from vegetations on the mitral or aortic valve.

Antiphospholipid antibodies are associated with pregnancy loss, both early spontaneous abortions and late intrauterine fetal death. The latter likely is due to placental vasculopathy or infarcts.

Some patients with antiphospholipid antibodies are thrombocytopenic. The reasons for thrombocytopenia are varied and include an autoimmune thrombocytopenia, platelet activation, or most worrisome, platelet consumption. Usually, the thrombocytopenia is mild, but on occasion it can be profound, potentially putting the patient at risk for both bleeding and clotting.

The most dire presentation of APS is the catastrophic form, in which thrombosis is occurring in multiple organs over a short period of time. Such patients may initially be given an incorrect diagnosis such as thrombotic thrombocytopenic purpura or disseminated intravascular coagulation. Precipitants of the catastrophic form of APS include infections, surgery, discontinuation of anticoagulation therapy, and hormonal factors such as oral contraceptives and pregnancy.

Obviously, not all persons with antiphospholipid antibodies clot. In a patient with systemic lupus erythematosus and lupus anticoagulant, the risk of a venous thrombosis is 50% over 20 years. In general, patients with a lupus anticoagulant, higher-titer anticardiolipin, and persistence of antibody over time are at greater risk for thrombosis. In addition, the presence of other risk factors for clotting, such as oral contraceptive pills, pregnancy, homocysteinemia, and so on, can increase the risk of thrombosis.

Clinical Findings

A. SYMPTOMS AND SIGNS

1. Cutaneous—Livedo reticularis is the classic cutaneous sign associated with antiphospholipid antibodies. It is not specific, because it can occur with lupus, vasculitis, cholesterol emboli, and cryoglobulinemia. Splinter hemorrhages, superficial thrombophlebitis, and leg ulcers are additional cutaneous manifestations.

2. Head, eyes, ears, nose, and throat—Optic neuropathy can occur as a thrombotic manifestation of APS.

3. Cardiopulmonary—Pulmonary emboli and pulmonary infarcts are thrombotic sequelae of APS. Rarely, pulmonary capillaritis can present in a patient. Myocardial infarction, even without atherosclerosis, can occur. Libman-Sacks endocarditis—sterile valve vegetations—can occur from APS, typically on the mitral or aortic

Table 20–1. Antiphospholipid antibody syndrome classification criteria.

Vascular thrombosis
 Arterial, venous, or small vessel
Pregnancy morbidity
 One or more fetal deaths
 One or more premature births due to severe preeclampsia
  or placental insufficiency
 Three or more first trimester losses
PLUS lupus anticoagulant
 Anticardiolipin IgG or IgM (medium to high titer) on
  two occasions 6 weeks (or more) apart

Ig, immunoglobulin.

valve. Valvular involvement can be severe enough to require valve replacement.

4. Gastrointestinal—Hepatic or splenic infarcts can occur as part of APS. Budd-Chiari syndrome can occur as well.

5. Neurologic—Transient ischemic attacks or strokes are the most common neurologic manifestations. Dementia can occur without infarcts. Cognitive impairment may be associated with antiphospholipid antibodies. Two neurologic manifestations, chorea and transverse myelitis, may represent nonthrombotic consequences of APS.

6. Endocrinologic—Adrenal insufficiency can occur in APS, either due to an infarct that turns hemorrhagic or as a primary hemorrhage.

7. Reproductive—In addition to pregnancy losses, antiphospholipid antibodies may be associated with other pregnancy morbidity, including severe preeclampsia, HELLP (hemolysis, elevated liver enzymes, and low platelet count) syndrome, and intrauterine growth restriction.

B. LABORATORY FINDINGS

1. Antiphospholipid antibody tests—

 a. False-positive test for syphilis—The FP-RPR is an antiphospholipid antibody. However, it is not as strongly associated with thrombosis as those antiphospholipid antibodies directed against negatively charged phospholipids.

 b. Lupus anticoagulant (LA)—The name LA is unfortunate, because only 50% of patients with the LA have lupus and because it is a procoagulant, not anticoagulant, in vivo. In vitro, though, the LA prolongs clotting times. The activated partial thromboplastin time is not a sensitive enough screening test. By international consensus, it is recommended that two sensitive screening tests should be done, such as a dilute Russell viper venom time and a sensitive partial thromboplastin time. The second step is to do a mix with normal plasma (1:1 and then 4:1 ratios) because there will be a lack of correction of the prolonged clotting time in the presence of an LA. The final confirming step is to add back phospholipids, such as with a platelet neutralization procedure.

 c. Anticardiolipin (aCL)—Anticardiolipin is a solid-phase enzyme-linked immunosorbent assay, usually of all three isotypes (IgG, IgM, IgA), although a polyclonal assay is also possible. International criteria for negative, low, medium, and high levels have been set, and standards are available for laboratory calibration.

 d. Anti-β_2 glycoprotein I (aβ_2 GPI)—β_2 GPI is the "cofactor" or target of aCL antibodies. Anti-β_2 GPI assay results, however, do not completely overlap with aCL results. There are no current international standards for anti-β_2 GPI.

2. Complete blood cell count—Thrombocytopenia is a common finding in patients with APS.

3. Urinalysis—Proteinuria, secondary to renal vasculopathy from APS, can be found.

C. IMAGING STUDIES

Imaging studies are frequently required in the evaluation of APS. Obviously, appropriate imaging studies will be done to diagnose a thrombotic event (duplex ultrasonogram or venogram for deep venous thrombosis, computed tomography or magnetic resonance imaging of the brain for stroke) or other APS manifestations (echocardiography for valve vegetations).

Arteriograms (coronary, mesenteric, and so on) may be necessary to ascertain the presence of thrombosis or vasculopathy in an organ.

Differential Diagnosis

Common genetic causes of hypercoagulability must be considered. The two most common are the factor V Leiden mutation (presenting predominantly as venous thrombosis) and the prothrombin mutation (usually venous, but some arterial thrombosis). Less common genetic hypercoagulable states include protein C, protein S, and antithrombin III deficiency, all of which are associated with venous thrombosis. Homocysteinemia, mediated by multiple genetic mutations, is a risk factor for both arterial thrombosis and atherosclerosis.

Acquired causes of hypercoagulability include pregnancy (especially the postpartum period), oral contraceptives, estrogen replacement therapy, bed rest, trauma, surgery, vasculitis, and malignancy.

The catastrophic form of APS may be confused with several entities. Thrombotic thrombocytopenia purpura—a disorder of von Willebrand monomers—often involves fever, and schistocytes will be seen on the peripheral blood smear. Disseminated intravascular coagulation will also be in the differential diagnosis.

Treatment

A. Venous and Arterial Thrombosis

The acute treatment of venous or arterial thrombosis does not change. Over the long term, two treatment caveats are important. First, because of the high risk of recurrence, long-term anticoagulation with warfarin is recommended. Second, based on retrospective studies, high-intensity warfarin (international normalized ratio goal of 3) was thought to be preferable, but a recent clinical trial found usual-intensity and high-intensity warfarin to be equally efficacious.

B. Pregnancy Loss

A landmark clinical trial showed that 40 mg of prednisone and low-dose aspirin versus 10,000 U of subcutaneous heparin twice daily and low-dose aspirin were equally successful in terms of live births; however, there was much more maternal morbidity (ie, preeclampsia and diabetes) in the prednisone arm. Heparin and aspirin have been the preferred therapy since then. Low-molecular-weight heparin may be substituted for unfractionated heparin, but twice-daily dosing is preferred in pregnant women. However, unfractionated heparin should be substituted for low-molecular-weight heparin before delivery. The long duration of action of low-molecular-weight heparin might lead to a bleeding complication during delivery.

In two trials, heparin plus aspirin were better than aspirin alone. In a third trial, there was no difference.

In women who continue to miscarry while receiving heparin plus aspirin, intravenous immunoglobulin has been used based on a strong scientific rationale that it binds antiphospholipid antibodies and may downregulate their production. However, no additional benefit was demonstrated in a small clinical trial.

C. Thrombocytopenia

Patients with APS and thrombosis cannot be given anticoagulant therapy safely if they are also profoundly (platelets < 50,000/μL) thrombocytopenic. Additional therapies (prednisone, intravenous immunoglobulin) should be added to keep the platelet count above 50,000/μL. A few patients have required splenectomies with variable success.

D. Chorea and Transverse Myelitis

Chorea and transverse myelitis are often not thrombotic manifestations of APS. They may respond to intravenous methylprednisolone, which should always be given promptly. Such patients are at risk, though, for APS-associated thrombosis elsewhere.

E. Catastrophic APS

The catastrophic form of APS has a high mortality of 50%. Essentials of treatment include heparin, intravenous methylprednisolone pulse therapy, and plasmapheresis to reduce the burden of circulating antiphospholipid antibodies.

F. Prophylactic Treatment

There is a strong case for using low-dose aspirin in patients with the lupus anticoagulant or medium- to high-titer aCL, or both. A retrospective study suggested that this reduced the thrombosis rate, but no clinical trials have been done.

Hydroxychloroquine has been shown to reduce the thrombosis rate in longitudinal studies in systemic lupus erythematosus and to prevent thrombosis in an animal model of a damaged femoral vein. Because 50% of patients with systemic lupus erythematosus make antiphospholipid antibodies, hydroxychloroquine may already be considered for its beneficial effect on disease activity.

Complications

An arterial or venous thrombotic event may lead to profound morbidity or even be fatal. APS patients have a high risk of recurrent thrombotic events if they do not receive long-term anticoagulant therapy.

Unfortunately, anticoagulation is not completely safe. Severe bleeding complications can occur. Monitoring the international normalized ratio every 2 weeks is recommended.

When to Refer to a Specialist

The initial diagnosis of APS may not be straightforward, given laboratory variability in quality. If a patient has already received anticoagulation therapy with warfarin, special mixing studies need to be set up to determine whether a lupus anticoagulant is present.

Patients who have recurrent thrombosis while taking warfarin should be referred to a rheumatologist, hematologist, or neurologist familiar with APS for additional therapeutic decisions.

Prognosis

With careful management of anticoagulation, recurrent thrombotic events can usually be prevented. Classic lupus may develop in a few patients who have APS.

REFERENCES

Alarcon-Segovia D, Cabral AR. The anti-phospholipid antibody syndrome: clinical and serological aspects. *Baillieres Best Pract Res Clin Rheumatol.* 2000;14:139. [PMID: 10882219] (A review of APS manifestations in a large Mexican SLE cohort.)

Asherson RA, et al. Catastrophic antiphospholipid syndrome: clues to the pathogenesis from a series of 80 patients. *Medicine (Baltimore)*. 2001;80:355. [PMID: 11704713] (Catastrophic antiphospholipid antibody syndrome carries a mortality of 50%.)

Cowchock FS, et al. Repeated fetal losses associated with antiphospholipid antibodies: a collaborative randomized trial comparing prednisone with low-dose heparin treatment. *Am J Obstet Gynecol.* 1992;166:1318. [PMID: 1595785]

Erkan D, et al. High thrombosis rate after fetal loss in antiphospholipid syndrome: effective prophylaxis with aspirin. *Arthritis Rheum.* 2001;44:1466. [PMID: 11407709] (A retrospective chart review study suggesting benefit of aspirin as prophylactic therapy.)

Exner T, et al. Guidelines for testing and revised criteria for lupus anticoagulants. SSC Subcommittee for the Standardization of Lupus Anticoagulants. *Thromb Haemost.* 1991;65:320. [PMID: 1904657] (A review of lupus anticoagulant testing.)

Harris EN, et al. The anti-cardiolipin assay. In: Harris EN, Exner T, Hughes GRV, Asherson RA, eds. *Phospholipid-Binding Antibodies.* CRC Press, 1991:175–187. (A review of anticardiolipin standardization and testing.)

Khamashta MA, et al. The management of thrombosis in the antiphospholipid antibody syndrome. *N Engl J Med.* 1995;332: 993. [PMID: 7885428] (A large retrospective study demonstrating that high-intensity warfarin therapy is the most successful treatment regimen.)

Schulman S, et al and the Duration of Anticoagulation Study Group. Anticardiolipin antibodies predict early recurrence of thromboembolism and death among patients with venous thromboembolism following anticoagulant therapy. *Am J Med.* 1998;104:332. [PMID: 9576405] (A prospective study proving the high risk of recurrent thrombosis in APS.)

Wilson WA, et al. International consensus statement on preliminary classification criteria for definite antiphospholipid syndrome: report of an international workshop. *Arthritis Rheum.* 1999;42:1309. [PMID: 10403256] (Classification criteria for APS were determined at a consensus conference.)

Raynaud Phenomenon

Sangeeta Dileep Sule, MD, & Fredrick M. Wigley, MD

ESSENTIALS OF DIAGNOSIS

- *An exaggerated response to cold temperatures that results in transient digital ischemia.*
- *Classified clinically into primary or secondary forms.*
- *Complications of digital tissue ischemia may occur in patients with secondary RP, leading to recurrent digital ulcerations, rapid deep tissue necrosis, and amputation.*
- *Avoidance of cold temperatures is crucial to the management of RP. The entire body must be kept comfortably warm.*
- *Medications are indicated if there are signs of critical tissue ischemia (eg, digital ulcers) or if the quality of life of the patient is so affected that normal function is restricted.*

General Considerations

When humans are exposed to cold temperatures, the body will sacrifice the viability of peripheral tissues by shifting blood flow from the skin and other organs to maintain a stable core body temperature. A unique circulatory system exists in the skin, especially in the hands, feet, and areas of the face that include both thermoregulatory and nutritional blood vessels. In these areas of the body, local blood flow is regulated by a complex interaction of neural signals, cellular mediators, and circulating vasoactive molecules. Temperature responses are principally mediated through the sympathetic nervous system by rapidly altering blood flow through arteriovenous shunts in the skin. During hot weather, these shunts open (vasodilate), allowing heat to dissipate. In cool weather, the shunts constrict, shifting blood centrally and helping maintain a stable core body temperature.

Raynaud phenomenon (RP) is an exaggerated response to cold temperatures that results in transient digital ischemia. The vasoconstriction of digital arteries, precapillary arterioles, and cutaneous arteriovenous shunts

leads to a sharp demarcation of skin pallor or cyanosis of the digits (Figure 21–1). This ischemic phase is followed by recovery of blood flow that appears as cutaneous erythema, secondary to rapid reperfusion of the digits.

RP is classified clinically into primary or secondary forms. Primary RP occurs in the absence of any associated disease or definable cause. In fact, most experts think that the primary form is merely an exaggeration of normal physiologic responses to cold environmental temperatures or emotional stress or both, rather than a disease. Secondary RP is associated with an underlying pathologic condition or disease that alters regional blood flow by damaging blood vessels, interfering with neural control of the circulation, or changing either the physical properties of the blood or the levels of circulating mediators that regulate the digital and cutaneous circulation. Although there are a large number of suspected causes of secondary RP, the primary care physician will most commonly encounter RP associated with a rheumatic or connective tissue disease, such as scleroderma, systemic lupus erythematosus (SLE), Sjögren syndrome, or dermatomyositis.

Clinical Findings

A. SYMPTOMS AND SIGNS

RP results from an exaggerated vascular response to cold temperatures or stress. This vascular constriction leads to color changes visible on the skin. The fingers are the most commonly affected, although attacks also occur in the toes and occasionally on areas of the face. A typical RP attack is characterized by the sudden onset of cold digits associated with a demarcation of skin pallor (white attack) or cyanosis (blue attack). After rewarming, the skin blushes from reperfusion, resulting in the erythema secondary to rebound of blood flow. Although many people in the general population (~ 30%) are "sensitive to the cold," a true RP attack is defined clinically by a history of both cold sensitivity and associated color changes of the skin (pallor or cyanosis or both) limited to the digits. RP attacks typically begin in a single finger and then spread to other digits of the same or both hands. The index, middle, and ring fingers are the most commonly involved digits. Primary RP occurs in the absence of a definable

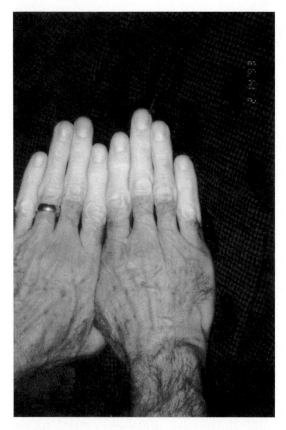

Figure 21–1. A typical Raynaud phenomenon attack characterized by a sharp demarcation of skin pallor.

Table 21–1. Criteria for the diagnosis of primary Raynaud phenomenon.[a]

Symmetric, intermittent RP attacks
No evidence of peripheral vascular disease
No evidence of tissue gangrene or digital pitting
No abnormal nailfold capillary microscopy
Negative antinuclear antibody test and normal erythrocyte
   sedimentation rate

[a]Adapted from LeRoy EC, Medsger TA Jr, Raynaud's phenomenon: a proposal for classification. *Clin Exp Rheumatol.* 1992; 10:485.

vere nature of the RP in these cases is due to secondary processes causing direct vessel damage. The clinical features that help distinguish primary from secondary RP are outlined in Table 21–3.

All patients with a history of RP should be asked about symptoms suggestive of an autoimmune disease, such as arthritis, dry eyes or dry mouth, myalgias, fevers, skin rash, or cardiopulmonary abnormalities. Careful

cause for the attacks. It is most common in otherwise healthy females with an age of onset between 15 and 30 years. A history that another first-degree family member is affected with RP is reported in about 30% of cases. Criteria for the diagnosis of primary RP are shown in Table 21–1.

Underlying causes of RP—usually connective tissue diseases—eventually emerge in 10–15% of patients in whom primary RP was initially diagnosed. If a patient meets criteria for primary RP and no new symptoms develop over 2 years of follow-up, the development of secondary disease is unlikely. The presence of abnormal nailfold capillaries on microscopy (see below) is the best predictor of secondary RP.

The most common causes of secondary RP are scleroderma, SLE, and other connective tissue disorders (Table 21–2). Patients with secondary RP generally have more severe RP, often accompanied by pain, which may herald an episode of serious digital ischemia, fingertip ulceration, and tissue loss. Tissue ischemia and digital ulceration may result. The more se-

Table 21–2. Secondary causes of Raynaud phenomenon.

Rheumatologic	Hematologic disorders
Systemic sclerosis (scleroderma)	Cryoglobulinemia
Systemic lupus erythematosus	Paraproteinemia
Rheumatoid arthritis	Polycythemia
Sjögren syndrome	Cold agglutinins
Dermatomyositis	
Polymyositis	
Vasculitis	
Mechanical	**Endocrine disorders**
Vibration injury	Hypothyroidism
Frostbite	Carcinoid syndrome
Thoracic outlet syndrome	Pheochromocytoma
Vascular embolus or occlusion	
Vasospasm	**Drugs**
Migraine headaches	Sympathomimetic drugs (decongestants, diet pills)
	Serotonin agonists (sumatriptan)
	Chemotherapeutic agents (bleomycin, cisplatin, carboplatin, vinblastine)
	Ergotamine tartrate
	Caffeine
	Nicotine

Table 21–3. Clinical features of secondary Raynaud phenomenon.

Male sex
Pain associated with attacks
Signs of tissue ischemia (digital ulcerations)
Age of onset > 40 years
Asymmetry of digits affected
Signs or symptoms of other diseases (rheumatic, endocrine, etc)
Abnormal laboratory tests (positive antinuclear antibodies, cryoglobulins)

examination for signs of a secondary process should include examination of the pulses, auscultation over large arteries, examination for evidence of tissue ischemia or inflammatory skin lesions, and nailfold capillary microscopy. If the clinician suspects an underlying autoimmune disease, the patient should be evaluated for the presence of specific autoantibodies (see Laboratory Findings).

B. LABORATORY FINDINGS

Patients who are young when symptoms begin; who have a normal history and physical examination, including normal nailfold capillaries and larger vessel examination; and who have no history of digital ischemic lesions can be considered to have primary RP. These patients can be monitored clinically, and no further laboratory testing is needed.

However, if a secondary cause of RP is suspected, appropriate testing is recommended, including serum chemistries, complete blood cell count, thyroid function tests, serum and urine protein electrophoresis, and testing for cryoglobulins or cryofibrinogens. In addition, inflammatory markers such as erythrocyte sedimentation rate or C-reactive protein are often elevated in patients with secondary RP.

Antinuclear antibody (ANA) assays are highly sensitive for the types of connective tissue disorders that are often associated with RP. However, positive ANAs are quite nonspecific and therefore should be followed by testing for autoantibodies with higher positive predictive values for such conditions. An anticentromere pattern detected on ANA testing is associated strongly with limited scleroderma (eg, the CREST [calcinosis, Raynaud phenomenon, esophageal dysmotility, sclerodactyly, telangiectasias] syndrome; see Chapter 22). Antitopoisomerase antibodies may be observed in patients with RP secondary to scleroderma. Anti-dsDNA, anti-Ro/SS-A, anti-La/SS-B, anti-Sm, and anti-RNP antibodies are detected in many patients with SLE. Anti-Jo-1 antibodies are often associated with inflammatory myopathies.

C. SPECIAL TESTS

Nailfold capillary microscopy can be used to examine the nailfold capillary bed of patients with RP. This can provide a clue for the classification of RP (primary versus secondary); patients with secondary RP may have capillary loop changes, including enlargement and dropout caused by the underlying vascular disease process (Figure 21–2). To perform nailfold capillary microscopy, a drop of grade B immersion oil is placed on the patient's skin at the base of the fingernail. This

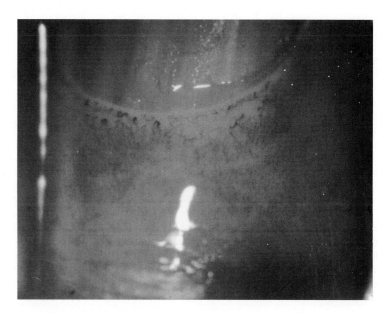

Figure 21–2. Nailfold capillary microscopy demonstrating nailfold capillary loop dilation and dropout.

area is then viewed using an ophthalmoscope set to 10–40 diopters or a stereoscopic microscope. Normal capillaries appear as symmetric, nondilated loops. In contrast, distorted, dilated, or absent capillaries suggest a secondary disease process.

Differential Diagnosis

The diagnosis of RP is clinical, based on a patient's report of sudden, episodic color changes of the digits provoked by cold temperature or emotional stress. However, many people without RP report an increased sensitivity to the cold. Thus, true RP should be distinguished from the nondemarcated mottling seen in a normal response to cool temperatures. True RP must also be distinguished from acrocyanosis—a condition seen when the patient has cool hands and feet with persistently cyanotic skin. Although acrocyanosis is aggravated by cold temperature, there are none of the episodic attacks or sharp demarcations of color changes observed in RP.

Repeated mechanical stress on the nerves or vessels in the hand or fingers may also cause sensitivity to the cold temperature. Vibration tool use, carpal tunnel syndrome, or neuropathy should be considered in a patient who complains of color changes of the hands and numbness with or without sensitivity to the cold. Paraproteinemias and hyperviscosity syndromes should also be considered in the differential diagnosis. RP in these patients results from sluggish blood flow through cutaneous and digital vessels. Patients may also have cold-sensitive proteins; RP is common among patients with cryoglobulinemia. The use of certain drugs (eg, sympathomimetic agents) that induce vasoconstriction can aggravate or cause RP. In addition, patients with hypothyroidism often have cold hands, acrocyanosis, or RP.

Distinguishing primary from secondary RP is critical. The connective tissue diseases are the most common secondary disorders that the internist will encounter. Thus, a thorough review of systems focusing on symptoms of a connective tissue disease is essential. Patients should be asked about dry eyes or mouth (Sjögren syndrome); painful joints or morning stiffness (arthritis); rashes, photosensitivity, or cardiopulmonary abnormalities (SLE); and skin tightening, respiratory distress, or gastrointestinal disease (scleroderma).

Most patients with RP report symmetric involvement of the digits. Therefore, if a patient reports asymmetric RP, a mechanical occlusion of the large vessels, either from atherosclerosis, emboli, or arterial occlusion, should be considered. In such cases, noninvasive vascular flow studies are helpful and vascular imaging such as a magnetic resonance arteriogram or arteriography may be appropriate. Although systemic vasculitides such as

polyarteritis nodosa, Wegener granulomatosis, and Buerger disease may cause critical digital ischemia and tissue necrosis, these patients do not have typical RP.

Treatment

A. PREVENTIVE STRATEGIES

Avoidance of cold temperatures is crucial to the management of RP. Although the importance of keeping the hands and feet warm is obvious, the whole body must be kept comfortably warm. Thus, wearing several layers of loose fitting clothing, mittens, stockings, and headwear in cold temperatures is very important. Damp windy weather or rapid shifts in ambient temperature are more likely to precipitate RP attacks. Air-conditioning during summer months can be a problem because of sudden shifts in temperature or uncontrolled drafts of cold air over the hands or body. Emotional stress can not only trigger a RP attack but also lower the threshold for cold-induced attacks. Therefore, stress control and relaxation techniques are helpful in preventing RP attacks.

Medications that have the potential to vasoconstrict the peripheral arteries should be avoided in patients with both primary and secondary RP. Sympathomimetic drugs (decongestants, diet pills, ephedra) and serotonin agonists such as sumatriptan should be avoided because they are vasoconstrictors and could aggravate RP. In addition, certain chemotherapeutic agents (bleomycin, cisplatin, carboplatin, and vinblastine) may cause vascular occlusion and trigger RP attacks. RP patients should avoid smoking because nicotine reduces cutaneous and digital blood flow. Nonselective β blockers were once thought to be contraindicated, but new studies refute this finding. Clonidine and narcotics also vasoconstrict the cutaneous circulation and should be used with caution. A recent warning has noted potential vasospasm with concomitant administration of ergotamine tartrate plus caffeine, a migraine medication, and CYP3A4 inhibitors such as macrolide antibiotics and protease inhibitors.

B. VASODILATOR THERAPY

Medications are indicated in the treatment of RP if there are signs of critical tissue ischemia (eg, digital ulcers) or if the quality of life of the patient is affected to the degree that normal functions are restricted. If preventive strategies fail, vasodilator therapy is the next available option. Calcium channel blockers are the most widely used vasodilators; however, other agents are rapidly becoming available. In general, no medication has proved to be more effective or safer than the calcium channel blockers. Although combinations of vasodilators are often used, there are no studies that address this strategy.

1. Calcium channel blockers—Calcium channel blockers are the most popular pharmacologic treatment for RP. Short-acting nifedipine reduces the frequency and severity of attacks by about one-third. The benefit is more robust in the patients with primary RP than in those with secondary RP. Calcium channel blockers differ in their peripheral vasodilatory properties. Nifedipine, amlodipine, felodipine, nisoldipine, and isradipine appear more effective than diltiazem and verapamil in the treatment of RP. The most significant side effects from calcium channel blockers are headache, hypotension, tachycardia, and lower extremity edema. However, aggravation of gastroesophageal reflux disease, constipation, and hypertrophy of the gums can also occur. In one study of sustained-release nifedipine, approximately 15% of healthy patients with primary RP had to stop taking the drug because of headache and lower extremity edema.

Slow-release preparations are preferred because they are as effective and safer than the rapid-release medications. Slow-release nifedipine may be used in the treatment of RP at doses from 30 to 180 mg/d. Currently, oral amlodipine at doses of 5–20 mg/d is preferred over nifedipine because amlodipine exerts less negative inotropy on the heart. Individual responses and tolerance to calcium channel blockers vary among patients. If one calcium channel blocker is ineffective, another calcium channel blocker may be tried. There is no evidence that combinations of calcium channel blockers are better than a single drug.

2. Angiotensin-converting enzyme (ACE) inhibitors—These drugs are used in the treatment of hypertension and scleroderma renal crisis. The role of ACE inhibitors in RP is debated and not well defined, but there is evidence that they may improve digital blood flow by increasing kinins and causing vasodilation. A small clinical trial using losartan, an angiotensin II receptor blocker, found a decrease in the number and severity of RP attacks in both primary and secondary RP. Captopril, a traditional ACE inhibitor, improved RP attacks in primary RP, but not RP secondary to scleroderma. Although the use of ACE inhibitors in RP needs further investigation, the use of these drugs alone in complex or refractory cases or in combination with calcium channel blockers is reasonable.

3. Sympatholytic agents—Sympathetic adrenergic stimulation, particularly α_2-adrenergic receptors on the digital arteries, is thought to play an important role in control of digital blood flow. Therefore, in severe RP, another option is to block sympathetic tone in the hope of inducing vasodilation of digital vessels. However, there are few controlled trials of sympatholytic agents in RP. The best studied is prazosin, an α_1-adrenergic receptor blocker. In two controlled trials, prazosin was more effective than placebo in primary and secondary RP. However, patients became resistant to prazosin after prolonged use. Thus, sympatholytic agents may be helpful in the treatment of RP, but the vasodilation lessens over time and side effects are often intolerable.

4. Nitrates and other topical therapy—Although not well studied in controlled trials, nitroglycerin ointment is frequently used in combination with a calcium channel blocker or alone in the treatment of both primary and secondary RP. There have been numerous anecdotal reports of improvement in RP with 0.25–0.5 inch of 2% nitroglycerin ointment applied daily to fingers, the forearms, or wrists of affected hands. The medication is systemically absorbed; thus, patients may still have such side effects as hypotension and headaches. Recently, topical application of prostaglandin E_1 was reported to reduce secondary RP attacks. The potential of topical prostaglandin therapy needs further investigation.

5. Prostaglandins/endothelin-receptor inhibitors—Prostacyclin and other prostaglandins are vasodilators and have been used in the treatment of RP in Europe. Iloprost, a stable prostacyclin analog, has been shown to be beneficial in the treatment of RP secondary to scleroderma. Therapy with iloprost (0.5–2 ng/kg/min intravenous infusion) can provide relief for several weeks following treatment. However, the drug is not currently available in the United States. Orally administered prostaglandins (oral iloprost, cicaprost, and beraprost) are not beneficial in RP, probably because of poor oral bioavailability.

Endothelin is a potent vasoconstrictor produced by a variety of cells including endothelial cells, smooth muscle cells, leukocytes, macrophages, and mesangial cells. Endothelin receptor antagonist drugs (ie, bosentan) have been developed to prevent this potent vasoconstriction. Currently, bosentan is used for the treatment of pulmonary hypertension. Anecdotal reports suggest an improvement in RP among patients with scleroderma. A recent study involving patients with scleroderma demonstrated that patients treated with bosentan had fewer new digital ulcers than those treated with the placebo. Liver toxicity, availability, and the expense of bosentan limit its use, but future studies may define its place in the treatment of difficult cases.

6. Sympathectomy—Surgical sympathectomy is used to ligate the sympathetic nerves that cause vasoconstriction. Both proximal (cervical) and localized (digital) sympathectomy can be used in the treatment of RP. Cervical sympathectomy is reported to be helpful in primary but not in secondary RP. However, a proximal sympathectomy may not be fully effective and this procedure is associated with significant risks including neuralgia, Horner syndrome, and decreased localized sweating. Therefore, a localized digital sympathectomy is the preferred procedure. Nevertheless, the procedure is limited to patients with severe RP, especially those who are in an active ischemic crisis and are not responding to medical management. Most of the available evidence shows that RP attacks recur several weeks to months following either proximal or digital sympathectomy.

7. Anticoagulation—Anticoagulation therapy with aspirin (81 mg/d) is recommended in selected patients with severe secondary RP who are at risk for digital ulceration or larger-artery thrombotic events. Heparin may be used acutely during an ischemic crisis to prevent further digital vessel thrombosis, but long-term anticoagulation with heparin or warfarin is not recommended unless there is evidence of a hypercoagulable disorder (eg, antiphospholipid syndrome, malignancy).

Complications

RP can be a mild nuisance to patients or it can alter their quality of life and prevent them from living in even cool temperatures. The primary form of RP is not associated with critical ischemia or tissue ulcerations, but cold sensitivity, digital numbness, and discomfort can alter hand function. Emotional problems can occur from the social stigma of cold hands with unsightly skin color changes.

Complications of digital tissue ischemia may occur in patients with secondary RP, leading to recurrent digital ulcerations, rapid deep tissue necrosis, and amputation. These patients, unlike patients with primary RP, have structurally abnormal digital vessels as the underlying problem.

A persistently demarcated ischemic digit with accompanying numbness and pain in the digit, hand, or arm characterizes critical digital ischemia. Pain is so severe that the patient seeks medical attention or is positioning the hand downward to improve blood flow, indicating that the tissue is ischemic and vulnerable to ulceration. Severe RP and signs or symptoms of critical tissue ischemia should be considered a medical emergency, and patients should be considered for hospitalization. They should be kept warm and at rest. Vasodilator therapy with a short-acting calcium channel blocker (eg, nifedipine 10–20 mg orally every 8 hours) should be started in combination with aspirin. If ischemia continues, a combination of vasodilators (eg, a calcium channel blocker plus a nitrate [topical nitroglycerin], a sympatholytic agent [prazosin], or an intravenous vasodilator such as prostaglandin infusion [eg, epoprostenol]) may be added. A temporary chemical digital sympathectomy (eg, xylocaine) may reverse vasospasm. Surgical digital sympathectomy may be considered if ischemia persists despite vasodilator therapy. Early intervention with hospitalization and vasodilator therapy is the key to preventing irreversible vessel occlusion and breaking the cycle of vasospasm and digital ischemia.

Digital ulcers from tissue ischemia often develop in patients with secondary RP. In order to avoid infection, it is important to keep these ulcers clean by washing with soap and water twice daily, followed by an appropriate protective dressing. Topical or systemic antibiotics are used if an infection develops.

When to Refer to a Specialist

Patients with primary RP may be treated by the family practitioner or internist with care focusing on preventive measures to keep the patient warm in order to avoid RP attacks. Patients with secondary RP due to a connective tissue disease or RP from an unknown cause should be referred to a rheumatologist for further diagnostic or management suggestions. Patients with RP and evidence of larger-vessel disease should be seen by a vascular specialist for consultation.

Any patient with critical digital ischemia or digital ulcerations should be referred to a specialist for hospitalization and further management as outlined earlier. A vascular surgeon should be consulted early in the hospitalization for chemical or surgical digital sympathectomy if the ischemia is unresponsive to vasodilators.

REFERENCES

LeRoy EC, Medsger TA Jr. Raynaud's phenomenon: a proposal for classification. *Clin Exp Rheumatol.* 1992;10:485. [PMID: 1458701]

Spencer-Green G. Outcomes in primary Raynaud phenomenon: a meta-analysis of the frequency, rates, and predictors of transition to secondary diseases. *Arch Intern Med.* 1998;158:595. [PMID: 9521223]

Thompson AE, et al. Calcium-channel blockers for Raynaud's phenomenon in systemic sclerosis. *Arthritis Rheum.* 2001;44: 1841. [PMID: 11508437]

Wigley FM. Clinical practice. Raynaud's phenomenon. *N Engl J Med.* 2002;347:1001. [PMID: 12324557]

Relevant World Wide Web Sites

[Arthritis Foundation]
http://www.arthritis.org
[Scleroderma Foundation]
http://www.scleroderma.org
[Scleroderma Research Foundation]
http://www.srfcure.org

Scleroderma

Laura K. Hummers, MD, & Fredrick M. Wigley, MD

ESSENTIALS OF DIAGNOSIS

- *The most frequent symptoms are (in descending order) Raynaud phenomenon, gastroesophageal reflux with or without dysmotility, swollen fingers, and arthralgias.*
- *Patients with Raynaud phenomenon and features atypical for primary disease should be evaluated for the possibility of scleroderma or another connective tissue disease.*
- *A negative antinuclear antibody test makes the diagnosis of scleroderma very unlikely.*
- *The degree of skin involvement is highly variable. Many patients with limited scleroderma have only subtle cutaneous findings (eg, mild sclerodactyly).*
- *The available diagnostic criteria do not include many patients with milder forms of scleroderma.*
- *Some patients may have overlapping clinical features with other systemic autoimmune rheumatic disorders such as polymyositis/dermatomyositis, Sjögren syndrome, systemic lupus erythematosus, and rheumatoid arthritis.*

General Considerations

Systemic sclerosis (scleroderma) is a chronic multisystem disease that belongs to the family of systemic autoimmune disorders. The word scleroderma literally means "hard skin" and describes the most dramatic clinical feature of the disease—namely, skin fibrosis. Scleroderma effects approximately 20 new patients per million per year and has an estimated prevalence of approximately 250 patients per million in the United States. As with many other autoimmune disorders, scleroderma is approximately 4–5 times more common in women than men. The average age at the time of diagnosis is approximately 50 years.

The prevalence and manifestations of scleroderma vary among racial and ethnic groups. For example, the disease is approximately 100 times more common

among the Choctaw Native Americans in Oklahoma, in whom the disease is characterized by diffuse skin disease and pulmonary fibrosis. Milder, "limited" disease is more common among white women, and African American patients are more likely to have severe lung disease. The finding of various subtypes of scleroderma among different ethnic or racial groups, the presence of familial clustering, and the appearance of specific autoantibodies that are associated with specific HLA types suggest genetic influences on disease expression. Certain environmental factors are also thought to play etiologic roles. For example, characteristic antibodies and scleroderma disease manifestations can develop in coal miners exposed to high levels of silica.

Clinical Findings

Scleroderma is a rare disorder but is characterized by symptoms that occur frequently in the general population, such as Raynaud phenomenon, gastroesophageal reflux, fatigue, and musculoskeletal pain. Therefore, it is important for primary care practitioners to be aware of scleroderma because early intervention can reduce morbidity and potentially prevent life-threatening complications.

The diagnostic criteria for scleroderma include either thickened (sclerodermatous) skin changes proximal to the metacarpophalangeal joints or at least two of the following:

1. Sclerodactyly.
2. Digital pitting (residual loss of tissue on the finger pads).
3. Bibasilar pulmonary fibrosis.

A diagnosis of limited scleroderma can be made if the patient has three of the five features of the CREST (calcinosis, Raynaud phenomenon, esophageal dysmotility, sclerodactyly, telangiectasias) syndrome. Table 22–1 outlines the classic presentations of limited and diffuse scleroderma.

Patients with definite Raynaud phenomenon who have abnormal nailfold capillary loops and the presence of autoantibodies known to be associated with scleroderma (see Laboratory Findings and Table 22–2) can be considered to have early scleroderma or a mild expression of the disease.

Table 22–1. Classic presentations of limited and diffuse scleroderma.

Limited
    Long history of Raynaud phenomenon
    Gastroesophageal reflux and dysphagia
    Swelling or skin thickening of the fingers
    Infrequent systemic symptoms such as arthralgias, weight
        loss, dyspnea
Diffuse
    New onset of Raynaud phenomenon
    Rapid change in skin texture with new onset of edema,
        pruritus, pain
    Significant systemic symptoms with severe arthralgias,
        weight loss, tendon friction rubs
    Early evidence of internal organ involvement such as
        dyspnea, hypertension

Although skin changes are usually the major diagnostic clues, scleroderma is a systemic disease that most commonly targets the peripheral circulation, muscles, joints, gastrointestinal tract, lung, heart, and kidney. Symptoms encountered in the early presentation of scleroderma include musculoskeletal discomfort, fatigue, weight loss, and heartburn associated with gastroesophageal reflux disease (GERD). When these symptoms are accompanied by the new onset of cold sensitivity or Raynaud phenomenon, then scleroderma should be considered and further diagnostic investigation is warranted.

A. SYMPTOMS AND SIGNS

1. Skin—Thickening of the skin is the most easily recognizable manifestation of scleroderma but is not prominent in all patients. Patients with scleroderma are typically classified based on the amount and location of skin involvement. Patients with "limited" disease have skin changes on the face and distal to the knees and el-

bows. One form of limited scleroderma, the CREST syndrome, typically only involves the skin of the fingers (sclerodactyly) distal to the metacarpophalangeal joints. In contrast, diffuse scleroderma refers to the group of patients with proximal extremity or truncal skin involvement (Figure 22–1). The amount of skin thickening can be quantified by performing a "skin score," in which the skin is pinched between the examiner's thumbs in 17 specified areas of the patient's body, scoring the thickness of the skin from 0 (normal) to 3 (very thick). The skin score provides a systematic approach to longitudinal disease evaluations. Moreover, epidemiologic studies indicate that higher skin scores correlate with greater degrees of internal organ involvement and worse overall prognosis.

Early in the course of diffuse scleroderma, the skin appears edematous and inflamed with erythema and pigmentary changes. Hyperpigmented areas alternating with vitiligo-like areas of depigmentation impart to the skin a "salt and pepper" appearance. The early inflammatory phase is associated with pruritus and discomfort that usually lasts for weeks to months. In vitro studies show that dermal fibroblasts derived from patients with scleroderma overproduce extracellular matrix that leads to increased tissue collagen deposition in the skin. Collagen cross-linking then causes progressive skin tightening. In the later stages of the disease, the involved skin becomes thickened, dry, and scaly because of the loss of its natural oils (sebaceous gland damage). These dry thickened areas of skin are often intensely pruritic, causing the patient to excoriate the skin.

Patients with the CREST syndrome often have other prominent skin changes, including marked telangiectasias (dilated capillaries) that occur on the skin of the face, the palmar surface of the hands, and the mucous membranes (Figure 22–2). A smaller proportion of patients with CREST syndrome have subcutaneous calcinosis, primarily on the fingers and along the extensor surfaces of the forearms.

Table 22–2. Autoantibodies associated with scleroderma.

Autoantibody	Prevalence	Associated Clinical Features
Antinuclear antibody	> 95%	—
Anti-topoisomerase I (Anti-Scl-70)	20–40%	Lung disease, diffuse skin involvement, African Americans, worse prognosis
Anticentromere	20–40%	CREST syndrome, digital ulcerations/digital loss
Anti-RNA polymerases	4–20%	Diffuse skin involvement, scleroderma renal crisis, cardiac disease, worse prognosis
Anti-U3-RNP (Anti-fibrillarin)	8%	Lung disease, diffuse skin involvement, African American males
Anti-U1-RNP	5%	Mixed connective tissue disease
Anti-Th/To	1–5%	Limited cutaneous involvement, pulmonary disease

CREST, calcinosis, Raynaud phenomenon, esophageal dysmotility, sclerodactyly, telangiectasias.

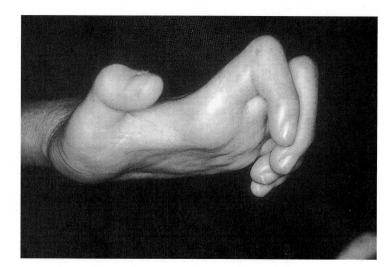

Figure 22–1. Skin thickening and contractures of the fingers in a patient with diffuse scleroderma.

2. Vascular disease—Involvement of the vasculature is ubiquitous among patients with scleroderma. A diffuse vasculopathy of peripheral arteries is manifested pathologically by intimal proliferation, activation of the arterial smooth muscle, and narrowing or occlusion of the vessel lumen. Critical ischemia occurs in the tissues when vasoconstriction occludes these diseased vessels. Evidence suggests that this vascular disease is fundamental to organ damage and subsequent malfunction of the heart (cardiomyopathy), lung (pulmonary hypertension), kidney (scleroderma renal crisis [SRC]), and other organs in scleroderma (see below).

Clinical features found to be predictive of an autoimmune rheumatic disease among patients with Raynaud phenomenon include the presence of antinuclear antibodies (ANAs) and abnormal nailfold capillaries (see Special Examinations below). Patients over the age of 30 in whom Raynaud phenomenon develops should be screened with an ANA test and nailfold capillary examination if they have severe, painful episodes, signs of digital ischemia, or any other systemic symptoms. Although patients with scleroderma almost always have a positive ANA, it is important to remember that the presence of a positive ANA does not, by itself, make the diagnosis of a connective tissue disorder (see Laboratory Findings below).

Raynaud phenomenon is the first manifestation of the disease in almost every patient. Stress and cold temperature induce an exaggerated vasoconstriction of the small arteries, arterioles, and arteriovenous shunts of the skin of the digits. This is manifested clinically as pallor and cyanosis of the digits, followed by a reactive hyperemia after rewarming. Unlike episodes of uncomplicated primary Raynaud phenomenon, attacks of Raynaud phenomenon in patients with scleroderma are often painful and frequently lead to digital ulcerations, gangrene, or amputation (Figure 22–3).

3. Lung involvement—Two main forms of lung disease occur in patients with scleroderma: inflammatory alveolitis leading to interstitial fibrosis and pulmonary hypertension. These two processes can occur independently or concomitantly. Lung involvement usually presents as dyspnea on exertion but can be asymptomatic early in the course of the disease. Therefore, routine screening tests for lung disease are important because early intervention may prevent progression. In the setting of interstitial fibrosis, physical examination reveals fine crackles at the lung bases. This finding, however, is not present in early disease. Pulmonary function testing (PFT) or high-resolution computed tomography (CT) scanning can detect very mild and early disease. Approximately 80% of patients with scleroderma have restrictive ventilatory defects on PFTs, consistent with interstitial lung disease. However, only about 10–20% suffer from progressive interstitial lung disease. In the late stages of aggressive interstitial lung disease, cor pulmonale with right heart failure can cause increasing dyspnea, hepatomegaly, and fluid retention with edema.

Pulmonary vascular disease with or without fibrosis can lead to pulmonary hypertension and ultimately right heart failure. Isolated pulmonary hypertension occurs more commonly in patients with limited scleroderma who have a long duration of disease. Pulmonary hypertension complicates the disease course in approximately 10% of patients with the CREST syndrome. Typically, patients with isolated pulmonary hypertension seek medical care complaining of dyspnea on exertion; however, signs of progressive, life-threatening right heart failure develop rapidly in later stages.

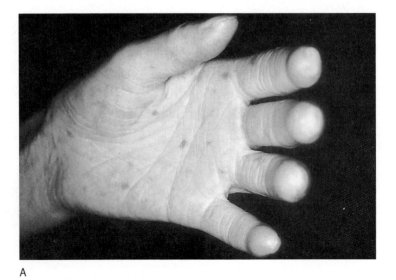

A

B

Figure 22–2. Raynaud phenomenon and telangiectasias of the skin (**A**) and of the tongue (**B**) in a patient with the CREST (calcinosis, Raynaud phenomenon, esophageal dysmotility, sclerodactyly, telangiectasias) syndrome.

4. Gastrointestinal involvement—Gastrointestinal disease in scleroderma usually involves both the upper and lower gastrointestinal tract but is highly variable in its clinical expression. Patients with measurable gastrointestinal involvement can be relatively asymptomatic (eg, mild constipation). Alternatively, they may have profound gastrointestinal tract dysfunction, with malnutrition and significant morbidity. The majority of patients with scleroderma have symptomatic GERD with dysphagia. Complaints include a sensation of food getting stuck in the mid-esophagus, atypical chest pain, or cough. Patients often complain that they must drink liquids to swallow solid food, particularly dry food such as meat or bread. Reflux and dysphagia occur because

of dysmotility of the esophagus and stomach (gastroparesis). This type of organ dysfunction results from atrophy of the esophageal smooth muscle that occurs in the absence of significant tissue fibrosis. If left untreated, the upper gastrointestinal disease can cause esophagitis, esophageal ulceration with bleeding, esophageal stricture, or Barrett esophagus.

The small and large intestines can also be affected by smooth muscle atrophy of the bowel wall causing abnormal motility of the gut. The most common symptom is the combination of constipation alternating with diarrhea. Severe disease causes recurrent bouts of pseudo-obstruction, bowel distention with leakage of air into the bowel wall (pneumatosis coli intestinalis),

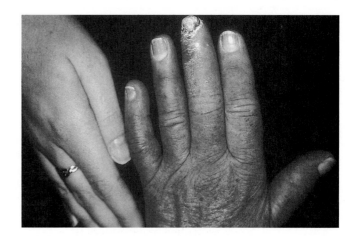

Figure 22–3. Digital ischemia with ulceration.

and even bowel rupture. Lower bowel dysmotility slows the movement of bowel contents severely, allowing bacterial overgrowth, diarrhea, and malabsorption. Fecal incontinence develops in a small subset of patients.

5. Renal involvement—Clinically important kidney disease occurs in only a minority of patients, but when it develops, renal disease poses a major threat to life. SRC develops in approximately 10% of patients. It is characterized by the sudden onset of malignant hypertension that, if untreated, can lead rapidly to renal failure and death. Prior to the discovery that angiotensin-converting enzyme (ACE) inhibitors can control hypertensive crises in scleroderma effectively, SRC was the leading cause of death. Patients in the early stages of diffuse scleroderma, particularly those treated with glucocorticoids, are at the greatest risk for SRC. Typically, patients in whom SRC develops have symptoms associated with the acute onset of severe hypertension, including headache, visual changes, or seizures. Some are asymptomatic and have undetected hypertension and an abrupt rise in creatinine; therefore, patients must have their blood pressure monitored frequently. Renal biopsy specimens reveal changes similar to malignant hypertension, thrombotic thrombocytopenic purpura/hemolytic uremic syndrome, and ecclampsia. There is intimal hyperplasia and vasospasm of cortical arteries. This leads to activation of the renin-angiotensin system and accelerated hypertension, proteinuria, microscopic hematuria, and microvascular hemolysis (schistocytes on peripheral blood smear).

6. Cardiac involvement—Cardiac involvement in scleroderma can frequently be demonstrated by objective testing (eg, echocardiography, thallium scan, or electrocardiogram), but is usually subclinical. Cardiopulmonary morbidity is seen primarily in the late stages of diffuse scleroderma. Ischemia-reperfusion injury secondary to small arterial disease of the my-

ocardium leads to contraction band necrosis and tissue fibrosis. This process can result in arrhythmias, a cardiomyopathy with diastolic dysfunction, or overt symptoms of heart failure. Although pericardial effusions are frequently detected by echocardiography, they are usually clinically silent. Large pericardial effusions are associated with a poor prognosis. Symptoms from scleroderma cardiac disease include chest pain from pericarditis, palpitations from arrhythmias, or dyspnea on exertion from heart failure.

7. Musculoskeletal involvement—Musculoskeletal symptoms range from mild arthralgias to frank nonerosive arthritis with synovitis resembling rheumatoid arthritis. The sclerosis of the skin of the fingers or limbs is often associated with contractures of the joints. Deeper tissue fibrosis can also involve the fascia and underlying muscle. If areas around the tendons are involved, active and passive range of motion of the joints are limited and painful. The physician can appreciate this on examination by feeling a "tendon friction rub" when placing the hand over the tendons as the patient flexes and extends the joint. Tendon friction rubs are found most commonly around the ankles, wrists, or knees.

Muscle weakness is a common complaint with a variety of causes including pain, prolonged muscle disuse, malnutrition, and a slowly progressive fibrosis of striated muscle. A true inflammatory myopathy is seen in a small subset of patients. Patients with "overlap" phenotypes who have scleroderma features (eg, Raynaud phenomenon, interstitial lung disease, and sclerodactyly) and a true inflammatory polyarthritis or polymyositis may be categorized as having mixed connective tissue disease. Patients with mixed connective tissue disease have high-titer anti-U1-RNP antibodies.

8. Other symptoms—Sicca complex (dry eyes and dry mouth) are common in patients with scleroderma but are usually not as severe as in patients with primary Sjö-gren syndrome (see Chapter 24).

Pain is very common and usually is associated with digital ulcers, fibrosis of tendons, joint contractures, or musculoskeletal disease. Rarely, neuropathic pain is present secondary to carpal tunnel syndrome or trigeminal neuralgia.

Depression is frequent among patients with scleroderma but does not correlate directly with disease severity. Depression probably reflects other factors such as degree of pain, personality traits, and social support systems.

Erectile dysfunction is very common among men with scleroderma and is often not detected or properly managed. Fortunately, erectile dysfunction in scleroderma patients can respond to conventional therapy such as sildenafil. Sexual dysfunction among women is also common; symptoms include vaginal dryness, dyspareunia, and vaginal tightness.

B. LABORATORY FINDINGS

There is no single laboratory study or test that confirms the diagnosis of scleroderma. The diagnosis is made by obtaining a careful history and performing a physical examination. However, autoantibodies are found in nearly every patient with scleroderma (sensitivity > 95%). ANAs are the most frequently detected, but they are not specific for scleroderma. ANAs can be detected in other connective tissue diseases, other diseases associated with autoimmunity (eg, Hashimoto thyroiditis), chronic infections (such as hepatitis C), and up to 10% of healthy individuals (at low titers). Anticentromere antibodies are detected in approximately 20–40% of patients with scleroderma and are associated specifically with the CREST syndrome and severe digital ischemia with digital loss. Anticentromere antibodies can also be found in patients with primary biliary cirrhosis and Sjö-gren syndrome. Antitopoisomerase I (anti-Scl-70) antibodies are also found in 20–40% of patients with scleroderma. Patients with antitopoisomerase I antibodies typically have diffuse skin changes, interstitial lung disease, and an overall worse prognosis. Antitopoisomerase I antibodies are highly specific for scleroderma. Antibodies to RNA polymerases (anti-RNAP I, II, III) are also associated with diffuse skin changes, cardiac and renal involvement, and increased mortality. Antibodies to other nucleolar proteins are found in a small percentage of scleroderma patients, but assays for these are generally not commercially available (Th, Nor-90, Fibrillarin, Pm-Scl, B23). The scleroderma-associated autoantibodies are outlined in Table 22–2.

C. IMAGING STUDIES

Chest films are an insensitive method to diagnose scleroderma lung disease. High-resolution CT scans of the chest have an increased sensitivity but do not determine disease activity. Radiographic testing for evaluation of upper gastrointestinal disease is not often required unless patients have atypical symptoms or do not respond to standard treatments. A CINE esophagram, however, will typically show a dilated esophagus, lower esophageal dysmotility, and gastroesophageal reflux.

D. SPECIAL TESTS

The use of specialized diagnostic testing depends on the organ system to be investigated. Every patient with scleroderma should be screened routinely at baseline and monitored for the development of pulmonary and cardiac disease. Patients should have PFTs (spirometry, lung volumes, and diffusing capacity) and an echocardiogram performed at baseline and then every 4–12 months depending on symptoms. PFTs provide the most sensitive measure for the development of interstitial lung disease, typically revealing a restrictive pattern with or without a reduction in diffusing capacity. PFTs can also suggest the presence of pulmonary hypertension by the finding of an isolated low diffusing capacity. The degree of pulmonary hypertension can be estimated on a two-dimensional echocardiogram by measuring the right ventricular systolic pressure. Additional specialized studies such as bronchoalveolar lavage or right heart catheterization may be performed to determine degree of activity or severity of disease in those patients with abnormal screening studies and cardiopulmonary symptoms.

Studies of the upper gastrointestinal tract are often unnecessary in a patient with scleroderma who has symptomatic gastroesophageal reflux alone. Patients with atypical symptoms, poor responses to proton pump inhibitors, or long-standing untreated symptoms warrant further studies such as a barium swallow or upper gastrointestinal endoscopy. The barium swallow is relatively insensitive to measure motility problems but is useful for the exclusion of other potentially treatable causes of dysphagia such as a stricture. Any patient with long-standing reflux should be referred for endoscopy to evaluate for the complications of GERD, including Barrett esophagus.

E. SPECIAL EXAMINATIONS

The capillaries of the skin can be visualized at the nail-fold by using simple tools available in a typical examination room, thus giving insight into a patient's microvasculature status. Nailfold capillary dropout and dilated capillary loops are seen in nearly every patient with scleroderma but are not specific for scleroderma because nailfold changes can also be seen in other connective tissue diseases. To examine the nailfold capillaries, a drop of either microscope oil or lubricant jelly is placed on the nail bed. An ophthalmoscope, set at minus 20–40 diopters (40 green) is used as a microscope to visualize the capillaries. Normally, the nailfold capillaries should be thin, linear, and uniform. In patients with scleroderma, these capillaries become dilated and areas of vessel dropout are apparent.

Differential Diagnosis

Given the multisystem nature of systemic sclerosis, the differential diagnosis is broad. Scleroderma is a rare disease but a protean one. Often, the diagnosis only becomes obvious after several evaluations over time.

Patients with symptoms compatible with early scleroderma are encountered frequently in the primary care office. For this reason, primary care providers should be aware of this potentially life-threatening disease and be able to distinguish it from other disorders with similar features so that appropriate referrals can be made. The differential diagnosis includes other disorders that are associated with Raynaud phenomenon, those with similar skin changes, and those with other components of systemic autoimmune rheumatic diseases, such as arthralgias and positive autoantibodies. This differential diagnosis is detailed in Table 22–3.

Table 22–3. Differential diagnosis of scleroderma.

Clinical Feature	Differential Diagnosis
Raynaud phenomenon	Primary Raynaud phenomenon
	Systemic lupus erythematosus
	Vibration-hand syndrome
	Medication-induced
	Chemotherapy (cisplatin,
	bleomycin, etc)
	Sympathomimetics
	Thoracic outlet syndrome
	Cryoglobulinemia/cryofibrino-
	genemia/cold agglutins
	Systemic vasculitis
Skin thickening	Scleredema
	Scleromyxedema
	POEMS syndrome
	Eosinophilic fasciitis
	Graft-versus-host disease
	Eosinophilia-myalgia syndrome
	Morphea
Overlapping clinical features	Systemic lupus erythematosus
	Sjögren syndrome
	Inflammatory myopathies
	Rheumatoid arthritis

POEMS, polyneuropathy, organomegaly, endocrinopathy, monoclonal gammopathy (in protein), skin changes.

Treatment

A. GENERAL PRINCIPLES

No single drug has been found to treat all of the manifestations of scleroderma, and no effective **disease-specific** therapy exists. Management, therefore, is based on the symptoms and disease manifestations of each individual patient and is often **organ-specific.** Recent therapeutic advances and improved screening tests have decreased the morbidity and mortality in scleroderma. For example, since the routine use of ACE inhibitors in the management of SRC, the incidence of end-stage renal disease and mortality from this once fatal complication has declined significantly.

Some important principles to keep in mind when treating patients with scleroderma follow:

- Each patient with scleroderma is unique with regard to disease features and prognosis (see below).
- No proven disease-modifying medication exists.
- Scleroderma skin disease tends to reach peak involvement over the first 18–24 months but then gradually improves with or without therapy.
- Routine screening and early intervention for internal organ manifestations may significantly reduce morbidity and mortality.

B. FIBROSIS

Although the pathogenesis of fibrosis is now understood better, this understanding has yet to translate into medications that treat cutaneous fibrosis effectively. Although some early, uncontrolled observations suggested that D-penicillamine may be beneficial, a recent controlled trial of low-dose versus high-dose D-penicillamine has cast doubt on the benefit of this drug (patients in the low-dose group had better outcomes). Most experts feel that until new antifibrotic drugs are available, the inflammatory process that triggers or causes the tissue injury and fibrosis needs to be controlled rapidly. Therefore, various immunosuppressive agents are used early in the disease course in an attempt to modify the course of skin fibrosis. Unfortunately, no convincing controlled trial using these agents is available to provide complete guidelines for their use. Agents that are currently used include glucocorticoids, methotrexate, cyclophosphamide, antithymocyte globulin, cyclosporine, and mycophenolate mofetil. Each drug has unique toxicities and risks. Great care and expert guidance should be sought when prescribing these medications.

C. VASCULAR DISEASE

While the vascular insult is common to all patients with scleroderma, the clinical expression varies widely. Many patients have only mildly symptomatic Raynaud phenomenon, whereas others can have recurrent digital ulcerations that can progress to gangrene and digital loss. In addition, the scleroderma vasculopathy (intimal proliferation of arteries) is often a contributing factor in the internal organ involvement that is the major cause of morbidity and mortality. Episodes of critical ischemia are multifactorial and are a culmination of severe vasospasm (with ischemia-reperfusion injury), progressive vascular intimal proliferation with narrowing of the vessel lumen, and microvascular thrombosis. A combined therapeutic approach that addresses each of these processes is often used. The management of Raynaud phenomenon is discussed in Chapter 21.

D. INFLAMMATION

In early diffuse scleroderma, biopsy specimens of the skin reveal inflammatory infiltrates, and patients often complain of pain and swelling and stiffness of skin, joints, and periarticular structures. Inflammation can also be demonstrated in the lungs of some patients with interstitial lung disease (see below). It is postulated, therefore, that an early inflammatory insult leads to the downstream processes of fibrosis, atrophy, and loss of function. Because of this, a variety of immunosuppressive agents have been tried in the treatment of scleroderma, including methotrexate, cyclophosphamide, antithymocyte globulin, cyclosporine, and mycophenolate mofetil. Unfortunately, data from rigorous clinical trials assessing the efficacy of these agents in scleroderma are limited. Regimens of intense immunosuppression are also currently being studied (bone marrow transplantation, immunoablative cyclophosphamide) in patients with severe, early disease. These interventions carry the risk of significant adverse events, and their use should be limited to patients at high risk for significant morbidity and mortality. Patients with early, potentially modifiable disease but features associated with poor prognoses are the ideal candidates for these experimental therapies.

E. ORGAN-SPECIFIC THERAPY

1. Scleroderma renal crisis—Scleroderma patients considered to be at high risk for the development of renal crisis (those with early diffuse skin changes, prednisone use) should have their blood pressure monitored several times a week. A physician should promptly evaluate any unexplained rise in blood pressure, and renal function should be checked (urinalysis and creatinine). If there is persistently elevated blood pressure or signs of renal insufficiency, SRC should be suspected. In this setting, further diagnostic work-up (such as a renal biopsy) may be unnecessary. Prompt institution of ACE inhibitor therapy is needed to control blood pressure, with a target blood pressure of 130/80 mm Hg or

lower. ACE inhibitors should be titrated upward to gain control of blood pressure as quickly as possible. If blood pressure remains high, patients may require hospitalization for the management of medications and close monitoring of blood pressure and renal function. It is not clear whether angiotensin II receptor blockers are as beneficial as ACE inhibitors in SRC. Despite the availability of effective therapy now and aggressive management, approximately 40% of patients with SRC have poor outcomes (death within 6 months or permanent dialysis).

2. Interstitial lung disease—All patients with scleroderma should be monitored for the development of lung disease. Patients with a restrictive pattern on PFTs or interstitial fibrosis on high-resolution CT scanning should be treated with immunosuppression if there is evidence of progression. Bronchoalveolar lavage should be performed to define the level of active disease in cases with suspected active alveolitis. There are data to suggest that cyclophosphamide is beneficial, particularly in those patients with evidence of an active alveolitis (increased neutrophils or eosinophils on bronchoalveolar lavage). Younger patients (under 60 years of age) with severe interstitial lung disease who do not respond to therapy should be considered for lung transplantation.

3. Pulmonary hypertension—Unlike the other significant organ involvement in scleroderma, isolated pulmonary hypertension is more commonly seen in those patients with limited scleroderma. All patients with scleroderma, however, should be evaluated with echocardiograms to screen for elevated pulmonary pressures. Patients with isolated pulmonary hypertension may also have a reduction in the diffusing capacity on PFTs.

In the past several years, new medications have been developed to treat patients with pulmonary hypertension. Prostaglandin therapy (delivered by continuous intravenous or subcutaneous infusion) is currently used for the management of severe pulmonary hypertension. In the United States, the only available formulations are intravenous epoprostenol, intravenous prostaglandin E_2 (PGE$_2$), and subcutaneous prostacyclin analog (treprostinil), usually given as a continuous infusion. The oral endothelin-1 antagonist, bosentan, has proved effective in a randomized trial to improve symptoms and exercise tolerance in scleroderma patients with pulmonary hypertension. Despite the encouraging results with prostaglandin therapy and the endothelin-1 antagonists, it is not yet clear whether a survival benefit will result in the management of severe pulmonary hypertension associated with scleroderma. Preliminary studies also suggest some therapeutic benefit of sildenafil, inhaled prostaglandins, or nitric oxide in the management of pulmonary hypertension. Further trials are necessary with these agents to define their role in the management of scleroderma. Patients with severe pulmonary hypertension are also candidates for lung transplantation (often performed simultaneously with heart transplantation). Scleroderma lung disease is quite complex and should be managed by those with expertise in pulmonary medicine.

4. Gastrointestinal disease—The gastrointestinal involvement in scleroderma is usually fairly easy to manage. The most frequent symptoms, gastroesophageal reflux and esophageal dysmotility, may be treated effectively with proton pump inhibitors (ie, omeprazole 20–40 mg twice daily). All patients with upper gastrointestinal symptoms should also be instructed in simple behavioral measures that can reduce symptoms:

- Eat small, frequent meals.
- Do not eat meals within 2 hours of bedtime.
- Keep the head of the bed elevated.
- Avoid aggravating factors (tobacco, alcohol, caffeine, etc).

Those with persistent symptoms may require the use of promotility agents such as metoclopramide. Any patient with severe dysphagia or symptoms unresponsive to the above measures should be referred to a gastroenterologist for an upper gastrointestinal endoscopy.

Lower gastrointestinal symptoms are less frequent but often more difficult to manage. Over-the-counter preparations such as loperamide and fiber supplements are used to treat mild symptoms. Persistent, frequent diarrhea may be a sign of bacterial overgrowth that requires treatment with antibiotics (eg, metronidazole). Promotility agents may also improve lower gastrointestinal symptoms. Severe dysmotility that is refractory to medical therapy and associated with either recurrent bouts of pseudo-obstruction or progressive weight loss and malnutrition is best treated with bowel rest and total parenteral nutrition.

Prognosis

The prognosis in scleroderma is highly dependent on the extent of major organ disease. This can be predicted by the degree of skin involvement. Patients with limited scleroderma have a normal life expectancy with approximately a 90% 5-year survival rate. Patients with diffuse skin disease have only about a 70–80% 5-year survival rate. Clinical features that predict poor outcomes include high skin scores, progressive lung disease, tendon friction rubs, evidence of heart disease, anemia, and SRC. Aggressive management early in the course of the disease can improve quality of life and reduce morbidity. In the future, new therapies and better methods of recognizing disease complications early will improve the prognosis of patients with scleroderma. In the meantime, primary care physicians are encouraged to refer scleroderma patients to a rheumatologist or specialty scleroderma treatment centers.

REFERENCES

Ferri C, et al. Systemic sclerosis: demographic, clinical, and serologic features and survival in 1,012 Italian patients. *Medicine (Baltimore)*. 2002;81:139. [PMID: 11889413]

Rubin LJ, et al. Bosentan therapy for pulmonary arterial hypertension. *N Engl J Med*. 2002;346:896. [PMID: 11907289]

Steen VD, Medsger TA Jr. Long-term outcomes of scleroderma renal crisis. *Ann Intern Med*. 2000;133:600. [PMID: 11033587]

White B. Evaluation and management of pulmonary fibrosis in scleroderma. *Curr Rheumatol Rep*. 2002;4:108. [PMID: 11890875]

Relevant World Wide Web Sites

[Scleroderma Foundation]
http://www.scleroderma.org
[Scleroderma Research Foundation]
http://www.srfcure.org
[Scleroderma Clinical Trials Consortium]
http://www.sctc-online.org
[American College of Rheumatology]
http://www.rheumatology.org

Adult Still Disease

Peggy Schlesinger, MD

ESSENTIALS OF DIAGNOSIS

- *Fever that spikes in "rabbit ears" pattern with daily return to normal.*
- *Salmon-colored macular rash only occurring with fever.*
- *Arthritis, splenomegaly, pleuritis, pericarditis, and marked leukocytosis common.*
- *Pharyngitis often initial symptom.*

General Considerations

Adult-onset Still disease (AOSD) is a multisystem inflammatory disease that typically begins with a sore throat. Nonsuppurative pharyngitis may develop days to weeks before the typical quotidian fever, evanescent rash, and joint pains begin. Other constitutional symptoms soon follow, including profound fatigue, weight loss, and anorexia. Malignancy and infectious causes of these symptoms must be excluded because AOSD is diagnosed mainly on clinical grounds.

The cause of AOSD has yet to be identified. The presence of daily spiking fevers has focused research efforts on the possibility that the cause of AOSD is infection related. To date, however, there has not been any infectious agent or genetic predisposition identified in patients with this disease.

Fortunately, AOSD is rare. One series reported an incidence of 0.16 cases per 100,000 population. Women and men are equally affected. The peak onset is between ages 20 and 45, although cases have been reported in all age groups. Pediatric patients with systemic-onset juvenile rheumatoid arthritis can have a recurrence of active Still disease at any age into adulthood.

Clinical Findings

There is no definitive laboratory test for AOSD, but a high serum ferritin and marked leukocytosis with fever, rash, and arthritis in the absence of other possible causes is highly suggestive of this diagnosis.

A. SYMPTOMS AND SIGNS

The fever of AOSD is relentless, often lasting weeks at a time before the diagnosis can be established. Temperature spikes occur daily in these patients, often in the afternoon or evening. These elevations in temperature can be preceded by shaking chills and followed by sweating as the temperature returns to normal. The daily return to baseline or normal temperature is a distinguishing feature that helps separate patients with AOSD from those with chronic infection. Typically, in patients with chronic infection, the temperature remains elevated between fever spikes.

The rash of AOSD is salmon-colored, macular, and can occur anywhere on the trunk and extremities. It is evanescent and manifests during the febrile episodes, but clears completely when the temperature returns to normal. It may be mildly pruritic and extend in areas that are scratched. Biopsy of involved skin, even with immunofluorescence, is usually not diagnostic. The presence of this particular rash in association with a daily quotidian fever is diagnostic of AOSD, even though the rash itself is nondescript and can easily be mistaken for a drug reaction or viral exanthem. In some patients, the rash may reappear in the identical location during subsequent flares of active disease. Usually the face, palms, and soles are spared.

Joint involvement is a common feature of AOSD, but true arthritis may be slow to develop. Initially, patients often have significant joint and muscle pain without true synovitis. Marked arthralgias and myalgias may be present initially and can develop into frank arthritis over time. Arthritis develops in large joints such as the hip, knee, ankle, shoulder, and wrist more often than the small joints of the hands and feet. Persistent synovitis and restricted range of motion in affected joints occasionally occur even after the fever has resolved. Destructive arthritis occurs in 20% of patients with AOSD. Carpal and cervical ankylosis can occur as a result of arthritis in both the adult- and childhood-onset forms of the disease. Avascular necrosis is a significant risk for those patients with AOSD who require glucocorticoids for control of the systemic symptoms or persistent arthritis, or both. Hip involvement and persistent synovitis are poor prognostic signs and justify an aggressive treatment approach.

Pleuritis, pericarditis, lymphadenopathy, hepatomegaly, and splenomegaly are common in AOSD (Table 23–1). Biopsy specimens of lymph nodes show reactive changes due to polyclonal B-cell hyperplasia.

B. LABORATORY FINDINGS

Mild elevations of liver function tests are a frequent but nonspecific finding, often associated with low serum albumin and the anemia of chronic disease. Marked leukocytosis (> 15,000) with a predominance of neutrophils (> 80%) is also common. The ANA and rheumatoid factor are negative in almost all cases (Table 23–2). There is no threat to renal function associated with AOSD, and creatinine and urinalysis typically remain normal.

Many of the laboratory findings seen in both acute and chronic inflammation can be seen in AOSD patients, including elevated C-reactive protein levels, elevated complement levels, and elevated erythrocyte sedimentation rate to > 90 mm/h in more than 50% of cases. Marked elevation of the serum ferritin (above 3000 mg/mL) is seen in over 70% of AOSD patients, as an acute phase response. The finding of a low percentage of glycosylated serum ferritin (< 20%) may be even more specific for AOSD.

Differential Diagnosis

When patients present with a sore throat, daily fever, rash, and muscle pain, infectious causes top the list of possible diagnoses. The more common causes of rash, fever, and arthritis are infectious, including viral infections such as rubella, parvovirus, hepatitis B and C, HIV, bacterial infections with *Borrelia burgdorferi* (Lyme disease), *Borrelia hermsii* (relapsing fever), streptococcal-associated arthritis and rheumatic fever recurrence, and endocarditis, among others. Most series that report clinical criteria of the diagnosis of AOSD will also list exclusions such as parvovirus, cytomegalovirus, lymphoma, and systemic lupus erythematosus or polyarteritis nodosa. It is vitally important to exclude infection before beginning treatment for AOSD.

Similarly, the combination of recurrent fever with enlarged lymph nodes and splenomegaly suggests a diagnosis of hematologic malignancy, granulomatous diseases, vasculitis, and other connective tissue disorders. Less common conditions such as sarcoidosis, familial Mediterranean fever, autoimmune neutropenia, inflammatory bowel disease, hemophagocytic syndromes, polyarteritis nodosa, and microscopic polyangiitis, as well as malignancy, can mimic the signs and symptoms of AOSD.

Diagnostic criteria have been proposed by several authors to help identify patients with AOSD. Several different classification systems exist with major and minor criteria taken from the list of clinical and laboratory findings in Tables 23–1 and 23–2. These proposed classification systems rely on different combinations of major and minor criteria once malignancy, infection, and other rheumatic disorders have been excluded.

Treatment

Treatment of this condition can be challenging. Early treatment with nonsteroidal anti-inflammatory drugs (NSAIDs) is useful to treat fever, joint pain, and muscle aches but can lead to markedly elevated liver function tests. Aspirin was previously considered to be the mainstay of therapy but frequently led to significant hepatitis. NSAIDs are less likely to cause similar problems, but the potential remains. Systemic glucocorticoids are indicated to control persistent synovitis and to treat life-threatening manifestations and constitutional symptoms that interfere with the activities of daily living. If arthritis persists, treatment with a disease-modifying agent, such as methotrexate or cyclosporine, or a biologic response modifier, such as anakinra or etanercept, can induce remission and minimize glucocorticoid ex-

Table 23–1. Clinical manifestations of adult-onset Still disease.

Fever
Acute pharyngitis
Arthritis/arthralgia
Severe myalgias
Lymphadenopathy
Splenomegaly
Hepatic dysfunction
Pleuritis
Pericarditis

Table 23–2. Common laboratory test abnormalities in adult-onset Still disease.

Elevated erythrocyte sedimentation rate
Elevated white blood cell count[a]
Elevated platelet count
Anemia
Elevated liver enzymes
Elevated ferritin
Negative antinuclear antibodies
Negative rheumatoid factor

[a]White blood cell count > 15,000 with > 80% polymorphonuclear neutrophils.

posure. Therapy should be continued until laboratory parameters show no signs of inflammation and clinical examination indicates no active disease is present. Medication can then be tapered slowly with the hope of maintaining a remission on the lowest effective dose. Disease-modifying agents should be continued for a 1-year disease-free interval before being discontinued altogether. Relapse is not uncommon and can occur after many years.

REFERENCES

Cush J. Adult-onset Still's disease. *Bull Rheum Dis.* 2000;49:1. [PMID: 11100625]

Esdaile JM. Adult Still's disease. In: Klippel JH, ed. *Primer on the Rheumatic Diseases,* 11th ed. Arthritis Foundation, 1997.

Fautrel B, et al. Proposal for new set of classification criteria for adult-onset Still's disease. *Medicine (Baltimore).* 2002;81:194. [PMID: 11997716]

Magadur-Joly G, et al. Epidemiology of adult Still's disease: estimate of the incidence by a retrospective study in west France. *Ann Rheum Dis.* 1995;54:587. [PMID: 7668903]

Mandl LE, Esdaile JM. Adult Still's disease. UpToDate Online 10.2, 2002 (www.uptodateonline.com).

Sjögren Syndrome

24

Kenneth H. Fye, MD

ESSENTIALS OF DIAGNOSIS

- *An autoimmune disorder that attacks exocrine glands and, in some patients, a wide variety of extraglandular organs.*
- *Principal feature of Sjögren syndrome (SS) is the sicca complex: dryness of the eyes, mouth, and other mucocutaneous tissues.*
- *May occur as either a primary disorder or secondary to a variety of other autoimmune disorders.*
- *Diagnosis often confirmed by biopsy of a minor salivary gland or suggested strongly by the presence of a positive Schirmer test or an abnormal Rose Bengal score.*
- *Often associated with antibodies to SS-A (Ro) and SS-B (La).*
- *Therapy is primarily symptomatic, although there are now medications that increase exocrine gland output.*

General Considerations

Sjögren syndrome (SS) is an autoimmune exocrinopathy first described fully by Henrik Sjögren in 1933. Although it is a systemic disorder, the primary targets of the inflammatory process are the exocrine glands. SS can occur either as a primary process or in association with other autoimmune disorders, such as rheumatoid arthritis, systemic lupus erythematosus, scleroderma, mixed connective tissue disease, dermatomyositis, or autoimmune thyroiditis. When it occurs in association with other diseases, the process is called "secondary" SS. The decrease in exocrine gland secretions seen in SS results in dryness that can affect virtually every mucocutaneous surface of the body. The set of symptoms associated with this dryness is termed "the sicca complex."

In pathologic terms, the disease is defined by the infiltration of lymphocytes, plasma cells, and macrophages into target tissues. The precise role of autoantibodies (see Laboratory Findings) in the pathophysiology of SS

is unclear, but anti-SS-A (Ro) and anti-SS-B (La) are a striking feature of many patients with this condition.

There are at least three major factors in the causation of SS. There is clearly a genetic predisposition to the development of the disease. A number of genes within the HLA-DR3 and HLA-DR4 loci have been associated with the development and the severity of SS. Because these genes are relatively common in populations of healthy individuals, however, environmental factors (eg, viral or retroviral infections) may also play a role, triggering the disease in genetically susceptible persons. However, no consistent environmental triggers have been identified. Finally, because the disease is up to 15 times more common in women than in men, hormonal factors must also be important in the development of SS. The precise role of female hormones in the cause of SS remains unclear.

Clinical Features

A. SYMPTOMS AND SIGNS

1. Oral—Adequate saliva production is crucial for the health of the mouth. Patients with SS complain of constant burning and dryness of oral mucosal surfaces. The lips, tongue, and roof of the mouth frequently stick together, making it difficult to talk without constantly sipping water. It is very difficult or impossible to chew or swallow dry foods such as crackers without consuming liquids at the same time. Most patients complain of burning discomfort in the mouth after eating acidic foods. A decrease in the amount of saliva can result in rampant dental caries, periodontitis with gum resorption, and atrophy of lingual papillae. Aggressive treatment of caries is crucial to prevent premature loss of the teeth in patients with SS.

Oral candidiasis is a common complication of the sicca complex. It is associated with angular cheilosis, accentuation of the lingual papillary atrophy already present in SS patients, and erythema of the tongue. Thrush, however, is unusual in adults with SS. Diffuse lymphocytic infiltration of the parotid and submandibular glands (Figure 24–1) can result in glandular enlargement, pain, and tenderness. Severe bilateral enlargement of the parotids may result in a typical "chipmunk" facies. Because of decreased salivary flow, patients with SS have increased susceptibility to bacter-

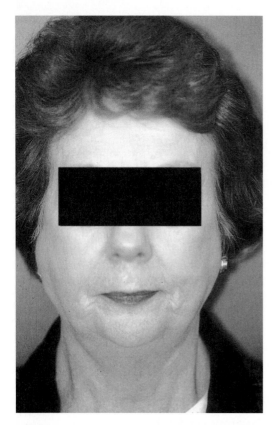

Figure 24–1. Parotid enlargement in a patient with Sjögren syndrome.

ial infections of the major salivary glands. The offending organisms are generally commensal oral flora such as *Staphylococcus* or *Streptococcus* species, including pneumococci. Appropriate antibiotic therapy rests upon the results of culture and sensitivity tests of the purulent material draining from Stensen or Wharton ducts.

2. Ocular—A normal tear film consists of layers of mucus, water, and oil. The ocular manifestations of SS are due to decreased production of the aqueous tear component. Dryness of the eyes (keratoconjunctivitis sicca) is usually associated with what is described as a "gritty" or "sandy" discomfort and the sensation of a foreign body in the eye. Symptoms are exacerbated by exposure to dry air. Physical examination reveals injection of the bulbar conjunctiva, particularly that surface exposed to the air. Lack of a normal tear film and accumulation of corneal debris can result in painful corneal filaments and blurred vision. Blepharitis secondary to abnormally thickened meibomian gland secretions de-

velops in some patients. The overnight accumulation of tenacious, inspissated secretions may bind the eyelids during sleep, making opening of the eyes difficult upon awakening. Photophobia is the result of corneal irritation caused by disruption of the protective tear film. Corneal denudation also heightens patients' susceptibility to ocular infections.

3. Cutaneous—The most common cutaneous manifestations of SS are due to a deficiency in the aqueous component of sweat. Dry skin with chronic scaling and pruritus is almost universal in well-established SS. The complications of chronic pruritus include lichenification and pigmentary changes of the skin. Leukocytoclastic vasculitis (often with a lymphocytic predominance) presenting with petechiae or palpable purpura can also be seen, usually associated with hypergammaglobulinemia (either polyclonal or monoclonal), cryoglobulinemia, or elevated circulating immune complexes.

4. Nasal—Dryness of the nares results in pain, tenderness, erythema, crusting, pruritus, and frequent anterior nose bleeds. Nasal dryness also leads to decreased smell and a consequent attenuation in the ability to taste food. Dryness of the sinuses is associated with an increased incidence of acute and chronic sinusitis.

5. Vaginal—Vaginal dryness is associated with pain, tenderness, pruritus, dyspareunia, and recurrent vaginal candidiasis. Dryness of the vulva frequently results in chronic vulvodynia and dysuria.

6. Musculoskeletal—Many patients with primary SS have an inflammatory, symmetric, nonerosive, arthralgic syndrome that affects small proximal joints. The proliferative synovitis typical of rheumatoid arthritis or systemic lupus erythematosus is not observed in SS. Arthritis typical of the underlying associated disorder can develop in patients with secondary SS. Fibromyalgia is very common in SS. Proximal muscle weakness caused by an inflammatory myopathy that is indistinguishable histologically from idiopathic polymyositis develops in some patients with SS. Most of these patients probably have secondary SS in association with a primary inflammatory myopathy (ie, polymyositis or dermatomyositis), mixed connective tissue disease, systemic lupus erythematosus, or another autoimmune process.

7. Pulmonary—Tracheobronchial dryness can lead to a chronic dry cough, typically worse on cool nights (when the air holds less moisture than during the warmth of daylight hours). The lymphocytic infiltration of tracheobronchial mucous membranes seen in SS can result in the signs and symptoms of acute and chronic obstructive pulmonary disease. Restrictive lung disease is due to aggressive lymphocytic infiltration into the pulmonary interstitium. Pulmonary manifestations include follicular bronchiolitis, lymphocytic interstitial pneumonitis, fibrosing alveolitis, interstitial fibrosis with restriction, pulmonary vasculitis, and pleuritis (with or without pleural effusions). Although rare, respiratory failure due to interstitial lung disease is a potentially fatal complication of SS.

8. Gastrointestinal—Oral discomfort as well as pharyngeal and upper esophageal dysphagia are frequent complaints in patients with SS, who cannot moisten their food adequately while chewing. Patients with SS are susceptible to reflux esophagitis, perhaps because of a decrease in the protective effects offered to the esophagus by continuous salivary flow. Acute and chronic pancreatitis may result from lymphocytic infiltration into the pancreas, the largest single exocrine gland in the body. Hepatic manifestations of SS include both chronic active hepatitis and primary biliary cirrhosis. Lymphocytic infiltration of the gastric mucosa is associated with chronic atrophic gastritis, while pernicious anemia, lymphocytic colitis, and even the malabsorption syndrome are seen in patients with intestinal mucosal infiltration.

9. Renal—Chronic lymphocytic interstitial nephritis is a well-described and common extraglandular complication of SS. Manifestations include decreased urinary concentrating ability, glycosuria, potassium wasting, renal tubular acidosis, and in patients with dense peritubular lymphocytic infiltration, light chain proteinuria. Renal tubular acidosis can lead to mobilization of calcium from bone with resultant hypercalciuria and nephrolithiasis. Membranous glomerulonephritis, perhaps related to the accumulation of immune complexes in the glomerulus, has also been described. Proliferative glomerulonephritis is unusual in SS and when present is generally associated with cryoglobulinemia.

10. Neurologic—Considerable controversy has existed in the past about the nature and extent of neurologic manifestations in SS. Reported central nervous system symptoms include decreased cognition, emotional lability, decreased memory, personality changes, and depression. However, confirmation of these many reports has been difficult. The true frequency of central nervous system disease in SS is believed now to be very low. On the other hand, symmetric stocking/glove peripheral neuropathies are clearly associated with hypergammaglobulinemic purpura and the mononuclear cell–mediated vasculitis of SS. Mononeuritis multiplex also has been described in SS patients with leukocytoclastic vasculitis. Much more debilitating is the demyelinating myelopathy reminiscent of multiple sclerosis (so-called "lupus sclerosis") that has been observed—albeit rarely—in patients with SS.

11. Other—The precise relationship of SS and thyroid disease is controversial, although most investigators believe the incidence of autoimmune thyroiditis, with or without resultant hypothyroidism, is increased in SS. "Pseudolymphoma" is a systemic disorder characterized by fever, diffuse lymphadenopathy, and prominent extraglandular internal organ involvement. As its name implies, this syndrome can mimic lymphoma in the nature of its systemic presentation, except that it is not malignant. Moreover, there is an increased incidence of true generalized histiocytic lymphoma in long-standing SS. (Lymphoma develops in ≤ 5% of patients with SS.) Serial biopsy studies have documented the progression from a benign polyclonal lymphocyte aggressive disorder into a lymphoma in some patients.

B. LABORATORY FINDINGS

Autoantibodies develop in most patients with SS at some time during the course of the disease. Rheumatoid factors develop in 90% of patients, over 80% have a positive antinuclear antibody assay (usually with a speckled pattern), and approximately 60% have anti-SS-A (Ro) or SS-B (La) antibodies. Anti-SS-A (Ro) antibodies are more likely to be seen in patients with primary SS or in those with SS and systemic lupus erythematosus. Anti-SS-B (La) antibodies are more specific for primary SS. A polyclonal hypergammaglobulinemia, detectable by immunoelectrophoresis and quantitative immunoglobulin assays, can be seen in up to 50% of patients; a benign monoclonal gammopathy, generally of the IgM kappa type, will develop in many of these patients. The erythrocyte sedimentation rate is commonly elevated due to the inflammation and hypergammaglobulinemia characteristic of the disease. Anemia, leukopenia, thrombocytopenia, hypocomplementemia, elevated circulating immune complexes, and cryoglobulinemia can all be seen in patients with extraglandular internal organ involvement. The cryoglobulinemia associated with SS is generally of the mixed type II variety, with a monoclonal IgM kappa rheumatoid factor.

C. IMAGING STUDIES

Bilateral or unilateral parotid gland enlargement can be seen as a manifestation of SS, but enlarged parotids can also seen in infections (particularly those related to parotid duct stones), local parotid neoplasia, endocrine disorders, and lymphomas. A number of imaging techniques are helpful in distinguishing SS from other disorders that cause parotid gland swelling. Sialography is fairly specific and sensitive, but the study requires an experienced radiology staff and is not universally available. Ultrasonography and magnetic resonance imaging are both sensitive in the detection of parotid masses, but any abnormalities that are of concern for malignancy should be evaluated further by tissue biopsy, if possible. Parotid gland scintigraphy using ^{99m}Tc-pertechnetate can be markedly abnormal in SS, but scintigraphy is very nonspecific, and normal parotid scintigraphy does not rule out SS.

D. SPECIAL TESTS

1. Minor salivary gland biopsy—Minor salivary gland biopsy is the single most specific and sensitive test for the diagnosis of SS. This test is performed routinely by dermatologists in the outpatient setting. The European Study Group Classification criteria for the diagnosis of SS (see below) include—but do not require—a positive minor salivary gland biopsy. Salivary gland biopsies are graded according to their "focus scores," ie, the number of foci of 50 or more mononuclear cells per 4 mm^2 of salivary gland tissue. Normal individuals have focus scores of zero.

2. Parotid sialography—This technique is used to define the anatomy of the parotid gland ductules. In SS, there is gross distortion of the finely arborized pattern normally observed with sialectasia.

3. Salivary gland scintigraphy—The scintigraphic findings in SS include decreased uptake and release of ^{99m}Tc-pertechnetate, generally paralleling the degree of oral sicca symptoms, sialography, and salivary flow rate studies.

4. Schirmer test—The Schirmer test is a simple test of the patient's ability to form tears. To perform the test (usually done by an ophthalmologist), a strip of Whatman No. 41 filter paper is folded and placed into the patient's lower conjunctival sacs bilaterally. In this painless test, normal persons produce sufficient tears to moisten at least 15 mm of the filter paper after 5 minutes. In contrast, < 5 mm of moisture indicates a positive test.

5. Rose Bengal test—The Rose Bengal test detects damage to the conjunctival epithelium. (In SS, this is caused by desiccation.) Twenty-five milliliters of Rose Bengal solution is placed in the inferior fornix of each eye, and the patient is asked to blink twice. Areas of destroyed conjunctival epithelium become temporarily red-spotted after this procedure, and the spots can be quantified as 1+ (sparsely scattered), 2+ (densely scattered), or 3+ (confluent) in three different areas of the eye. The totals for the three areas are added to achieve the Rose Bengal score (> 4 in at least one eye is abnormal).

Differential Diagnosis

The diagnosis begins with a history of sicca symptoms. However, the differential diagnosis of mucocutaneous dryness is extensive and includes aging, the effects of medications, menopause, diabetes mellitus, hypothyroidism, nutritional deficiencies, postradiation dryness, lymphoma, amyloidosis, sarcoidosis, and a number of viral infections, such as hepatitis C or HIV infections. Uveoparotid fever (Heerfordt disease) is a form of sarcoidosis that affects only the salivary and lacrimal glands. Sometimes SS can only be distinguished from uveoparotid fever by minor salivary gland biopsy.

Because of the numerous disorders associated with dryness, two different groups of investigators have devised diagnostic criteria to help clinicians make the distinction between SS and other causes of the sicca complex. The criteria created by these two groups, known respectively as the European Study Group and the San Diego Classifications, have been merged into the Revised International Classification Criteria for SS (Table 24–1). The rules for applying these criteria to the diagnoses of primary and secondary SS are shown in Table 24–2. These criteria were devised to ensure that investigators at different institutions would be evaluating comparable patients. Although they were not meant to be used in the diagnosis of individual patients in routine clinical settings, these criteria do provide a diagnostic framework that will help clinicians recognize and prioritize characteristic manifestations of SS.

Treatment

A. ORAL

Fastidious dental care is crucial if patients are to retain their teeth. Patients should brush their teeth with fluoride toothpaste and perform flossing after every meal. Regular dental check-ups for cleaning and fluoride treatments should be scheduled at least 3 times a year. Chewing sugar-free gum or sucking on sugar-free candies can increase salivary flow and reduce the discomfort of xerostomia in many patients. Sugar-free breath mints will help alleviate the halitosis that plagues most patients with severe xerostomia.

During the daytime, frequent small sips of water relieve dry mouth symptoms. Patients should avoid drinking copious amounts of free water, since a full glass of water offers no more symptomatic relief than a small sip. Moreover, because of their craving for water, SS patients are at risk for the development of polydipsia, polyuria, and dilutional hyponatremia. Patients should be encouraged to keep artificial saliva by the bedside at night. The use of artificial saliva at night can reduce the need for water intake, thereby decreasing nocturia and improving sleep. There are a number of commercial artificial saliva products on the market. Some come in individual squeeze packets, some in bottles, some in atomizers, and still others come as a gel that can be applied directly to the tongue. Personal preferences vary widely, so each patient needs to be en-

Table 24–1. Revised International Classification Criteria for Sjögren syndrome.

I. Ocular symptoms: a positive response to at least one of the following questions:
  a. Have you had daily, persistent, troublesome dry eyes for more than 3 months?
  b. Do you have a recurrent sensation of sand or gravel in the eyes?
  c. Do you use tear substitutes more than 3 times a day?
II. Oral symptoms: a positive response to at least one of the following questions:
  a. Have you had a daily feeling of dry mouth for more than 3 months?
  b. Have you had recurrently or persistently swollen salivary glands as an adult?
  c. Do you frequently drink liquids to aid in swallowing dry food?
III. Ocular signs: objective evidence of ocular involvement defined as a positive result for at least one of the following two tests:
  a. Schirmer test, performed without anesthesia (< 5 mm in 5 minutes).
  b. Rose Bengal score or other ocular dye score (> 4 according to van Bijsterveld scoring system).
IV. Histopathology: In minor salivary glands (obtained through normal-appearing mucosa) focal lymphocytic sialoadenitis, evaluated by an expert histopathologist, with a focus score ≥ 1, defined as the number of lymphocytic foci that are adjacent to normal-appearing mucous acini and contain more than 50 lymphocytes per 4 mm^2 of examined glandular tissue.
V. Salivary gland involvement: objective evidence of salivary gland involvement, defined by a positive result for at least one of the following diagnostic tests:
  a. Unstimulated whole salivary flow (< 1.5 mL in 15 minutes).
  b. Parotid sialography showing the presence of diffuse sialectasias (punctate, cavitary, or destructive pattern), without evidence of obstruction in the major ducts.
  c. Salivary scintigraphy showing delayed uptake, reduced concentration, and/or delayed excretion of tracer.
VI. Autoantibodies: presence of at least one of the following serum autoantibodies:
  a. Antibodies to SS-A (Ro) or SS-B (La) antigens, or both.

Table 24–2. Revised rules for the classification of Sjögren syndrome (SS).[a]

For primary SS
a. "4 of 6 criteria are present provided that criteria from histopathology or autoantibodies sections are positive" The presence of any four of the six items, provided that either item IV (Histopathology) or VI (Autoantibodies) is positive.
b. The presence of any three of the four objective criteria items (ie, items III, IV, V, VI).
For secondary SS
In patients with a potentially associated disease, the presence of item I or II plus any two from among III–V may be considered indicative of secondary SS.
Exclusion criteria
Past history of head and neck radiation therapy, hepatitis C infection, AIDS, preexisting lymphoma, sarcoidosis, graft-versus-host disease, or use of anticholinergic drugs.

[a]See Table 24–1.

couraged to experiment with a variety of products. Oral candidiasis is responsible for many of the unpleasant oral symptoms of SS. Sucking on nystatin lozenges twice a day will ensure enough direct mucosal contact to eliminate the infection.

B. OCULAR

Artificial tears are the mainstay treatment for the ocular manifestations of SS. Preparations with high levels of mucopolysaccharides are preferred because long chain polysaccharides adhere to the surface of the cornea and conjunctiva, providing a tear film that lasts much longer than that seen with the use of aqueous preparations. Artificial tears should be used as often as necessary to relieve the symptoms of keratoconjunctivitis sicca. Some patients derive benefit from the use of hydroxypropylcellulose pellets placed under the lower eyelid. These pellets dissolve slowly, providing a fairly long-lasting artificial tear film. However, they are only effective in patients with enough aqueous tear production to dissolve the pellets.

The application of artificial tears at night is problematic. Bedtime use of an ophthalmologic ointment such as lacrilube helps maintain ocular moisture during sleep, and decreases the discomfort of opening the eyelids in the morning. Sometimes keratoconjunctivitis sicca does not respond to conservative treatment with artificial tears and ophthalmologic ointment. In such patients, lacrimal duct occlusion, using reversible plugs or irreversible cauterization, will prevent drainage of both artificial and natural tears and help maintain a more effective tear film. In patients with severe disease, painful filaments consisting of inspissated corneal epithelial debris become adhered to the corneal surface, resulting in pain, photophobia, and blurred vision. These filaments may require surgical debridement.

C. MUCOSAL

Relief of nasal and vaginal dryness can often be accomplished with water-miscible lubricants, such as lubafax. These lubricants are hygienic, easy to apply, and easy to wash off. Saline nasal sprays are sometimes helpful in alleviating dryness in deep nasal passages. Unfortunately, in patients with severe disease, the relief offered by water-based products is short lived. When water-based lubricants are inadequate, petroleum-based products can be used. Although greasy, they adhere to mucosal surfaces more efficiently and for longer periods of time. Dryness of the vagina is associated with an increased susceptibility to vaginal candidiasis. Vaginal nystatin tablets or suppositories are effective but may have to be used frequently. The prophylactic use of suppositories twice a week can sometimes prevent recurrent infection. In recalcitrant cases, oral ketoconazole or fluconazole may be necessary. Dryness of the tracheal or bronchial mucosa is associated with a chronic cough. A room humidifier in the bedroom, turned on only at night, will increase the humidity of nighttime air and ameliorate the nocturnal cough suffered by many patients with SS. Because increased humidity is associated with the growth of molds, patients with an allergy to molds cannot use this treatment.

D. CUTANEOUS

Dryness and flaking of the skin are common complaints. Aloe- or lanolin-based creams can help maintain skin moisture in many patients. Patients need to be warned that daily showers or baths will increase dryness of the skin and cause chronic pruritus. They should be encouraged to bathe every other day and apply baby oil to the skin while it is still moist from the bath. Patients should still use aloe or lanolin creams on the days they do not bathe or shower. Using pharmacologic agents such as hydroxyzine hydrochloride or diphenhydramine hydrochloride to treat pruritus should be avoided, as these medications can actually exacerbate increased dryness.

E. PHARMACOLOGIC THERAPY

Oral cholinergic parasympathomimetic agents capable of increasing exocrine gland function can be of significant clinical benefit in many patients with the sicca complex. The two agents now available are pilocarpine hydrochloride and cevimeline. To a certain degree, salivary, lacrimal, sweat, gastrointestinal, pancreatic, and respiratory mucosal secretions all can be increased using these agents. Unfortunately, muscarinic effects on smooth muscle can also be seen at doses used in the treatment of SS. Therefore, potential side effects of these drugs include decreased visual acuity, nausea, vomiting, diarrhea, bradycardia, tachycardia, heart block, hypotension or hypertension, biliary or renal colic, urinary urgency, decreased cognition, tremors, bronchospasm, flushing, and diaphoresis. Increased sweating is the most common side effect, occurring in up to 40% of patients. The recommended dose of pilocarpine hydrochloride is 5 mg 3 or 4 times daily. The dose of cevimeline is 30 mg 3 times daily. These agents offer substantial relief to patients whose sicca symptoms cannot be controlled by conservative measures.

Treatment of the arthritis of SS rests on the judicious use of anti-inflammatory medicines. Fast-acting, nonsteroidal anti-inflammatory drugs (NSAIDs) or cyclooxygenase-2 (COX-2) inhibitors are the cornerstone of therapy. Because SS is more frequent in the elderly who are particularly susceptible to the gastrointestinal toxicities of NSAIDs, patients frequently require H_2 blockers (such as misoprostol) or proton pump inhibitors to treat NSAID-induced gastrointestinal symptoms. In patients who do not respond to anti-inflammatory doses of nonselective NSAIDs or COX-2 inhibitors, the use of disease-modifying antirheumatic drugs (DMARDs) should be considered. Hydroxychloroquine (200 mg twice daily) is effective in the treatment of the arthritis and can help alleviate fatigue in many patients. Methotrexate (15–20 mg/wk) can also be useful in patients with severe articular disease.

Severe inflammation of major salivary glands or the presence of extraglandular involvement, such as interstitial lung disease, renal disease, or vasculitis, may require the use of systemic glucocorticoids. Low-dose prednisone (less than 10 mg/d) can be used to treat the arthritis of SS and will also frequently result in decreased pain and swelling in major salivary glands. Systemic glucocorticoids may also result in increased energy and a sense of well-being. High-dose glucocorticoids or cytotoxic therapy with such drugs as azathioprine, methotrexate, mycophenolate mofetil, cyclosporine, chlorambucil, or cyclophosphamide is useful in the treatment of life-threatening complications that develop in some patients.

Prognosis

SS is usually a chronic, slowly progressive, sometimes debilitating but benign disorder that affects elderly women. In patients with extraglandular involvement, SS may be an aggressive disorder with potentially life-threatening complications that can affect the lungs, kidneys, gastrointestinal tract, neuromuscular system, and vasculature. SS in these patients is not a slowly progressive, benign lymphocyte disorder but an aggressive, life-threatening affliction that challenges the skills of the most accomplished clinician. These manifestations of extraglandular disease warrant the use of systemic glucocorticoids or cytotoxic drugs. Finally, lymphoid malignancies develop in some patients ($\leq$ 5%), who will need the expertise of the oncologist.

REFERENCES

Fox RI, et al. Use of muscarinic agonists in the treatment of Sjögren's syndrome. *Clin Immunol.* 2001;101:249. [PMID: 11726216] (Reviews the use of pilocarpine and cevimeline to treat xerostomia.)

Garcia-Carrasco M, et al. Primary Sjögren syndrome: clinical and immunologic disease patterns in a cohort of 400 patients. *Medicine (Baltimore)*. 2002;81:270. [PMID: 12169882] (There are two subsets of primary SS: The first is disease limited to glandular involvement, with a lower frequency of immunologic and extraglandular manifestations, and a second is systemic involvement and a greater likelihood of complications in other organs. There are few or no distinguishing features between these subsets on most diagnostic tests.)

Ramos-Casals M, et al. Primary Sjögren syndrome: hematologic patterns of disease expression. *Medicine (Baltimore)*. 2002;81: 281. [PMID: 12169883] (Among a cohort of 380 patients, 22% had a monoclonal IgG gammopathy. Only one of these patients had overt lymphoma, suggesting that the presence of an IgG monoclonal gammopathy is a frequent and probably benign feature of SS.)

Polymyositis & Dermatomyositis

25

Robert L. Wortmann, MD

ESSENTIALS OF DIAGNOSIS

- *Proximal muscle weakness, elevated serum levels of enzymes derived from skeletal muscle, myopathic changes demonstrated by electromyography, and muscle biopsy evidence of inflammation are diagnostic criteria for polymyositis and other idiopathic inflammatory myopathies.*
- *The addition of a skin rash indicates dermatomyositis.*
- *These manifestations can occur in a variety of combinations or patterns, and no single feature is specific or diagnostic.*
- *Diagnosis is made by finding these criteria in combination and excluding all other causes for these abnormalities.*

General Considerations

Inflammatory myopathies are rare diseases. Estimates of incidence range from 0.5 to 8.4 cases per million. The incidence does appear to be increasing, although this may simply reflect increased awareness and more accurate diagnosing. Table 25–1 lists the clinical classification of the idiopathic inflammatory myopathies.

These diseases are seen in all age groups, but overall, the age at onset has a bimodal distribution with peaks observed between ages 10 and 15 years in children and between 45 and 60 years in adults. However, the mean ages for specific groups differ. Both myositis associated with malignancy and inclusion body myositis are more common after age 50 years. The age at onset for myositis occurring with another collagen vascular disease is similar to that for the associated condition. Women are twice as commonly affected as men, with the exception of inclusion body myositis, which affects men more often.

Clinical Features

A. SYMPTOMS AND SIGNS

The clinical features of polymyositis in the adult are representative of all the inflammatory myopathies. Typically, polymyositis begins insidiously over 3–6 months with no identifiable precipitating event. Pelvic and shoulder girdle musculature are most affected, but weakness of neck muscles, particularly the flexors, is also common. Ocular and facial muscles are virtually never involved. Dysphagia may develop secondary to esophageal dysfunction or cricopharyngeal obstruction. Pharyngeal muscle weakness may cause dysphonia and difficulty swallowing. Myalgias and arthralgias are not uncommon, but severe muscle tenderness and frank synovitis are unusual. Raynaud phenomenon is sometimes present, and periorbital edema may be noted.

Pulmonary and cardiac manifestations may precede the onset of muscle weakness or develop at any time during the course of disease. Velcro-like crackles may be heard on chest auscultation of patients with interstitial fibrosis or interstitial pneumonitis. Cardiac involvement is usually limited to asymptomatic electrocardiographic abnormalities. However, supraventricular arrhythmia, cardiomyopathy, and congestive heart failure can occur.

The clinical features of dermatomyositis include all those described for polymyositis plus a variety of cutaneous manifestations. Skin involvement varies widely from patient to patient. Rashes can antedate the onset of muscle weakness or follow its development by more than a year. Furthermore, the characteristics of the rash may change over time. Two cutaneous manifestations are considered pathognomonic. These include Gottron papules (symmetric lacy pink or violaceous raised areas typically found on the dorsal aspect of interphalangeal joints, elbows, patellae, and medial malleoli) and heliotrope (violaceous) discoloration of the eyelids. The latter is often with associated periorbital edema. Other characteristic cutaneous findings include macular erythema of the posterior shoulders and neck (shawl sign), anterior neck and upper chest (V-sign), malar region, forehead, or small joints of the fingers; dystrophic cuti-

Table 25–1. Clinical classification
of the idiopathic inflammatory myopathies.[a]

Polymyositis
Dermatomyositis
Juvenile dermatomyositis
Myositis associated with neoplasia
Myositis associated with collagen vascular disease
Inclusion body myositis

[a]In the past, the terms "idiopathic inflammatory myopathy" and "polymyositis" have been used interchangeably. Today, idiopathic inflammatory myopathy is used to represent the spectrum of these conditions; polymyositis represents one of these diseases.

cles; and mechanic's hands (darkened or dirty-appearing horizontal lines and fissures that are seen across the lateral and palmar aspects of the fingers). Periungual telangiectasias and nailfold capillary changes similar to those observed in patients with scleroderma or systemic lupus erythematosus and Raynaud phenomenon can be seen.

The inflammatory myopathy that affects children tends to have a highly characteristic pattern, although a disease similar to adult polymyositis does occur. In juvenile dermatomyositis, the skin lesions and weakness are almost always coincidental, but the severity and progression of each varies greatly from patient to patient. In some patients, remission is complete with little or no therapy. The juvenile variant differs from the adult form because of the coexistence of vasculitis, ectopic calcification, and lipodystrophy. Unfortunately, in dermatomyositis accompanied by vasculitis, progression may be devastating despite therapy. Gastrointestinal ulcerations resulting from vasculitis can cause hemorrhage or perforation of a viscus. Ectopic calcifications may occur in the subcutaneous tissues or in the muscles.

Some patients with biopsy-confirmed, classic cutaneous findings of dermatomyositis have normal motor function, muscle enzyme, electromyograms (EMGs), and muscle histology. The terms "amyotrophic dermatomyositis" and "dermatomyositis sine myositis" have been used to describe these patients. Although there is no evidence of myopathy, fatigue may be a dominant complaint. Some patients with this presentation continue to have skin disease only, whereas others progress over time, becoming weak and developing typical dermatomyositis. There may be an increased prevalence of neoplasia associated with this presentation.

Muscle weakness is a common finding in patients with collagen vascular diseases. The features of idiopathic inflammatory myopathy may dominate the clinical picture in some patients with scleroderma, systemic lupus erythematosus, mixed connective tissue disease, and Sjögren's syndrome, but the classic picture of polymyositis is less common in rheumatoid arthritis, Wegener granulomatosis, polyarteritis nodosa, and adult Still disease. Weakness in these latter conditions is more commonly the result of vasculitis.

Muscle weakness associated with an underlying malignancy develops in a subset of patients with inflammatory myopathies. The true incidence of this relationship is not clear. Although malignancy may precede, or develop after, the onset of muscle weakness, usually the two are diagnosed within a 1-year period. The association occurs in patients of all ages but is rare in childhood. Although an associated malignancy may be more common with dermatomyositis, cancer can be found in association with each subset. The sites or types of malignancy that occur in association with myositis are those that are expected for the age and gender of the patient. Ovarian cancer may prove the exception; it appears to be overrepresented in women with dermatomyositis.

Inclusion body myositis mainly affects older persons. The symptoms begin most insidiously and progress slowly. Symptoms are often present for 5–8 years before the diagnosis is made. The clinical picture in some patients is identical to that of typical polymyositis. In others, however, focal, distal, or asymmetric weakness is present. Dysphagia is not infrequent in this disease. As the muscle weakness becomes severe, it can be accompanied by atrophy and diminished deep tendon reflexes. In some patients, inclusion body myositis follows a slow, steadily progressing course. In others, the weakness seems to plateau, leaving the person with fixed weakness and atrophy of the involved musculature.

B. Laboratory Findings

An abnormal creatine kinase (CK) level is possibly the most sensitive indicator of skeletal muscle damage. The serum level of this enzyme is elevated at some time during the course of an inflammatory myopathy and, in most instances, the serum CK level reasonably correlates with disease activity. Normal levels of CK may be found very early in the course of polymyosits or dermatomyositis, in advanced cases with significant muscle atrophy, or in myositis associated with a malignancy. CK levels are often only minimally elevated or can be normal in inclusion body myositis. Other enzymes derived from diseased skeletal muscle include aldolase, aspartate aminotransferase (AST), alanine aminotransferase (ALT), and lactate dehydrogenase (LDH). Accordingly, these enzymes may also be elevated in the course of the disease.

Tests of acute phase reactants, the erythrocyte sedimentation rate (ESR) and C-reactive protein levels, are abnormal in only some patients with myositis. The ESR is normal in about half of patients with polymyositis and is elevated above 50 mm/h (Westergren method) in only 20%.

Antinuclear antibodies (ANAs) may be found in the serum of over 50% of patients with inflammatory muscle disease. The presence of a high-titer ANA may indicate the presence of an associated collagen-vascular disease (for example, anti-Sm or anti-dsDNA in systemic lupus erythematosus or anti-Scl-70 antibodies in scleroderma). In the other forms of myositis, the ANA tends to be present in low titer and is nonspecific in nature.

Certain autoantibodies are found almost exclusively in patients with idiopathic inflammatory myopathies and, therefore, are termed myositis-specific autoantibodies (Table 25–2). With extremely rare exceptions, an individual patient will have only one myositis-specific autoantibody, and the particular autoantibody present appears to identify relatively homogeneous groups of patients with regard to clinical manifestations and prognosis.

Most myositis-specific autoantibodies are directed against amino acyl-tRNA synthetase activities. The most common of these is anti-histidyl-tRNA synthetase, called anti-Jo-1. Patients with these autoantibodies typically manifest myositis (polymyositis more commonly than dermatomyositis) plus several extramuscular features including interstitial lung disease, arthritis, mechanic's hands, and Raynaud phenomenon. The combination of these features and an inflammatory myopathy

Table 25–2. Myositis-specific autoantibodies.

Autoantibody	Clinical Features	Treatment Response
Antisynthetase[a]	Polymyositis or dermatomyositis with interstitial lung disease Fever Arthritis Raynaud phenomenon	Moderate with disease persistence
Anti-SRP	Polymyositis with very acute onset Often in fall Severe weakness Palpitations	Typically poor
Anti-Mi-2	Dermatomyositis with V sign and shawl disease Cuticular overgrowth	Good in most cases

[a]Anti-Jo-1 is the most common myositits-specific antibody. Other antisynthetase antibodies are anti-PL-7, anti-PL-12, anti-EJ, and anti-OJ.
SRP, signal recognition particle.

has been termed "antisynthetase syndrome." Patients with this syndrome have a variable response to therapy and often are difficult to treat because they tend not to sustain complete remission. Anti-Mi-2 antibodies are directed against helicase activities. These autoantibodies are found almost exclusively in patients with dermatomyositis and most respond very well to treatment. In contrast, but with some exceptions, polymyositis of sudden onset develops in patients with antibodies to signal recognition particle (SRP); these patients are relatively resistant to treatment. Cardiomyopathy and distal muscle weakness are also associated with the presence of anti-SRP antibodies.

C. IMAGING STUDIES

Although neither conventional radiography nor radionuclide imaging have proved particularly useful in patients with muscle diseases, computer-based image analysis using ultrasonography, computed tomography, and magnetic resonance imaging (MRI) can be helpful. Of these, MRI with T2-weighted images and fat suppression or STIR technique offers the best imaging of soft tissue and muscle. MRI can detect early or subtle disease changes as well as identify patchy muscle involvement. Because of these capacities and the fact that it is noninvasive, MRI may prove superior to EMG in determining the site for muscle biopsy. Furthermore, MRI can be used to semiquantitatively grade muscle involvement and, therefore, can be used to monitor the response to therapy. This may be particularly useful when trying to differentiate between active myositis and glucocorticoid myopathy.

D. SPECIAL TESTS

EMG is a valuable technique for determining the classification, distribution, and severity of diseases affecting skeletal muscle. Although the changes identified with this technique are not specific, EMG is quite effective for (1) differentiating between myopathic and neuropathic conditions, and (2) in the case of neurologic abnormalities, localizing the lesion to the central nervous system, spinal cord anterior horn cell, peripheral nerves, or neuromuscular junction. In addition, knowledge of the distribution and severity of abnormalities can guide selection of the most appropriate site to biopsy if MRI is not available.

In polymyositis and dermatomyositis, EMG classically reveals the following triad: 1) increased insertional activity, fibrillations, and sharp positive waves; 2) spontaneous, bizarre high-frequency discharges; and 3) polyphasic motor unit potentials of low amplitude and short duration. This triad is characteristic but not diagnostic. The complete triad is seen in approximately 40% of patients, whereas 10–15% of patients will have completely normal EMGs. In a small number of patients, abnormalities are limited to the paraspinal muscle. In patients with inclusion body myositis, EMG may also reveal neurogenic or mixed neurogenic and myopathic changes, especially in those with distal or asymmetric muscle weakness.

Muscle histology is useful for making the diagnosis of an inflammatory myopathy. It is also helps determine the specific disease type because there are characteristic changes seen in polymyositis, dermatomyositis, and inclusion body myositis. In classic polymyositis, muscle fibers are in varying stages of necrosis and regeneration. The lymphocytic cell infiltrate is found predominantly in focal and endomysial locations. T lymphocytes, especially CD8+ cytotoxic T cells, accompanied by a smaller number of macrophages surround and then invade the initially nonnecrotic fibers. In other cases, however, changes are minimal with fiber atrophy or degeneration observed in the absence of inflammatory cells. With disease progression, muscle fibers are replaced by fibrous connective tissue and fat. However, in some cases, no fiber necrosis is observed, and the only recognized change is that of type 2 fiber atrophy.

The histopathology of muscle biopsies of classic adult or juvenile dermatomyositis shows a perivascular infiltration of inflammatory cells composed largely of B lymphocytes and CD4+ T helper lymphocytes. Biopsies also characteristically reveal plugged capillaries and perifascicular atrophy.

The characteristic change in inclusion body myositis is the presence of intracellular lined (rimmed) vacuoles. Electron microscopy reveals either intracytoplasmic or intranuclear tubular or filamentous inclusions. These structures are straight and rigid-appearing with periodic transverse and longitudinal striations. Myelin figures (also called myeloid bodies) and membranous whorls are also common. Neither the lined vacuoles or changes seen with electon microscopy are specific for inclusion body myositis, but they may prove diagnostic in the appropriate clinical setting.

Differential Diagnosis

Although polymyositis and dermatomyositis are relatively rare, the list of diseases that can cause similar clinical manifestations is long (Table 25–3). When encountering a patient with proximal muscle weakness, the initial step is to determine whether the process is myopathic or neuropathic in origin. Neurologic diseases can generally be identified by the additional presence of distal or asymmetric weakness or abnormalities on other components of the neurologic examination (ie, altered sensorium, cranial defects, abnormal deep tendon reflexes). Typically, the weakness in myopathy is limited to proximal muscles, and the remainder of the physical examination of the nervous system is nor-

mal. Exceptions include inclusion body myositis, myositis with circulating anti-SRP antibodies, and myositis with neoplastic disease.

Neoplasia should also be considered in the evaluation of patients with myopathic symptoms. Although generalized weakness and fatigue can occur in these diseases from the systemic effects of cytokines released by tumor cells or as a result of immune response to the malignancy, prominent neuromuscular changes can also develop as features of paraneoplastic syndromes.

Numerous infections can cause a myopathy, with viruses being the most common. Children with influenza infections can experience severe myalgias associated with very high CK levels. Weakness is a common finding in patients suffering from AIDS and may be due to cachexia, central or peripheral nervous system diseases, polymyositis emerging as a consequence of altered immune function, zidovudine toxicity, or opportunistic infections (eg, cytomegalovirus, *Mycobacterium avium-intracellulare, Cryptococcus, Trichinella,* or *Toxoplasma*)(see Chapter 47).

Metabolic myopathies are diseases caused by abnormalities in muscle energy metabolism that result in skeletal muscle dysfunction. These diseases, which can be primary or inherited or secondary or acquired, are more prevalent than previously appreciated. Secondary metabolic myopathies may be caused by various endocrine disorders such as thyroid or adrenal diseases, electrolyte abnormalities, or drugs. Patients with a variety of these diseases can fulfill the criteria for the diagnosis of polymyositis.

The glycogen storage diseases, such as myophosphorylase deficiency (McArdle disease), share an underlying defect that blocks the ability of tissues to use carbohydrate to produce energy and that often causes abnormal accumulation of glycogen in skeletal muscle. The clinical manifestations of a glycogen storage disease include exercise intolerance that is attributed to pain, fatigue, stiffness, weakness, or intense cramping; severe rhabdomyolysis with myoglobinuria; or progressive proximal muscle weakness. In adults, the latter presentation can be difficult to distinguish from polymyositis because it is accompanied by an elevated CK level and myopathic changes on EMG. The diagnosis of glycogen storage diseases may be suggested by finding increased glycogen deposition on muscle histochemistry and is established by enzyme analyses in muscle tissue.

The recognized disorders of lipid metabolism that cause myopathic problems are due to abnormalities in the transport and processing of fatty acids for energy in mitochondria. Patients with muscle carnitine deficiency present with chronic muscle weakness in late childhood, adolescence, or early adulthood. Muscle carnitine deficiency can also be confused with polymyositis because serum CK levels are elevated in more than half

Table 25–3. Differential diagnosis of muscle weakness.[a]

Neuropathic diseases	Cytomegalovirus
Muscular dystrophies	Echovirus
Denervating conditions	Epstein-Barr virus
Neuromuscular junction disorders	HIV
Proximal neuropathies	Influenza viruses
Myotonic diseases	Rubella virus
Neoplasm	Spirochetal
Paraneoplastic syndromes	*Borrelia burgdorferi* (Lyme spirochete)
Eaton-Lambert syndrome	Fungal
Drug-related conditions	*Cryptococcus*
Alcohol	Parasitic
Cocaine	*Toxoplasma gondii*
Colchicine	Helminthic
Cyclosporine	*Trichinella*
Fibrates	Inborn errors of metabolism
Gemfibrozil	Muscle glycogenoses
Glucocorticoids	Lipid storage disorders
Heroin	Mitochondrial myopathies
Hydroxychloroquine	Endocrine disorders
Ketoconazole	Acromegaly
Nicotinic acid	Cushing syndrome
D-Penicillamine	Hypothyroidism
Phenytoin	Hyperthyroidism
Statins	Hyperparathyroidism
Valproic acid	Miscellaneous causes
Zidovudine	Sarcoidosis
Infections	Atherosclerotic emboli
Viral	Behçet disease
Advenovirus	Fibromyalgia
Coxsackievirus	Psychosomatic

[a]Does not include inflammatory diseases described in the text.

the patients, and EMG often reveals myopathic changes. Patients with other lipid storage disorders or mitochondrial defects also can have presentations that mimic inflammatory muscle disease.

Numerous drugs can cause myopathic changes by a variety of mechanisms. Some, such as alcohol, may have direct toxic effects. Other drugs may cause metabolic or electrolyte abnormalities. For example, thiazide diuretics induce hypokalemia, which can cause weakness, myalgias, and cramps; clofibrate, lovastatin, gemfibrozil, and other lipid-lowering agents probably alter muscle fiber energetics; and zidovudine can induce a mitochondrial myopathy. D-Penicillamine can actually trigger polymyositis through altered immunity.

Finally, the finding of an elevated CK level is not specific for an inflammatory myopathy. Elevated CK levels can result from any disease or factor that causes muscle necrosis or membrane damage. Trauma is a well-recognized cause of high CK levels, as are isometric and aerobic exercise (especially in poorly condi-

tioned persons). Occasionally, elevated CK levels are observed in asymptomatic persons. Racial differences in normal CK levels must be considered in this context; healthy black males have higher CK levels than whites or Hispanics, with the majority of values appearing abnormal by usual laboratory values. Some asymptomatic persons with high CK levels are carriers for disease, such as one of the glycogen storage diseases, malignant hyperthermia, or muscular dystrophy. Over time, symptomatic myopathy may develop in some patients, but others remain asymptomatic for years. This latter condition has been termed "benign hyper-CK-emia."

Treatment

Before initiating medications, it is recommended that the patient's clinical status be evaluated as objectively as possible. Assessing the strength of individual muscle groups provides valuable information because these measures can be compared with those obtained after therapy is initiated. Chest radiography, pulmonary function studies, and swallowing studies may be indicated. Muscle enzymes, including CK, aldolase, AST, ALT, and LDH, should be measured in addition to other laboratory values that might be affected by therapy. The tests chosen to screen for cancer are those indicated by the patient's age and gender, as well as those that would address any areas of concern identified through the review of systems or physical examination. Women with dermatomyositis should have pelvic imaging to rule out ovarian cancer.

Physical therapy has an important role. Bed rest may be required during intervals of severe inflammation. Passive range of motion exercise is encouraged during these intervals to maintain movement and prevent contractures. With improvement, therapy should include active-assisted and then active exercises. The head of the bed should be elevated in patients with dysphagia or dysphonia in an attempt to reduce the risk of aspiration.

The choice of medications used to treat polymyositis and dermatomyositis is determined empirically because randomized trials are few and evaluate only small numbers of patients. Glucocorticoids are the standard first-line medication for any idiopathic inflammatory myopathy. Initially, prednisone is usually given in a single dose of 1 mg/kg/d, but in severe cases, the daily dose can be divided or intravenous methylprednisolone can be used. Clinical improvement may be noted in the first weeks or gradually over 3–6 months. In general, the earlier in the course of disease that prednisone is started, the faster and more effectively it works. As many as 90% of patients attain some response with glucocorticoid therapy and 50–75% of those achieve complete remission.

If a patient does not respond to glucocorticoid therapy, another agent is added, usually either azathioprine or methotrexate. Methotrexate is generally given on a weekly schedule at doses of 5–15 mg orally or 15–50 mg subcutaneously or intravenously. The typical dose of azathioprine is 2–3 mg/kg/d (maximum of 150 mg/d). Other immunosuppressive agents have been used in glucocorticoid-resistant patients. Cyclophosphamide, 6-mercaptopurine, chlorambucil, cyclosporine, etanercept, infliximab, mycophenolate, plasmapheresis, lymphapheresis, total-body (or total-nodal) irradiation, and intravenous immunoglobulin have also been used. Oral hydroxychloroquine and topical glucocorticoids can be used to treat the cutaneous lesions of dermatomyositis, although they have no recognized effect on the myositis.

Complications

Progression of the underlying disease process produces the major complications that develop in patients with inflammatory muscle diseases. These are more likely to be seen in patients in whom the diagnosis was delayed or in patients with refractory disease. Persistent or progressive muscle weakness can result in the patient becoming wheelchair-dependent. Severe disease may be associated with loss of deep tendon reflexes, muscle atrophy, and especially in children, joint contractures. Patients with dysphagia or dysphonia are at great risk for aspiration pneumonia. Those with interstitial lung disease may progress to respiratory failure, and acute respiratory distress syndrome has been described. Cardiomyopathy with congestive heart failure can develop in the few patients with cardiac involvement.

Complications also result from therapy. Of major concern are the side effects and toxicities of glucocorticoid use. Although patients treated with these agents can manifest all of the features of iatrogenic Cushing syndrome, two of the more troubling complications are opportunistic infections and glucocorticoid-induced proximal muscle weakness. Opportunistic pulmonary infections such as *Pneumocystis carinii* pneumonia can be rapidly fatal. Glucocorticoid myopathy can be particulary frustrating because it can complicate the course of a patient who is getting stronger in response to therapy. Clinically, this is often observed in patients who show improvement with glucocorticoid therapy and then suddenly plateau or deteriorate. In this setting, it is difficult to determine whether the decrease in muscle strength is due to a disease flare or glucorticoid toxicity. The only method of distinguishing between these two possibilities is a provocative test of significantly increasing or decreasing the glucocorticoid dosage and assessing the response.

When to Refer to the Specialist

Because the inflammatory myopathies are rare, it is prudent to refer each patient in whom the diagnosis is suspected (or made) to a specialist familiar with the natural history and therapies for these diseases. Once the diagnosis is confirmed, a physician comfortable prescribing high-dose glucocorticoids and other immunosuppressive agents can manage the patient's treatment. Referral back to the specialist is warranted if the patient does not respond to therapy as predicted or a complication of the disease or its therapies develops.

REFERENCES

Bohan A, Peter JB. Polymyositis and dermatomyositis: first of two parts. *N Engl J Med.* 1975;292:344. [PMID: 1090839] (Remains the classic description of diagnostic criteria used for the diagnosis and established the foundation for our current understanding of the idiopathic inflammatory myopathies.)

Buchbinder R, Hill CL. Malignancy in patients with inflammatory myopathy. *Curr Rheumatol Rep.* 2002;4:415. [PMID: 12217247] (Extensive review of the current information on the relation between these diseases with annotated bibliography.)

Callen JP. Dermatomyositis. *Lancet.* 2000;355:53. [PMID: 10615903] (Authoritative review of this disease from a dermatologist's perspective.)

Dion E, et al. Magnetic resonance imaging criteria for distinguishing between inclusion body myositis and polymyositis. *J Rheumatol.* 2002;29:1897. [PMID: 12233884] (Describes the findings in the various forms of myositis using the most recently developed evaluative tool, one that is becoming more and more important in the evaluation of patients with these diseases.)

Wortmann RL, ed. *Diseases of Skeletal Muscle.* Lippincott Williams & Wilkins, 2000. (Comprehensive text on myopathies with chapters devoted to adult and childhood inflammatory muscle diseases, their pathogenesis, and the evaluations used to diagnose and manage these disorders, including the myositis-specific autoantibodies as well as other diseases in the differential diagnosis of myositis.)

Relevant World Wide Web Site

[The Myositis Association]
http://www.myositis.org

Relapsing Polychondritis

26

John H. Stone, MD, MPH

ESSENTIALS OF DIAGNOSIS

- *Auricular chondritis (spares the earlobe).*
- *Inflammation in other cartilaginous areas (eg, the nose, joints, trachea, ribcage, and airways) and in tissues rich in proteoglycans, such as the eyes and heart valves.*
- *Frequently associated with an underlying disorder such as systemic vasculitis, connective tissue disease, or myelodysplastic syndrome.*

General Considerations

Relapsing polychondritis (RP) is an immune-mediated condition associated with inflammation in cartilaginous structures and other connective tissues throughout the body, including the ears, nose, joints, respiratory tract, and others. Thirty percent of RP cases occur in association with another disease, usually some form of systemic vasculitis (particularly Wegener granulomatosis), connective tissue disorder (eg, rheumatoid arthritis), or a myelodysplastic syndrome. RP is often assumed to be "autoimmune" in nature, but the evidence for a true autoimmune pathogenesis is relatively weak. Some patients have been reported to have antibodies to type 2 collagen, but these assays are not widely available and their poor sensitivities and specificities make them inappropriate for general clinical use. In general, the diagnosis of RP is a clinical one, based on the identification of cartilaginous inflammation in typical areas and the exclusion of other possible causes.

Clinical Findings

Table 26–1 lists the major clinical manifestations of RP.

A. SYMPTOMS AND SIGNS

1. Ears—Unilateral or bilateral auricular chondritis is often the first symptom of the disease. The inflammation may be confused with cellulitis of the ear, but a major clue to the diagnosis of RP is confinement of the inflammation to the auricular part of the ear, with sparing of the earlobe (Figure 26–1). The ears are erythematous and tender to touch. Swelling of the external ear canal may cause conductive hearing loss. RP may also be associated with sensorineural hearing loss, the mechanism of which remains obscure (vasculitis is often implicated, without proof).

2. Nose—Inflammation of the nasal cartilage leads to tenderness of the nasal bridge and often to epistaxis. In severe cases, "saddle-nose" deformities develop through collapse of the nasal bridge. This is usually preceded by the development of a nasal septal perforation.

3. Trachea—Subglottic stenosis results from tracheal inflammation and scarring inferior to the vocal cords. Early subglottic involvement often has minimal symptoms and may manifest itself as only subtle changes in voice. With time, however, substantial airway scarring may occur, leading to potentially life-threatening tracheal narrowing. In addition to the subglottic region, other parts of the tracheal wall may be softened by cartilaginous inflammation, leading to a tendency of the airway to collapse. Tracheal inflammation may be associated with tenderness to palpation of the anterior cervical trachea, the thyroid cartilage, and larynx.

4. Bronchi and airways—Cartilaginous inflammation may extend to the lower respiratory tract, with bronchial involvement. This manifestation, unlike the tracheal disease, may have a lengthy subclinical period but is usually detectable by investigations such as pulmonary function testing. Lower airway disease and its associated mucociliary dysfunction may heighten patients' susceptibility to infections.

5. Eyes—Nearly any part of the eye may be involved in RP. Scleritis causes photophobia and painful, often raised, scleral erythema. If unchecked, necrotizing scleritis may lead to scleral thinning, scleromalacia perforans, and visual loss. Peripheral keratitis may cause ulcerations on the margin of the cornea and lead to the syndrome of "corneal melt." Episcleritis and conjunctivitis are very common in RP. Extraocular involvement may include periorbital edema, chemosis, and proptosis.

6. Heart—Cartilaginous inflammation within the heart valve rings may lead to valvular dysfunction. The usual lesions are aortic and mitral regurgitation; aortic

215

Table 26–1. Major clinical manifestations of relapsing polychondritis.

Feature	Data
Mean age at diagnosis	47 years
Auricular chondritis	90%
Reduced hearing	37%
Nasal chondritis	60%
Saddle-nose deformities	25%
Laryngotracheal involvement	52%
Ocular inflammation	54%
Arthritis	69%
Skin involvement	25%
Aortic or mitral regurgitation	8%
Vasculitis	12%

Adapted from Molina JF, Espinoza LR. *Baillieres Best Pract Res Clin Rheumatol.* 2000;14:97, which summarizes the findings of four studies:
McAdam LP, et al. *Medicine (Baltimore).* 1976;55:193.
Michet CJ Jr., et al. *Ann Intern Med.* 1986;104:74.
Zeuner M, et al. *J Rheumatol.* 1997;24:96.
Trentham DE, Le CH. *Ann Intern Med.* 1998;129:114.

valve disease is more common. The proximity of the conduction system to some areas of valve ring inflammation may lead to cardiac conduction abnormalities. Pericarditis and rare cases of coronary arteritis have also been described in RP.

7. Joints—Articular lesions are often the first nonspecific manifestation of RP. The pattern of joint involvement at presentation is typically a migratory oligoarthritis, but symmetric polyarticular presentations are also seen. In general, the arthritis associated with RP is nondestructive, unless there is underlying rheumatoid arthritis. Joint symptoms tend to correlate very well with activity of disease at other sites.

8. Skin—Patients with RP may demonstrate a panoply of cutaneous lesions, none of which is specific for the disorder. Cutaneous findings are particularly common in cases of RP that are associated with myelodysplasia but occur frequently in other cases as well. Among patients with primary RP, the most common skin findings are aphthous ulcers, nodules (erythema nodosum–like lesions), purpura, papules, and sterile pustules. The cutaneous lesions of RP may resemble those of Behçet disease. An overlap syndrome of these two disorders—MAGIC (mouth and genital ulcers with inflamed cartilage)—has been described.

9. Kidneys—Renal lesions in RP range from pauci-immune glomerulonephritis to mild mesangial expansion and cellular proliferation. Distinguishing RP from Wegener granulomatosis is difficult in the setting of pauci-immune glomerulonephritis.

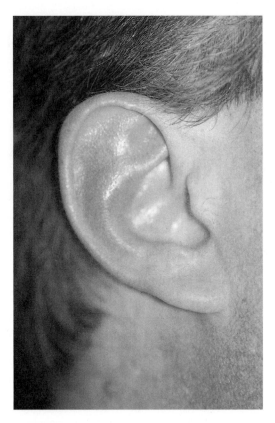

Figure 26–1. Auricular chondritis in a patient with relapsing polychondritis. Note the sparing of the earlobe (a noncartilaginous portion of the ear).

B. LABORATORY FINDINGS

There are no specific laboratory findings in RP. Mild normochromic, normocytic anemias and mild degrees of thrombocytosis may be observed. Major cytopenias should trigger suspicion of myelodysplasia. Mild to moderate elevations of acute phase reactants are expected. Antinuclear antibodies and rheumatoid factor are usually negative, and complement levels are normal. In the setting of antineutrophil cytoplasmic antibody (ANCA) positivity, underlying Wegener granulomatosis should be suspected, particularly if the antibody specificity is to proteinase-3 or, less commonly, to myeloperoxidase.

C. IMAGING STUDIES

Advances in computed tomography make these studies increasingly useful in the evaluation of airway disease. Computed tomography findings include edema, wall thickening, granulation tissue, and fibrosis.

D. SPECIAL TESTS

1. Biopsy—Given the proper constellation of clinical symptoms and signs, tissue biopsy is rarely required to establish the diagnosis of RP. (Biopsy may be more important, however, in the exclusion of RP mimickers.) In contrast to Wegener granulomatosis, RP is not associated with granulomatous inflammation. Biopsy of the trachea or larynx should be performed only with great caution because acute airway narrowing may result from additional damage to already compromised tissues.

2. Pulmonary function tests—Full sets of pulmonary function tests, including inspiratory and expiratory flow-volume loops, are useful in RP.

Differential Diagnosis

Aural chondritis is often confused initially with infectious processes, particularly cellulitis of the ear. Other infections in the differential diagnosis include tuberculous laryngitis, now rare in developed countries.

"Pure" RP must be distinguished from RP associated with an underlying condition because the complications of the underlying disorder may greatly affect the patient's prognosis. The major underlying disorders of concern are systemic vasculitides (particularly Wegener granulomatosis), connective tissue diseases (such as rheumatoid arthritis and systemic lupus erythematosus), and myelodysplastic syndromes.

Treatment

Glucocorticoids are the treatment of choice for reducing major inflammation in cartilaginous areas. In order to limit glucocorticoid exposure, dapsone, colchicine, and nonsteroidal anti-inflammatory drugs have all been used empirically. For patients with sustained disease, however, methotrexate is the most commonly used glucocorticoid-sparing agent. Cyclophosphamide is required for glomerulonephritis and other disease manifestations that are refractory to glucocorticoid alone. In the case of airway disease, it is essential to distinguish dysfunction secondary to active cartilaginous inflammation from that caused by damage from previously active disease.

The management of upper airway problems in RP requires collaboration with an experienced otolaryngologist or pulmonologist or both. Some upper airway disease manifestations (eg, subglottic stenosis) respond better to mechanical interventions and glucocorticoid injections than to systemic therapies. Stenting may also be required for cases in which the tracheal or bronchial walls have lost their integrity, provided that the regions of tracheomalacia or bronchomalacia are not too long. Continuous positive airway pressure may help some patients during sleep.

Complications

Prolonged or repeated bouts of aural chondritis may lead to deformation of the ear cartilage and "cauliflower ear." Similarly, nasal chondritis may cause nasal septal perforation and "saddle-nose" deformities.

Tracheomalacia may lead to extrathoracic airway obstruction and sometimes requires tracheostomy. Collapsible airways may be associated with postobstructive infections. Cardiac valvular regurgitation in RP may lead to valve replacement.

When to Refer to a Specialist

Voice huskiness and subtle signs of stridorous breathing may indicate impending critical stenosis of the subglottic region and should prompt a consultation with an otolaryngologist. Subacute respiratory stridor presents in some patients. Severe cases may require tracheostomies. Pulmonary function tests (flow-volume loops) provide a useful noninvasive means of quantifying and following the degree of extrathoracic airway obstruction. However, thin-cut computed tomography scans of the trachea are more sensitive for these lesions. In some cases, direct visualization with fiberoptic laryngoscopy is required to make the diagnosis.

Sensorineural hearing loss, which is often associated with other symptoms of inner ear dysfunction, such as vertigo, tinnitus, and nausea, may proceed quickly to irreversible hearing loss. Sensorineural hearing loss requires the prompt institution of treatment and consultation with an otolaryngologist to ensure that no other causes of hearing loss are present.

REFERENCES

Frances C, et al. Dermatologic manifestations of relapsing polychondritis. *Medicine (Baltimore)*. 2001;80:173. [PMID: 11388093] (Examines both the skin lesions associated with primary RP and those potentially associated with underlying conditions. Aphthous ulcers, skin nodules, and purpura were the most common cutaneous lesions in primary RP.)

Molina JF, Espinoza LR. Relapsing polychondritis. *Baillieres Best Pract Res Clin Rheumatol*. 2000;14:97. [PMID: 10882216] (Concise clinical summary with literature review.)

Tillie-Leblond I, et al. Respiratory involvement in relapsing polychondritis. Clinical, functional, endoscopic, and radiographic evaluations. *Medicine (Baltimore)*. 1998;77:168. [PMID: 9653428]

Pregnancy & Rheumatic Diseases 27

Phyllis N. Bonaminio, MD, & Rosalind Ramsey-Goldman, MD, DrPH

SYSTEMIC LUPUS ERYTHEMATOSUS

 ESSENTIAL FEATURES

- *Systemic lupus erythematosus (SLE) increases risk of spontaneous abortion, intrauterine fetal death, intrauterine growth restriction, and prematurity.*
- *Patients should not become pregnant when SLE is active.*
- *Pregnancy should be planned.*
- *Distinguishing SLE flare from preeclampsia is difficult.*
- *A multidisciplinary approach to patient care is essential for optimal outcome.*

General Considerations

SLE primarily affects women of childbearing age. Typical clinical symptoms include fatigue, fever, arthralgias, arthritis, photosensitive rash, serositis, Raynaud phenomenon, glomerulonephritis, vasculitis, and hematologic abnormalities (see Chapter 19).

SLE increases the risk of spontaneous abortion, intrauterine fetal death, preeclampsia, intrauterine growth restriction, and preterm birth. SLE not only affects pregnancy outcome, but the pregnancy can potentially affect disease activity. Optimizing care of the mother and fetus requires a coordinated team approach among internists, rheumatologists, obstetricians specializing in high-risk pregnancies, and in some instances, nephrologists and neonatologists.

Family Planning

Since SLE does not decrease fertility and since both maternal and fetal outcomes improve when maternal disease activity is quiescent for at least 6–12 months before pregnancy, great emphasis should be placed on contraception and timing of conception.

A. CONTRACEPTION

Barrier methods, such as condoms and foam or a diaphragm with spermicidal jelly, are the safest means of preventing conception because these strategies do not increase the risk of causing an SLE flare. However, the efficacy of these methods depends on the attentiveness of the woman and her partner.

Many patients may already be taking a combination pill when SLE is first diagnosed. Estrogen has been associated with an increased risk of an SLE flare developing or thromboembolic events. As long as there is no history of hypercoaguable risk, a pill with the lowest estrogen dose could be considered. If there is a risk of thromboembolism, then a combination hormone pill containing estrogen and progesterone is contraindicated.

An alternative hormonal medication for contraception is a single agent, progesterone, which is available in an oral or injectable form. Progesterone alone has not been associated with precipitating SLE flares or thromboembolic events. However, women often complain of breakthrough bleeding while on the progesterone-only preparation, thus limiting compliance. Fortunately, irregular bleeding usually subsides after the patient has been taking this medication for a few months.

Since SLE patients may be at increased risk for infection, an intrauterine device is not a preferred method of contraception. However, if the woman is not taking immunosuppressive drugs (including prednisone) and does not have a history of frequent genitourinary infections, then the intrauterine device may be considered.

B. RISKS

There is still debate about whether pregnancy increases SLE activity. On the one hand, most studies suggest that the chance of flare during pregnancy and postpartum is minimal if the patient has controlled or inactive disease at the time of conception. On the other hand, women with active disease at conception appear more likely to have a disease flare during or after pregnancy. For instance, women with active nephritis at conception have approximately a 50–60% chance of having a renal flare during pregnancy or postpartum; however, they only have a 7–10% chance of a renal flare if they conceive during a period of inactive disease.

Women with established SLE have approximately an 80% chance of having a live birth. However, women with SLE should also be counseled about increased risk of adverse fetal outcome risks such as preterm birth, pregnancy loss, and intrauterine growth restriction. Risk of preterm birth, birth before 37 weeks of gestation, is approximately 33% compared with 5–15% of the general population. Risk factors for preterm birth include increased maternal SLE activity, nephrotic range proteinuria, maternal hypertension, and premature rupture of membranes. Women with SLE have a higher incidence of pregnancy loss, including spontaneous abortion and intrauterine fetal death (stillbirths). Risk of spontaneous abortion—spontaneous termination of pregnancy before the 20th week of gestation—is approximately 15%, compared with 7–13% of the general obstetric population. Risk of intrauterine fetal death—spontaneous termination of pregnancy after the 20th week of gestation—is approximately 4%. Risk of intrauterine growth restriction—weight below the 10th percentile for gestational age—is approximately 17%, compared with 10% of the general obstetric population. Active maternal lupus, nephritis or renal impairment, the presence of anti-Ro/SS-A antibodies which can cause neonatal lupus erythematosus (NLE), and antiphospholipid antibodies have all been associated with fetal loss.

C. CONTRAINDICATIONS

Women with active disease or a flare within the last 6 months should delay becoming pregnant for at least 1 year while women with newly diagnosed SLE should delay becoming pregnant for at least 2 years.

Women with new, recurrent, or persistent renal disease indicated by an active urinary sediment, proteinuria > 3 g/24 h, moderate to severe hypertension, and creatinine levels > 2 mg/dL should be discouraged from becoming pregnant.

Women with pulmonary hypertension (pulmonary artery pressure > 40 mm Hg) or decreased cardiac output may not be able to tolerate the increase in intravascular volume and should be discouraged from becoming pregnant.

Women with active central nervous system disease such as cerebritis, uncontrolled seizure activity, and active psychosis and a history of cerebral vascular accidents should also be discouraged from getting pregnant.

Patients who are taking cyclophosphamide, methotrexate, warfarin, leflunomide, angiotensin-converting enzyme (ACE) inhibitors (captopril, lisinopril, or equivalent), angiotensin receptor blockers (valsartan or losartan), or anticonvulsants (diphenylhydantoin, valproic acid, and carbamazepine) must be discouraged from becoming pregnant until these medications have been discontinued at least 3–6 months before conceiving because the risk is high for drug-associated fetal abnormalities. Alternative medications that can be used during pregnancy are discussed below.

Leflunomide requires a special drug elimination procedure once a woman has discontinued the medication and desires to become pregnant. The elimination procedure involves administering cholestyramine at 8 g 3 times daily for 11 days (the days do not have to be consecutive unless there is a need to rapidly lower the plasma levels). Afterward, plasma levels must be verified by two separate tests at least 14 days apart. Levels should be < 0.02 mg/L; if the levels are not at the required level, additional cholestyramine should be considered.

Prenatal Evaluation

A. HISTORY

The physician should begin by closely reviewing the patient's original presenting symptoms of SLE, frequency and severity pattern of flare signs and symptoms, and any laboratory abnormalities since presentation. Knowing how a disease flare manifested in the past may help the physician distinguish an SLE flare from changes that normally occur during pregnancy.

Medications should be reviewed; those with teratogenic potential must be stopped and alternatives should be selected.

B. PHYSICAL EXAMINATION

The physical examination should include height, weight, blood pressure, and a general physical examination with a special focus on the heart, lungs, joints, oral ulcers, lymphadenopathy or rash, and the presence of edema.

C. LABORATORY FINDINGS

The recommended initial work-up is detailed in Table 27–1. A few of the tests deserve further comment. If the spot urine ratio of protein to creatinine is abnormal (> 0.3), then perform a 24-hour urine for protein, creatinine, and creatinine clearance. If a woman has had poor obstetric outcomes in the past, usually defined as three prior fetal losses, β_2 glycoprotein I antibody should be ordered.

Anti-SS-A/Ro and anti-SS-B/La antibodies help determine whether a woman's infant is at risk for NLE including congenital heart block (CHB) (see Special Circumstances section below).

Monitoring for disease activity by general examination and laboratory values should be continued until 3–6 months postpartum. The SS-A/Ro and SS-B/La antibodies need only be tested at the initial visit.

D. FETAL MONITORING

Women with SLE are at increased risk for intrauterine growth restriction and preterm births (< 37 weeks of gestation dated from the last menstrual period). Therefore, it is important to confirm menstrual dating with ultrasonography at the first prenatal visit to accurately estimate gestational age.

During the first trimester, fetal heart tones should be ascultated by Doppler or ultrasonogram at each office visit, starting as early as 10 weeks.

Table 27–1. Suggested laboratory evaluation schedule for monitoring pregnancy in a patient with systemic lupus erythematosus.

Laboratory Evaluation on Initial Visit	Frequency After Initial Visit
CBC with differential and platelets	Every 1–3 months
Liver function tests including albumin	Initial visit
Chemistry panel including BUN, creatinine, and glucose	Every 1–3 months
Urinalysis with microscopic examination	Monthly
Spot or 24-hour urine for protein and creatinine	Each trimester
C3, C4, and CH50	Each trimester
dsDNA antibody	Each trimester
Antiphospholipid antibodies and lupus anticoagulant	Initial visit
Anti-SS-A/Ro and anti-SS-B/La antibodies	First trimester

CBC, complete blood cell count; BUN, blood urea nitrogen.

During the second trimester, a level 2 ultrasonography should be done between 18 and 20 weeks of gestation to assess fetal anatomy, with a special focus on cardiac function to access for the presence of CHB if the mother is SS-A/SS-B antibody positive. During this time, the obstetrician continues monitoring fetal heart tones and fundal height. A delay in fundal height growth may indicate growth restriction and require more frequent monitoring.

At 24 weeks of gestation, the fetus has reached an age of potential viability. Any evidence suggesting imminent fetal demise may require delivery after this time period.

During the third trimester, monitoring of fundal height is continued and an ultrasonogram should be done frequently if the mother is SS-A/Ro or SS-B/La antibody positive. At 28 weeks of gestation, a weekly biophysical profile, consisting of a nonstress test and an ultrasonogram examination that assesses amniotic fluid volume, fetal body movements, fetal tone, and breathing movements should be performed. If amniotic fluid volume is low, this may indicate decreased placental perfusion. A Doppler or pulse wave of the umbilical artery should be done if placental abnormalities are suspected. If any of these tests results are abnormal, early delivery may be indicated.

E. Special Circumstances

The NLE syndrome includes photosensitivity, rash, cytopenias, and hepatomegaly or splenomegaly, and these are usually transient manifestations. CHB is a rare manifestation of this syndrome, which is usually permanent, and the infant may require a pacemaker. Unfortunately, in some instances, CHB may result in fetal or neonatal demise. Mothers who have SS-A/Ro and/or SS-B/La antibodies have a 2–5% risk of having a baby with NLE.

Special Problems

A. SLE Flare versus Normal Changes of Pregnancy

A particular challenge facing physicians who care for patients with SLE is how to distinguish an SLE flare from the normal changes of pregnancy (Table 27–2).

1. Musculoskeletal and cutaneous manifestations—Normal pregnancy is associated with alopecia, facial or palmar erythema, arthralgias, and edema.

Low back pain and pelvic pain are common complaints and are usually due to the softening and stretching of the ligaments from hormonal changes in preparation for delivery and from the added weight gain straining the lower back. Women may experience bland knee effusions, which must be distinguished from true arthritis that may be attributed to an SLE flare.

Skin changes associated with normal pregnancy can often be mistaken for SLE exacerbations. Alopecia is due to a fluctuation in the amount of estrogen. Whereas alopecia associated with pregnancy tends to be diffuse and usually occurs postpartum when the level of estrogen is at its lowest, hair loss associated with SLE can be either diffuse or occur in patches and occur at any time during pregnancy. The pregnancy facial mask called chloasma or melasma gravidarum is irregular, hyperpigmented, and patchy in appearance; located on forehead, cheeks, and the bridge of the nose; and is due to increased melanin deposition in skin macrophages. In SLE, the malar or butterfly rash extends over the cheeks and can involve the bridge of the nose; however, it typically spares the nasolabial folds. This rash can be macular but is usually erythematous and raised and can have papules or plaques.

2. Cardiovascular, renal, and pulmonary systems—The normal physiologic effects on the cardiovascular system in pregnancy include an increase in resting heart rate up to 90 beats per minute, lower blood pressure, and a crescendo-decrescendo systolic murmur. In contrast, pericardial chest pain may be associated with an SLE flare.

The renal system also undergoes normal physiologic alterations in the pregnant patient including a lowering

Table 27–2. Lupus manifestations versus the normal changes of pregnancy.

System	SLE	Normal Pregnancy
Cutaneous	Raised inflammatory rash often sparing the nasolabial folds	Irregular, hyperpigmented, and patchy rash (chloasma)
Musculoskeletal	True arthritis	Arthralgias, bland knee effusions
Cardiovascular	Pericarditis	Increased resting heart rate, low blood pressure, murmur
Renal	Increased creatinine or proteinuria compared with baseline or active urinary sediment	Decreased BUN, increased CrCl, slight increase in proteinuria
Pulmonary	Pleuritic chest pain	Shortness of breath, hyperventilation
Hematologic	Cytopenias	Anemia (iron deficient), decreased platelets, elevated WBC without a left shift
Serologic	Unchanged or decreasing C3 and C4 levels, rising dsDNA	Increased ESR
Constitutional	Fever not due to infection	Fatigue

BUN, blood urea nitrogen; CrCl, creatinine clearance; WBC, white blood cell count; ESR, erythrocyte sedimentation rate.

of the blood urea nitrogen and creatinine with an increase in creatinine clearance. There may also be a slight increase in proteinuria due to the increase in glomerular filtration rate that normally accompanies pregnancy. If the serum creatinine increases compared with baseline instead of decreasing and the urinary sediment is active (red or white cell casts or hematuria), then an SLE flare should be considered.

Finally, the pulmonary system changes in pregnancy are manifested as shortness of breath and hyperventilation. These are common complaints and are secondary to the increased level of progesterone. Pleuritic chest pain or pain with deep inspiration can be a sign of active SLE.

3. Hematologic and immunologic changes—An increase in intravascular volume of up to 50% causing mild anemia with a hematocrit ranging from 30% to 35% occurs during pregnancy. Iron deficiency may also contribute to anemia due to increased demand for iron stores by both the mother and fetus. Thrombocytopenia ranging from 100,000 to 150,000/µL can develop and is believed to be due to increased platelet turnover. Other hematologic abnormalities include an elevated white blood cell count without a left shift ranging from 10,000 to 15,000/µL. Cytopenias must be considered in the context of other symptoms and laboratory data before attributing them to an SLE flare.

The erythrocyte sedimentation rate (ESR) increases in normal pregnancy and cannot be used to detect SLE disease activity. The ESR level can reach > 40 mm/h by the Westergren method during normal pregnancy, and the elevated ESR is due to an increase in protein, especially fibrinogen, in pregnancy and should not be mistaken as an acute phase reactant supporting an SLE flare.

Serum complement levels normally increase during pregnancy. Levels of C3, C4, or both that are unchanged or begin to fall may indicate an SLE exacerbation.

An SLE flare can therefore be suggested when a raised inflammatory rash, arthritis, lymphadenopathy, fever not due to infection, or pleuritic chest pain is present. Laboratory tests that have been helpful in distinguishing a flare include leukopenia, hematuria and red cell casts, falling C3 or C4 or both complement levels, and rising titers of dsDNA antibody.

B. Lupus Nephritis versus Preeclampsia

Preeclampsia is defined as the abrupt onset of hypertension and proteinuria after 20 weeks of gestation and is most commonly found in the primagravida. Pregnant patients with SLE are at increased risk for preeclampsia, especially if the patient has a prior history of renal disease or hypertension, or has positive antiphospholipid antibodies. The risk of developing preeclampsia in a woman with lupus nephritis is as high as 38% versus 0.5–10% of the normal population. Consequently, there is an increased risk for preterm delivery and fetal death if active nephritis or preeclampsia is present.

Distinguishing between a lupus nephritis flare and preeclampsia is a challenging clinical problem during pregnancy (Table 27–3). During the second half of pregnancy, significant proteinuria and hypertension develop in up to 25% of women with SLE, but this may be due to either preeclampsia or lupus nephritis. By definition, normal blood pressure excludes preeclampsia. However, both lupus nephritis and preeclampsia can have hypertension, proteinuria, or edema. Thrombocytopenia and hemolytic anemia can be seen in an SLE flare; however, both are also features of the HELLP

Table 27–3. How to differentiate between lupus nephritis and preeclampsia.

Manifestation	Lupus Nephritis	Preeclampsia
Gravidity	Any pregnancy	Usually prima-gravida
Hypertension	Present/absent	DBP > 90 mm Hg
Proteinuria	Before 3rd trimester	After 3rd trimester
Active urinary sediment (RBC or WBC casts)	Present	Absent
C3, C4	Low or failure to rise	Normal or rising
Anti-dsDNA antibodies	Rising	Absent
Uric acid levels	Normal	High
Impaired calcium excretion	Absent	Present

RBC, red blood cell; WBC, white blood cell; DBP, diastolic blood pressure.

syndrome (hemolytic anemia, elevated liver enzymes, and low platelets), which is a variant of preeclampsia.

The laboratory features that suggest an SLE flare include the development of proteinuria before the third trimester; active urinary sediment with red blood cell or white blood cell casts or both, a fall or failure to increase complement levels (C3, C4, or CH50), and a rise in titer of dsDNA antibodies. Two other tests that may be used because they are more indicative of preeclampsia are impaired calcium excretion (levels below 11.5 mg/dL by spot urine testing or below 195 mg in a 24-hour urine test) and elevated uric acid levels.

Distinguishing between lupus nephritis and preeclampsia is important because treatment options are completely different. A lupus nephritis flare is treated with glucocorticoids and possibly remittive drugs, whereas preeclampsia is treated with antihypertensive medication to control the blood pressure and immediate delivery.

Managing the SLE Flare

A general guideline in choosing a medication to use during pregnancy is that the risk of flare must outweigh the risk of toxicity to the fetus.

A. GLUCOCORTICOIDS

Any signs of a SLE flare should be aggressively treated with the lowest possible dose of glucocorticoids (prednisone or methylprednisolone) needed to control the disease (Table 27–4). For most patients, this may be as little as 10 mg/d of prednisone, but for active disease the dose of glucocorticoids may be as high as 1 mg/kg/d.

The US Food and Drug Administration (FDA) categorizes glucocorticoids as category B drugs. A category B drug means that there have been no controlled studies in pregnant women, and no fetal risks have been documented in animal studies; or there have been adverse effects shown in animal studies, but there have been no controlled studies in pregnant women to confirm the findings.

Glucocorticoids have not been found to be teratogenic in humans, although there have been reports of cleft palate in rabbits and mice. The fetus is protected from the effect of prednisone or hydrocortisone because of the placental enzyme, 11-β-dehydrogenase, which oxidizes these glucocorticoids into the inactive form. In contrast, dexamethasone and betamethasone cross the placenta and are used for fetal indications if preterm delivery is imminent. Other risks associated with glucocorticoid use include premature rupture of membranes, intrauterine growth restriction or low birth weight, and preterm delivery. Complications from these medications include maternal gestational diabetes mellitus, hypertension, osteoporosis, and infection. However, if maternal disease is uncontrolled, the risks of using glucocorticoids outweigh the drug toxicity risks to the mother and fetus.

The use of glucocorticoids as prophylactic treatment to prevent SLE exacerbations is generally not accepted as routine practice. However, if a woman has been taking glucocorticoids within the last year, then stress dose glucocorticoids at delivery are required. The usual recommended dose of hydrocortisone is 100 mg intravenously every 8 hours (or equivalent) for a period of 24 hours. Predelivery dosages of glucocorticoids, if any, may be started day 1 postpartum if normal oral intake resumes.

B. HYDROXYCHLOROQUINE

The antimalarial hydroxychloroquine may be administered to control SLE disease activity. The usual dose is between 200 and 400 mg/d or up to 6 mg/kg/d. The exact mechanism of action is unclear. Although regarded as an FDA category C medication with animal studies showing fetal effects and no controlled human studies, there are only rare reports of congenital malformations or ophthalmologic abnormalities in babies

Table 27–4. Medications used to treat rheumatic diseases during pregnancy.

Drug	FDA Risk Category	Fetal Effects	Use in Lactation	Other Comments
Glucocorticoids (prednisone, methylprednis-olone, hydrocor-tisone)	B	Premature rupture of membranes, intrauterine growth restriction, preterm delivery in human studies. No congenital defects in humans. Animal studies show cleft palate.	Yes	Watch for maternal gestational diabetes, elevated blood pressure, and osteoporosis; women may need stress doses at delivery.
Sulfasalazine	B	Increased risk of neonatal jaundice during third trimester	Yes	Folic acid supplementation recommended.
Heparin	C	Thrombocytopenia and osteo-porosis	Yes	Calcium supplementation is recommended.
NSAIDs including selective COX-2 inhibitors	C	Premature closure of the ductus arteriosus, prolongation of labor and delivery; and, hemorrhage when used during the third tri-mester	Some	Low-dose aspirin (< 325 mg/d) has no ad-verse effects on fetal renal function, ductus arteriosus, or hemorrhage risk.
Hydroxychloroquine	C	Very rare congenital anomalies attributed to this drug.	Yes	Long acting. Discontinue at least 3 months before conception if patient does not want this medication.
Cyclosporine A	C	Preterm delivery, low birth weight, hypertension, and pregnancy-induced hypertension	No	Monitor maternal blood pressure and renal function.
Mycophenolate mofetil	C	Limited information indicates no fetal abnormalities.	No	Limited information available in the renal transplant literature.
Azathioprine	D	Rare neonatal immunosuppression	No	Used if major organ involvement or as a glucocorticoid-sparing agent to control disease
TNF-α inhibitors	B	Limited information in animals indicates no fetal abnormalities.	No	Limited information in humans.
Interleukin-1 receptor antag-onists (IL1-Ra)	B	Limited information in animals indicates no fetal abnormalities.	No	Limited information in humans.

born to mothers while taking this medication. The use of hydroxychloroquine during pregnancy remains controversial.

Hydroxychloroquine is a long-acting drug and remains in the system between 2 and 4 months following its discontinuation. If a woman becomes pregnant while taking hydroxychloroquine, there is no rationale to stop the medication since therapeutic levels remain in the body for 2–4 months, which is during the period of organogenesis for the fetus. However, discontinuation of this medication may cause a subsequent SLE exacerbation. Therefore, if a mother conceives while on this medication, the benefit of continuing hydroxychloroquine throughout the pregnancy and preventing

a flare outweighs the very minimal risk to the fetus. The decision to continue hydroxychloroquine should be based on a discussion between the specialist and the patient and her partner.

C. AZATHIOPRINE

Azathioprine is a medication used for the treatment of SLE associated with major organ involvement or as a glucocorticoid-sparing drug. The usual dose of this medication ranges between 1 and 2.5 mg/kg/d. Azathioprine is a prodrug that gets converted to 6-mercaptopurine. Both azathioprine and 6-mercaptopurine interfere with the synthesis of purine nucleotides, resulting in cytotoxicity and decreased cell proliferation. Folic acid supplementation at 1 mg/d is recommended while taking azathioprine and 6-mercaptopurine.

Azathioprine and 6-mercaptopurine are FDA category D drugs, which means that there has been evidence of human fetal risk, but the benefit of use in a pregnant woman may outweigh the risk. The fetal liver lacks the enzyme inosinate phosphorylase, which converts azathioprine to its active metabolite, 6-mercaptopurine. Although azathioprine readily crosses the placenta, only trace amounts of 6-mercaptopurine are found in cord blood. Therefore, this fetal enzyme deficiency should protect the fetus from the adverse effects of azathioprine. The rare adverse effects that have been reported in infants exposed to azathioprine in utero include neonatal immunosuppression characterized by leukopenia, lymphopenia, and absence or decreased levels of immunoglobulins and intrauterine growth restriction. Azathioprine is contraindicated during breastfeeding.

D. Nonsteroidal Anti-Inflammatory Drugs

Nonsteroidal anti-inflammatory drugs (NSAIDs) are FDA category C drugs and do not appear to be teratogenic. NSAIDs variably inhibit the enzyme cyclooxygenase (COX) and decrease prostaglandin production. Adverse fetal effects observed following third-trimester ingestion of NSAIDs include premature closure of the ductus arteriosus, which can lead to primary pulmonary hypertension and prolongation of gestation and labor. Other potential fetal side effects include excessive maternal and neonatal hemorrhage during delivery because of the antiplatelet effects of NSAIDs. Oligohydramnios may occur due to the effect of NSAIDs on the fetal renal output. It is generally recommended that NSAIDs be discontinued during the last trimester of pregnancy; if they are needed, low-dose prednisone can be used as a safer alternative. Low-dose aspirin, which is used for the treatment of antiphospholipid antibody syndrome, is the exception and can be continued throughout pregnancy.

COX-2 inhibitors, a relatively new class of NSAIDs, include rofecoxib, celecoxib, valdecoxib, and meloxicam. These medications are FDA category C drugs. Risks are similar to traditional NSAIDs, and they should be discontinued during the last trimester of pregnancy.

E. Cyclosporine A

Cyclosporine A is an FDA category C drug. The usual dose is 2.5 mg/kg/d, with the maximum dose not exceeding 5 mg/kg/d. The mechanism of action involves the inhibition of cytotoxic T cells, thus decreasing the production of interleukin-2. Most of the information regarding cyclosporine and pregnancy comes from data on pregnant renal transplant patients. Cyclosporine has been associated with the risk of preterm delivery, low birth weight, hypertension, and pregnancy-induced hypertension. This medication has not been found to be teratogenic in animals or humans; however, there was one isolated case of proximal renal damage in fetal rat kidney. Cyclosporine A is secreted in breast milk and is contraindicated during breastfeeding.

F. Mycophenolate Mofetil

Mycophenolate mofetil is a prodrug that is enzymatically broken down into the active metabolite mycophenolic acid. Mycophenolic acid is a purine synthesis inhibitor that causes a decrease in lymphocyte production and adhesion.

This medication has been used in renal transplant patients and most recently incorporated in the treatment of lupus nephritis and cutaneous lupus.

Although regarded as a category C medication by the FDA, the limited information available on its use during pregnancy indicates no reports of malformations in infants exposed in utero. This medication should not be used during breastfeeding.

G. Other Disease-Modifying Medications

Medications such as cyclophosphamide, leflunomide, penicillamine, methotrexate, and chlorambucil are not recommended for use during pregnancy, with an FDA category D or X rating because of their teratogenic potential (Table 27–5). Occasionally, these cytotoxic medications are used in life-threatening instances during the second or third trimester of pregnancy, but a qualified specialist should determine appropriate dosages of these medications. Women should continue folic acid even after discontinuation of methotrexate to prevent the occurrence of folate deficiency.

H. Nonrheumatic Medications Needed During Pregnancy

1. Antihypertensives—Antihypertensive medication may be required during pregnancy to control blood pressure. Methyldopa (FDA Category B) and hydralazine (FDA Category C) have been used by obstetricians for many years and are considered safe to use during pregnancy (Table 27–6).

β-Blockers such as atenolol, labetolol, or metoprolol and thiazide diuretics have been shown to cause decreased placental perfusion leading to fetal growth restriction. Despite this concern, qualified physicians have used both medications in high-risk pregnant patients. Ultrasonographic assessment for fetal growth while taking this medication is recommended.

Calcium channel blockers are generally considered safe during pregnancy.

ACE inhibitors are contraindicated during pregnancy because of the association with fetal renal abnormalities.

Table 27–5. Contraindicated rheuamtic disease medications during pregnancy.

Drug	FDA Risk Category	Fetal Effects	Use in Lactation	Other Comments
Cyclophosphamide	D	Myelosuppression	No	May be used if maternal disease is life-threatening.
Leflunomide	X	May increase risk of fetal death or have teratogenic effects.	No	Need cholestyramine washout prior to conception. Check the serum level after washout.
Penicillamine	D	Cutis laxis	No	Discontinue 6 months before conception.
Chlorambucil	D	Unknown	No	Discontinue 6 months before conception.
Methotrexate	X	Myelosuppression, desquamating fibrosing alveolitis, chromosome abnormalities in clinicially normal infants	No	Discontinue 3–6 months before conception. Continue folic acid supplementation after this medication is discontinued.

2. Anticonvulsants—All anticonvulsants have teratogenic potential. A qualified physician should decide whether use of these medications is essential for maternal health.

3. Antidepressants—Antidepressants may be required for symptoms of depression or chronic pain. Tricyclic antidepressants such as amitriptyline and imipramine are FDA category C drugs. There are no well-controlled studies conducted in pregnant women to determine the effect of these medications on the fetus. There have been animal studies involving amitriptyline given at higher than normal human dosing showing teratogenic effects in mice and hamsters. There were also studies in rats that showed delayed ossification of fetal vertebral bodies. Therefore, tricyclic antidepressants should only be used if necessary.

Selective serotonin reuptake inhibitors such as sertraline, fluoxetine, and citalopram are FDA category C drugs. There are also no well-controlled studies in pregnant women to determine the effect of these medications on the fetus. Reproduction studies in rats have generally shown an increase in stillborn pups, a decrease in pup weight, and an increase in pup deaths during the first few days postpartum following maternal exposure to higher than normal human dosing of these selective serotonin reuptake inhibitors. Only sertraline showed evidence of delayed ossification when pregnant rats were exposed to higher than normal human doses of this medication during organogenesis.

Buyon JP, et al. Assessing disease activity in SLE patients during pregnancy. *Lupus.* 1999;8:677. [PMID: 10568906]

Chang E, Ramsey-Goldman R. Managing systemic lupus erythematosus during pregnancy. *Womens Health.* 2001;1:53.

Esplin MS, Branch DW. Immunosuppressive drugs and pregnancy. *Obstet Gynecol Clin North Am.* 1997;24:601. [PMID: 9266581]

Khamashta MA, et al. Systemic lupus erythematosus flares during pregnancy. *Rheum Dis Clin North Am.* 1997;23:15. [PMID: 9031372]

Kitridou RC. The mother in systemic lupus erythematosus. And, The fetus in systemic lupus erythematosus. In: Wallace DJ, Hahn BH, ed. *Dubois' Lupus Erythematosus.* Lippincott Williams & Wilkins, 2002.

Mascola MA, Repke JT. Obstetric management of the high-risk lupus pregnancy. *Rheum Dis Clin North Am.* 1997;23:119. [PMID: 9031378]

Parke AL. Anti-rheumatic drugs in pregnancy. *Bull Rheum Dis.* 2002;51(9).

Petri M. Hopkins Lupus Pregnancy Center: 1987 to 1996. *Rheum Dis Clin North Am.* 1997;23:1. [PMID: 9031371]

Ramsey-Goldman R, Schilling E. Immunosuppressive drug use during pregnancy. *Rheum Dis Clin North Am.* 1997;23:149. [PMID: 9031380]

Ramsey-Goldman R, Schilling E. Optimum use of disease-modifying and immunosuppressive antirheumatic agents during pregnancy and lactation. *Clin Immunother.* 1996;5:40.

ANTIPHOSPHOLIPID ANTIBODY SYNDROME

 ESSENTIAL FEATURES

- *May be a primary syndrome or secondary to SLE or other underlying disorders.*
- *Includes the anticardiolipin antibodies, lupus anticoagulant, and occasionally β_2 glycoprotein I antibodies.*

Table 27–6. Nonrheumatic disease medications used during pregnancy.

Drug	FDA Risk Category	Fetal Effects	Other Comments
Antihypertensives			
Methyldopa	B	Reproduction studies performed in rats revealed no evidence of harm to the fetus. There are no well-controlled human studies, but published reports of the use of this drug during all trimesters of pregnancy indicate that fetal harm is remote.	Considered safe to use during pregnancy.
Hydralazine	C	Teratogenic effects observed in studies involving mice and rabbits using higher than normal human doses included cleft palate and malformations of facial and cranial bones. There are no well-controlled human studies.	Despite the animal studies, this medication is considered safe to use during pregnancy.
β-Blockers	C	Decreased placental perfusion leading to fetal growth restriction.	Use only if necessary.
Calcium channel blockers (nifedipine)	C	Studies using various animals including rats, mice, and rabbits showed anomalies such as cleft palate, rib deformities, fetal death, and prolonged pregnancy.	Despite animal studies this medication is considered safe to use during pregnancy.
Angiotensin-converting enzyme inhibitors (captopril or lisinopril) and angiotensin receptor blockers (valsartan or losartan)	D	Renal effects.	Contraindicated.
Anticonvulsants (all)		Teratogenic.	Use only if necessary.
Tricyclic antidepressants (amitriptyline or imipramine)	C	Teratogen in animal studies. Delayed ossification of fetal vertebral bodies.	Use only if necessary.
Selective serotonin reuptake inhibitors (sertraline, fluoxetine, or citalopram)	C	Animal studies showing increase in stillbirth, decreased weight, and increased death.	Use only if necessary.

- *Antiphospholipid antibody syndrome has been linked to recurrent fetal loss, intravascular clotting with venous or arterial thrombosis, and thrombocytopenia.*

General Considerations

Antiphospholipid antibody syndrome (APS) can occur as a primary syndrome with no previous diagnosis of a connective tissue disorder and includes a history of recurrent arterial or venous thrombosis, recurrent fetal loss, or thrombocytopenia (50,000 to 100,000 platelets/μL). Secondary APS is associated with an underlying connective tissue disorder such as SLE or rheumatoid arthritis (RA). Both primary and secondary APS also include the antibodies anticardiolipin antibodies (aCL), lupus anticoagulant (LAC), or occasionally β_2 glycoprotein I (see Chapter 20).

Patients with APS may have recurrent arterial or venous thrombotic events including deep venous thrombosis, pulmonary emboli, transient ischemic attacks, cerebral vascular accident, and myocardial infarction. Thrombocytopenia and livedo reticularis, a lacy-looking rash over the trunk and extremities, are also common findings in patients with APS. The presence of these antibodies during pregnancy may increase the risk of fetal loss, including spontaneous miscarriages in the second and third trimester, midpregnancy fetal distress, intrauterine growth restriction, prematurity, and preeclampsia. The mechanism of fetal loss may be related to abnormal implantation and placentation.

Laboratory Findings

Healthy women with no history of SLE, thrombosis, thrombocytopenia, repeated fetal loss during any gestational period, or preeclampsia do not need to be screened for APS.

Laboratory tests positive for aCL and LAC support the diagnosis of APS in the appropriate clinical setting.

The enzyme-linked immunosorbent assay (ELISA) for aCL is widely available and standardized. Normal levels are usually less than 16 GPL U/mL and IgM less than 10 MPL U/mL. (GPL is the abbreviation for immunoglobulin G and phospholipid, and MPL is the abbreviation for immunoglobulin M and phospholipid.) High positive values are above 80 GPL U/mL or 40 MPL U/mL.

The presence of LAC may initially be indicated by an elevated activated partial thromboplastin time (aPTT) or a false-positive rapid plasma reagin test for syphilis. Abnormal results in either test should warrant further investigation. In patients with the presence of circulating LAC, the aPTT will not correct when normal plasma is added in a 1:1 mix. The aPTT will normalize in patients with a factor deficiency. Another test to aid in the recognition and confirmation for LAC is the dilute Russell viper venom time.

Patients in whom both aCL and LAC are negative but who have a clinical history consistent with APS should be screened using ELISA for β_2 glycoprotein I.

Treatment

Treatment of APS depends on the patient's history. Prophylactic use of heparin or aspirin in asymptomatic women with no history of thrombosis or pregnancy loss is not recommended. However, a baby aspirin may occasionally be used if antibody titers are elevated in an asymptomatic woman.

A combination of low-dose aspirin (80 mg/d) and unfractionated heparin (5000 IU every 12 hours) or low-molecular-weight heparin (enoxaparin or dalteparin) has been successful in the treatment of APS. Treatment should commence once conception is confirmed and be continued until delivery. Anticoagulation should be continued for 6 weeks postpartum, using either form of heparin or switching to warfarin. Glucocorticoids are reserved for the treatment of inflammatory-based symptoms such as thrombocytopenia or an SLE flare and are generally not recommended for use in the treatment of APS when anticoagulation or antiplatelet agents are used.

Low-molecular-weight heparin and heparin are FDA category B and C drugs, respectively. These medications do not cross the placenta and do not cause harm to the fetus, but both have been associated with maternal thrombocytopenia, and heparin, more than low-molecular-weight heparin, has been associated with osteoporosis. Supplementation with 1500 mg/d of calcium is highly recommended.

Chang E, Ramsey-Goldman R. Antiphospholipid antibodies and RA: barriers to successful pregnancy? *Womens Health.* 2001; 1:97.

Cuadrado MJ, Hughes GRV. Hughes (antiphospholipid) syndrome. Clinical features. *Rheum Dis Clin North Am.* 2001;27: 507. [PMID: 11534257]

RHEUMATOID ARTHRITIS

 ESSENTIAL FEATURES

- *Arthritis usually improves during pregnancy.*
- *Adverse pregnancy outcomes are not increased.*
- *Postpartum joint flares are common.*

General Considerations

Pregnancy is associated with improvement of clinical signs and symptoms of RA in up to 75% of patients. Most women with RA see a reduction in disease activity by the end of the first trimester. Approximately 20–30% of pregnant patients with RA will need medications to control disease activity. However, it is important to monitor all postpartum patients with RA closely because there is approximately a 90% risk of flare by 3–6 months after delivery.

RA does not increase adverse pregnancy outcomes including, stillbirth, prematurity, or low birth weight.

Special Problems

Special care must be taken in patients with cervical spine disease who need surgical delivery by cesarean section if general anesthesia is needed because of the risk associated with atlantoaxial subluxation. Women may require cervical bracing to prevent hyperextension or nasotracheal intubation instead of orotracheal intubation.

Women with severe hip disease or hip replacement may not have adequate range of motion to allow normal vaginal delivery, and thus will require surgical delivery. The patient who requires surgical delivery may need antibiotics if an artificial joint is present to prevent bacterial seeding.

Management of the RA Flare

Treatment of a patient with RA who is having a flare depends on the type of complaint, either localized or systemic symptoms and signs. If only one or two joints are involved, intra-articular injections with glucocorticoids may be the best option. If a woman requires systemic treatment for multiple joint complaints or extra-articular manifestations, oral glucocorticoids are among the safest alternative medications. As mentioned previously in the SLE section, the lowest possible dose of glucocorticoids to control symptoms is recommended. Other medications, such as NSAIDs, hydroxychloroquine, and azathioprine, may also be used and are discussed in the SLE section above and in Table 27–4.

Sulfasalazine, which has been used extensively to treat inflammatory bowel disease, is another alternative medication safely used during pregnancy. The preferable dose is usually < 3 g/d. Sulfasalazine is classified as an FDA category B drug. However, there is a theoretical risk of the infant developing kernicterus during the neonatal period. Despite this risk, sulfasalazine is often continued during pregnancy if indicated. There is no evidence that sulfasalazine causes congenital malforma-

tions. Folic acid supplementation is recommended because sulfasalazine may cause folate deficiency.

The biologic agents approved for the treatment of RA include tumor necrosis factor-α (TNF-α) inhibitors and interleukin-1 receptor antagonist (IL-1Ra). Although the FDA regards the TNF agents etanercept, infliximab, and adalimumab and the IL-1Ra agent anakinra as category B drugs, there are minimal human data to reassure safety of their use during pregnancy.

Gold, an older medication, that has limited use in the current era, is regarded as a category C drug by the FDA classification system. There are insufficient data on the safety of gold when used during pregnancy (Table 27–7).

Within the first 3–6 months postpartum, flares are common in mothers with RA. If the mother is nursing, then glucocorticoids at the lowest dose necessary to control symptoms are recommended. However, the mother should be encouraged to resume her prepregnancy therapeutic regimen as soon as possible to minimize joint damage.

Belilos E, Carsons S. Rheumatologic disorders in women. *Med Clin North Am.* 1998;82:77. [PMID: 9457152]

Johnson MJ. Obstetric complications and rheumatic disease. *Rheum Dis Clin North Am.* 1997;23:169. [PMID: 9031381]

Nelson JL, Ostensen M. Pregnancy and rheumatoid arthritis. *Rheum Dis Clin North Am.* 1997;23:195. [PMID: 9031383]

Ostensen M, Ramsey-Goldman R: Treatment of inflammatory rheumatic disorders in pregnancy: what are the safest treatment options? *Drug Saf.* 1998;19:389. [PMID: 9825952]

SPONDYLOARTHROPATHIES

 ESSENTIAL FEATURES

- *Disorders including psoriatic arthritis, ankylosing spondylitis, reactive arthritis, and arthritis secondary to inflammatory bowel disease (IBD).*
- *Patients with psoriatic arthritis often improve symptomatically; however, patients with ankylosing spondylitis may have flares.*

General Considerations

There is limited information regarding these diseases and pregnancy. Women with ankylosing spondylitis often get an exacerbation of spinal symptoms or peripheral arthritis mid-gestation. However, 80% of women with psoriatic arthritis tend to improve beginning in

Table 27–7. Medications used in various rheumatic diseases.

Drug	Systemic Lupus Erythematosus	Rheumatoid Arthritis	Spondyloarthropathy	Antiphospholipid Antibody Syndrome
Glucocorticoids	X	X	X	X
NSAIDs	X	X	X	X
Hydroxychloroquine	X	X		
Sulfasalazine	X	X	X	
Azathioprine	X	X	X	
Cyclosporine A	X	X		
Mycophenolate mofetil	X			
TNF-α blockers		X	X	
IL-1-Ra		X		
Gold		X		
Cyclophosphamide	X	X		
Leflunomide	X	X	X	
Methotrexate	X	X	X	
Chlorambucil	X (rare)			
Heparin/LMWH				X

NSAIDs, nonsteroidal anti-inflammatory drugs; TNF-α, tumor necrosis factor-α; IL-1-Ra, interleukin-1 receptor antagonist; LMWH, low-molecular-weight heparin.

the first trimester and then continuing throughout pregnancy. Women with IBD, regardless of arthritic disease, are at increased risk for preterm birth and lower birth weight independent of disease activity. Patients with active bowel symptoms are at increased risk for spontaneous abortion, stillbirth, and developmental defects; therefore, active IBD must be treated aggressively during pregnancy. There is no information regarding reactive arthritis and pregnancy outcome in the literature.

Managing a Spondyloarthropathy Flare

Since women with psoriatic arthritis improve, most joint flares will involve patients with ankylosing spondylitis and IBD. Symptoms of pain and stiffness may be treated with NSAIDs or glucocorticoids with similar precautions as mentioned previously. Women with active bowel symptoms must be treated aggressively with glucocorticoids for the acute flare. Sulfasalazine, azathioprine, or 6-mercaptopurine may be used for maintenance. Higher doses of folic acid are needed in the pregnant patient with IBD.

SCLERODERMA

 ESSENTIAL FEATURES

- *Pregnancy risks are chiefly seen with diffuse scleroderma.*
- *Pregnancy risks are small with limited scleroderma.*

General Considerations

There are two types of systemic scleroderma: limited and diffuse. The limited form is characterized by cutaneous changes with some internal organ involvement, while diffuse scleroderma not only affects the skin but is more likely to have life-threatening internal organ involvement (see Chapter 22).

Pregnancy does not seem to affect the course of scleroderma in women with limited disease; however, some women with diffuse disease have increased skin thickening postpartum. Gastrointestinal reflux, constipation, and arthralgias were the most common complaints that worsened during pregnancy; however, Raynaud phenomenon often improved. There is evidence that women with both limited and diffuse scleroderma are at increased risk for preterm birth; however, the risk of miscarriage was increased in women with long-standing diffuse disease only. The reported cases of renal crisis during pregnancy occurred in women with early diffuse disease. Therefore, women with diffuse scleroderma should wait until their disease is stable before getting pregnant to decrease the risk of renal crisis. Women with pulmonary hypertension (pulmonary artery pressure > 40 mm Hg) should be discouraged from becoming pregnant.

Managing the Symptoms Caused by Scleroderma

There are no medications proven to be effective in modifying the course of scleroderma. Most complaints are symptomatic in nature and management is directed toward relieving the symptoms. Raynaud disease can be treated conservatively with avoidance of cold temperatures. If symptoms persist, vasodilators such as nifedipine have been successfully used during pregnancy. Gastroesophageal reflux disease is treated with lifestyle modifications such as avoiding lying down within 3 hours after meals, elevating the head of the bed, avoiding acidic food such as coffee or spicy food, and avoiding foods that relax the lower esophageal sphincter such as fatty foods, peppermint, alcohol, and chocolate. Medications such as antacids may also be considered if lifestyle modifications are not successful. Proton pump inhibitors are FDA category B drugs and include lansoprazole, pantoprazole, rabeprazole, and esomeprazole. The only FDA category C drug is omeprazole because high doses in rabbits resulted in embryo lethality, fetal resorptions, and pregnancy disruptions. Since there are no adequate or well-controlled studies in pregnant women regarding proton pump inhibitors, these medications should be used only if necessary during pregnancy. ACE inhibitors are contraindicated during pregnancy unless there is a life-threatening situation such as a renal crisis.

Lautenbach GL, Petri M. Women's health. *Rheum Dis Clin North Am.* 1999;25:539. [PMID: 10467628]

Steen VD. Pregnancy in women with systemic sclerosis. *Obstet Gynecol.* 1999;94:15. [PMID: 10389711]

OTHER RHEUMATIC DISEASES

Dermatomyositis (DM) & Polymyositis (PM)

There are few data regarding pregnancy outcome in women with these diseases because the pregnancy experience for women during the reproductive years is minimal. As with other rheumatic diseases, conception should be planned during a period of remission. If a woman develops DM or PM during pregnancy, approximately 50% of pregnancies may be complicated by fetal loss or neonatal death. However, pregnancies in most women with established disease resulted in live births. The most common complications of pregnancy in women with established disease were intrauterine growth restriction or preterm birth.

DM or PM flares are managed in a similar manner to patients with SLE. See the section Managing the SLE Flare for further details.

Vasculitis

There are few data regarding pregnancy outcome, since vasculitis tends to affect men more than women, and this disease tends to occur in female patients after their childbearing years. Flares should be managed similar to patients with SLE.

SECTION IV

Vasculitis

<table>
<tr><td>

Introduction to Vasculitis: Classification & Clinical Clues

</td><td>

28

</td></tr>
</table>

David B. Hellmann, MD

General Considerations

Vasculitis refers to a heterogeneous group of disorders that is characterized by inflammatory destruction of blood vessels. Inflamed blood vessels are liable to occlude or rupture or develop a thrombus, and thereby lose the ability to deliver oxygen and other nutrients to tissues and organs. Depending on the size, distribution, and severity of the affected vessels, vasculitis can result in clinical syndromes that vary in severity from a minor, self-limited rash to a life-threatening multisystem disorder.

Because it often begins with nonspecific symptoms and signs and unfolds slowly over weeks or months, vasculitis is one of the great diagnostic challenges in all of medicine. Yet, physicians who know the general and specific clinical clues for vasculitis can often learn to suspect when vasculitis is present at the bedside. Establishing the diagnosis of vasculitis requires confirmation by laboratory tests, usually a biopsy of an involved artery but sometimes an angiogram or a serologic test.

Treating vasculitis has become as rewarding as establishing the diagnosis. In the absence of treatment, most patients with systemic vasculitis will suffer and die. With treatment, the vast majority of patients will improve, many will achieve remission, and a few will be cured.

Classification

Because the causes of most forms of vasculitis are not known, the vasculitides are classified according to their clinicopathologic features. Although no schema has been accepted universally, one frequently used classification system separates the vasculitides based first on whether the process is primary (ie, of unknown cause) or secondary to some other condition (eg, a connective tissue disease or infection). The vasculitides can then be further separated by the size of vessels usually affected—large-sized, medium-sized, or small-sized arteries (Table 28–1). Finer distinctions among forms of vasculitis affecting the same size vessel can be made by other clinicopathologic characteristics. For example, Takayasu arteritis and giant cell arteritis are grouped together because they both can affect the aorta and other large arteries. However, they are distinguished from each other by their clinical differences, such as the age of onset. Takayasu arteritis is chiefly a disease of young women, while giant cell arteritis almost never occurs before age 50. To take another example, both Wegener granulomatosis and Churg-Strauss syndrome affect small-sized vessels and are associated with antineutrophil cytoplasmic antibodies (ANCA). But only Churg-Strauss syndrome is associated with asthma and striking levels of eosinophilia.

Although classification systems are useful in highlighting differences among the vasculitides, the arbitrary categories suggest neater lines of demarcation than nature always recognizes. Despite being classified as a form of primary, medium-vessel vasculitis group, polyarteritis nodosa results from chronic hepatitis B or C infection in about 20% of cases and can affect small vessels. Until the causes of all forms of vasculitis are known, exceptions in the classification schema will be common.

Epidemiology

The epidemiology of individual forms of vasculitis is covered in the relevant chapters. In general, the vasculitides are relatively uncommon but not rare in Western countries: about 1 out of 2000 adults has some form of

Table 28–1. Classification of the primary vasculitides: Major examples.

Large artery vasculitis
  Giant cell arteritis
  Takayasu arteritis
  Cogan syndrome
Medium-vessel vasculitis
  Polyarteritis nodosa
  Primary central nervous system disease
  Buerger disease
Small-vessel vasculitis
  ANCA-associated small-vessel vasculitis
  • Wegener granulomatosis
  • Microscopic polyangiitis
  • Churg-Strauss syndrome
  • Drug-induced ANCA-associated vasculitis
  Behçet disease
  Hypersensitivity vasculitis
  Urticarial vasculitis

ANCA, antineutrophil cytoplasmic antibodies.

Table 28–3. General clinical clues suggesting the presence of systemic vasculitis.

---

1. Constitutional symptoms prominent
2. Subacute onset
3. Symptoms and signs of inflammation common
4. Pain common
5. Multisystem disease evident

---

vasculitis, and each year vasculitis develops in approximately 1 in 7000 adults. In the United States, the most common forms of primary systemic vasculitis are giant cell arteritis, Wegener granulomatosis, and microscopic polyangiitis (Table 28–2).

Clinical Findings

Although the presenting manifestations of vasculitis are protean, they can be grouped into five categories of clinical clues (Table 28–3). The first general clue is that most forms of systemic vasculitis begin with constitutional symptoms (such as malaise, fever, sweats, fatigue, decreased appetite, and weight loss). These nonspecific symptoms, in the absence of more specific signs, usually effectively camouflage the vasculitic nature of the patient's illness. A second clue is that most forms of vasculitis unfold subacutely over weeks or months. In contrast to many patients with acute infections, patients

Table 28–2. Average annual incidence rates of different forms of vasculitis.

Form of Vasculitis	Incidence Per Million
Giant cell arteritis	170[a]
Wegener granulomatosis	4–15
Polyarteritis nodosa	9
Microscopic polyangiitis	1–24
Takayasu arteritis	2

[a]Population 50 years of age or older.

with vasculitis usually cannot pinpoint the hour or the day that their illness began. More typically, patients with vasculitis will struggle to define the month or the season in which their nonspecific symptoms accumulated sufficiently to become memorable. A corollary of the subacute course typical of vasculitis is that the initial diagnosis of vasculitis is rarely made (correctly) in the intensive care unit. Although pulmonary hemorrhage, bowel infarction, or other devastating complications of vasculitis frequently result in a patient being admitted to the intensive care unit, these catastrophic events usually develop late, weeks or months after other clinical clues have suggested or established the patient's diagnosis.

The tendency of most forms of vasculitis to produce striking signs of inflammation constitutes a third general clue. Manifestations of inflammation can include fever, arthritis, rash, pericarditis, anemia of chronic disease, or a markedly elevated erythrocyte sedimentation rate. Pain is a fourth common feature of the vasculitides and can originate from many different sources, such as arthritis; myalgia; or infarction of a digit, nerve, bowel, or testicle. The fifth general clinical clue is that vasculitis tends to cause multisystem disease. The skin, joints, nervous system, kidneys, lung, and gastrointestinal tract are especially favorite targets of many different forms of vasculitis. Although specific forms of vasculitis can defy generalization, most vasculitides start with constitutional symptoms that evolve over weeks and months to a painful disorder marked by signs of inflammation and multiorgan injury.

A. SYMPTOMS AND SIGNS

The signs and symptoms of specific forms of vasculitis are detailed in the individual chapters. The signs and symptoms common to many forms of systemic vasculitis are found in Table 28–4.

In general, the skin and the peripheral nervous system signs are especially useful because they often develop early in the course of the disease and because they can be detected at the bedside. The onset of small-vessel vasculitis (eg, hepatitis C–associated vasculitis) is often heralded by palpable purpura, usually on the lower extremities, whereas medium-vessel diseases (eg, poly-

Table 28–4. Organ- or tissue-specific manifestations of vasculitis.

Organ or Tissue	Manifestation
Skin	Livedo reticularis, palpable purpura, nodules, ulcers, gangrene
Peripheral nervous system	Mononeuritis multiplex, polyneuropathy
Central nervous system	Stroke, seizure, encephalopathy
Kidney	Hypertension, proteinuria, hematuria, renal failure
Heart	Myocardial infarction, cardiomyopathy, pericarditis, arrhythmia
Lung	Cough, chest pain, hemoptysis, breathlessness
Eyes	Blindness, scleritis
Gastrointestinal tract	Pain, bleeding, perforation
Genitals	Testicular infarction, ovarian mass

arteritis nodosa) more commonly produce nodules, ulcers, or digital gangrene.

The most characteristic nervous system manifestation of vasculitis is mononeuritis multiplex, which is defined as a distinctive peripheral neuropathy in which named peripheral nerves are infarcted one at a time. The nerve infarctions result from vasculitis of the vessels of the vasa nervorum, causing ischemia of a nerve. Clinically, the two features that characterize this neuropathy are the **asynchrony** and **asymmetry** of the symptoms and findings. These features are best illustrated by comparing mononeuritis multiplex with other peripheral neuropathies. With most forms of nonspecific neuropathy the patient experiences numbness and tingling in a symmetric, stocking or glove distribution, which develop so slowly that the patient cannot accurately date the onset of the neuropathy. Examination of these patients usually fails to identify the involvement of large, named nerves. In sharp contrast, the onset of mononeuritis multiplex is strikingly memorable: The patient will often recall the day that his foot drop or wrist drop began. The patient will also often vividly recall how the neuropathy progressed asynchronously so that each month or so a new area of the body (usually an extremity) became involved. On examination, the damage from mononeuritis multiplex can be mapped to individual, named nerves (eg, the peroneal, tibial, ulnar, radial, or median nerves). Almost all will have sensory abnormalities and about half will have weakness as well. Although mononeuritis multiplex is often bilat-

eral, the lesions are usually asymmetric: The right hand may demonstrate a median nerve infarct while the left hand has an ulnar nerve lesion.

Mononeuritis multiplex produces such a characteristic clinical picture that usually it can be diagnosed at the bedside. Occasionally, identifying mononeuritis multiplex becomes difficult late in the course when the infarctions of so many nerves can coalesce to produce an unusually symmetric pattern of deficits. In most cases, the early history of sequential peripheral nerve lesions supports the diagnosis of vasculitic neuropathy. In some cases, proof of mononeuritis multiplex will require electrodiagnostic studies.

Mononeuritis multiplex is one of the physical findings in medicine of great differential diagnostic value. In the absence of diabetes or multiple compression injuries, mononeuritis multiplex usually means the patient has some form of vasculitis. Polyarteritis nodosa, microscopic polyangiitis (MPA), Churg-Strauss syndrome, and Wegener granulomatosis are the forms of vasculitis most likely to cause mononeuritis multiplex.

B. LABORATORY FINDINGS

Laboratory abnormalities accompany virtually every form of vasculitis (Table 28–5). Some abnormalities, such as anemia and an elevated erythrocyte sedimenta-

Table 28–5. Common laboratory tests in vasculitis.

Test Result	Disease Association
Hematocrit	Low in many forms
Erythrocyte sedimentation rate	Usually high, especially in giant cell arteritis
Creatinine	Elevated by renal forms of vasculitis
Urinalysis	Often abnormal, red blood cell casts caused by vasculitis of the glomeruli
Liver function tests	Abnormal in hepatitis B– or C–associated polyarteritis
Serum cryoglobulins	Present in cryoglobulinemia
Complement levels	Low in SLE, cryoglobulinemia
Immunoelectrophoresis	Monoclonal gammopathies common in hepatitis C–related vasculitis
Antineutrophil cytoplasmic antibodies (ANCA)	Positive in WG, MPA, Churg-Strauss syndrome

SLE, systemic lupus erythematosus; WG, Wegener granulomatosis; MPA, microscopic polyangiitis.

tion rate, are very nonspecific and can be seen with many other diseases. Other findings, such as red blood cell casts in the urine (indicating vasculitis of the glomerulus) or antineutrophil cytoplasmic antibodies (associated with Wegener granulomatosis), have much greater specificity.

C. IMAGING TESTS

The role of imaging tests depends greatly on the form of vasculitis suspected. Plain radiographs infrequently provide important clues except in Wegener granulomatosis, where views of the sinuses and chest may yield findings (albeit usually not specific ones). Computed tomography scans of the chest are more sensitive in Wegener granulomatosis. Angiograms are especially helpful in supporting or establishing the diagnosis of Takayasu arteritis, polyarteritis nodosa, and primary central nervous system vasculitis.

D. SPECIAL TESTS

Biopsy of involved tissues is the most common method for establishing definitively the diagnosis of vasculitis. Skin, peripheral nerves, airways, arteries, kidney, and gut are the most common sampled tissues. In general, biopsies of symptomatic areas have a yield of about 66%, whereas biopsy of sites with no symptoms or findings have low yield. Special stains are sometimes required to reveal the degree of damage to particular arterial layers (such as the internal elastic lamina) or the extent of immune complex deposition.

Differential Diagnosis

Specific diagnostic criteria have been established for most forms of vasculitis and are detailed in subsequent chapters. In general, the diagnosis of vasculitis requires a compatible clinical picture and a laboratory test—usually a biopsy but sometimes an angiogram or a specific serologic test (such as ANCA for Wegener granulomatosis). It is also important to consider, and to exclude where appropriate, other diseases that can mimic primary systemic vasculitis. Cholesterol emboli, drug reactions, Whipple disease, syphilis, HIV, endocarditis, antiphospholipid antibody syndrome, and atrial myxoma are particularly common mimickers of primary vasculitis. Indeed, endocarditis and syphilis can cause vasculitis. In the appropriate setting, these conditions may need to be considered.

Treatment

An important general principle in the treatment of vasculitis is to make sure that the intensity of treatment fits the severity of vasculitis. Although most forms of vasculitis require aggressive treatment to prevent morbidity and mortality, some do not. Minor vasculitis limited to the skin and caused by drug reactions requires no therapy other than stopping the offending drug. In contrast, rapid and intensive therapy is required to prevent blindness from developing in giant cell arteritis or renal failure from complicating Wegener granulomatosis.

Another important principle of treatment is to limit the toxicity of therapy. When long-term prednisone is required, for example, appropriate measures to prevent osteoporosis should be initiated. If immunosuppression will result (as occurs with high-dose prednisone or immunosuppressive drugs), then prophylaxis against *Pneumocystis carinii* pneumonia should be started. Other potential toxicities of therapies must be monitored closely.

When to Refer to a Specialist

Given that vasculitis is relatively uncommon in general practice, most patients in whom vasculitis is suspected should be referred to a specialist. Depending on the manifestations, patients may be referred to a rheumatologist, nephrologist, pulmonologist, ophthalmologist, or another specialist.

REFERENCES

González-Gay MA, García-Porrúa C. Epidemiology of the vasculitides. In: Stone JH, Hellmann DB, eds. *Rheumatic Disease Clinics of North America.* WB Saunders; 2001:729–749.

Hellmann DB, Stone J. Small and medium vessel primary vasculitis. In: Rich RR, et al, eds. *Clinical Immunology.* 2nd ed. Mosby, 2001:67.1–67.24.

Relevant World Wide Web Sites

[Johns Hopkins Vasculitis Center]
http://vasculitis.med.jhu.edu

Giant Cell Arteritis & Polymyalgia Rheumatica

David B. Hellmann, MD

Giant cell arteritis (GCA)—also known as temporal arteritis—is the most common form of systemic vasculitis in adults. GCA is a panarteritis that occurs almost exclusively in older people and preferentially affects the extracranial branches of the carotid artery. The most feared complication of GCA is blindness, which usually can be prevented by early diagnosis and treatment with glucocorticoids. Polymyalgia rheumatica (PMR) is an aching and stiffness of the shoulders, neck, and hip-girdle area that can occur with GCA or, more commonly, by itself.

ESSENTIALS OF DIAGNOSIS

- *For GCA, headache, PMR, jaw claudication, and visual symptoms.*
- *The gold standard for diagnosing GCA is temporal artery biopsy.*
- *For PMR, stiffness and aching of the shoulders, neck, and hip region.*
- *PMR is a clinical diagnosis. The only common laboratory abnormality is an elevated erythrocyte sedimentation rate (ESR).*
- *Markedly elevated ESR.*

General Considerations

Although the causes of PMR and GCA are unknown, the disorders share many risk factors and probably mechanisms of pathogenesis. Age is the greatest risk factor for developing either condition. Almost all patients who have GCA are older than 50 years (the average age of onset is 72). The incidence of GCA rises from 1.54 cases per 100,000 people in the sixth decade to 20.7 per 100,000 in the eighth decade.

PMR is 2–4 times more common than GCA, and its incidence also rises with age. Women are twice as likely as men to have GCA or PMR. Both conditions develop most often in Scandinavians and in Americans of Scandinavian origin. GCA develops rarely in black men.

GCA and PMR are associated with the same HLA genes as those seen in patients with rheumatoid arthritis (ie, HLA-DR4 variants *0401 and *0404). The pathogenesis of GCA appears to be initiated by T cells in the adventitia responding to an unknown antigen, which prompts other T cells and macrophages to infiltrate all layers of the affected artery and to elaborate cytokines that mediate both local damage to the vessel and systemic effects. Magnetic resonance imaging and ultrasonography show that PMR is caused by inflammation of the synovial lining of the bursa and joints around the neck, shoulders, and hips.

Although GCA may develop later in some patients with PMR, patients who have only PMR are not at risk for losing their vision and usually require small doses of prednisone (ie, < 20 mg/d). In contrast, patients with GCA are at risk for losing their vision and require higher doses of prednisone (≥ 40 mg/d) to prevent blindness. Because patients who have GCA and PMR require treatment with glucocorticoids for months or years, it is important to minimize the likelihood of adverse effects from therapy (eg, osteoporosis, hypertension, and cataracts).

Clinical Findings

A. SYMPTOMS AND SIGNS

The classic symptoms of GCA include headache, jaw claudication, PMR, visual symptoms, and malaise (Table 29–1). The onset may be gradual or sudden. Three of the following five criteria must be met to diagnosis GCA: (1) age greater than 50 years, (2) new headaches, (3) abnormal temporal artery, (4) ESR ≥ 50 mm/h, and (5) positive temporal artery biopsy results for vasculitis (Figure 29–1).

The most frequent finding during a physical examination is an abnormal temporal artery, which develops in only 50% of the patients; thus, a normal temporal artery does not exclude the diagnosis of GCA. The temporal artery may be enlarged, difficult to compress,

Table 29–1. Classic presenting manifestations of giant cell arteritis.

Symptoms	Percentage of Cases
Headache	70
Jaw claudication	50
Constitutional symptoms	50
Polymyalgia rheumatica	40
Visual loss	20
Abnormal temporal artery	50
Anemia	80
ESR > 50 mm/h	90
Arthritis	15

ESR, erythrocyte sedimentation rate.

nodular, or pulseless. About 10–15% of patients will have axillary or subclavian disease, which manifests as diminished pulses, unequal arm blood pressures, or bruits heard above or below the clavicle or along the upper arm. Tongue ulcers, mass lesions of the breast and ovaries, and aortic regurgitation are other signs of GCA.

1. Headache—The intensity and location of the headache, the most common symptom, varies greatly

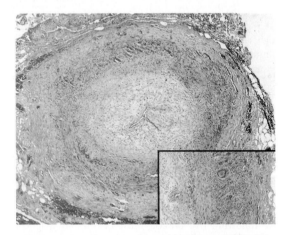

Figure 29–1. Giant cell arteritis. Temporal artery biopsy showing endothelial proliferation, fragmentation of internal elastic lamina, and infiltration of the adventitia and media by inflammatory cells. Giant cells are especially well seen in the inset. (Reprinted from Hellmann DB. Vasculitis. In: Stobo J, et al, eds. *Principles and Practice of Medicine.* Appleton & Lange, 1996.)

from patient to patient. The headache is typically described as a dull, aching pain of moderate severity, localized over the temporal area, but variations in location, quality, and severity occur often. The most striking feature of the headache is that the patient notices that it is new or different. Even if the patient has had migraine or other headache problems in the past, features of the new headache are different. Patients frequently describe tenderness of the scalp, especially when they comb or brush their hair. Some patients will localize the tenderness to the temporal arteries, which may be enlarged or nodular in only a minority of cases.

2. Jaw claudication—Jaw claudication, defined as pain in the masseter muscles associated with protracted chewing, develops when the oxygen demand of the masseter muscles exceeds the supply provided by narrowed and inflamed arteries. Typically, patients with jaw claudication notice pain when eating foods that require vigorous chewing, such as meats, and little or no pain when chewing soft foods. Of all the possible symptoms of GCA, jaw claudication is the most specific for this disease. Many patients do not provide such a classic description of jaw claudication, and instead report a vague sense of discomfort along the jaw or face, with or without protracted chewing. Atypical manifestations of jaw claudication include discomfort over the ear or around the nose.

3. PMR and joints—PMR is defined as pain and stiffness in the neck, shoulders, and hip-girdle area that are usually much worse in the morning. All of the following criteria must be met to diagnose PMR: (1) age greater than 50 years; (2) aching and stiffness for at least 1 month, affecting at least two of the three abovementioned areas (ie, shoulders, neck, and pelvic girdle); (3) morning stiffness lasting at least 1 hour; (4) ESR > 40 mm/h; (5) exclusion of other diseases except GCA; and (6) rapid response to prednisone (≤ 20 mg/d).

The shoulders are more commonly involved (70–95%) than the hips (50–70%). Shoulder pain in PMR may begin unilaterally but quickly becomes bilateral. Patients with PMR may report great difficulty getting out of bed, arising from the toilet, or brushing their teeth. People in whom GCA develops frequently describe feeling "old" for the first time at the onset of the disease. The stiffness is especially severe in the morning but may improve, usually a little but sometimes markedly, during the day. When asked to localize the pain, patients often say the pain is "in the flesh" rather than in the joints. Examination of the shoulders and hips is usually unremarkable except for decreased active and passive range of motion. Swelling, erythema, and heat are usually absent. However, some patients with PMR or GCA experience arthralgia or arthritis of the sternoclavicular joint, wrists, fingers, knees, or ankles. Rarely, pitting edema develops in the patient's hands or feet.

4. Visual symptoms—About one-third of patients present with visual symptoms, chiefly diplopia or visual loss. Visual hallucinations occur rarely. The visual loss may be transient or permanent or monocular or binocular. Visual loss is the most feared complication of GCA because it is usually irreversible. Blindness can develop abruptly but more often is preceded by episodes of blurred vision or amaurosis fugax. Rarely is visual loss the first manifestation of GCA: On average, visual loss develops 5 months after the onset of other GCA symptoms. The direct cause of visual loss in GCA is usually occlusion of the posterior ciliary artery, a branch of the ophthalmic artery, which is a branch of the carotid artery. The posterior ciliary artery supplies blood to the optic nerve head. Interruption of that flow leads to anterior ischemic optic neuropathy.

When visual loss occurs, it usually is profound. Patients often cannot detect a hand waving directly in front of the affected eye. In the first few hours after infarction, the disc generally appears normal on fundoscopic examination, even in the presence of profound visual loss. Later, disc pallor (Figure 29–2) and swelling, cotton-wool spots, and flame-shaped intraretinal hemorrhages may develop. Over weeks or months, the disc becomes atrophic. Most patients with visual loss also demonstrate a relative afferent pupillary defect, demonstrated by moving a shining light from the normal eye to the blind eye and noting that both pupils dilate.

5. Other features—Almost all patients with the classic features of GCA also have nonspecific manifestations such as malaise, fatigue, and loss of appetite. Weight loss of 2–10 kg is common. Some patients also experience depression.

B. ATYPICAL MANIFESTATIONS

GCA presents with atypical features in 40% of cases. Awareness of these atypical presentations (Table 29–2) maximizes the physician's chance of diagnosing GCA before blindness develops.

1. Fever of unknown origin—Fever develops in about 40% of patients with GCA; of those, 10–15% are fevers of unknown origin (FUO). Although GCA causes only 2% of all cases of FUO, it accounts for 16% of all FUO cases in patients over the age of 65. Fevers in GCA may reach nearly 40 °C, and average about 39 °C. About two-thirds of patients with fevers also have rigors and drenching sweats. Despite these manifestations of a robust inflammatory response, the white blood cell count is almost always normal (at least before prednisone is started).

2. Respiratory—Respiratory symptoms develop in 1 of 10 patients and constitute the presenting complaint in 1 of 25. The most common symptom is a dry cough, resembling that seen in some patients taking angiotensin-converting enzyme inhibitors. The cause of the cough is obscure because chest imaging studies are normal. The cough may reflect inflammation within the arteries adjacent to cough centers, which are distributed throughout various sites in the respiratory apparatus, including the diaphragm, the bronchi, and the

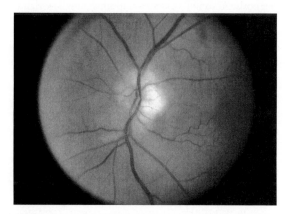

Figure 29–2. Early fundoscopic appearance in a patient with giant cell arteritis in whom blindness has developed.

Table 29–2. Atypical manifestations of giant cell arteritis.

Fever of unknown origin
Respiratory tract symptoms
    Dry cough
    Throat pain
    Tongue pain
Neurologic symptoms
    Mononeuritis multiplex
    Stroke
    Transient ischemic attack
    Dementia
    Hallucinations
Large artery involvement
    Claudication, arms or legs
    Unequal arm blood pressure
    Thoracic aortic aneurysm
Tumor-like lesions
    Especially of breasts, ovaries
Syndrome of inappropriate antidiuretic hormone
   secretion

mid-brain. Other respiratory or otolaryngeal manifestations include tongue pain, glossitis, dental pain, and posterior or anterior pharyngeal pain. These symptoms reflect ischemia caused by arteritis of nearby vessels; tongue ulceration and gangrene may also occur.

3. Neurologic—The most common neurologic manifestation of GCA is mononeuritis multiplex. Unlike mononeuritis multiplex in other forms of vasculitis, which most commonly affects the foot or the hand, mononeuritis multiplex in GCA most commonly affects the shoulder, producing sudden weakness and pain that mimics a C5 radiculopathy. Central nervous system disease, outside of the eye, also occurs. Delirium, dementia, transient ischemic attacks (TIAs), and cerebral vascular accidents (CVAs) have been reported. GCA preferentially affects the posterior circulation of the brain: Whereas the ratio of anterior to posterior circulation CVAs is about 3:2 in the general population, the ratio is reversed in GCA. Intracranial disease does not occur in GCA, perhaps because arteries lose their elastic lamina almost as soon as they penetrate the dura. TIAs and CVAs complicating GCA, therefore, are attributed to occlusion of extracranial vessels or to thromboemboli.

4. Large-artery disease—Involvement of large arteries—the aorta and its major branches—develops in at least 15% of patients. The most commonly affected vessels include the vertebral, carotid, subclavian, axillary, axillary arteries, and the aorta. Involvement of large arteries in the lower extremities has also been described. Presenting symptoms may include TIA, CVA, hand ischemia, and arm or leg claudication. Aortic involvement may lead to thoracic aortic aneurysm (TAA), which is increased 17-fold in patients with GCA. TAA develops an average of 7 years after the diagnosis of GCA. TAA may be asymptomatic or cause aortic regurgitation, myocardial infarction, or dissection. Abdominal aortic aneurysms, although less common than thoracic lesions, also occur. Involvement of the pulmonary or mesenteric arteries virtually never occurs.

5. Other atypical manifestations—The protean manifestations of GCA include tumor-like lesions localized to the breast or ovaries, mimicking cancer at those sites. Other manifestations include the syndrome of inappropriate antidiuretic hormone secretion and hemolytic anemia (Table 29–2).

C. LABORATORY FINDINGS

The laboratory hallmarks of GCA and PMR are a markedly elevated ESR and anemia (Table 29–1). An ESR > 30 mm/h is present in 96% of patients with GCA, and an ESR of > 50 mm/h is seen in 87% of patients with GCA. A normal ESR may be seen in a slightly higher percentage of patients with PMR. The ESR averages about 100 mm/h in GCA and slightly

lower in isolated PMR. The C-reactive protein is also usually elevated and may be more sensitive than the ESR. The anemia, typically normochromic and normocytic, is usually mild with a hematocrit often in the 32 to 35 range. Occasionally, the anemia may be profound with hematocrits in the 20s. Approximately 20% of patients with GCA demonstrate a mildly elevated alkaline phosphatase (of liver origin). The platelet count, often elevated nonspecifically by inflammatory disorders, is frequently increased in GCA and PMR.

D. IMAGING STUDIES

Radiographs of shoulders and hips are invariably unhelpful. However, magnetic resonance imaging and ultrasonography of shoulders and hips in patients with PMR show inflammation of the bursa and the synovium of nearby joints. Color duplex ultrasonography of affected temporal arteries can show a characteristic "halo" of edema, but this technology is no more sensitive for the diagnosis of GCA than a careful physical examination of the temporal artery.

Making the Diagnosis

The diagnosis of PMR rests almost entirely on clinical grounds, namely symptoms of proximal limb stiffness associated with an elevated ESR and a dramatic response to prednisone. While MRI and ultrasonographic images are abnormal in PMR, their sensitivity and specificity have not been established and usually are not obtained.

Classification criteria have also been proposed for GCA, but their predictive value in clinical settings is not well established. Since GCA is uncommon, clinicians have to maintain a high index of suspicion for the diagnosis. Among its classic symptoms, only jaw claudication has been shown to increase the odds (by about three-fold) that a patient in whom GCA is suspected actually has the disease. The only physical finding with a high positive predictive value for diagnosing GCA is an abnormal temporal artery. Although strikingly elevated ESR (eg, > 100 mm/h) strongly suggest the diagnosis in the proper setting, moderate elevations of the ESR are quite nonspecific. A normal ESR substantially reduces the likelihood of GCA, but does not eliminate it altogether.

Two guidelines may help determine when to suspect GCA. First, one should consider the composite clinical picture when trying to decide whether a patient could have GCA. A comprehensive review of systems may be especially helpful since most patients with GCA have multiple symptoms. For example, vasculitis should not be suspected in most patients with a dry cough, one of the atypical symptoms of GCA. However, GCA should be considered in a 72-year-old patient with a dry cough, PMR, headache, weight loss, fever, anemia, and a ESR of 105 mm/h. Second, because many of the atypical symptoms involve some type of pain above the neck—headache, vague discomfort around the jaw, throat, ear, tongue, or teeth—it may be prudent to consider the diagnosis of GCA in any patient over the age of 50 who has pain in any of these areas without another explanation. Thus, the elderly patient with ear pain and a normal ear examination does not benefit from a diagnosis of otitis media and antibiotics, but may benefit from a comprehensive review of systems and an ESR.

In practice, then, the diagnosis of GCA is suggested by the clinical picture combined with an elevated ESR, and proven by a positive temporal artery biopsy. Rarely, patients with large-artery involvement, such as subclavian disease, are diagnosed by angiography showing long, smooth arterial taperings uncharacteristic of atherosclerosis. Although some have proposed using color duplex ultrasonography of the temporal artery, experience with that technique is not sufficient to replace temporal artery biopsy as the gold standard for diagnosing GCA.

Differential Diagnosis

It is important to distinguish patients who have PMR alone from those who have PMR plus GCA. Patients are classified as having PMR alone if they have no "above-the-neck symptoms," namely headache, jaw claudication, scalp tenderness, or visual symptoms. Although about 20% of patients with symptoms of PMR have positive temporal artery biopsy results, practice has shown that patients who have symptoms of PMR alone respond well to low-dose prednisone (see following section on Treatment).

Distinguishing PMR from rheumatoid arthritis in an older person can be difficult, especially in those patients with PMR who have distal polyarthritis. Severe erosive arthritis, rheumatoid nodules, and a positive rheumatoid factor make rheumatoid arthritis the more likely diagnosis. Because both conditions can respond well to low-dose prednisone, differentiating the two disorders may not be possible during the early months of treatment.

Polymyositis causes much more proximal weakness than pain. In contrast, patients with PMR always rate their pain greater than any weakness. The creatine phosphokinase is usually elevated in polymyositis but normal in PMR. Proximal limb pain or stiffness can occur with a variety of endocrine disorders, including hypothyroidism and panhypopituitarism. PMR is usually easily distinguished from fibromyalgia, which is a condition of diffuse pain—both proximal and distal—typically occurring in young women in the absence of

objective findings or abnormal laboratory tests. Solid tumors, especially renal cell carcinoma, can produce musculoskeletal pain that resembles PMR. However, patients with malignancy usually have some atypical feature such as pain that affects the distal limbs as much as the proximal portions, clubbing, or a requirement for more than 20 mg of prednisone per day.

Other conditions that can mimic PMR include early Parkinson syndrome, amyloidosis, late-onset systemic lupus erythematosus, endocarditis, myelodysplastic syndrome, and drug reactions (eg, myositis from "statin" drugs). Since absence of shoulder involvement is rare in PMR, patients thought to have "below the waist" PMR are more likely to have lumbar spinal stenosis, which can cause stiffness and pain restricted to the hip-girdle region.

Transient nonocular loss of vision (amaurosis fugax) or permanent nonocular blindness can also occur from atherosclerotic cerebrovascular or cardiovascular disease. The nonarteritis patients may be distinguished by their lack of other symptoms and a normal ESR. Both atherosclerosis and GCA can also cause upper or lower extremity claudication. Angiography can usually differentiate these conditions. GCA produces isolated long segments of smooth narrowing in the mid-portions of arteries, whereas atherosclerosis tends to be diffuse and favors branch points.

Some of the clinical features of GCA can be produced by other forms of systemic vasculitis. Wegener granulomatosis and polyarteritis nodosa, for example, can cause jaw claudication. Takayasu arteritis can affect the large vessels as GCA does, but Takayasu arteritis is usually seen in young women. Multiple myeloma, Waldenström macroglobulinemia, and osteomyelitis can produce systemic features with markedly elevated ESRs. Endocarditis should also be considered in a patient with symptoms resembling GCA and a new heart murmur. Many patients with diabetes in whom proteinuria has developed feel poorly and have very high ESRs, as do patients with other forms of renal failure. For example, about 20% of all patients receiving hemodialysis have ESRs > 100 mm/h. Although many of these patients also suffer from malaise, they rarely have symptoms strongly suggestive of GCA. Those who do have symptoms suggesting GCA will require temporal artery biopsy. Other mimickers of GCA include myelodysplastic syndromes and systemic amyloidosis.

Treatment

Prednisone (40–60 mg/d) should be given to any patient in whom GCA is strongly suspected. Then, the patient should be referred for a temporal artery biopsy. Temporal artery biopsy has almost zero mortality and very low morbidity. It is the only test that can confirm the diagnosis of GCA, so it is recommended in all suspected cases. Although it is traditional to obtain the temporal artery biopsy quickly, evidence suggests that the pathologic features persist for at least 2 weeks after the start of glucocorticoid treatment. GCA does not involve arteries continuously, so skip areas may occur. Consequently, the greatest yields will come from biopsies of large segments of artery (eg, 3–5 cm) that have multiple sections examined pathologically. Positive biopsy results demonstrate chiefly mononuclear cells infiltrating all the layers of the artery with varying degrees of intimal proliferation and disruption of the internal elastic lamina. About 50% of positive specimens show multinucleated giant cells. It is intuitively appealing to biopsy the temporal artery that is abnormal on physical examination or that corresponds to the side of the head with symptoms. Unilateral temporal artery biopsy is about 90% sensitive and bilateral biopsies about 95% sensitive. These figures come from centers where GCA is studied frequently and may not be as high in other communities. In any setting, some patients with a convincing story of GCA may have a negative biopsy result.

Patients with suspected GCA who have experienced transient visual loss for a few hours should be admitted and given high-dose intravenous methylprednisolone (eg, 1000 mg/d) for 3–5 days, as a few patients have recovered some vision with this regimen. Visual loss of more than 1 day's duration is almost always permanent.

Patients with PMR alone are treated usually with 10–20 mg/d of prednisone. Nonsteroidal anti-inflammatory drugs can help alleviate PMR symptoms but rarely obviate the need for glucocorticoids.

Patients with PMR or GCA respond dramatically to initial treatment. Some report improvement within hours of taking the first dose of prednisone, and most describe a "miraculous" improvement within 2 days. However, about 10% will require a week of therapy before feeling better. Dividing the dose of prednisone into a morning and evening dose for the first 1–2 weeks helps some patients. If the patient does not improve within the first week, doubt should be cast on the diagnosis of PMR or of biopsy-negative GCA. Every-other-day prednisone is not effective initial treatment.

To prevent osteoporosis, patients starting prednisone therapy should take 1500–1800 mg of calcium daily with 400–800 U of vitamin D. Bone density scans should be performed, and those with osteopenia or osteoporosis should be started on bisphosphonates.

After the first month of treatment, almost all patients will have a normal ESR. At this point, the prednisone can begin to be tapered by 10% every week or two. The rate of prednisone tapering should be determined by the total clinical picture produced by the patient's symptoms (most important), physical findings, and some laboratory measure of inflammation, such as the ESR or C-reactive protein (least important). Once patients with GCA reach 15 mg of prednisone or patients with PMR reach 10 mg, decrements of 1 mg every 2 or so weeks may reduce the chance of flare.

Complications

Unfortunately, 50–80% of patients with PMR or GCA relapse during the first year as prednisone is tapered. Flares are defined clinically: Isolated elevations of ESR do not require alteration of therapy. The only exception to this rule is that very rare case when visual loss develops in a patient with biopsy-proven GCA in the absence of other symptoms. Patients who experience renewed symptoms usually respond to increasing the prednisone dose 5–10 mg above the last dose at which the patient was asymptomatic. Most patients are unable to completely taper off of prednisone for 1–2 years, and a substantial minority will require some prednisone—usually in the range of 5 to 10 mg—for longer periods. No glucocorticoid-sparing agent has been proved consistently effective. Reports of the efficacy of methotrexate for GCA have been conflicting.

Complications from prednisone therapy develop in most patients being treated for PMR or GCA (Table 29–3). For example, diabetes or osteoporosis is 2–5 time more likely to develop in patients treated with prednisone than in others of the same age not receiving therapy. Important measures for limiting the toxicity of prednisone therapy include slow but steady tapering of prednisone as suggested above, protecting against early osteoporosis, and avoiding making the dose of prednisone a slave of an isolated ESR elevation.

Table 29–3. Possible side effects of long-term glucocorticoid therapy.

Weight gain
Diabetes
Cataracts
Insomnia
Fluid retention
Hypertension
Proximal weakness
Alopecia
Sweats
Osteoporosis
Infection
Psychiatric disturbance (eg, depression, mania, psychosis)
Easy bruising of the skin
Stress
Tremor
Peptic ulcer disease

When to Refer to a Specialist

All patients with visual loss should be referred to an ophthalmologist to make certain the visual loss is caused by vasculitis and not by another treatable cause such as acute glaucoma.

Patients whose symptoms persist or recur despite appropriate prednisone therapy and a slow taper should be referred to a rheumatologist.

REFERENCES

Chuang TY, et al. Polymyalgia rheumatica: a 10-year epidemiologic and clinical study. *Ann Intern Med.* 1982;97:672. [PMID: 6982645]

Healey LA. Long-term follow-up of polymyalgia rheumatica: evidence for synovitis. *Semin Arthritis Rheum.* 1984;13:322. [PMID: 6729485]

Hunder GG, et al. The American College of Rheumatology 1990 criteria for the classification of giant cell arteritis. *Arthritis Rheum.* 1990;33:1122. [PMID: 2202311]

Huston KA, et al. Temporal arteritis: a 24-year epidemiologic, clinical, and pathologic study. *Ann Intern Med.* 1978;88:162. [PMID: 626444]

Levine SM, Hellmann DB. Giant cell arteritis. *Curr Opin Rheumatol.* 2002;14:3. [PMID: 11790989]

Miller NR. Visual manifestations of temporal arteritis. *Rheum Dis Clin North Am.* 2001;27:781. [PMID: 11723764]

Salvarani C, et al. Polymyalgia rheumatica and giant-cell arteritis. *N Engl J Med.* 2002;347:261. [PMID: 12140303]

Relevant World Wide Web Sites

[The Johns Hopkins Vasculitis Center]
http://vasculitis.med.jhu.edu
[The International Network for the Study of the Systemic Vasculitides]
http://www.2.ccf.org/inssys/
[The Cleveland Clinic Foundation Center for Vasculitis]
http:www.clevelandclinic.org/arthritis/vasculitis/default.htm
[The National Institute of Allergy and Infectious Disease]
http://www.niaid.nih.gov/dir/general.htm

Takayasu Arteritis

David B. Hellmann, MD

Takayasu arteritis, named for the Japanese ophthalmologist who first described the ocular manifestations in 1908, is a large-vessel vasculitis of unknown cause that chiefly affects women during their reproductive years. The disease often presents two challenges. First, the diagnosis can be delayed for months or even years due to the rarity of the disease, the young age of the (typical) patient, and the protean presenting manifestations. Second, treatment is a challenge. Although Takayasu arteritis is a chronic disease, it usually pursues a waxing and waning course that requires careful monitoring to determine when the disease is active and medical therapy is needed. Treatment with glucocorticoids usually succeeds in halting progression of the vasculitis. Indeed, because of the advances in medical therapy and surgical treatment of vascular complications, such as aortic regurgitation, survival of patients with Takayasu arteritis has increased dramatically.

ESSENTIALS OF DIAGNOSIS

- *Causes vasculitis of the aorta and its major branches.*
- *Preferentially affects young women.*
- *Often presents with absent pulse, bruit, claudication, hypertension, or fever of unknown origin.*
- *Erythrocyte sedimentation rate is usually elevated.*
- *Most patients respond to prednisone.*

General Considerations

Although Takayasu arteritis has been most extensively reported in Japan, Korea, China, Southeast Asia, and Mexico, cases have been described worldwide. In North America, the annual incidence is about 1–3 cases per million people. Takayasu arteritis affects women 8 times more frequently than men. The average age of diagnosis is in the mid-20s but the disease may begin as early as age 7 or as late as age 70. Symptoms develop before age 20 in nearly one-third of patients and after age 40 in about 10%. The age of onset tends to be older in European countries.

Pathogenesis

The cause of Takayasu arteritis remains elusive. The geographic clustering of cases suggests important genetic or environmental factors, but few have been identified. HLA associations have been found in Japanese patients (who preferentially express Bw52, DR2, Dw12, and DQw1) but not in other populations. The predominance of Takayasu arteritis in women of childbearing age suggests that female hormones may play a permissive role, as in systemic lupus erythematosus. An animal model of Takayasu arteritis has been produced with a herpes virus. In that model, the media of the aorta provide an immunoprivileged site for persistent herpes virus infection, which results in chronic inflammation (arteritis).

However initiated, Takayasu arteritis appears to be propagated by a T-cell-driven immune response that results in a granulomatous inflammation affecting all layers of the vessel. Indeed, the histopathology of Takayasu arteritis cannot be distinguished from that of temporal arteritis (also called giant cell arteritis; see Chapter 29). The inflammatory injury mediated by activated T cells, macrophages, and cytokines often results in proliferation of the intima and of smooth muscle cells in the media, leading to occlusion and stenosis of the artery. Transmural inflammation can also cause aneurysmal dilation of the vessel. Overproduction of inflammatory cytokines, such as interleukin-6, results in fever and other constitutional symptoms.

Clinical Findings

A. SYMPTOMS AND SIGNS

Although the presenting features of Takayasu arteritis vary greatly, they can be categorized into two broad groups: those caused by vascular damage (ie, occlusion, stenosis, or dilation of blood vessels), and those caused by systemic inflammation (Table 30–1). The separation of these presenting features is not always neatly maintained; many patients have both vascular complications and constitutional symptoms, and others have a biphasic presentation, with constitutional symptoms domi-

Table 30–1. Clinical features of Takayasu arteritis.

Feature	At Presentation (%)	Ever Present (%)
Vascular	50	100
Bruit		80
Claudication (upper extremity)	30	62
Claudication (lower extremity)	15	32
Hypertension	20	33
Unequal arm blood pressures	15	50
Carotodynia	15	32
Aortic regurgitation		20
Central nervous system	30	57
Light-headedness	20	35
Visual abnormality	10	30
Stroke	5	10
Musculoskeletal	20	53
Chest wall pain	10	30
Joint pain	10	30
Myalgia	5	15
Constitutional	33	43
Malaise	20	30
Fever	20	25
Weight loss	15	20
Cardiac	15	38
Aortic regurgitation	8	20
Angina	2	12
CHF	2	10

CHF, congestive heart failure.
Data based on studying 60 patients reported by Kerr GS, et al. Takayasu arteritis. *Ann Intern Med.* 1994;120:919.

nating early and vascular features becoming more salient later.

Among the vascular manifestations, bruit, claudication, hypertension, light-headedness (associated with vertebral or carotid artery disease), unequal blood pressures in the extremities, carotodynia, aortic regurgitation, and loss of a pulse are most common. Bruits develop most frequently over the carotid arteries but also often develop in the supraclavicular or infraclavicular space (reflecting subclavian disease), along the flexor surface of the upper arm (from axillary artery disease), or in the abdomen (from renal or mesenteric artery vasculitis). Many patients have multiple bruits. Upper extremity claudication—commonly manifested in young women by fatigue and pain in the arm while exercising or blow-drying hair—develops more often than lower extremity claudication. A widened pulse pressure and diastolic murmur along the right sternal border may signal the aortic regurgitation that develops in 20% of patients. Stroke, angina, and congestive heart failure affect a significant minority of patients.

The visual symptoms that were first described in 1908 occur rarely today. When present, visual symptoms chiefly result from retinal ischemia produced by narrowing or occlusion of the carotid arteries. Some patients may have such limited blood flow through their carotids and vertebral arteries that merely turning and tilting their head causes light-headedness, dizziness, or visual loss.

Almost half of patients experience constitutional or musculoskeletal symptoms. These constitutional and musculoskeletal features dominate the presentation in approximately one-third of all cases of Takayasu arteritis. Aethenia, weight loss, fever, myalgia, and arthralgia occur commonly. Prominent back pain, especially in the thoracic region, develops in a few patients. This pain resembles that seen in older patients with thoracic dissection and probably results from stimulation of nociceptive nerve fibers along the inflamed aorta.

B. LABORATORY FINDINGS

Takayasu arteritis does not cause any specific blood test or urinary abnormalities but usually produces nonspecific findings of inflammation. Nearly 80% of patients have elevated erythrocyte sedimentation rates, especially during phases of active disease. Anemia develops in 50% of patients, with hematocrits typically in the high 20s or low 30s. Anemic patients commonly have slightly low mean corpuscular volume (MCV) (eg, high 70s). Thrombocytosis, which develops in one-third of patients, is often mild but may exceed 800,000/μL. Fewer than 10% of patients with Takayasu arteritis have an elevated serum creatinine. About one-quarter will have mild proteinuria or hematuria. Renal abnormalities usually result from hypertension; glomerulonephritis from Takayasu arteritis very rarely occurs.

C. IMAGING STUDIES

Magnetic resonance imaging (MRI), computed tomography, vascular ultrasonography, and conventional aortography will be abnormal in virtually all patients with Takayasu arteritis. MRI appears most sensitive in that it can detect the inflammatory thickening of the aorta or its branches (Figure 30–1) that precedes changes in the caliber of the vessels' lumen. Conventional angiography, although agnostic about the thickness of the vessel wall, provides the most detailed images of the stenoses, occlusions, dilatation, and other vascular wall irregularities characteristic of Takayasu arteritis (Figure 30–2).

The most frequently affected vessels are the subclavian arteries, carotid arteries, and aorta (Table 30–2). Involvement of the aorta above and below the diaphragm occurs most commonly. In the extra-aortic vessels, long segments of stenosis are more frequent than dilation or aneurysm. Takayasu arteritis is one of the few forms of vasculitis that can affect, albeit rarely, the pulmonary arteries.

D. SPECIFIC TESTS

Biopsies of the aorta or other actively affected arteries show a granulomatous vasculitis with giant cells.

Differential Diagnosis

The biggest impediment to diagnosing Takayasu arteritis is that few physicians are familiar enough with this rare disease to recognize its presenting manifestations. The American College of Rheumatology has developed six criteria for classification of Takayasu arteritis (Table 30–3). In practice, the diagnosis of Takayasu arteritis requires demonstrating vasculitis of the aorta or its major branches by imaging tests (Figures 30–1 through 30–3)

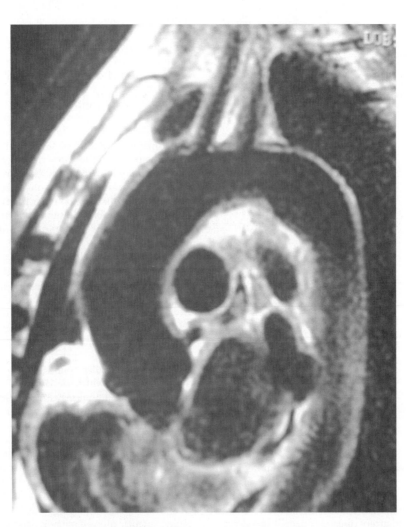

Figure 30–1. Magnetic resonance image showing thickening of the wall of the ascending and descending thoracic aorta in a 26-year-old woman with Takayasu arteritis.

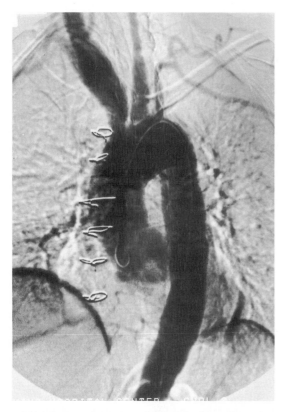

Figure 30–2. Angiogram showing multiple changes of Takayasu arteritis, including dilatations of the ascending aorta (with surgical wires from aortic valve replacement surgery) and the brachiocephalic and proximal right common carotid arteries. The left common carotid artery is occluded distal to its origin. (From Hellmann DB, Flynn JA. Clinical presentation and natural history of Takayasu's arteritis and other inflammatory arteritides. In: Perler BA, Becker GJ, eds. *Vascular Intervention. A Clinical Approach.* Thieme Medical and Scientific Publisher, 1998:249-256. Reprinted by permission.)

Table 30–2. Frequency of blood vessel involvement in Takayasu arteritis.

Blood Vessel	% Abnormal
Aorta	65
Aortic arch or root	35
Abdominal aorta	47
Thoracic aorta	17
Subclavian	93
Common carotid	58
Renal artery	38
Vertebral artery	35
Celiac axes	18
Common iliac	17
Pulmonary artery	5

Data based on studying 60 patients reported by Kerr GS, et al. Takayasu arteritis. *Ann Intern Med.* 1994;120:919.

inflammation (especially keratitis or inflammation of the cornea). A minority of patients with Cogan syndrome have medium- or large-vessel vasculitis, or both. A few other diseases can affect the aorta or its branches, but almost never do they convincingly mimic Takayasu arteritis (Table 30–4). Relapsing polychrondritis, which results in characteristic changes in cartilage, may also affect the aorta. Rheumatoid arthritis and ankylosing spondylitis rarely affect the thoracic root. Buerger disease—a form of medium-vessel vasculitis associated with smoking—may affect the femoral, brachial, and axillary arteries, as can ergotism. Syphilitic aortitis can be excluded by appropriate serologic studies. Neurofibromatosis and congenital coarctation may affect the abdominal

Table 30–3. American College of Rheumatology classification criteria for Takayasu arteritis.[a]

1. Onset at age < 40 yrs
2. Limb claudication
3. Decreased brachial artery pulse
4. Unequal arm BP (> 10 mm Hg)
5. Subclavian or aortic bruit
6. Angiographic evidence of narrowing or occlusion of aorta, or its primary branches, or large limb arteritis

[a]The presence of three or more of the six criteria was sensitive (91%) and specific (98%) for the diagnosis of Takayasu arteritis. The American College of Rheumatology 1990 Criteria for the Classification of Takayasu Arteritis. *Arthritis Rheum.* 1990;33:1129.

or biopsy, and excluding the diseases that can produce similar abnormalities (Table 30–4).

Of the other vasculitides, temporal arteritis (see Chapter 29) is the form most likely to be confused with Takayasu arteritis. Both diseases cause a granulomatous panarteritis and an elevated erythrocyte sedimentation rate. In contrast to Takayasu arteritis, temporal arteritis exclusively affects patients over the age of 50 and chiefly involves extracranial branches of the carotid artery (such as the temporal artery). Cogan syndrome is a rare disease characterized by vestibular-auditory abnormalities (often producing deafness and vertigo) and ocular

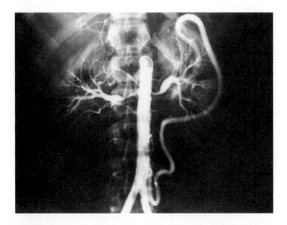

Figure 30–3. Angiogram showing bilateral renal artery stenosis in Takayasu arteritis. A large left colic branch of the inferior mesenteric artery provides collateral circulation. (From Hellmann DB, Flynn JA. Clinical presentation and natural history of Takayasu's arteritis and other inflammatory arteritides. In: Perler BA, Becker GJ, eds. *Vascular Intervention. A Clinical Approach.* Thieme Medical and Scientific Publisher, 1998:249-256. Reprinted by permission.)

aorta and mesenteric great vessels. Radiation-induced damage can affect any vessel including the aorta. Atherosclerosis of the aorta and major branches rarely develops before age 50 and does not produce the long, smoothly tapered and stenotic segments of arteries that are so characteristic of Takayasu arteritis. Marfan syndrome does not produce inflammatory symptoms or signs.

Patients with predominantly constitutional symptoms are often evaluated for other conditions. For example, a woman with a hematocrit of 28, an MCV of

Table 30–4. Differential diagnosis of Takayasu arteritis: Other diseases that can affect the aorta.

Rheumatic diseases	Temporal arteritis, Cogan syndrome, relapsing polychrondritis, ankylosing spondylitis, rheumatoid arthritis, systemic lupus erythematosus, Buerger disease, Behçet disease
Infectious disease	Syphilis
Other	Atherosclerosis, ergotism, radiation-induced damage, retroperitoneal fibrosis, inflammatory bowel disease, sarcoidosis, neurofibromatosis, congenital coarctation, Marfan syndrome

78 (reflecting anemia of chronic disease), and a platelet count of 980,000/μL (nonspecifically reflecting inflammation)—not uncommon findings in Takayasu arteritis—will often unproductively undergo evaluation for gastrointestinal hemorrhage, iron deficiency anemia, or another hematologic disorder. Fatigue and weight loss might erroneously suggest a diagnosis of depression. Transient ischemic attacks in a young woman can be wrongly attributed to migraine. Fever and aortic regurgitation may initially suggest bacterial endocarditis. Measuring blood pressure in both arms, carefully palpating pulses in all extremities, and listening for bruits in the abdomen and chest and along the carotids and supraclavicular and axillary areas provide the best clinical tools in early diagnosis of Takayasu arteritis.

Treatment

Although glucocorticoid therapy for Takayasu arteritis has not been tested in controlled trials, it appears very effective in suppressing vascular inflammation. Initial therapy consists of prednisone (1 mg/kg) for 1 month and then tapered to 10 mg/d over 4–6 months. This treatment nearly universally succeeds in eliminating constitutional and musculoskeletal symptoms within days to a few weeks. Anemia, thrombocytosis, and elevated erythrocyte sedimentation rates also usually respond promptly. Remission, defined as resolution of signs, symptoms, and laboratory markers of inflammation as well as lack of progression of angiographic abnormalities, is seen in most patients who receive glucocorticoid therapy. Unfortunately, many patients with Takayasu arteritis experience relapses of symptoms or progression of vascular disease that necessitate restarting high-dose prednisone therapy. Open studies suggest that methotrexate plus prednisone or mycophenolate plus prednisone may be more effective than prednisone alone in some patients. Because of its toxicity, cyclophosphamide is rarely used to treat Takayasu arteritis.

Complications of Takayasu arteritis, such as hypertension, congestive heart failure, angina, or aortic regurgitation, may benefit from other forms of medical therapy. Treating hypertension is especially tricky in patients with extensive Takayasu arteritis who may have two or more arterial beds with substantially different blood pressures. Reducing blood pressure to achieve a "normal blood pressure" in the legs may aggravate or cause upper extremity claudication. Often the physician must accept compromises in blood pressures that sustain perfusion of critical organs or tissues. Other complications that can be prevented or treated include osteoporosis. Patients taking prednisone long term can guard against osteoporosis by performing weight-bearing exercises and taking 400–800 U of vitamin D and

1200–1800 mg of calcium daily, and a bisphosphonate (see Chapter 56).

Interventional radiologists and surgeons also often play important roles in treatment. Angioplasty and stenting have been successful in treating some cases of hypertension caused by renal artery stenosis. However, restenosis is common. Aortic valve replacement, replacement of severely damaged vessels with Dacron grafts, and coronary artery bypass surgery can be lifesaving. Whenever possible, angioplasty or vascular surgery should be deferred until medical therapy has suppressed the inflammation.

When to Refer to a Specialist

Almost all patients with Takayasu arteritis should be referred to a rheumatologist for diagnosis and treatment. Depending on the manifestations, consultation may be needed with an ophthalmologist, nephrologist, cardiologist, or vascular surgeon.

Prognosis

Most patients have a chronic relapsing and remitting course requiring careful monitoring and adjusting of suppressive therapy. Judging the level of inflammation can be difficult and requires monitoring symptoms, signs, and laboratory markers of inflammation (eg, hematocrit, erythrocyte sedimentation rate). Some experts advocate annual MRI of the aorta and its branches since some patients show progression in the absence obvious symptoms or signs of active disease. Pregnancy appears surprisingly well tolerated if the patient has inactive disease, is taking low doses of prednisone (ie, < 15 mg), and has normal renal function.

Almost all patients experience permanent morbidity from Takayasu arteritis. Because of the morbidity, only about half of the patients are able to work. Survival rates have increased greatly recently so that 10-year survival rates of 80–90% have become common. Advances in diagnosis, medical and surgical treatment, and monitoring augur even better prognosis in the near future. Mortality has been caused chiefly by renal failure, stroke, cardiac failure, or infectious complications of immunosuppressive treatment.

REFERENCES

Daina E, et al. Mycophenolate mofetil for the treatment of Takayasu arteritis: report of three cases. *Ann Intern Med.* 1999;130:422. [PMID: 10068416]

Kerr GS, et al. Takayasu arteritis. *Ann Intern Med.* 1994;120:919. [PMID: 7909656]

Ronthal M, et al. Case records of the Massachusetts General Hospital weekly clinicopathological exercises Case 21—2003. A 72-year-old man with repetitive strokes in the posterior circulation. *N Engl J Med.* 2003;349:170. [PMID: 12853591]

Salvarani C, et al. Polymyalgia rheumatica and giant cell arteritis. *N Engl J Med.* 2002;347:261. [PMID: 12140303]

Weyand CM, Goronzy JJ. Medium- and large-vessel vasculitis. *N Engl J Med.* 2003;349:160. [PMID: 12853590]

Relevant World Wide Web Site

[Johns Hopkins Vasculitis Center]
http://vasculitis.med.jhu.edu

Wegener Granulomatosis

John H. Stone, MD, MPH

ESSENTIALS OF DIAGNOSIS

- *Three pathologic hallmarks of Wegener granulomatosis (WG) are granulomatous inflammation, vasculitis, and necrosis.*
- *Classic clinical features include persistent upper respiratory tract and ear infections that do not respond to antibiotic therapy.*
- *Nonspecific constitutional symptoms, such as fatigue, myalgias, weight loss, and fevers.*
- *Migratory pauciarticular or polyarticular arthritis.*
- *Orbital pseudotumor, nearly always associated with chronic nasosinus conditions.*
- *Nodular or cavitary lung lesions that are initially misdiagnosed as malignancies or infections.*
- *Rapidly progressive glomerulonephritis.*
- *Antineutrophil cytoplasmic antibodies (ANCAs) are helpful in diagnosis if positive (by both immunofluorescence and enzyme immunoassay), but a significant number of patients with WG are ANCA-negative.*

General Considerations

WG is one of the most common forms of systemic vasculitis, with a reported annual incidence of 10 cases per million. The disease involves small- to medium-sized blood vessels (small-sized vessels more often than medium-sized vessels). It affects both the arterial and venous circulations. The cause of WG is not known, but the prominence of upper and lower airway involvement suggests a response to an inhaled antigen. The disease is the prototype of conditions associated with ANCAs. These antibodies are believed to amplify rather than initiate the inflammatory process. WG occurs in people of all ethnic backgrounds but demonstrates a strong predominance for whites, particularly those of northern European ancestry. The male:female ratio is approximately 1:1. Although the mean age at diagnosis is 50 years, the disease also affects the elderly and (occasionally) children.

WG typically presents in a subacute fashion. Patients complain of apparently innocuous symptoms such as nasal stuffiness, "sinusitis," and decreases in hearing. During this "prodrome," attentive primary care physicians may suspect and diagnose the disease before the onset of generalized WG. Such early recognition of WG may prevent the disfiguring and devastating end-organ complications of this disorder, such as collapse of the nasal bridge, renal failure, diffuse alveolar hemorrhage, and widespread infarctions of peripheral nerves.

Therapies for WG are associated with substantial treatment-induced morbidity in both the short and long term (see the following section on Complications and Chapter 56, Cyclophosphamide). Careful follow-up and monitoring of basic laboratory tests (eg, regularly obtaining complete blood cell counts) may prevent some adverse effects of treatment or minimize their impact.

Because of the often chronic nature of WG and its tendency to recur during or after the taper of treatment, primary care physicians play an important role in the early detection of disease flares.

Clinical Findings

A. Symptoms and Signs

1. Nose, sinuses, and ears—Approximately 90% of patients with WG have nasal involvement, often as the first manifestation of disease. The typical symptoms include persistent rhinorrhea, unusually severe nasal obstruction, epistaxis, and bloody or brown nasal crusts (Table 31–1). Cartilaginous inflammation may lead to perforation of the nasal septum and collapse of the nasal bridge (a "saddle-nose" deformity) (Figure 31–1). Bony erosions of the sinus cavities are characteristic of WG but only develop after long-standing disease (months).

Both conductive and sensorineural forms of hearing loss occur in WG. Conductive hearing loss results from granulomatous involvement of the middle ear, most often leading to serous otitis media. Granulomatous inflammation in the middle ear may also compress the seventh cranial nerve as it courses through the middle ear cavity, leading to a peripheral facial nerve palsy. Sensorineural hearing loss results from inner ear (cochlear) involvement and may also be associated with

Table 31–1. Major clinical manifestations of Wegener granulomatosis.

Organ	Manifestation
Nose	Persistent rhinorrhea; bloody, brown nasal crusts; nasal obstruction; nasal septal perforation; saddle-nose deformity
Sinuses	Sinusitis with radiologic evidence of bony erosions
Ears	Conductive hearing loss due to granulomatous inflammation in the middle ear; sensorineural hearing loss; mixed hearing loss common
Mouth	Strawberry gums; tongue or other oral ulcers; occasional purpuric lesions on palate
Eyes	Orbital pseudotumor; scleritis (often necrotizing); episcleritis; conjunctivitis; keratitis (risk of corneal melt); uveitis (anterior)
Trachea	Subglottic stenosis
Lungs	Nodular, cavitary lesions; nonspecific pulmonary infiltrates; alveolar hemorrhage; bronchial lesions
Heart	Occasional valvular lesions, usually not evident during life; pericarditis
Gastrointestinal	Mesenteric vasculitis uncommon; splenic involvement quite common but usually subclinical (detected as splenic infarcts on cross-sectional imaging)
Kidneys	Glomerulonephritis (small-vessel vasculitis of the kidney). Medium-vessel vasculitis occasionally evident on renal biopsy.
Skin	Palpable purpura, subcutaneous nodules (Churg-Strauss granulomas), ulcers, vesiculobullous lesions, splinter hemorrhages
Joints	Migratory pauciarthritis or polyarthritis or arthralgias. Arthritis is nondestructive.
Peripheral nerve	Sensory or motor mononeuritis multiplex
Central nervous system	True central nervous system vasculitis rare but reported. More common is granulomatous involvement of the meninges, with a clinical picture of chronic meningitis.

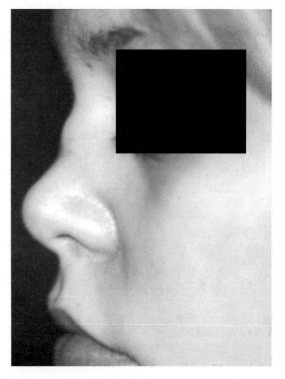

Figure 31–1. Cartilaginous inflammation of the nose in Wegener granulomatosis may lead to nasal septal perforation and ultimately to collapse of the nasal bridge ("saddle-nose" deformity).

vestibular dysfunction (eg, nausea, vertigo, tinnitus). "Mixed" hearing loss, the simultaneous occurrence of both conductive and sensorineural hearing loss, is common in WG.

2. Eyes—WG may present with a variety of inflammatory lesions of the eye (Figure 31–2). Orbital pseudotumors behind the eye may lead to proptosis and visual loss through ischemia of the optic nerve. Scleritis causes photophobia and painful, often raised, scleral erythema. If unchecked, necrotizing scleritis may lead to scleral thinning, scleromalacia perforans, and visual loss. Peripheral keratitis may cause ulcerations on the margin of the cornea and lead to the syndrome of "corneal melt." Although episcleritis and conjunctivitis constitute less serious ocular complications, they are very common in WG. Their occurrence may be the presenting symptom of the disease or the first manifestation of a flare. Other ocular complications of WG are anterior uveitis and nasolacrimal duct obstruction. Retinal lesions (posterior uveitis) are rare in WG.

3. Trachea—Subglottic stenosis, the result of tracheal inflammation and scarring below the vocal cords, is a

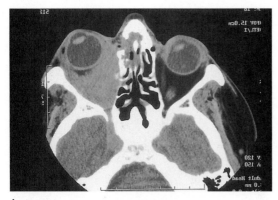

A

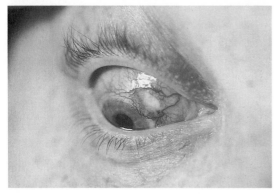

B

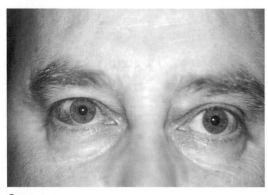

C

Figure 31–2. **A:** Computed tomography scan of the orbit showing an orbital pseudotumor, leading to proptosis and visual loss. **B:** Scleritis with a marginal corneal ulceration. **C:** Painless erythema of the superficial surface of the eye—episcleritis—the most common ocular complication of Wegener granulomatosis.

potentially disabling manifestation largely specific to WG (relapsing polychondritis can also cause this lesion). Subglottic involvement is often asymptomatic and may manifest itself only as a subtle hoarseness. With time, however, airway scarring and profound tracheal narrowing may occur.

4. Lungs—Approximately 80% of patients with WG have pulmonary lesions during the course of their disease. Pulmonary symptoms include cough, hemoptysis, dyspnea, and sometimes pleuritic chest pain. Lung lesions are often asymptomatic, however, and may be detected only if chest imaging is performed. The most common radiographic findings are pulmonary infiltrates and nodules. The infiltrates, which may wax and wane, are often misdiagnosed initially as pneumonia. Nodules are usually multiple and bilateral and often cavitary. Pulmonary capillaritis may lead to hemoptysis and rapidly changing alveolar infiltrates.

5. Kidneys—Renal disease is the most ominous clinical manifestation of WG. While renal involvement is present in approximately 20% of patients with WG at the time of diagnosis, this manifestation develops in nearly 80% of patients at some point during the course of the disease. The clinical presentation of renal disease in WG is rapidly progressive glomerulonephritis: hematuria, red blood cell casts, proteinuria (usually nonnephrotic), and rising serum creatinine. Without appropriate therapy, loss of renal function may ensue within days or weeks.

6. Other organs—Nonspecific arthralgias and frank arthritis often occur early in the course of WG. The arthritis of WG is migratory in nature and may assume a variety of joint patterns, from a pauciarticular syndrome of lower extremity joints to a polyarthritis of the small joints of the hands. Splinter hemorrhages and digital ischemia and gangrene resulting from inflammation in medium-sized digital arteries are occasionally the presenting feature of WG. The skin manifestations of WG include the full array of findings associated with cutaneous vasculitis: palpable purpura, papules, ulcers, and vesiculobullous lesions. Examination of the skin should include careful inspection for the nodular lesions of "Churg-Strauss granulomas" (cutaneous extravascular necrotizing granulomas), typically located on the extensor surfaces of the elbows and other pressure points (Figure 31–3). Lesions resembling pyoderma gangrenosum may also occur. Although involvement of the brain parenchyma with WG has been reported, meningeal inflammation (presenting as excruciating headaches and cranial neuropathies) is a more typical central nervous system disease manifestation. Mononeuritis multiplex may also accompany WG but is less characteristic of this disease than others (eg, poly-

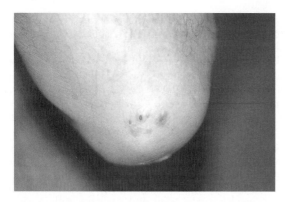

Figure 31–3. The patient has Wegener granulomatosis and has a positive test result for rheumatoid factor. The nodule over the extensor surface of the elbow was initially misdiagnosed as a rheumatoid nodule instead of a "Churg-Strauss granuloma" (cutaneous extravascular necrotizing granuloma).

arteritis nodosa, microscopic polyangiitis, and the Churg-Strauss syndrome).

B. Laboratory Findings

The results of routine laboratory tests and more specialized assays in WG are shown in Table 31–2. All of these tests are appropriate at the initial evaluation of a patient with possible WG. The exclusion of renal disease through the careful performance of a urinalysis is essential in the evaluation and follow-up of all patients with WG. The erythrocyte sedimentation rate and serum C-reactive protein level are useful in the longitudinal evaluation of disease activity.

C. Imaging Studies

Up to one-third of patients with WG have asymptomatic pulmonary lesions on radiologic imaging. Computed tomography is superior to chest radiography in demonstrating the extent of pulmonary disease (Figure 31–4). Consequently, patients with confirmed or strongly suspected diagnoses of WG should have computed tomography scans of the chest as baseline studies. Virtually any finding (with the rare exception of hilar and mediastinal adenopathy) may be present on chest imaging in WG, including pleural effusions and nonspecific infiltrates. Lung nodules are typically multiple and bilateral and have a tendency to cavitate. The pulmonary lesions are often located in the periphery of the lung and may appear to be wedge-shaped and pleural-based. They may therefore be mistaken for pulmonary emboli or lung malignancies.

Table 31–2. The laboratory evaluation in Wegener granulomatosis.

Test	Typical Result
Complete blood cell count	• Normochromic, normocytic anemia; acute, severe anemias possible in alveolar hemorrhage • Mild to moderate leukocytosis common, usually not exceeding 18×10^9/L • Moderate to pronounced thrombocytosis typical, ranging from platelet counts of 400×10^9/L to occasionally $> 1000 \times 10^9$/L
Electrolytes	Hyperkalemia in the setting of advanced renal dysfunction
Liver function tests	Hepatic involvement quite unusual in WG; when present, there can be elevations of transaminases (AST/ALT) in excess of 1000 mg/dL
Urinalysis with microscopy	• Hematuria (ranging from mild to so high that red blood cells are too numerous to count) • Red blood cell casts • Proteinuria (nephritic range proteinuria in a small minority)
Erythrocyte sedimentation rate/C-reactive protein	Dramatic elevations of acute phase reactants are typical, generally with good correlation to disease activity
ANA	Negative
Rheumatoid factor	Positive in 40–50% of patients, often leading to diagnostic confusion with rheumatoid arthritis
C3, C4	Complement levels are normal to elevated in WG, in contrast to systemic lupus erythematosus, cryoglobulinemia, and other diseases in which immune complexes appear to play major roles
ANCA	Positive in 60–90% of patients with WG
Anti-GBM	A minority of patients with WG also have anti-GBM antibodies

WG, Wegener granulomatosis; AST/ALT aspartate aminotransferase/alanine aminotransferase; ANA, antinuclear antibody; ANCA, antineutrophil cytoplasmic antibody; anti-GBM, antiglomerular basement membrane antibody.

D. Special Tests

1. Biopsy—Because of the numerous potential mimickers of WG and the frequent shortcomings of ANCA (see next section on ANCA testing), the diagnosis of WG is most secure when established through biopsy of an involved organ. Among the organs commonly involved in WG, those most likely to yield tissue that permits a diagnosis are (in descending order): lung, kidney,

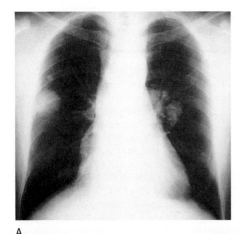

A

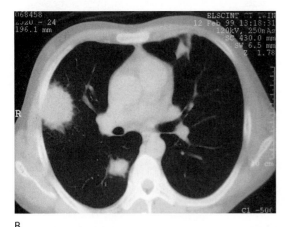

B

Figure 31–4. Chest radiograph and computed to-mography scan show multiple bilateral nodules. **A:** Posterior-anterior view of the chest shows bilateral lung nodules. **B:** Computed tomography scan of the chest in the same patient shows additional lesions not evident on the radiograph.

and upper respiratory tract (nose or sinuses). The tissue necrosis associated with WG is frequently so extensive within diseased tissues that it is termed "geographic necrosis." Even when all three pathologic hallmarks (granulomatous inflammation, vasculitis, and necrosis) are present, the diagnosis of WG requires the careful integration of pathologic findings with clinical, laboratory, and radiologic data. Acid-fast and fungal pathogens must be excluded by special stains and cultures.

Biopsies of the upper respiratory tract (nose, sinuses, and subglottic region) are frequently nondiagnostic, yielding only nonspecific acute and chronic inflamma-

tion. Upper respiratory tract biopsies demonstrate the complete diagnostic triad in only about 15% of cases. However, these biopsies are generally safer than lung or kidney biopsies, and the finding of even parts of this triad in a nose or sinus biopsy may serve as compelling evidence for the diagnosis of WG, provided that other manifestations of the disease are present elsewhere.

WG finds its fullest pathologic expression in the lung, where the large amounts of tissue obtained at open or thoracoscopic lung biopsy may capture the entire spectrum of disease. Transbronchial and radiologically guided needle biopsies usually fail to yield diagnostic tissue specimens. The leukocytoclastic vasculitis of WG may involve arteries, veins, and capillaries, with or without granulomatous features. Vascular necrosis begins as clusters of neutrophils within the blood vessel wall (microabscesses) that degenerate and become surrounded by palisading histiocytes. Coalescence of such neutrophilic microabscesses leads to geographic necrosis.

Although renal biopsy findings are not specific for WG (other pauci-immune forms of glomerulonephritis may have identical findings), renal biopsy results are sufficiently characteristic to establish the diagnosis in appropriate clinical settings. The typical renal lesion of WG is segmental necrotizing glomerulonephritis, with or without crescent formation. Thrombotic changes in the glomerular capillary loops are among the earliest histologic lesions. Immunofluorescence studies of renal biopsies in WG confirm the "pauci-immune" nature of the renal involvement (ie, the relatively sparse immunoglobulin and complement deposition found in this disorder compared with such diseases as systemic lupus erythematosus, Henoch-Schönlein purpura, and Goodpasture syndrome).

2. Serologic testing for ANCA—ANCAs are directed against antigens that reside within the primary granules of neutrophils and monocytes. Positive ANCA assays are often instrumental in suggesting the diagnosis, but the titers of these antibodies correlate poorly in time with disease flares. The two types of ANCA tests now in common use are immunofluorescence assays and enzyme immunoassays. These two tests are complementary in the diagnosis of WG, and both should be used in evaluating patients in whom this disease is suspected. Negative ANCA assays do not preclude the diagnosis of WG: most series indicate that 10–20% of patients with active, "disseminated," untreated WG do not have ANCA. For patients with "limited" disease (see Treatment section), 30% or more of patients may lack ANCA.

With immunofluorescence, three principal patterns are recognized: cytoplasmic (C-ANCA), perinuclear (P-ANCA), and atypical. Immunofluorescence testing alone has low specificity and a low positive predictive value for WG. Hence, the diagnosis of WG should never rest largely on a positive immunofluorescence assay, regardless of whether the pattern is C-ANCA or P-ANCA. In patients with vasculitis, the C-ANCA pattern usually corresponds to the presence of antiproteinase-3 antibodies, detected by enzyme immunoassay. The presence of both a C-ANCA pattern on immunofluorescence testing and antiproteinase-3 antibodies has a high positive predictive value for WG.

The P-ANCA pattern, which (in patients with vasculitis) usually corresponds to the presence of anti-myeloperoxidase antibodies, occurs in approximately 10% of patients with WG but is more typical of microscopic polyangiitis, the Churg-Strauss syndrome, and necrotizing crescentic glomerulonephritis. Atypical immunofluorescence ANCA patterns, which may occur in association with a wide variety of diseases such as inflammatory bowel disease and connective tissue disorders, are not directed against either proteinase-3 or myeloperoxidase and do not imply the presence of a primary vasculitis.

Differential Diagnosis

The protean nature of WG dictates that an all-inclusive differential diagnosis for the varied presentations of this disease is enormously broad. It encompasses sinusitis and pneumonia caused by microbial pathogens, other forms of vasculitis often associated with ANCA, and the confluence of several common medical problems in the same patient (eg, the simultaneous occurrence of pneumonia and interstitial nephritis caused by antibiotics). The major disease entities in the differential diagnosis of WG are shown in Table 31–3.

WG may smolder in the upper respiratory tract for months or even years before becoming a generalized, life-threatening illness. Recognition of the systemic disorder underlying the repeated ear infections, allergies, musculoskeletal symptoms, and other complaints is often delayed. Patients with WG frequently endure multiple courses of antibiotics, myringotomies, and other largely ineffectual interventions before physicians make the correct diagnosis. In short, WG should be suspected when mundane complaints persist long enough to become unusual.

Limited WG may pose difficult diagnostic problems. The destructive upper airway disease that occurs in limited WG may also be caused by infection (eg, mycobacteria, fungi, actinomycosis, and syphilis), malignancy (eg, squamous cell carcinoma and extranodal lymphoma), or illicit drug use (eg, intranasal cocaine or smoking crack). The sinus destruction of WG may be mimicked by nonvasculitic disorders such as "lethal midline granuloma," now known to be an angioproliferative T-cell lymphoma.

Table 31–3. Differential diagnosis of Wegener granulomatosis.

Other vasculitides
Polyarteritis nodosa
Microscopic polyangiitis
Churg-Strauss syndrome
Henoch-Schönlein purpura
Mixed cryoglobulinemia
Goodpasture syndrome
Giant cell arteritis

Infections
Mycobacterial diseases
Fungal infections (histoplasmosis, blastomycosis, coccidioidomycosis)
Streptococcal pneumonia with glomerulonephritis

Malignancies
Nasopharyngeal carcinoma
Hodgkin disease
Non-Hodgkin lymphoma
Angiocentric lymphoma ("lymphomatoid granulomatosis")
Castleman disease

Granulomatous disorders
Sarcoidosis
Berylliosis

Systemic autoimmune conditions
Systemic lupus erythematosus
Rheumatoid arthritis
Relapsing polychondritis

Chronic infections such as those caused by mycobacterial and fungal pathogens are essential to exclude through special stains and cultures of tissue biopsies. Because granulomatous infections of the lung may also cause vasculitis and necrosis, special stains and cultures for infection should show negative results before the diagnosis of WG is made. Infections are especially important to consider in patients with established diagnoses of WG who have been treated with immunosuppressive medications.

Rheumatoid arthritis is a common misdiagnosis because arthritis is a frequent finding at presentation and approximately half of all patients with WG have positive test results for rheumatoid factor. Churg-Strauss granulomas often occur at precisely the most frequent sites for rheumatoid nodules—the elbows—further heightening the diagnostic confusion. (Patients are usually unaware of these lesions, as they may be unaware of rheumatoid nodules.) Other systemic inflammatory conditions associated with autoimmunity (eg, lupus) also affect multiple organ systems and must be distinguished from WG. Sarcoidosis is an excellent mimicker of WG because of the frequency with which it involves many of the same organs.

Finally, many other forms of systemic vasculitis are high on the differential diagnosis for WG. Accurate distinction among WG, polyarteritis nodosa, giant cell arteritis, Goodpasture syndrome, microscopic polyangiitis, Churg-Strauss syndrome, Henoch-Schönlein purpura, relapsing polychondritis, and cryoglobulinemia is essential because their complications, treatments, and prognoses vary widely. ANCA-associated vasculitis can also be induced by certain medications, particularly propylthiouracil and hydralazine. Cutaneous vasculitis is usually the predominant manifestation of drug-induced ANCA-associated vasculitis, and the antigen specificity is usually for myeloperoxidase rather than for proteinase-3.

Treatment

The management of WG should be stratified according to whether the patient has severe or limited disease. Severe disease (defined as an immediate threat to either the function of a vital organ or to the patient's life) requires treatment with cyclophosphamide and high doses of glucocorticoids. The combination of cyclophosphamide (2 mg/kg/d for those with normal renal function) and glucocorticoids (1 mg/kg/d of prednisone, perhaps preceded by a 3-day intravenous "pulse" of methylprednisolone) leads to excellent initial therapeutic responses (and dramatic improvement) in 90% or more of patients and to complete remission in 75%. Daily cyclophosphamide administration is more likely to result in durable remissions than intermittent (ie, monthly) dosing.

Limited disease by definition includes all cases of WG that are not severe. Because patients with limited WG are more likely to have nasosinus disease, arthritis, nodular pulmonary lesions, cutaneous findings, minor ocular complications, and mild renal disease as their principal manifestions, they may benefit from a less dangerous approach to therapy. Patients with limited WG may respond to the combination of methotrexate (up to 25 mg/wk) and glucocorticoids, thus sparing patients the potential side effects of cyclophosphamide. Methotrexate is not an appropriate first-line treatment for patients with severe involvement of the kidney, lung, or other vital organs and should not be used in patients with significant renal dysfunction (eg, a serum creatinine of > 2.0 mg/dL). Regardless of whether cyclophosphamide or methotrexate is used in the remission induction regimen, all patients with WG should receive prophylaxis against *Pneumocystis jiroveci* pneumonia with either single-strength trimethoprim-sulfamethoxazole or 100 mg/d of dapsone. The higher doses of prednisone and methotrexate used to treat WG (compared with other systemic inflammatory conditions) justify the use of *P jiroveci* pneumonia prophylaxis in WG.

Contrary to widespread beliefs, the induction of neutropenia is not necessary for the achievement of remission and control of the disease. By opening the door to opportunistic infections, the induction of neutropenia is far more likely to cause harm than good. One strategy for the avoidance of such infections is to keep the white blood cell count > 4.0×10^9/L. Reducing the dose of cyclophosphamide, azathioprine, or methotrexate is appropriate when the total white blood cell count begins to decline.

In attempting to control the disease and avoid the side effects of long-term cyclophosphamide therapy, shorter courses (eg, 3–6 months) of induction treatment with cyclophosphamide are now used followed by longer-term treatment for the maintenance of remission with either azathioprine (up to 2 mg/kg/d) or methotrexate. A wide array of other therapies (eg, plasmapheresis and intravenous immunoglobulin) have been considered as adjunct approaches for the induction of remission. These treatments have been used in small numbers of patients, so data are insufficient to judge their efficacy.

Patients with subglottic stenosis comprise a unique subset of WG, with a disease complication that often responds better to mechanical interventions (eg, surgical dilatation accomplished through noninvasive approaches and glucocorticoid injections) than to immunosuppressive therapy. Laser techniques should be avoided during these procedures because they may exacerbate tissue injury.

Complications

Regimens of cytotoxic agents and glucocorticoids have converted this once nearly always fatal disease into one that responds well to treatment and enters remission (for variable lengths of time) in most cases. Unfortunately, WG is marked by a pronounced tendency to flare during the tapering of medications or after the cessation of treatment. The requirement of treating disease flares with additional courses of therapy frequently leads to mounting treatment-related morbidity.

Under the original regimen established by the National Institutes of Health (NIH), patients were treated with cyclophosphamide for a mean period of approximately 2 years (for 1 full year after the achievement of remission). Although many patients had remissions that lasted for up to several years, less than 40% of the patients in the NIH series achieved "cures" following their initial courses of therapy. Repeated administration of these potentially toxic treatments to patients with disease recurrences led to substantial long-term morbidity.

Forty-two percent of patients treated under the NIH regimen suffered permanent medication-induced morbidity. The major complications of treating WG with cytotoxic agents (not including the multiple and often severe side effects of prolonged glucocorticoid treatment) follow:

Bone marrow suppression

Myelodysplastic syndromes

Opportunistic infection

Drug-induced injury to the lungs, bladder, and liver

Infertility

Long-term risk of malignancies, particularly lymphoma and bladder cancers

When to Refer to a Specialist

The overall disease process frequently appears to accelerate once renal involvement becomes evident. Thus, the finding of an active urine sediment or a rise in serum creatinine in WG signals a matter of utmost urgency.

Gross hematuria may indicate drug-induced cystitis in patients treated with cyclophosphamide. This complication may be associated with dysuria but not always. Cystoscopy is required to confirm the diagnosis in patients with drug-induced cystitis. Upon the diagnosis of cyclophosphamide-induced bladder injury, further treatment with this medication is contraindicated. Alternatively, gross hematuria is sometimes a presenting feature of active glomerulonephritis. The occurrence of hematuria months to years after a course of cyclophosphamide may indicate the development of bladder cancer and should prompt a cystoscopic evaluation by a urologist.

Hemoptysis, shortness of breath, rapidly changing pulmonary infiltrates, and abrupt declines in hematocrit may all indicate active pulmonary capillaritis. Hemoptysis may be an insensitive indicator of diffuse alveolar hemorrhage. This WG complication requires rapid intervention with immunosuppressive medications (cyclophosphamide and glucocorticoids) and perhaps observation or management in an intensive care unit.

The occurrence of thrush should prompt reevaluation of the patient's immunosuppressive regimen.

A fever in a patient who is receiving therapy for WG signals a potential medical emergency, indicating the possibility of infection in immunocompromised patients.

The complaint of ocular pain, photophobia, or visual loss should prompt a swift referral to an ophthalmologist. Orbital pseudotumor, necrotizing scleritis, and marginal ulcers of the cornea may all lead quickly to vision-threatening ocular events.

Voice huskiness and subtle signs of stridorous breathing may indicate impending critical stenosis of the subglottic region. Some patients present with subacute respiratory stridor. Severe cases may require tracheostomies. Pulmonary function tests (flow-volume loops) provide a useful noninvasive means of quantifying and following the degree of extrathoracic airway obstruction. However, thin-cut computed tomography scans of the trachea are more sensitive for these lesions. In some cases, direct visualization with fiberoptic laryngoscopy is required to make the diagnosis.

Sensorineural hearing loss, which is often associated with other symptoms of inner ear dysfunction such as vertigo, tinnitus, and nausea, may proceed quickly to irreversible hearing loss. The cochlea should be regarded (along with the glomerulus) as an integral part of a vital organ that may suffer permanent damage in relatively short order. Sensorineural hearing loss requires the prompt institution of treatment and consultation with an otolaryngologist to ensure that no other causes of hearing loss are present.

REFERENCES

Hoffman G, et al. Wegener's granulomatosis: an analysis of 158 patients. *Ann Intern Med.* 1992;116:488. [PMID: 1739240] (Report of the long-term follow-up of patients treated under the NIH regimen of daily cyclophosphamide and glucocorticoids.)

Hoffman G, Specks U. Antineutrophil cytoplasmic antibodies. *Arthritis Rheum.* 1998;41:1521. [PMID: 9751084] (An instant classic, even though still not very old.)

Regan MJ, et al. Treatment of Wegener's granulomatosis. *Rheum Dis Clin North Am.* 2001;27:863. [PMID: 11723769] (Up-to-date thinking on the best current regimens for remission induction and maintenance for patients with severe and limited disease.)

Reinhold-Keller E, et al. An interdisciplinary approach to the care of patients with Wegener's granulomatosis: long-term outcome in 155 patients. *Arthritis Rheum.* 2000;43:1021. [PMID: 10817555] (Long-term follow-up of a large patient cohort in Germany, emphasizing the high rate of disease flares following remission. Less bladder toxicity observed than in the National Institutes of Health cohort, perhaps because of the concomitant use of oral MESNA [not currently available in the United States].)

Relevant World Wide Web Sites

[The Johns Hopkins Vasculitis Center]

http://vasculitis.med.jhu.edu

[The Wegener's Granulomatosis Association]

http://www.wgsg.org

[The International Network for the Study of the Systemic Vasculitides]

http://www2.ccf.org/inssys

[The Cleveland Clinic Foundation Center for Vasculitis]

http://www.clevelandclinic.org/arthritis/vasculitis/default.htm

[The National Institute of Allergy and Infectious Disease]

http://niaid.nih.gov/dir/general.htm

Microscopic Polyangiitis

John H. Stone, MD, MPH

ESSENTIALS OF DIAGNOSIS

- *Microscopic polyangiitis is the most common cause of the pulmonary-renal syndrome of alveolar hemorrhage and glomerulonephritis (several times more common than Goodpasture disease, ie, antiglomerular basement membrane disease).*
- *Usually includes combinations of two or more of the following:*
  - *Nonspecific constitutional symptoms, including fatigue, myalgias, weight loss, and fevers*
  - *Migratory arthralgias or arthritis, either pauci-articular or polyarticular*
  - *Palpable purpura, sometimes with skin ulcerations*
  - *Sensorimotor mononeuritis multiplex*
  - *Hemoptysis and dyspnea associated with alveolar hemorrhage*
  - *Glomerulonephritis*
- *Antineutrophil cytoplasmic antibodies (ANCAs) are an important adjunct to diagnosis, but serologic testing for these antibodies has many pitfalls. These tests seldom obviate the need to confirm the diagnosis by tissue biopsy.*

General Considerations

Microscopic polyangiitis (MPA) is a form of systemic vasculitis that may affect many major organs in a crippling or even fatal fashion. Seventy percent of patients with MPA have antineutrophil cytoplasmic antibodies (ANCAs). There has been increasing recognition of this disorder in the United States since the 1994 Chapel Hill Consensus Conference on the nomenclature of systemic vasculitides. Many cases before then were considered to be forms of polyarteritis nodosa, a disease with which MPA shares substantial overlap. An even closer disease relative is Wegener granulomatosis, which is often very difficult to distinguish from MPA on clinical grounds alone. However, there are significant differences among MPA, polyarteritis nodosa, and Wegener granulomatosis in organ involvement, treatment, response to therapy, and prognosis; thus, it is important

to distinguish among these major forms of systemic vasculitis. Table 32–1 compares the features of MPA with these other two diseases.

The term "polyangiitis" is preferred over "polyarteritis" for MPA because of its tendency to involve both arteries and veins. The Chapel Hill Consensus Conference defined MPA as a process that (1) involves necrotizing vasculitis with few or no immune deposits, (2) affects small blood vessels (capillaries, arterioles, or venules) and possibly medium-sized vessels as well, and (3) demonstrates a tropism for the kidneys and lungs. With an estimated incidence of 4 cases per million per year, MPA is more common than classic polyarteritis nodosa but slightly less common than Wegener granulomatosis.

MPA occurs in people of all ethnic backgrounds, but epidemiologic studies in the United States demonstrate a predilection for whites. The male:female ratio is approximately 1:1. The typical patient is middle-aged, but the disease may affect people of all ages.

Clinical Findings

A. SYMPTOMS AND SIGNS

Regarding MPA exclusively as a disease that affects the kidneys and lungs is a major clinical error potentially, resulting in the failure to diagnose the disease until the patient is very ill and advanced features are present in other organs, eg, the peripheral nerves. The five most common clinical manifestations of MPA are glomerulonephritis (nearly 80% of patients), weight loss (> 70%), mononeuritis multiplex (60%), fevers (55%), and a variety of cutaneous findings (> 60%). The major clinical manifestations of MPA are shown in Table 32–2.

1. Head, eyes, ears, nose, and throat—Upper respiratory tract involvement in MPA is limited to rhinitis or mild cases of nondestructive sinusitis. Serous otitis media may occur in MPA but unlike in Wegener granulomatosis, granulomatous inflammation is absent. Ocular lesions in MPA (eg, episcleritis, conjunctivitis, keratitis, and occasionally scleritis) have been reported.

2. Lungs—The principal pulmonary manifestation of MPA is capillaritis, which leads to alveolar hemorrhage and often to hemoptysis (although the latter may be only a late indication of hemorrhage). The typical radiologic features of alveolar hemorrhage are shown in Figure 32–1. Even though alveolar hemorrhage is a hall-

Table 32–1. Comparison of the features of MPA, WG, and PAN.

	MPA	WG	PAN
Vessel size	Small to medium	Small to medium	Medium
Vessel type	Capillaries, venules, and arterioles; sometimes arteries and veins	Capillaries, venules, and arterioles; sometimes arteries and veins	Muscular arteries
Granulomatous inflammation	No	Yes	No
Lung involvement	Yes (pulmonary capillaritis)	Yes (pulmonary nodules, often cavitary)	No
Glomerulonephritis	Yes	Yes	No
Renin-mediated hypertension	No	No	Yes
ANCA-positive	75%	60–90%	No
Hepatitis B association	No	No	Yes (< 10% of cases now)
Microaneurysms	Rarely	Rarely	Typically
Mononeuritis multiplex	Commonly (60%)	Occasionally	Commonly (60%)
Likelihood of disease recurrence	33%	> 50%	≤ 10%

MPA, microscopic polyangiitis; WG, Wegener granulomatosis; PAN, polyarteritis nodosa; ANCA, antineutrophil cytoplasmic antibody.

Table 32–2. Major clinical manifestations of microscopic polyangiitis.

Organ	Manifestation
Constitutional	Weight loss, anorexia, fevers
HEENT	Rhinitis, tongue or other oral ulcers; occasional purpuric lesions on palate; ocular inflammation (eg, sclerouveitis) reported but rare
Lungs	Alveolar hemorrhage; nonspecific infiltrates; pulmonary fibrosis; pleural effusions
Gastrointestinal	Mesenteric vasculitis with microaneurysms in some patients
Kidneys	Glomerulonephritis (small-vessel vasculitis of the kidney); medium-vessel vasculitis occasionally evident on renal biopsy or demonstrated by cross-sectional imaging studies (renal infarcts)
Skin	Palpable purpura, ulcers, vesiculobullous lesions, splinter hemorrhages
Joints	Migratory pauciarthritis or polyarthritis or arthralgias; arthritis is nondestructive
Peripheral nerve	Sensory or motor mononeuritis multiplex
Central nervous system	True central nervous system vasculitis rare but reported

HEENT, head, eyes, ears, nose, throat.

mark of MPA, this complication occurs in only a minority of patients (12%). Interstitial fibrosis and pleuritis occur in some patients with MPA.

3. Kidneys—The clinical presentation of renal disease in MPA is glomerulonephritis. Some patients demonstrate rapidly progressive glomerulonephritis reminiscent of Wegener granulomatosis (Figure 32–2A). Others, however, have renal deterioration that progresses more slowly, over many months. The pathologic features of renal disease in MPA are indistinguishable from other forms of pauci-immune glomerulonephritis, namely a necrotizing, crescentic lesion (Figure 32–2B).

4. Peripheral nerve—Vasculitic neuropathy may be a devastating complication of MPA. The nerve involvement typically occurs in the pattern of a distal, asymmetric, axonal polyneuropathy (mononeuritis multiplex). The first symptoms of vasculitic neuropathy are usually sensory, with numbness, tingling, and dysesthesias. Muscle weakness and wasting follows the infarction of motor nerves (Figure 32–3). Recovery from vasculitic neuropathy may take months; some patients have residual nerve damage after the disease is controlled.

5. Skin—The skin manifestations of MPA include all of the cutaneous lesions associated with small-vessel vasculitis (palpable purpura, papules, vesiculobullous lesions, splinter hemorrhages). In the presence of medium-vessel involvement, ulcers, nodules, livedo reticularis, and digital gangrene may occur. As with most forms of cutaneous vasculitis, the lesions favor the lower extremities.

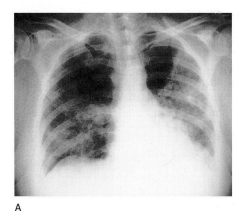

A

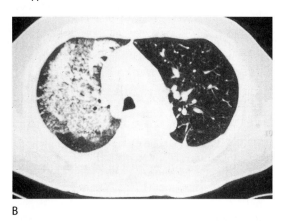

B

Figure 32–1. Radiologic features of alveolar hemorrhage. **A:** Chest radiograph. **B:** Computed tomography scan of the chest.

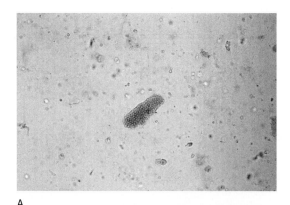

A

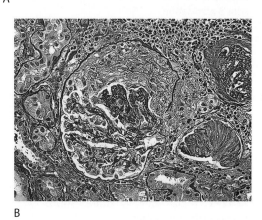

B

Figure 32–2. Renal manifestations of microscopic polyangiitis. **A:** Red blood cell cast in a patient with glomerulonephritis secondary to microscopic polyangiitis. (Reproduced, with permission, from Stone JH, et al. Vasculitis. A collection of pearls and myths. *Rheum Dis Clin North Am.* 2001;27:677.) **B:** Glomerular crescent in a patient with microscopic polyangiitis.

6. Musculoskeletal system—Nonspecific arthralgias and frank arthritis usually present early in the course of MPA and respond very quickly to therapy. Musculoskeletal symptoms may also herald disease flares. The arthritis of MPA is migratory in nature and may assume a variety of joint patterns, from a pauci-articular syndrome of large joints to a polyarthritis of small joints. Destructive joint lesions do not occur in MPA.

B. LABORATORY FINDINGS

The results of routine laboratory tests and specialized assays in MPA are shown in Table 32–3. All of these tests are appropriate at the initial evaluation in patients who demonstrate features consistent with MPA. The exclusion of renal disease through the careful performance of a urinalysis is essential in the evaluation and follow-up of all patients with MPA. The erythrocyte sedimentation rate and serum C-reactive protein level are useful in the longitudinal evaluation of disease activity. Positive ANCA assays are often instrumental in

suggesting the diagnosis, but the titers of these antibodies correlate poorly in time with disease flares. The diffusion capacity of carbon monoxide (DLCO) may be used as an indicator of alveolar hemorrhage, because bleeding into the alveoli leads to elevated DLCO measurements. However, because of the increased sensitivity of thin-cut computed tomography scans, this test has largely been supplanted as a screen for active lung hemorrhage.

C. SPECIAL TESTS

1. Tissue biopsy—By definition, MPA involves small blood vessels: arterioles, venules, and capillaries. Glomerulonephritis is considered the renal equivalent of small-vessel vasculitis (akin to palpable purpura in the skin and capillaritis in the lung). Renal biopsy find-

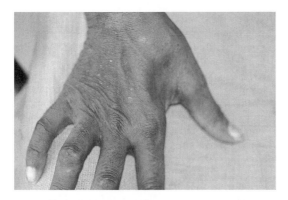

Figure 32–3. Muscle wasting caused by vasculitic neuropathy (mononeuritis multiplex) associated with microscopic polyangiitis.

ings, although not specific for MPA, are sufficiently characteristic to establish the diagnosis in appropriate clinical settings. Immunofluorescence studies of renal biopsies in MPA confirm the "pauci-immune" nature of the renal involvement. MPA may also involve medium-sized arteries and veins, but such medium-vessel involvement is not essential to the diagnosis.

MPA is high on the differential diagnosis of leukocytoclastic vasculitis within the small blood vessels of skin lesions. The presence of extracutaneous findings and ANCA (particularly if directed against myeloperoxidase) increase the likelihood of MPA. If sufficiently deep, skin biopsies may also demonstrate the involvement of medium-sized vessels in the deep dermis subcutaneous tissue layer. The finding of medium-vessel involvement eliminates certain forms of cutaneous vasculitis limited to small-vessel disease, eg, hypersensitivity vasculitis (cutaneous leukocytoclastic angiitis) and Henoch-Schönlein purpura. The involvement of both veins and arteries distinguishes MPA from classic polyarteritis nodosa, which is confined to arterial lesions.

2. Nerve conduction studies—Nerve conduction studies are an important part of the work-up for patients with neuropathic symptoms. Nerve conduction studies may reveal the characteristic asymmetric, axonal sensorimotor neuropathy. Nerves shown to be involved in this fashion are prime candidates for biopsy, along with the adjacent muscle, for confirmation of the diagnosis.

Although lung involvement can be a florid manifestation of MPA, demonstration of vasculitis on thoracoscopic or open lung biopsy is often challenging; frank capillaritis may be difficult to demonstrate. Nevertheless, lung biopsies are often essential to exclude other processes (eg, infections or malignancies) if no other tissue options exist for biopsy.

Table 32–3. The laboratory evaluation in microscopic polyangiitis.

Test	Typical Result
Complete blood cell count	• Normochromic, normocytic anemia; acute, severe anemias possible in alveolar hemorrhage • Mild to moderate leukocytosis common, usually not exceeding 18×10^9/L • Moderate to pronounced thrombocytosis typical, ranging from platelet counts of 400×10^9/L to occasionally $> 1000 \times 10^9$/L
Electrolytes	Hyperkalemia in the setting of advanced renal dysfunction
Liver function tests	Hepatic involvement unusual in MPA When present, there can be elevations of transaminases (AST/ALT) in excess of 1000 mg/dL
Urinalysis with microscopy	• Hematuria (ranging from mild to so high that red blood cells are too numerous to count) • Red blood cell casts • Proteinuria (nephritic range proteinuria in a small minority)
Erythrocyte sedimentation rate/C-reactive protein	• Dramatic elevations of acute phase reactants are typical, generally with good correlation to disease activity
ANA	Negative
Rheumatoid factor	Positive in 40–50% of patients, often leading to diagnostic confusion with rheumatoid arthritis
C3, C4	Usually normal (or increased, because complement proteins are acute phase reactants)
ANCA	Positive in 70% of patients with MPA (and probably a higher percentage of patients with generalized disease)
Anti-GBM	A small number of patients have both ANCA and anti-GBM antibodies

MPA, microscopic polyangiitis; AST/ALT, aspartate aminotransferase and alanine aminotransferase; ANA, antinuclear antibody; ANCA, antineutrophil cytoplasmic antibody; anti-GBM, antiglomerular basement membrane antibodies.

3. Serologic testing for ANCA—Three fourths of all patients with clinical diagnoses of MPA are ANCA-positive. A full discussion of ANCA is found in the chapter on Wegener granulomatosis (see Chapter 31). In MPA, the classic pattern of serum reactivity upon immunofluorescence testing (with human neutrophils as the substrate) is perinuclear staining (P-ANCA). In MPA, the P-ANCA pattern is usually caused by antibodies to myeloperoxidase, a constituent of the primary granules of neutrophils. A variety of nonvasculitic conditions (Table 32–4) can also cause P-ANCA immunofluorescence, but these results are usually caused by antibodies to antigens not associated with vasculitis (ie, antimyeloperoxidase and antiproteinase-3 antibodies). The presence of both a P-ANCA pattern on immunofluorescence testing and antimyeloperoxidase antibodies has a high positive predictive value for ANCA-associated vasculitis, most commonly MPA. Some patients with MPA are PR3-ANCA (and therefore usually cytoplasmic-ANCA)-positive. Despite advances in ANCA testing techniques, histopathology remains the cornerstone of diagnosis in MPA. When the diagnosis is unconfirmed, all reasonable attempts to obtain a "tissue diagnosis" should be pursued.

Differential Diagnosis

The greatest mimickers of MPA are other forms of vasculitis (Table 32–4). Henoch-Schönlein purpura and hypersensitivity vasculitis (also known as cutaneous leukocytoclastic angiitis) can cause identical skin lesions, as can Wegener granulomatosis, the Churg-Strauss syndrome, mixed cryoglobulinemia, and polyarteritis nodosa. The delineation of MPA from these disorders comes from the pattern recognition of extra-cutaneous involvement (kidneys, lung, nerve), the biopsy of involved organs, and ANCA testing. The difficulties of distinguishing MPA from Wegener granulomatosis and from polyarteritis nodosa are illustrated in Table 32–1. Goodpasture disease may present in an identical fashion and may benefit from plasmapheresis or plasma exchange in addition to glucocorticoids and cytotoxic agents. MPA may sometimes cause headaches as one of its principal manifestations and has been known to affect the temporal arteries, leading to its mimicking giant cell arteritis. In addition, some medications, particularly those for thyroiditis, can cause a drug-induced, ANCA-associated vasculitis associated with high titers of antibodies to myeloperoxidase.

A variety of pulmonary, renal, and peripheral nerve disorders must be distinguished from MPA by imaging studies, tissue biopsy, nerve conduction studies, and serologic testing. Systemic autoimmune conditions such as systemic lupus erythematosus and rheumatoid arthritis are also prone to imitating MPA because of their abilities to involve multiple organ systems. These multisystem and single-organ autoimmune disorders may mimic MPA serologically by causing positive P-ANCA results on immunofluorescence testing (see above).

Treatment

The essentials of management for MPA are shown in Table 32–5. MPA is one of a handful of vasculitic conditions that usually requires both glucocorticoids and a cytotoxic agent to control. The usual regimen to induce remission in those patients with severe organ involvement includes high doses of prednisone (often preceded by a 3-day "pulse" of methylprednisolone, 1 g/d) plus cyclophosphamide. Cyclophosphamide may be administered either daily (orally) or intermittently (eg,

Table 32–4. Differential diagnosis of microscopic polyangiitis.

Other vasculitides
  Polyarteritis nodosa
  Wegener granulomatosis
  Churg-Strauss syndrome
  Henoch-Schönlein purpura
  Hypersensitivity vasculitis
  Mixed cryoglobulinemia
  Goodpasture disease
  Giant cell arteritis
  Drug-induced, ANCA-associated vasculitis
Infections
  Endocarditis
Pulmonary conditions
  Interstitial pulmonary fibrosis
  Idiopathic pulmonary hemosiderosis
Systemic autoimmune conditions
  Systemic lupus erythematosus
  Rheumatoid arthritis
Miscellaneous nonvasculitic conditions associated with P-ANCA
  Inflammatory bowel disease
  Autoimmune hepatitis
  Sclerosing cholangitis

ANCA, antineutrophilic cytoplasmic antibody; P-ANCA, perinuclear antineutrophilic cytoplasmic antibody.

Table 32–5. Essentials of MPA management.

- Because most patients with MPA have major organ involvement such as glomerulonephritis, alveolar hemorrhage, or vasculitic neuropathy, the combination of cyclophosphamide and glucocorticoids is the cornerstone of most treatment regimens.
- Cyclophosphamide may be administered on either a daily or intermittent basis.
- "Pulse" methylprednisolone (1 g/d for 3 days) may be considered for patients with severe organ involvement at diagnosis.
- Alternative medications such as azathioprine or methotrexate should be considered after 4–6 months of cyclophosphamide therapy.

MPA, microscopic polyangiitis.

monthly). Daily cyclophosphamide may be more effective in the induction of durable remissions but may also be more toxic; neither of these issues has been tested in clinical trials of sufficient power. Both means of cyclophosphamide administration are successful in the induction of remission if used carefully. The important points are that the medication be used promptly and with appropriate cautions (see Chapter 56). For example, all patients who are receiving treatment for MPA should be given either single-strength trimethoprim-sulfamethoxazole or 100 mg/d of dapsone as prophylaxis against *Pneumocystis jiroveci* pneumonia.

Following the induction of remission, patients may be switched to either azathioprine (up to 2 mg/kg/d) or methotrexate (up to 25 mg/wk, assuming that residual renal dysfunction does not preclude this medication). The optimal duration of these remission maintenance agents is not clear. In general, the continuation of azathioprine or methotrexate for a period of 1 year after the achievement of remission is a reasonable recommendation.

Once the inflammatory process has been controlled with immunosuppressive therapy, primary care physicians may institute renal preservation therapies for patients with renal damage (blood pressure control, angiotensin-converting enzyme inhibition, salt restriction).

Complications

If MPA is diagnosed early and treated promptly, patients have a high likelihood (> 90%) of achieving disease remissions. Approximately one-third of patients suffer disease flares after the achievement of remission. Unfortunately, significant damage frequently ensues before recognition of the disease. One study indicated that the 5-year renal survival for patients with this disease was only 55%. This prognosis may have improved somewhat since the widespread availability of ANCA testing. The other major disability associated with MPA results from nerve damage and consequent muscle weakness caused by vasculitic neuropathy.

When to Refer to a Specialist

Glomerulonephritis in MPA often progresses rapidly. Thus, the finding of an active urine sediment or a rise in serum creatinine signals a matter of utmost urgency. The renal prognosis in MPA may be worse than that of Wegener granulomatosis, perhaps because of a greater likelihood of delay in diagnosis in MPA.

Hemoptysis, shortness of breath, rapidly changing pulmonary infiltrates, and abrupt declines in hematocrit may all herald the presence of active pulmonary capillaritis. Hemoptysis may be an insensitive indicator of diffuse alveolar hemorrhage. This complication of MPA requires rapid intervention with immunosuppressive medications (cyclophosphamide and glucocorticoids).

Nerve infarctions resulting from vasculitis neuropathy may be permanent and crippling. Swift institution of therapy may prevent this complication.

REFERENCES

Guillevin L, et al. Microscopic polyangiitis: clinical and laboratory findings in eighty-five patients. *Arthritis Rheum.* 1999;42: 421. [PMID: 10088763] (Only 70–75% of patients with microscopic polyangiitis are ANCA-positive and only 12% have alveolar hemorrhage.)

Guillevin L, Lhote F. Treatment of polyarteritis nodosa and microscopic polyangiitis. *Arthritis Rheum.* 1998;41:2100. [PMID: 9870866] (Because of its propensity to cause glomerulonephritis, pulmonary hemorrhage, and other life- or organ-threatening complications, microscopic polyangiitis should be treated with cyclophosphamide and prednisone.)

Jennette JC, et al. Nomenclature of systemic vasculitides. Proposal of an international consensus conference. *Arthritis Rheum.* 1994;37:187. [PMID: 8129773] (This paper framed the current thinking about vasculitis classification, and clearly differentiated microscopic polyangiitis from classic polyarteritis nodosa.)

Niles JL, et al. The syndrome of lung hemorrhage and nephritis is usually an ANCA-associated condition. *Arch Intern Med.* 1996;156:440. [PMID: 8607730] (ANCA-associated diseases [eg, microscopic polyangiitis and Wegener granulomatosis] were several times more common than Goodpasture disease.)

Savage CO, et al. Microscopic polyarteritis: presentation, pathology, and prognosis. *Q J Med.* 1985;56:467. [PMID: 4048389]

Relevant World Wide Web Sites

[The Johns Hopkins Vasculitis Center]
http://vasculitis.med.jhu.edu
[The International Network for the Study of the Systemic Vasculitides]
http://www2.ccf.org/inssys
[The Cleveland Clinic Foundation Center for Vasculitis]
http://www.clevelandclinic.org/arthritis/vasculitis/default.htm

Churg-Strauss Syndrome

33

John H. Stone, MD, MPH

ESSENTIALS OF DIAGNOSIS

- *Asthma, eosinophilia, and systemic vasculitis are the three hallmarks of Churg-Strauss syndrome.*
- *Classic clinical features include the following:*
  - *Allergic rhinitis/nasal polyposis*
  - *Obstructive airway disease*
  - *Peripheral eosinophilia (10–60% of all circulating leukocytes)*
  - *Fleeting pulmonary infiltrates and occasional alveolar hemorrhage*
  - *Vasculitic neuropathy*
  - *Congestive heart failure*
- *Approximately 50% of patients with Churg-Strauss syndrome have antineutrophil cytoplasmic antibodies (ANCAs), usually with a specificity for myeloperoxidase (MPO).*

General Considerations

In 1951, Churg and Strauss reported a series of 13 patients with "periarteritis nodosa" (see Chapter 34) who demonstrated severe asthma and an unusual constellation of other symptoms: "fever. . . hypereosinophilia, symptoms of cardiac failure, renal damage, and peripheral neuropathy, resulting from vascular embarrassment. . . ." The investigators termed this new disease "allergic angiitis and allergic granulomatosis," and specified three histologic criteria for the diagnosis: (1) the presence of necrotizing vasculitis, (2) tissue infiltration by eosinophils, and (3) extravascular granulomas.

In 1990, an American College of Rheumatology panel liberalized the criteria for the classification of this disease, dropping the requirements for histopathologically proven vasculitis and granulomas (Table 33–1). The Chapel Hill Consensus Conference on nomenclature of the vasculitides subsequently defined Churg-Strauss syndrome (CSS) as a disorder characterized by eosinophil-rich, granulomatous inflammation of the respiratory tract and necrotizing vasculitis of small- to medium-sized vessels, associated with asthma and eosinophilia.

CSS is a rare disease—significantly more rare than Wegener granulomatosis, a related disease. The annual incidence of CSS is approximately 2.4 cases per million individuals. The distribution of cases is roughly equal between males and females. In recent years, associations between the use of leukotriene antagonists and CSS have been reported. Rather than causing the disease, however, it is more likely that these highly effective asthma medications permit the tapering of glucocorticoids for obstructive airway disease, thereby "unmasking" underlying CSS.

Clinical Findings

A. SYMPTOMS AND SIGNS

After the diagnosis of CSS has been made, three disease phases are often recognizable:

- *Prodrome:* Characterized by the presence of allergic disease (typically asthma or allergic rhinitis). This phase often lasts for several years.
- *Eosinophilia/tissue infiltration:* Remarkably high peripheral eosinophilia may occur and tissue infiltration by eosinophils is observed in the lung, gastrointestinal tract, and other tissues.
- *Vasculitis:* Systemic necrotizing vasculitis afflicts a wide range of organs, ranging from the heart and lungs to peripheral nerves and skin (Figure 33–1).

1. Nose and sinuses—Upper airway disease in CSS usually takes the form of nasal polyps or allergic rhinitis. A surprisingly high percentage of patients with CSS have histories of nasal polypectomies, usually long before suspicion of an underlying disease is raised. Although pansinusitis occurs frequently, destructive upper airway disease is not characteristic of CSS.

2. Ears—Middle ear granulation tissue with eosinophilic infiltrates occurs in some patients, leading to conductive hearing loss. Cases of sensorineural hearing loss have also been reported.

3. Lungs—More than 90% of patients with CSS have histories of asthma. Typically, the asthma represents either obstructive pulmonary disease of new onset or a significant worsening of long-standing disease. Upon encroachment of the vasculitis phase of CSS, patients'

Table 33–1. American College of Rheumatology 1990 criteria for the classification of Churg-Strauss syndrome.[a]

Criterion	Definition
Asthma	History of wheezing or diffuse high-pitched rales on expiration
Eosinophilia	Eosinophilia > 10% on white blood cell differential count
Mononeuropathy or polyneuropathy	Development of mononeuropathy, multiple mononeuropathies, or polyneuropathy (ie, stocking/glove distribution)
Pulmonary infiltrates, nonfixed	Migratory or transitory pulmonary infiltrates on radiographs
Paranasal sinus abnormality	History of acute or chronic paranasal sinus pain or tenderness, or radiographic opacification of the paranasal sinuses
Extravascular eosinophils	Biopsy including artery, arteriole, or venule, showing accumulations of eosinophils in extravascular areas

[a]To be classified has having Churg-Strauss syndrome, a patient must have at least four of these six criteria. Among patients with various forms of systemic vasculitis, the sensitivity of these criteria for the classification of an individual patient as having the Churg-Strauss syndrome was estimated to be 85%.
Adapted from Masi AT, et al. *Arthritis Rheum.* 1990.

asthma may improve substantially, even before therapy for vasculitis has begun. Following successful treatment of the vasculitic phase, however, glucocorticoid-dependent asthma persists in many patients.

The pathologic features of lung disease in CSS vary according to the disease phase. In the early phases, there may be extensive eosinophilic infiltration of the alveoli and interstitium. During the vasculitic phase, necrotizing vasculitis and granulomas may be evident. In the current era, when many patients with asthma are treated with varying doses of systemic glucocorticoids, lung biopsy specimens showing all three histologic hallmarks of this disease are unusual.

4. Peripheral nerves—Mononeuritis multiplex occurs with a remarkable frequency in CSS, with often devastating effects. Vasculitic neuropathy was evident in 74 (77%) of the 96 patients in one series. Nerve infarctions may appear several weeks after the start of appropriate treatment. This may be due to continued disease activity but is more likely secondary to thrombosis of vessels that have become severely compromised by previously active inflammation. Nerve infarctions clinically are heralded by the abrupt occurrence of a foot drop, wrist drop, or some other focal nerve lesion. Muscle wasting secondary to nerve infarctions may continue to appear for weeks after the disease has been brought under control (Figure 33–2).

5. Heart—Cardiac involvement also occurs with a disproportionate frequency in CSS. Some form of cardiac involvement, usually congestive heart failure, occurred in 12.5% of patients in one large series. Cardiac complications are a common cause of death in CSS.

6. Skin—Skin disease in CSS takes many forms, none of which is specific: Palpable purpura, papules, ulcers, and vesiculobullous lesions are common. Nodular skin lesions are usually "Churg-Strauss granulomas" (cutaneous extravascular necrotizing granulomas). These tend to occur on the extensor surfaces of the elbows and other pressure points. Skin biopsy specimens in CSS reveal eosinophilic infiltration of blood vessel walls. Splinter hemorrhages, digital ischemia, and gangrene associated with inflammation in medium-sized digital arteries are often present at the time of diagnosis.

7. Kidneys—Renal disease in CSS has been described as less common and less likely to cause end-stage renal disease compared with the glomerulonephritis observed in other forms of ANCA-associated vasculitis. However, the histopathologic findings are often indistinguishable from those of other pauci-immune vasculitides (Wegener granulomatosis, microscopic polyangiitis, and renal-limited vasculitis), and aggressive renal lesions in CSS have been reported.

8. Joints—Nonspecific arthralgias and frank arthritis often occur early in the course of CSS. The arthritis of CSS is migratory in nature and may assume a variety of joint patterns, from a pauciarticular syndrome of lower extremity joints to a polyarthritis of the small joints of the hands.

B. LABORATORY FINDINGS

Eosinophilia (before treatment) is a sine qua non of CSS. Eosinophil counts may comprise as much as 60% of the total white blood cell count. Eosinophil counts are usually sensitive markers of disease flares, but respond very quickly—within 24 hours—to treatment with high doses of glucocorticoids. Most patients with CSS also have elevated serum IgE levels. Serum complement levels are usually normal. (Immune complexes are not believed to play a primary role in this disease.) The erythrocyte sedimentation rate and serum C-reactive protein level are useful in the longitudinal evaluation of disease activity. Standardized assays for other biomarkers that correlate well with clinical disease activity, eg, interleukin-5 and eosinophil cationic protein, are not widely available.

The reported percentages of CSS patients with ANCA are somewhat variable, with most figures in the literature in the range of 50% (see Chapter 31, Wegener Granulomatosis, for a full discussion of ANCA).

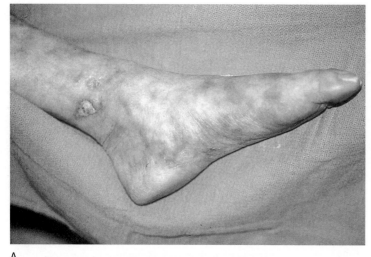

A

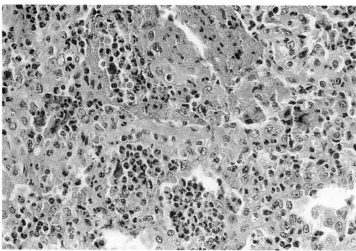

B

Figure 33–1. **A:** Foot of a patient with Churg-Strauss syndrome showing livedo reticularis and a cutaneous ulcer just superior to the medial malleolus. The patient's foot is held in extension because of a left foot drop (vasculitis neuropathy of the left peroneal nerve). **B:** Eosinophilic pneumonia in a patient with Churg-Strauss syndrome. Biopsy shows dense clusters of eosinophils within the lung parenchyma.

Antibodies to either proteinase-3 or MPO (but not to both) may be found. Of the two vasculitis-specific ANCAs, which include antibodies to MPO and proteinase-3, those to MPO are more common in CSS. MPO-ANCAs usually produce a perinuclear-ANCA pattern on serum immunofluorescence testing.

C. Imaging Studies

Pulmonary infiltrates are evident in approximately one-third of patients with CSS. These lesions are usually migratory infiltrates that occur bilaterally. Pulmonary hemorrhage is unusual but reported. Nodular or cavitary lesions suggest the alternative diagnoses of Wegener granulomatosis or an infection. Among patients

with cardiac involvement, echocardiography may confirm poor cardiac function consistent with cardiomyopathy or demonstrate findings compatible with regional myocardial fibrosis.

Differential Diagnosis

The major disease entities in the differential diagnosis of CSS are shown in Table 33–2. There are many diseases in which patients occasionally demonstrate mild eosinophilia (eg, a peripheral blood eosinophilia on the order of 10% or so in asthma or parasitic infections); few disorders cause eosinophilias as high as 20–60%, as occasionally observed with CSS and its related conditions.

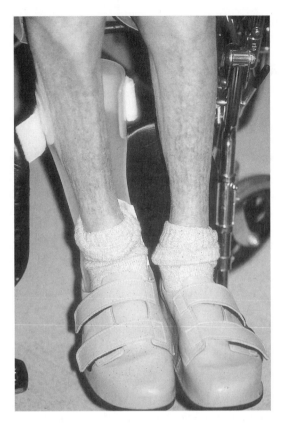

Figure 33–2. The ravages of vasculitic neuropathy. Bilateral ankle-foot orthoses required because of bilateral foot drop. Note severe muscle wasting in both legs.

In particular, CSS must be distinguished from a group of hypereosinophilic disorders: Löffler syndrome, chronic eosinophilic pneumonia (CEP), eosinophilic gastroenteritis, hypereosinophilic syndrome (HES), and eosinophilic leukemia.

The fleeting pulmonary infiltrates of the Löffler syndrome and the peripheral infiltrates of CEP may both mimic CSS closely. Differentiating CSS from HES may

Table 33–2. Differential diagnosis of the Churg-Strauss syndrome.

Eosinophilic Disorders	Other Vasculitides
Löffler syndrome	Wegener granulomatosis
Chronic eosinophilic pneumonia	Microscopic polyangiitis
	Polyarteritis nodosa
Eosinophilic gastroenteritis	Mixed cryoglobulinemia
Hypereosinophil syndrome	Goodpasture syndrome
Eosinophilic leukemia	

be the biggest challenge, however. HES may cause even higher elevations of the peripheral eosinophil count than CSS (counts in excess of 100×10^9/L are not unusual in HES), and HES is often more refractory to treatment.

Many other forms of systemic vasculitis are high on the differential diagnosis for CSS. Wegener granulomatosis, polyarteritis nodosa, microscopic polyangiitis, Goodpasture syndrome (antiglomerular basement membrane disease), cryoglobulinemia, and other vasculitic disorders have clinical features that overlap with those of CSS. However, the finding of eosinophilia superimposed upon a history of allergy or asthma usually permits the clear distinction of CSS from these other disorders.

Treatment

Many patients with CSS may be treated effectively with glucocorticoids alone. (This is in contrast to the related diseases, Wegener granulomatosis and microscopic polyangiitis, which nearly always require an additional immunosuppressive agent.) Nevertheless, certain disease complications, particularly the presence of vasculitic neuropathy, should trigger the use of cyclophosphamide (2 mg/kg/d, decreased in the setting of renal dysfunction or advanced age) as part of the remission induction strategy. Cyclophosphamide should also be considered with other complications of CSS that pose immediate threats to the function of vital organs (eg, the heart). Appropriate cautions are paramount when using this medication (see Chapter 56). Whenever possible, the duration of cyclophosphamide therapy should be limited to 6 months or less. Milder cases may be treated with azathioprine (2 mg/kg/d) or methotrexate (15–25 mg/wk), provided that appropriate precautions are observed (see Chapter 56). For patients whose disease remains active despite the combination of glucocorticoids and a cytotoxic agent, interferon-α has been used with some success in a limited number of cases.

Complications

Substantial morbidity and death may result from CSS. The major sources of morbidity are the disease itself and its therapies. Because the disease begins with a long prodrome of comparatively mundane problems (atopic symptoms, asthma), the diagnosis is often overlooked until the occurrence of significant damage. The complications of vasculitic neuropathy are particularly devastating in this regard. Crippling nerve dysfunction occurs to varying degrees in all four distal extremities, leading to enormous disabilities. The recovery of function in infarcted nerves generally requires months, and in many cases the return of function is minimal. Recovery is likely dependent partly on the age of the patient and on the severity and extent of nerve damage.

Treatment regimens for CSS that include prolonged courses of high-dose glucocorticoids and (often) cyclophosphamide are associated with a high incidence of adverse effects, some of which may be permanent or fatal. Following the remission of vasculitis, many patients have persistent, glucocorticoid-dependent asthma. The long-term use of even moderately low-dose glucocorticoids brings many unwanted side effects. More dangerous, however, is the intensive immunosuppression associated with the combination of glucocorticoids and cytotoxic agents. Even with careful monitoring, opportunistic infections, myelosuppression, infertility, bladder toxicity, and (in the long term) an increased risk of certain malignancies are all major concerns.

Although clinical remissions may be obtained in more than 90% of patients with CSS, disease recurrences are common upon cessation of therapy (as with other ANCA-associated vasculitides). In the largest series reported to date, flares were detected in more than 25% of the patients. In most cases, relapses are heralded by the return of eosinophilia.

When to Refer to a Specialist

All patients with CSS should be comanaged by a rheumatologist and an internist. The input of pulmonologists for optimal management of asthmatic symptoms is also important. Patients with vasculitic neuropathy benefit from individually designed programs of physical and occupational therapy and may require consultation with a specialist in rehabilitative medicine.

REFERENCES

Churg A. Recent advances in the diagnosis of Churg-Strauss syndrome. *Mod Pathol.* 2001;14:1284. [PMID: 11743052] (Enlightened discussion of the pathologic approach to diagnosis in the modern era of glucocorticoid therapy and leukotriene antagonists.)

Gross WL. Churg-Strauss syndrome: update on recent developments. *Curr Opin Rheumatol.* 2002;14:11. [PMID: 11790990] (Current, concise update.)

Guillevin L, et al. Churg-Strauss syndrome. Clinical study and long-term follow-up of 96 patients. *Medicine (Baltimore).* 1999;78:26. [PMID: 9990352] (Largest and most comprehensive clinical report on this disease to date.)

Masi AT, et al. The American College of Rheumatology 1990 criteria for the classification of Churg-Strauss syndrome (allergic granulomatosis and angiitis). *Arthritis Rheum.* 1990;33:1094. [PMID: 2202307] (Discussion of clinical and laboratory features that distinguish CSS from other forms of vasculitis.)

Relevant World Wide Web Sites

[The Johns Hopkins Vasculitis Center]
http://vasculitis.med.jhu.edu
[The International Network for the Study of the Systemic Vasculitides]
http://www2.ccf.org/inssys
[The Cleveland Clinic Foundation Center for Vasculitis]
http://www.clevelandclinic.org/arthritis/vasculitis/default.htm
[The National Institute of Allergy and Infectious Disease]
http://niaid.nih.gov/dir/general.htm

Polyarteritis Nodosa

34

John H. Stone, MD, MPH

ESSENTIALS OF DIAGNOSIS

- *Subacute onset of constitutional complaints (eg, fever, weight loss, malaise, arthralgias), lower extremity nodules and ulcerations, mononeuritis multiplex, and intestinal angina (postprandial pain caused by the involvement of mesenteric vessels).*
- *Angiogram or biopsy of an involved organ required for diagnosis.*
- *Angiography may reveal microaneurysms in the kidneys or gastrointestinal tract.*
- *Biopsies of the skin and peripheral nerves (with sampling of the adjacent muscle) are the least invasive ways of confirming the diagnosis histopathologically.*

General Considerations

Classic polyarteritis nodosa (PAN), as defined by a 1994 Consensus Conference, is a disorder characterized by necrotizing inflammation of small or medium arteries that spares the smallest blood vessels (eg, arterioles or capillaries) and is not associated with glomerulonephritis. Additional distinguishing features of PAN include the confinement of the disease to the arterial circulation (as opposed to the venous) and the absence of granulomatous inflammation.

Reported annual incidence rates of PAN range from 2 to 9 cases per million people per year. A higher incidence (77 cases/million) was reported in an Alaskan area hyperendemic for hepatitis B virus (HBV). With the availability of the HBV vaccine, however, the percentage of cases associated with HBV has declined substantially (now < 10% of all cases in the developed world). PAN appears to affect men and women with approximately equal frequencies and to occur in all ethnic groups.

Clinical Findings

A. SYMPTOMS AND SIGNS

PAN can involve virtually any organ system, with the exception of the lungs. The disease, however, demonstrates a predilection for certain organs, particularly the skin, peripheral nerves, gastrointestinal tract, and kidneys. A nearly universal complaint among patients is pain caused by myalgias, arthritis, peripheral nerve infarction, testicular ischemia, or mesenteric vasculitis.

1. Constitutional symptoms—Fevers are a common feature of PAN. The characteristics of the fever vary substantially among patients, ranging from periods of low-grade temperature elevation to spiking febrile episodes accompanied by chills. Malaise, weight loss, and myalgias are also common in PAN.

2. Skin and joints—Vasculitis of medium-size arteries may produce several types of skin lesions. These cutaneous findings include livedo reticularis, nodules, papules, ulcerations, and digital ischemia leading to gangrene. All of these findings or combinations of them may occur in the same patient. The livedo reticularis, which may have a diffuse distribution over the extremities and buttocks, does not blanch with the application of pressure to the skin. Nodules, papules, and ulcers tend to occur on the lower extremities, particularly near the malleoli, in the fleshy parts of the calf, and over the dorsal surfaces of the feet. Nodules frequently evolve into ulcerations that have scalloped borders (Figure 34–1). Digital ischemia, often accompanied by splinter hemorrhages, sometimes leads to tissue loss. Arthralgias of large joints (knees, ankles, elbows, wrists) occur in up to 50% of patients; however, true synovitis is seen in many fewer patients.

3. Peripheral nerves—Mononeuritis multiplex, the infarction of named nerves by inflammation in the vasa nervorum, occurs in approximately 60% of patients with PAN. The most commonly involved nerves are the sural, peroneal, radial, and ulnar. Vasculitic neuropathy tends to involve the longest (ie, distal) nerves first and usually begins asymmetrically. Thus, the first motor symptoms of vasculitic neuropathy may be a foot or wrist drop (resulting from infarctions of the peroneal

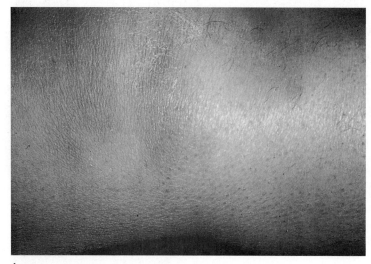

A

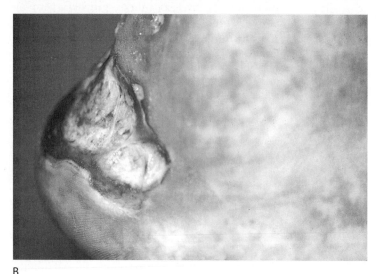

B

Figure 34–1. Cutaneous manifestations of polyarteritis nodosa. **A:** A nodular lesion. **B:** An ulcer with scalloped borders. (Reproduced, with permission, from Williams & Wilkins.)

and radial nerves, respectively). In advanced stages, the neuropathy may mimic a confluent, symmetric polyneuropathy. Careful history taking, however, may unmask its initial asymmetry.

4. Gastrointestinal tract—The gastrointestinal manifestations of PAN occur in approximately half of all patients and are among the most challenging symptoms to diagnose correctly because of their nonspecific nature. Postprandial abdominal pain ("intestinal angina") is common. Involvement of the mesenteric arteries in PAN may lead to the disastrous complications of mesenteric infarction or aneurysmal rupture, each of

which is associated with high mortality rates. Angiography of the mesenteric vessels reveals multiple microaneurysms (Figure 34–2A). These range in size from lesions that are barely visible to the naked eye to those large enough to rupture. Sometimes PAN is detected at cholecystectomy or appendectomy in the absence of other disease manifestations. In such cases, surgical removal of the involved organ may be curative.

5. Intraparenchymal renal inflammation—This major feature of PAN is found in 40% of patients. The inflammatory process targets the renal and interlobar arteries (the medium-size, muscular arteries within the

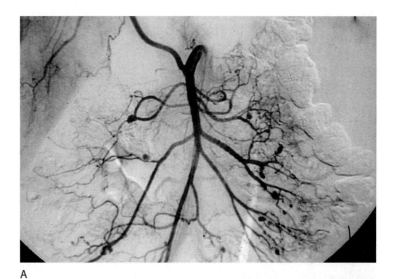

A

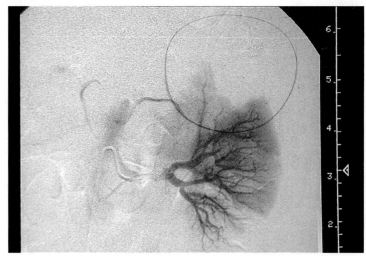

Figure 34–2. Angiographic features of polyarteritis nodosa. **A:** Mesenteric angiogram showing multiple microaneurysms. **B:** A wedge-shaped renal infarction. (Reproduced, with permission, from Elsevier.)

B

kidney) and occasionally also involves the smaller arcuate and interlobular arteries. Angiography may reveal microaneurysms within the kidney or large, wedge-shaped renal infarctions (Figure 34–2B). Red blood cell casts on urinalysis imply glomerulonephritis and thus usually implicate another disease (eg, microscopic polyangiitis). However, both proteinuria and hematuria may be observed in PAN.

6. Cardiac symptoms—Patchy necrosis of the myocardium caused by subclinical arteriolar involvement is a frequent finding. Tachycardia is common, either as a manifestation of direct cardiac involvement or a reflection of the general inflammatory state. Congestive

heart failure and myocardial infarction sometimes occur. Specific heart lesions are rarely diagnosed while the patient is alive; however, autopsy series indicate that cardiac involvement is present in a majority of patients with PAN.

7. Miscellaneous—Central nervous system involvement occurs in a small percentage of patients with PAN. The usual presentations are encephalopathy and strokes. Renin-mediated hypertension may contribute to both of these neurologic complications. Other unusual presentations of PAN include involvement of the eyes (scleritis), pancreas, testicles, ureters, breasts, and ovaries.

B. LABORATORY FINDINGS

Although the laboratory features of PAN are often strikingly abnormal and help characterize the disease process as inflammatory, they do not distinguish PAN from a host of other inflammatory diseases. Anemia, thrombocytosis, and elevation of acute phase reactants are typical (Table 34–1). Erythrocyte sedimentation rate and C-reactive protein are often useful in longitudinal evaluations of disease activity but are imperfect for this purpose. Assays for antinuclear antibodies and rheumatoid factor are also generally negative in patients with PAN, but low titers of these antibodies are detected in a few patients. Patients with HBV-associated PAN are generally hypocomplementemic, regardless of whether they have demonstrable cryoglobulins. When associated with HBV, PAN usually develops within weeks to months of the acute viral infection.

When tested by immunofluorescence, the sera of some patients with PAN are positive for antineutrophil cytoplasmic antibodies (ANCAs). However, specific enzyme immunoassays for antibodies to proteinase-3 or myeloperoxidase (the two antigens known to be associated with systemic vasculitis) are negative. Thus, PAN is not considered to be an ANCA-associated vasculitis.

C. SPECIAL TESTS

The diagnosis of PAN requires either a tissue biopsy or an angiogram that demonstrates microaneurysms.

1. Biopsy—In the skin, medium-size arteries lie within the deep dermis and in the subdermal adipose tissue. Thus, the diagnosis of PAN can be made by obtaining biopsy specimens of the skin that capture lobules of subcutaneous fat. Biopsies of nodules, papules, and ulcer edges have higher yields than biopsies of livedo reticularis. Nerve conduction studies are useful in detecting the typical axonal pattern of nerve injury and identifying involved nerves for biopsy. Because muscle tissue is highly vascular and may harbor involved vessels even in the absence of symptoms or signs of muscle involvement, biopsies of adjacent muscle should be performed simultaneously (eg, the gastrocnemius, if the sural nerve is biopsied). Blind biopsies of asymptomatic organs such as the testicle, however, are rarely diagnostic.

2. Angiography—PAN is a panarteritis characterized by transmural necrosis and a homogeneous, eosinophilic appearance of the blood vessel wall (fibrinoid necrosis). The cellular infiltrate is pleomorphic, with both polymorphonuclear cells and lymphocytes present in varying degrees at different stages. Degranulation of neutrophils within and around the arterial wall leads to leukocytoclasis. The vascular wall inflammation in PAN may be strikingly segmental, affecting only part of

Table 34–1. Laboratory and radiologic evaluation in PAN.

Test	Typical Results
Complete blood cell count	• Normochromic, normocytic anemia. • Mild to moderate leukocytosis common, usually not exceeding 18×10^9/L. • Moderate to pronounced thrombocytosis typical, ranging from platelet counts of 400×10^9/L to occasionally $> 1000 \times 10^9$/L.
Renal function	Renal artery involvement may cause elevated serum creatinines and, occasionally, end-stage renal disease.
Serum hepatic transaminases	Hepatic artery involvement common in PAN. Can lead to mild to moderate elevations in serum hepatic transaminases.
Urinalysis with microscopy	• Hematuria (ranging from mild to severe). • Red blood cell casts suggest glomerulonephritis and are therefore atypical. • Proteinuria (nephritic range proteinuria distinctly unusual).
ESR/CRP	Dramatic elevations of acute phase reactants are typical. ESRs in excess of 100 mm/h are frequently found.
ANA	Negative.
Antiprecipitin antibodies (anti-Ro, -La, -Sm, -RNP)	Negative.
Rheumatoid factor	Negative.
C3, C4	Low in patients with PAN associated with HBV. In patients with idiopathic PAN, serum complement levels may be elevated (as acute phase reactants).
ANCA	Occasionally positive on immunofluorescence testing (low titers of perinuclear [P-ANCA] immunofluorescence, but specific antibodies to serine proteinase-3 and myeloperoxidases are negative).
Hepatitis B and C serologies	Hepatitis B causes a minority of cases (< 10% in the developed world).
Chest radiography	Normal. PAN spares the lungs.

PAN, polyarteritis nodosa; ESR, erythrocyte sedimentation rate; CRP, C-reactive protein; ANA, antinuclear antibody; HBV, hepatitis B virus; ANCA, antineutrophil cytoplasmic antibody.

the circumference of a given artery. Segmental necrosis, in turn, leads to aneurysm formation. During later stages, complete occlusion may occur secondary to endothelial proliferation and thrombosis. Throughout involved tissues, the coexistence of acute and healed lesions is typical. Even in patients without gastrointestinal symptoms, mesenteric angiography may demonstrate telltale microaneurysms.

Differential Diagnosis

Even when flagrant inflammation is present, PAN may elude diagnosis for weeks or months. Except for evidence obtained from angiography or biopsy, the disease has no individual features that are pathognomonic. Many connective tissue diseases must be considered in the differential diagnosis of PAN (Table 34–2). However, systemic lupus erythematosus, mixed connective tissue disease, and undifferentiated connective tissue disorders usually can be distinguished from PAN by the presence of autoantibodies (eg, anti-Ro/SS-A, anti-La/SS-B, anti-Sm, anti-RNP). These are absent in PAN.

In its early phases, rheumatoid arthritis may mimic PAN, but the arthritis of PAN is usually migratory and

Table 34–2. Differential diagnosis of polyarteritis nodosa.

Systemic disorders associated with autoimmunity
  Systemic lupus erythematosus
  Mixed connective tissue disease
  Catastrophic antiphospholipid antibody syndrome
  Rheumatoid arthritis (with rheumatoid vasculitis)
  Still disease
Systemic vasculitides
  Wegener granulomatosis
  Microscopic polyangiitis
  Churg-Strauss syndrome
  Cryoglobulinemia
  Isolated vasculitis of peripheral nerves
Infections
  Endocarditis
  Deep fungal infections (histoplasmosis, coccidioidomycosis, blastomycosis)
Miscellaneous
  Inflammatory bowel disease
  Sarcoidosis
  Erythema nodosum
  Atrophie blanche
  Cholesterol emboli
  Fibromuscular dysplasia
  Lymphoma

always nondestructive. Similarly, although the fever pattern of PAN may recall Still disease, the evanescent, salmon-colored rash in that disorder is atypical of PAN. Moreover, diffuse polyarthritis develops in 95% of patients with Still disease within 1 year (or earlier) of disease onset. The catastrophic antiphospholipid syndrome, which causes digital ischemia, strokes, and other arterial thrombotic events, may be confused with PAN. However, venous events, which are even more common than arterial events in most patients with the antiphospholipid syndrome, are not characteristic of PAN.

The lack of pulmonary involvement in PAN helps distinguish it from most cases of ANCA-associated vasculitis. The occurrence of pulmonary lesions (pulmonary nodules, cavities, infiltrates, or alveolar hemorrhage) in combination with systemic vasculitis shifts the differential diagnosis in favor of other vasculitides, such as Wegener granulomatosis, microscopic polyangiitis, and Churg-Strauss syndrome. In addition, features of small-vessel disease (eg, purpura) are absent in PAN. Isolated peripheral nervous system vasculitis, a form of vasculitis that involves the peripheral nervous system alone, may mimic PAN and require similar therapy. In addition, in a subset of cases, the predominant features of PAN imitate the presentation of giant cell arteritis (eg, headache, jaw claudication, fever, and polymyalgias). Findings of histopathologic features of PAN on temporal artery biopsy specimens have been reported.

The multiorgan system inflammatory nature of PAN may be mimicked by numerous bacterial, mycobacterial, or fungal infections. These must be excluded with great caution before beginning a treatment course for vasculitis. Finally, a host of other systemic or single-organ diseases may mimic PAN in their individual organ features. These include inflammatory bowel disease, sarcoidosis, erythema nodosum, atrophie blanche (livedoid vasculitis), cholesterol emboli, fibromuscular dysplasia, and malignancies (particularly lymphoma). PAN may occur as a complication of hairy cell leukemia.

Treatment

In patients with idiopathic PAN, glucocorticoids and cytotoxic agents remain the cornerstones of treatment. Approximately half of patients with PAN achieve remissions or cures with high doses of glucocorticoids alone. Cyclophosphamide (eg, 2 mg/kg/d orally or 0.6 g/m^2/mo intravenously, decreased in the setting of renal dysfunction) is indicated for patients whose disease is refractory to corticosteroids or who have serious involvement of major organs. Prophylaxis against *Pneumocystis jiroveci* pneumonia is an important consideration in patients treated with these medications.

Treatment of HBV-associated PAN with immunosuppressive agents has deleterious long-term effects on the liver. Fortunately, the availability of effective antiviral agents has revolutionized the treatment of HBV-associated cases in recent years. One effective strategy involves the initial use of prednisone (1 mg/kg/d) to suppress the inflammation. Patients begin 6-week courses of plasma exchange (approximately three exchanges per week) simultaneously with the start of prednisone. The doses of glucocorticoids are tapered rapidly (over approximately 2 weeks), followed by the initiation of antiviral therapy (eg, lamivudine 100 mg/d).

Complications

Advanced mononeuritis multiplex can be a severely disabling problem from which recuperation is measured in months or years, if at all. Residual nerve dysfunction in the form of muscle weakness or painful neuropathy is common. The patient's ultimate degree of recovery is difficult to predict. The occurrence of bowel perforation and rupture of a mesenteric microaneurysm are potentially catastrophic events in PAN, requiring emergency surgical intervention and associated with high mortality rates. Patients treated with levels of immunosuppression required for PAN are at substantial risk for opportunistic infection and other complications of treatment (see Chapter 56 under Cyclophosphamide and Glucocorticoids).

When to Refer to a Specialist

Appearance of symptoms suggesting mononeuritis multiplex may signal the need for cyclophosphamide and thereby trigger a prompt consultation with the neurologist (electrophysiologist) for diagnostic confirmation and with the rheumatologist for treatment.

Postprandial abdominal pain may be a symptom of intestinal angina. A period of bowel rest, hospitalization for the exclusion of other causes, surgical consultation, and consideration of intensified immunosuppression may be necessary.

Fever in a patient receiving or recently treated with high doses of glucocorticoids and/or cyclophosphamide is considered to be an infection until proven otherwise.

Prognosis

In contrast to the ANCA-associated vasculitides, which are more prone to recurrences, PAN is generally considered to be a "one-shot" disease. For patients with HBV-associated PAN, seroconversion to anti-HBe antigen antibody usually signals the end of the active phase of vasculitis. Among those with idiopathic PAN, disease recurrences are observed in perhaps 10% of cases.

REFERENCES

Guillevin L, Lhote F. Treatment of polyarteritis nodosa and microscopic polyangiitis. *Arthritis Rheum.* 1998;41:2100. [PMID: 9870866]

Matteson EL. A history of early investigation of polyarteritis nodosa. *Arthritis Care Res.* 1999;12:294. [PMID: 10689994]

Matteson EL. *Commemorative Translation of the 130-Year Anniversary of the Original Article by Adolf Kussmaul and Rudolf Maier.* Mayo Foundation, 1996.

Stone JH. Polyarteritis nodosa. *JAMA.* 2002;288:1632. [PMID: 12350194]

Relevant World Wide Web Sites

[The Cleveland Clinic. Center for Vasculitis]
http://www.clevelandclinic.org/arthritis/vasculitis/default.htm
[The International Network for the Study of the Systemic Vasculitides]
http://www2.ccf.org/inssys/
[The Johns Hopkins Vasculitis Center]
http://vasculitis.med. jhu.edu

Mixed Cryoglobulinemia

John H. Stone, MD, MPH

ESSENTIALS OF DIAGNOSIS

- *Vasculitis associated with mixed cryoglobuline-mia (MC) involves both small- and medium-sized vessels. The skin is the most commonly involved organ.*
- *Other frequently affected organs include the joints, peripheral nerves, kidneys, and liver. The central nervous system, gastrointestinal tract, and lungs are involved rarely or very rarely in MC.*
- *Virtually all patients are rheumatoid factor positive.*

General Considerations

Cryoglobulins are immunoglobulins (Ig) that precipitate from serum at temperatures of < 37 °C and redissolve upon rewarming.

Formerly referred to as "essential" MC, hepatitis C virus (HCV) infections are now known to be associated with approximately 90% of all cases of MC. Latency periods of up to 15 years between the occurrence of HCV infection and the development of clinical signs of MC have been reported. In some cases, the presentation of HCV may be the development of the clinical features of MC (usually palpable purpura). Cryoglobulins also occur in the setting of other types of infections as well as in connective tissue disorders and hematopoietic malignancies.

The presence of cryoglobulins is not always associated with clinical disease, but these proteins may result in a wide variety of immune complex–mediated complications. The term "mixed cryoglobulinemia" was coined to differentiate types II and III (both of which contain mixtures of both IgG and IgM) from type I (which contains only a single monoclonal antibody).

Cryoglobulinemia is divided into three clinical subtypes based on two features: the clonality of the IgM component and the presence of rheumatoid factor (RF) activity (Table 35–1). RF activity, by definition, is the reactivity of an IgM component with the Fc portion of IgG. This chapter focuses on cryoglobulinemia types II and III. (Type I cryoglobulinemia is usually not "mixed," being associated with only a monoclonal IgG or IgM in the setting of a malignancy.)

When an underlying infection, autoimmune disorder, or malignancy can be identified, the preferred treatment approach is to direct therapy toward the underlying condition. Occasionally, in patients with rampant systemic vasculitis, generalized immunosuppression or measures designed to remove immune complexes (ie, plasmapheresis) may be required for limited periods.

Clinical Findings

The symptoms and signs of MC-associated vasculitis are caused by the vascular deposition of cryoprecipitate components. In type II MC, the cryoprecipitate contains IgG, a highly restricted monoclonal IgM that has RF activity, low-density lipoprotein and, in cases of HCV-associated disease, HCV RNA. In general, the diagnosis of MC is made by some combination of the following: (1) recognition of a compatible clinical syndrome, accompanied nearly invariably by cutaneous vasculitis of small blood vessels (Figure 35–1); (2) isolation of cryoglobulins from serum; (3) detection of antibodies to HCV or HCV RNA; and (4) biopsy of other apparently involved organs as necessary to exclude other diagnoses. Because assays for cryoglobulins are not 100% sensitive and because HCV does not cause all cases of MC, all four of these conditions are not required.

A. Symptoms and Signs

1. Skin—A major hallmark of MC is a small-vessel vasculitis of the skin. Medium-vessel vasculitis may also be present, but this type of involvement does not occur without small-vessel disease. Biopsy of the skin with immunofluorescence studies shows an immune complex–mediated leukocytoclastic vasculitis, with deposition of IgG, IgM, C3, and other immunoreactants in and around the walls of small- and medium-sized vessels. Vascular thrombi are also prominent in many cases. Palpable purpura with a predilection for the lower extremities is the typical skin rash, but the rash is also found sometimes on the upper extremities, trunk,

Table 35–1. Types of cryoglobulinemia.

Subtype	Rheumatoid Factor Positivity	Monoclonality	Associated Diseases
Type I	No	Yes (IgG or IgM)	Hematopoietic malignancy (multiple myeloma, Waldenström macroglobulinemia)
Type II	Yes	Yes (polyclonal IgG, monoclonal IgM)	Hepatitis C (other infection, Sjögren syndrome, systemic lupus erythematosus)
Type III	Yes	No (polyclonal IgG and IgM)	Hepatitis C (other infection, Sjögren syndrome, systemic lupus erythematosus)

or buttocks. In addition, a host of other types of vasculitic rashes may be encountered, depending on the size of blood vessel involved. Such findings may include macules, papules, vesiculobullous lesions, urticarial lesions in the setting of small-vessel involvement, and ulcers—potentially extensive—in the context of medium-vessel disease.

2. Extremities—Arthralgias are a prominent symptom in most cases of MC. The typically involved joints are the proximal interphalangeal and metacarpophalangeal joints and the knees. Frank arthritis is much less common than arthralgias but does occur. When present, the arthritis of MC is nondeforming. Raynaud phenomenon may also complicate MC.

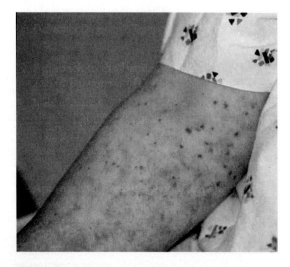

Figure 35–1. Small- and medium-vessel vasculitis in a patient with mixed cryoglobulinemia. Palpable purpura, a feature of small-vessel vasculitis, coexists with florid livedo reticularis, a manifestation of medium-vessel disease.

3. Peripheral nerve—In the peripheral neuropathy of MC, sensory involvement predominates over motor nerve disease. The typical presentation is an axonal sensory neuropathy, associated with pain and paresthesias for years before the development of motor deficits. In unusual cases, motor mononeuritis multiplex occurs but never in the absence of sensory symptoms.

4. Kidney—Renal involvement, which occurs in approximately one-third of MC patients, is typically a membranous glomerulonephritis. As with the other manifestations of MC, the glomerulonephritis typically demonstrates periods of exacerbation and remission. In its renal histopathology, MC resembles lupus nephritis. MC-related renal disease may lead to nephrotic-range proteinuria, but progression to end-stage renal disease is uncommon. Rapidly progressive glomerulonephritis occurs in only a small number of patients.

5. Liver—Although HCV is an obviously hepatotropic virus, the clinical manifestations of liver disease in MC are few. Furthermore, correlations between clinical liver disease and histology are poor, with most patients who have HCV-related MC demonstrating various degrees of periportal inflammation, fibrosis, and even cirrhosis. The formation of lymphoid follicles in the liver is a characteristic histologic feature of chronic HCV infection. Within these follicles (and in the bone marrow), most of the IgM RF is formed. Immunophenotyping of mononuclear cells within liver biopsy specimens from patients with HCV-associated MC reveals that they are mostly B cells that express IgM.

6. Hematopoietic system—In many cases, MC is truly a lymphoproliferative condition. In addition to its hepatotropism, HCV also tends to infect lymphocytes. Infections of these cells often lead to lymphoproliferation and a type III (polyclonal) MC. If a dominant B-cell clone emerges, a type II (monoclonal) MC is produced. In some cases, the emergence of a dominant B-cell clone results from a genetic alteration that favors

B-cell survival, eg, a *bcl-2* gene mutation (translocation of the *bcl-2* gene from chromosome 18 to chromosome 14). Such a mutation leads to overexpression of the antiapoptotic *bcl-2*.

7. Central nervous system (CNS)—CNS disease in MC usually results from hyperviscosity and symptoms secondary to "sludging" of blood within the brain. Hyperviscosity, a rare complication of types II or III MC, is more common in type I cryoglobulinemia, a condition in which the levels of cryoglobulinemia are often substantially higher. The occurrence of a hyperviscosity syndrome is an indication for plasmapheresis. In addition to hyperviscosity syndromes, "true" CNS vasculitis also occurs in a very small number of patients with MC.

8. Gastrointestinal tract—Clinically evident gastrointestinal tract involvement is uncommon, but patients with MC present occasionally with acute abdomens. For example, cases of acute cholecystitis secondary to MC have been reported.

9. Miscellaneous organ involvement in MC—Pulmonary disease, consisting chiefly of interstitial lung lesions, has been described in MC. This manifestation remains poorly understood; cases are usually mild or even asymptomatic. Dryness of the mouth and eyes caused by lymphocytic salivary gland infiltration is not uncommon in MC. This type of organ involvement occurs in the absence of specific serologic evidence of Sjögren syndrome, ie, the finding of anti-Ro/SS-A or anti-La/SS-B antibodies. Bilateral parotid swelling and lymphadenopathy have also been described.

B. LABORATORY FINDINGS

MC is associated with a number of laboratory findings that offer clues to the diagnosis. These tests are of very limited usefulness in the assessment of disease activity, however, because in general their levels correlate very poorly with disease. An overview of laboratory test results is shown in Table 35–2.

1. Cryoglobulins—Assays for cryoglobulins are associated with a high false-negative rate, caused principally by insufficient care in handling. After phlebotomy, the blood sample must be transported to the laboratory at 37 °C and allowed to clot at that same temperature. Specimens are then centrifuged at 37 °C and stored at 4 °C for up to 1 week. The presence of cryoglobulins is indicated by the development of a white precipitate at the bottom of the tube.

2. Cryocrit—The percentage of serum comprised by cryoglobulins may be determined by the centrifugation of serum at 4 °C. The **cryocrit** may then be measured in precisely the same fashion as a hematocrit. As with

Table 35–2. Laboratory and radiologic evaluation in possible mixed cryoglobulinemia (MC).

Test	Typical Results
Complete blood cell count	Mild anemia common. Thrombocytopenia may be present if liver disease is advanced.
Renal and hepatic function	Renal function may be impaired in patients with glomerulonephritis. Hepatic dysfunction often subclinical but evident in most cases on liver biopsy. Liver transaminases may be normal.
Urinalysis with microscopy	Abnormal in cases with renal involvement. Proteinuria may reach nephritic range.
Erythrocyte sedimentation rate/ C-reactive protein	Moderate to severe elevations common, generally reflecting disease activity when very high.
ANA	Positive in the majority of cases.
Rheumatoid factor	Positive in types 2 and 3.
C3, C4	Low, particularly C4 levels.
ANCA	Negative.
Hepatitis B and C serologies	Hepatitis C serologies positive in approximately 90% of patients.
Antiphospholipid antibodies	Negative rapid plasma reagin and anticardiolipin antibody assays. Normal Russell viper venom time (for lupus anticoagulant).
Blood cultures	Negative.

ANA, antinuclear antibody; ANCA, antineutrophil cytoplasmic antibody.

other laboratory indicators, the cryocrit correlates poorly with clinical status and treatment. Cryocrit levels should not dictate therapeutic decisions, which are driven more appropriately by patients' clinical condition.

3. Hypocomplementemia—Because complement proteins are involved in the formation of immune complexes, C3 and C1q are often found on specific immunofluorescence testing of biopsy specimens. Serum complement levels—C3, C4, and CH50—are also low in MC. The finding of a very low serum C4 level in the setting of a normal or only moderately reduced level of C3 is a strong clue to the presence of MC.

4. Rheumatoid factor positivity—Eighty percent of the monoclonal IgMs found in HCV-associated MC share a major complementarity region termed "WA." ("WA" refers to the initials of the patient in whom it was initially reported.) This cross idiotype has a high degree of RF activity. Virtually all patients with type II MC are RF positive.

5. Anti-HCV antibodies and quantification of HCV RNA—Anti-HCV assays are typically performed by enzyme immunoassay or immunoblotting. Levels of HCV RNA may be used to follow the treatment response to specific antiviral therapies. HCV genotyping may also be performed by polymerase chain reaction, but no specific viral genotype has been associated with a predisposition to the development of MC.

Differential Diagnosis

MC develops in up to one-third of patients with Sjögren syndrome, but manifestations of vasculitis are present in only a small subset of these patients. Clinical and laboratory features of MC and SS also overlap. In both disorders, patients may have sicca symptoms of the eyes and mouth and have RF, antinuclear antibodies (ANAs), and hypocomplementemia. In general, patients with MC not associated with SS do not have antibodies to the Ro- and La- antigens.

Patients with systemic lupus erythematosus (SLE) and MC patients share tendencies for ANA positivity and hypocomplementemia as well as the clinical features of Raynaud phenomenon, joint complaints, and an immune complex–mediated glomerulonephritis. The two disorders are usually distinguishable through the presence of other clinical and laboratory features (eg, specific antibody testing for antibodies to double-stranded DNA or precipitins). Some patients with SLE have positive test results for cryoglobulins, but the attribution of disease to these proteins in the setting of SLE is often difficult.

RF positivity and joint complaints among patients with MC often lead to the misdiagnosis of rheumatoid arthritis (RA). True synovitis in MC is the exception, however; when the arthritis associated with MC is present, it is nondestructive.

Other forms of systemic vasculitis must also be distinguished from MC. There may be considerable overlap in the clinical features of polyarteritis nodosa (see Chapter 34), microscopic polyangiitis (see Chapter 32), Wegener granulomatosis (see Chapter 31), and Henoch-Schönlein purpura (see Chapter 38). The reader is referred to these specific chapters for further details.

Treatment

Although certain laboratory tests (see above) are useful in making the diagnosis, there remain no laboratory values—apart from acute phase reactants such as the erythrocyte sedimentation rate and C-reactive protein

levels—that are generally reliable in attempts to ascertain levels of disease activity. As a rule, treatment decisions must be based on the presence of other clinical manifestations of the disease and on the determination by the physician that the symptoms or signs are the result of active disease rather than damage.

MC is characterized by periods of remission and exacerbation. There is also a wide range of disease severity, from mild purpura to severe necrotizing vasculitis. Consequently, all treatment decisions must be individualized, based on the patient's particular circumstances, considerations of organs at risk, and the potential for adverse effects of therapy. The tendency for cutaneous vasculitis to develop in dependent areas may be exacerbated by venous stasis. Support stockings may reduce the number of cutaneous vasculitis flares.

Under ideal circumstances, the treatment of MC is based on the identification and treatment of the underlying cause, such as a viral infection. For HCV, the sustained response rates to interferon-α are poor (15–20%) but improved somewhat by the addition of ribavirin. Pegylated preparations of interferon-α are more effective for the treatment of HCV and presumably, therefore, for HCV-associated MC, as well.

When direct antiviral approaches are not possible or not sufficiently effective, treatment options include nonsteroidal anti-inflammatory drugs for arthralgias and arthritis, low-dose glucocorticoids for cutaneous vasculitis and peripheral neuropathy, and higher-dose glucocorticoids plus cytotoxic therapy for necrotizing vasculitis involving vital organs in a dangerous fashion. Because of heightened rates of viral replication among patients treated with immunosuppression, these treatment approaches should be used for circumscribed periods. Patients with severe necrotizing vasculitis may also benefit from plasmapheresis.

Complications

Hyperpigmentation over the involved areas of skin often develops in patients with long-standing, recurrent cutaneous vasculitis (Figure 35–2). Cutaneous ulcers may heal with scarring. End-stage renal disease results in glomerulonephritis in a small number of patients, particularly those who are not treated adequately. Vasculitic neuropathy may lead to permanent sensory or motor neurologic sequelae. In 10% or less of type II MC cases, the disease evolves into a malignant B-cell lymphoma. The portion of HCV-related non-Hodgkin lymphomas ranges widely in different studies, from 0% to 40%. Low-grade B-cell lymphomas may regress with effective treatment of the underlying HCV infection (ie, interferon), but high-grade malignancies require chemotherapy.

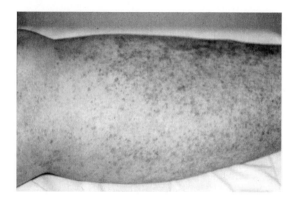

Figure 35–2. Hyperpigmentation of the lower extremities resulting from recurrent bouts of purpura in a patient with mixed cryoglobulinemia.

When to Refer to a Specialist

Many patients with HCV have MC with no overt clinical manifestations of vasculitis. Such patients require no treatment except for that dictated by the liver disease, which should be managed in consultation with a hepatologist. Rheumatologists should be involved in the care of patients with vasculitis, and nephrology consultation is appropriate for those with glomerulonephritis.

REFERENCES

Della Rossa A, et al. Treatment of chronic hepatitis C infection with cryoglobulinemia. *Curr Opin Rheumatol.* 2002;14:231. [PMID: 11981318] (Aggressive use of cytotoxic agents is discouraged in favor of treatments related to the underlying cause, eg, HCV.)

Kjaergard LL, et al. Interferon alpha with or without ribavirin for chronic hepatitis C: systematic review of randomized trials. *BMJ* 2001;323:1151. [PMID: 11711405] (Compared with interferon-α alone, the combination of that agent plus ribavirin reduced the risk of not having a sustained virologic response for 6 months by 26% in naïve patients, 33% in relapsers, and 11% in previous nonresponders.)

Relevant World Wide Web Sites

[The Johns Hopkins Vasculitis Center]
http://vasculitis.med.jhu.edu
[The International Network for the Study of the Systemic Vasculitides]
http://www2.ccf.org/inssys
[The Cleveland Clinic Foundation Center for Vasculitis]
http://www.clevelandclinic.org/arthritis/vasculitis/default.htm

Hypersensitivity Vasculitis

36

John H. Stone, MD, MPH

ESSENTIALS OF DIAGNOSIS

- *Small-vessel vasculitis of the skin, with no apparent involvement of other organs (with the exception of joint symptoms in many patients).*
- *Known by a variety of other names, including cutaneous leukocytoclastic angiitis.*
- *Not associated with any primary form of vasculitis such as Henoch-Schönlein purpura, microscopic polyangiitis, or Wegener granulomatosis; also not associated with well-recognized forms of secondary vasculitis, such as mixed cryoglobulinemia caused by hepatitis C.*
- *Precipitants such as medications and infections are often identifiable, but approximately 40% of cases have no definable cause.*
- *Most cases are self-limited if the precipitant can be identified and removed. Colchicine, dapsone, or glucocorticoids are required in other cases.*

General Considerations

Hypersensitivity vasculitis refers to small-vessel vasculitis that is restricted to the skin and not associated with any other form of primary or secondary vasculitis. Implicit in this definition is that the condition is not associated with large-vessel disease at other sites nor with small-vessel disease in other organs (eg, the glomeruli or pulmonary capillaries). In many cases, an identifiable precipitant such as a drug or an accompanying infection is present—hence the term "hypersensitivity." In up to 40% of cases, however, no specific cause is identified.

The term "hypersensitivity vasculitis" has been associated with much confusion ever since it became incorporated into the first vasculitis classification scheme in the early 1950s, partly because small-vessel vasculitis of the skin may occur in a host of disorders. The condition's name derives from the fact that by the 1950s,

both human and animal models of hypersensitivity—reactions of the immune system to foreign antigens—had been shown to cause small-vessel vasculitis involving the kidneys, lungs, and other organs besides the skin. Consequently, even microscopic polyangiitis (see Chapter 32), a disorder that commonly affects internal organs as well as the skin and is often associated with antineutrophil cytoplasmic antibodies (ANCAs), was grouped initially under the heading of hypersensitivity vasculitis. Because of the confusion surrounding its name, many clinicians have suggested that hypersensitivity vasculitis be replaced, but no entirely suitable alternative has been found. Terms used synonymously with hypersensitivity vasculitis have included **leukocytoclastic vasculitis, cutaneous leukocytoclastic angiitis, and cutaneous small-vessel vasculitis,** among others.

In most cases of hypersensitivity vasculitis, the problem is believed to have an immune complex–mediated pathophysiology. Histopathology generally shows a leukocytoclastic vasculitis, with features of necrosis in some cases but not granulomatous inflammation. Biopsies very early in the course of disease may show a lymphocytic predominance.

Clinical Findings

Table 36–1 outlines the classification criteria for hypersensitivity vasculitis established in 1990 by the American College of Rheumatology.

A. SYMPTOMS AND SIGNS

1. Skin—The lesions of small-vessel vasculitis of the skin include purpura (either palpable or nonpalpable) (Figure 36–1), papules, urticaria/angioedema, erythema multiforme, vesicles, pustules, ulcers, and necrosis. The lesions typically occur first and most prominently in dependent regions, ie, the lower extremities or buttocks. The lesions tend to occur in cohorts or "crops" that are the same age. The occurrence of the lesions may be asymptomatic but is usually accompanied by a burning or tingling sensation.

2. Joints—Hypersensitivity vasculitis is sometimes accompanied by arthralgias and even frank arthritis, with a predominance for large joints.

Table 36–1. American College of Rheumatology 1990 criteria for the classification of hypersensitivity vasculitis.[a]

1. Age at disease onset > 16 years
2. Medication at disease onset
3. Palpable purpura
4. Maculopapular rash
5. Biopsy including arteriole and venule, showing granulocytes in a perivascular or extravascular location

[a]For purposes of classification, hypersensitivity vasculitis may be diagnosed if the patient meets at least three of these five criteria. Sensitivity = 71%; specificity = 83.9%.
Adapted from Calabrese LH et al. The American College of Rheumatology 1990 criteria for the classification of hypersensitivity vasculitis. *Arthritis Rheum.* 1990; 33(8): 1108.

B. LABORATORY FINDINGS

The results of routine laboratory tests and more specialized assays in hypersensitivity vasculitis are shown in Table 36–2. All of these tests are appropriate at the time of initial patient evaluation, primarily for the purpose of excluding other forms of vasculitis that may mimic hypersensitivity vasculitis.

C. SPECIAL TESTS

1. Biopsy—The pleiomorphic lesions of cutaneous vasculitis and the large number of vasculitis mimickers make histopathologic confirmation of the diagnosis by skin biopsy important in most cases. A biopsy specimen of an active lesion (< 48 hours old, if possible) usually demonstrates leukocytoclastic vasculitis of the postcapillary venules. Direct immunofluorescence (DIF) studies show variable quantities of immunoglobulin and complement deposition, with a nondiagnostic pattern. The performance of DIF studies, however, is an important (and often neglected) part of the work-up,

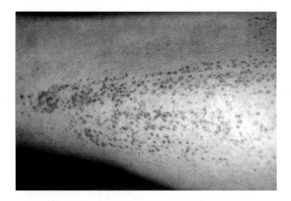

Figure 36–1. Palpable purpura.

Table 36–2. Laboratory and radiographic work-up of patients with possible hypersensitivity vasculitis.

Test	Typical Result
Complete blood cell count, with differential	Normal
Electrolytes	Normal
Liver function tests	Normal
Urinalysis with microscopy	Normal
Erythrocyte sedimentation rate/ C-reactive protein	Mild to moderate elevations in < 50% of patients
ANA	Negative
Rheumatoid factor	Negative
C3, C4	Normal
ANCA	Negative
Antihepatitis B and C assays	Negative
Cryoglobulins	Negative
Chest radiography	Normal

ANA, antinuclear antibody; ANCA, antineutrophil cytoplasmic antibody.

critical for the exclusion of Henoch-Schönlein purpura, cryoglobulinemia, and other conditions.

Differential Diagnosis

The differential diagnosis of hypersensitivity vasculitis is shown in Table 36–3. Hypersensitivity vasculitis must be distinguished primarily from other small-vessel vasculitides, from autoimmune inflammatory conditions associated with joint disease and rashes, and from other cutaneous reactions to medications.

Table 36–3. Differential diagnosis of hypersensitivity vasculitis.

Other vasculitides
Henoch-Schönlein purpura
Microscopic polyangiitis
Churg-Strauss syndrome
Wegener granulomatosis
Mixed cryoglobulinemia
Polyarteritis nodosa

Systemic autoimmune conditions
Systemic lupus erythematosus (including urticarial vasculitis)
Rheumatoid arthritis

Miscellaneous
Acute hemorrhagic edema of infancy
Other types of drug eruptions

Treatment

Treatment strategies for hypersensitivity vasculitis are largely empiric. The type, intensity, and duration of therapy are based on the degree of disease severity in individual cases. For patients in whom a precipitant can be identified, removal of the offending agent usually leads to resolution of the vasculitis within days to weeks. Mild cases may be treated simply with leg elevation and the administration of nonsteroidal anti-inflammatory drugs (or H_1 antihistamines). For persistent disease that does not lead to cutaneous ulcers or gangrene, colchicine (0.6 mg 2 or 3 times daily), hydroxychloroquine (200 mg twice daily), or dapsone (100 mg/d) may be used. For refractory or more severe cases, immunosuppressive agents may be indicated, generally beginning with a moderate dose of glucocorticoids (eg, prednisone 20–40 mg/d). When a patient cannot tolerate a glucocorticoid taper over weeks or even several months, the addition of an immunosuppressive agent may be necessary. Azathioprine (2 mg/kg/d) is used most commonly for this purpose (see Chapter 56 for appropriate precautions with this drug).

Complications

Most cases with a clearly identified precipitant resolve over 1 to 4 weeks, often with some residual hyperpigmentation or (in the case of ulcerated lesions) scars. A subset of patients, however, have recurrent disease that remains confined to the skin and requires prolonged therapy.

When to Refer to a Specialist

Except in cases that are unequivocally associated with a precipitant such as a medication, consultation with a dermatologist or rheumatologist or both is important to help exclude other forms of vasculitis.

REFERENCES

Fiorentino D. Cutaneous vasculitis. *J Am Acad Dermatol.* 2003; 48:311. [PMID: 12637912] (A comprehensive review that places hypersensitivity vasculitis in the context of other causes of small-vessel vasculitis of the skin.)

Relevant World Wide Web Sites

[The Johns Hopkins Vasculitis Center]
http://vasculitis.med.jhu.edu
[The Cleveland Clinic Foundation Center for Vasculitis]
http://www.clevelandclinic.org/arthritis/vasculitis/default.htm

Behçet Disease

37

David B. Hellmann, MD

ESSENTIALS OF DIAGNOSIS

- *Recurrent attacks of oral aphthous ulcers, genital ulcers, uveitis, and skin lesions.*
- *Onset usually in young adults, aged 25–35 years.*
- *Prevalent in parts of Asia and Europe; rare in North America.*
- *Blindness, central nervous system disease, and large-vessel events most serious complications.*
- *Glucocorticoids, immunosuppressive drugs, or both required for severe disease.*

General Considerations

Behçet disease, a form of vasculitis of unknown cause, is named for the Turkish dermatologist who in 1937 described the syndrome as a triad of recurrent oral aphthous ulcers, genital ulcers, and ocular inflammation. Although these features are often the most salient, Behçet disease can cause inflammation in almost any organ. Indeed, involvement of the central nervous system, gastrointestinal tract, and large vessels can be life-threatening. Except for eye disease, most of the manifestations of Behçet disease do not persist chronically but recur in attacks, which usually become less frequent over time. Disability stems most often from ocular inflammation, which causes blindness, and less often from central nervous system disease. Mortality results chiefly from major vascular events, including thrombosis, aneurysm, and rupture of large vessels.

Epidemiology

One of the most striking features of Behçet disease is how common it is in countries along the ancient Silk Road and how rarely it develops elsewhere. Most prevalent in Turkey (up to nearly 400 cases per 100,000 people), Behçet disease also occurs frequently in Iran, Saudi Arabia, Greece, Japan, Korea, and China. In contrast, Behçet disease rarely develops in Western coun-

tries such as the United States, where the disease affects about 1 of every 170,000 people.

Behçet disease is chiefly a disease of young people: typically, patients are in their 20s or 30s when symptoms first develop. Although males are more commonly affected than females in the Middle Eastern countries, female patients predominate in Japan.

Etiology & Pathogenesis

Although the cause of Behçet disease is unknown, the distinct geographic clustering of cases suggest the importance of environment, genes, or both. Genetic studies have revealed a strikingly high prevalence of the HLA-B51 allele in patients living along the Silk Road, reaching nearly 80% of Asian patients. However, this allele is not associated with Behçet disease in Western countries.

Much of the damage in Behçet disease results from blood vessel inflammation, justifying the disease being classified as a form of vasculitis. Although Behçet disease typically affects the small- and medium-sized vessels, it is one of the rare forms of vasculitis capable of also affecting large arteries. Arterial inflammation can lead to occlusion, aneurysm, or rupture. Behçet disease joins Wegener granulomatosis and Buerger disease in being a form of vasculitis that has a predilection for involving veins and causing venous thrombosis.

Vasculitis does not appear to account for all of the pathologic changes in Behçet disease. Many of the pathologic changes—including ulceration of the mouth and gut—may be more attributable to an abnormal reactivity of neutrophils and lymphocytes.

Clinical Findings

A. SYMPTOMS AND SIGNS

Oral ulceration is the hallmark of the disease, tends to be the earliest manifestation, and is required for the diagnosis of Behçet disease. Typically, the ulcers are small, shallow, aphthous-like, and painful, and affect the tongue, buccal mucosa, and palate. During an attack, patients usually have two to five lesions, but some patients may have a single ulcer or too many to count. The aphthae may be so painful that the patient has trouble eating or drinking. Usually, the aphthous lesions heal without scarring over 10–20 days.

Genital aphthae occur slightly less often than oral ulceration. However, genital ulcers tend to be larger, deeper, and often heal with scarring. In men, the ulcers develop most commonly on the scrotum and penis, and in women ulcers affect the vagina and vulva. Genital lesions in men are often associated with epididymitis.

Cutaneous manifestations of Behçet disease, which develop in 60–90% of patients, are protean. Erythema nodosum occurs most commonly, especially in women. Erythema nodosum in Behçet disease tends to ulcerate and heal with scarring and hyperpigmentation, compared with erythema nodosum associated with sarcoidosis and inflammatory bowel disease, which does not ulcerate and heals without scarring. In men, pseudofolliculitis and acneiform nodules develop frequently over the neck and face. Pathergy—the phenomenon of developing an aseptic nodule or ulcer larger than 2 mm in diameter 24–48 hours following a sterile needle prick to the forearm—occurs frequently in Turks but in only approximately one-third of Americans with Behçet disease. Migratory thrombophlebitis also commonly occurs in Behçet disease.

Ocular inflammation, one of the hallmark manifestations of Behçet disease, tends to occur early in the course. Recurrent or persistent ocular inflammation frequently leads to visual loss, making eye inflammation one of the most common causes of disability in Behçet disease. Behçet disease is one of the few autoimmune diseases that can cause both anterior and posterior uveitis. Anterior uveitis typically presents with a red eye, intense photophobia, and blurred vision. The anterior uveitis may be so intense that a grossly visible layer of pus in the anterior chamber (hypopyon) develops. The posterior uveitis and vasculitis of the carotid and retina occur less commonly but pose a greater threat to vision.

Peripheral arthritis or spondylitis develops in approximately half of patients with Behçet disease. The peripheral arthritis may be monarticular or polyarticular, while the spondylitis usually presents as sacroiliitis (with low back or buttock pain). The peripheral arthritis is usually not deforming.

Gastrointestinal involvement develops in about one-quarter of patients. Although gastrointestinal involvement can appear at any time, it typically emerges several years after the onset of oral ulcers. Behçet disease of the gastrointestinal tract most commonly presents as aphthous ulcers affecting the ileum and cecum. However, any portion of the gut from the mouth to the anus can be involved. The most frequent manifestations of bowel involvement are pain, anorexia, rectal bleeding, vomiting, and diarrhea. In American patients, esophageal ulceration appears especially common. In addition, ischemia of the bowel may result from vasculitis of the medium- and large-sized mesenteric arteries. The unusual predilection for Behçet disease to involve veins explains why the Budd-Chiari syndrome develops in some patients.

Central nervous system disease, which develops in 10–20% of patients, resembles gastrointestinal involvement in following oral ulceration by 3–5 years. The neurologic features are variable and include headache and confusion (from recurrent sterile meningitis) and meningoencephalitis. Other complications are thrombotic or hemorrhagic hemispherical stroke, seizures, hearing and vestibular involvement, progressive dementia, and psychiatric disease including personality changes.

Large-vessel vasculitis explains why bruits develop in some patients' chest or abdomen. Affected vessels—especially in the pulmonary and mesenteric circulation—may occlude, develop aneurysm swelling, or rupture. Clinically important cardiac disease develops infrequently, and renal disease occurs rarely.

B. LABORATORY FINDINGS

Behçet disease produces no specific blood test abnormalities. Nonspecific markers of inflammation, such as

Table 37–1. Criteria for the diagnosis of Behçet's disease.

Clinical Feature	Definition
Recurrent oral ulceration	Minor aphthous, major aphthous, or herpetiform ulcerations observed by physician or patient that recurred at least three times over a 12-month period
Plus two of the following criteria:	
Recurrent genital ulceration	Aphthous ulceration or scarring observed by patient or physician
Ocular lesions	Anterior uveitis, posterior uveitis, or cells in vitreous on slit-lamp examination, or retinal vasculitis observed by ophthalmologist
Skin lesions	Erythema nodosum observed by patient or physician, pseudofolliculitis or papulopustular lesions, or acneiform nodules observed by physician in a postadolescent patient not taking glucocorticoids
Positive pathergy test	Interpreted by physician at 24–48 hours

Criteria from International Study Group for Behçet's Disease: Criteria for the diagnosis of Behçet's Disease. *Lancet.* 1990;335:1078.

Table 37–2. Treatment for Behçet disease.

Treatment	Dose	Used as First-Line Therapy	Used as Alternative Therapy
Topical corticosteroids			
Triamcinolone acetonide ointment	3 times a day topically	Oral ulcers	
Betamethasone ointment	3 times a day topically	Genital ulcers	
Betamethasone drops	1–2 drops 3 times daily topically	Anterior uveitis, retinal vasculitis	
Dexamethasone	1–1.5 mg injected below Tenon capsule for an ocular attack	Retinal vasculitis	
Systemic corticosteroids			
Prednisone	5–20 mg/d orally		Erythema nodosum, anterior uveitis, retinal vasculitis, arthritis
	20–100 mg/d orally	Gastrointestinal lesions, acute meningoencephalitis, chronic progressive central nervous system lesions, arteritis	Retinal vasculitis, venous thrombosis
Methylprednisolone	1000 mg/d for 3 days IV	Acute meningoencephalitis, chronic progressive central nervous system lesions, arteritis	Gastrointestinal lesions, venous thrombosis
Tropicamide drops	1–2 drops once or twice daily topically	Anterior uveitis	
Tetracycline	250 mg in water solution once a day topically		Oral ulcers
Colchicine	0.5–1.5 mg/d orally	Oral ulcers,[a] genital ulcers,[a] pseudofolliculitis,[a] erythema nodosum, anterior uveitis, retinal vasculitis	Arthritis
Thalidomide	100–300 mg/d orally		Oral ulcers,[a] genital ulcers,[a] pseudofolliculitis[a]
Dapsone	100 mg/d orally		Oral ulcers, genital ulcers, pseudofolliculitis, erythema nodosum
Pentoxifylline	300 mg/d orally		Oral ulcers, genital ulcers, pseudofolliculitis, erythema nodosum
Azathioprine	100 mg/d orally		Retinal vasculitis,[a] arthritis,[a] chronic progressive central nervous system lesions, arteritis, venous thrombosis

(continued)

Table 37–2. Treatment for Behçet disease. *Continued*

Treatment	Dose	Used as First-Line Therapy	Used as Alternative Therapy
Chlorambucil	5 mg/d orally		Retinal vasculitis, acute meningoencephalitis, chronic progressive central nervous system lesions, arteritis, venous thrombosis
Cyclophosphamide	50–100 mg/d orally		Retinal vasculitis, acute meningoencephalitis, chronic progressive central nervous system lesions, arteritis, venous thrombosis
	700–1000 mg/mo intravenously		Retinal vasculitis, acute meningoencephalitis, chronic progressive central nervous system lesions, arteritis, venous thrombosis
Methotrexate	7.5–15 mg/wk orally		Retinal vasculitis, arthritis, chronic progressive central nervous system lesions
Cyclosporine[b]	5 mg/kg of body weight/day orally	Retinal vasculitis[a]	
Interferon-α	5 million U/day intramuscularly or subcutaneously		Retinal vasculitis, arthritis
Indomethacin	50–75 mg/d	Arthritis orally	
Sulfasalazine	1–3 g/d orally	Gastrointestinal lesions	Arthritis
Warfarin[c]	2–10 mg/d orally	Venous thrombosis	Arteritis
Heparin[c]	5000–20,000 U/d subcutaneously	Venous thrombosis	Arteritis
Aspirin[d]	50–100 mg/d orally	Arteritis, venous thrombosis	Chronic progressive central nervous system lesions
Dipyridamole	300 mg/d orally	Arteritis, venous thrombosis	Chronic progressive central nervous system lesions
Surgery	—		Gastrointestinal lesions, arteritis, venous thrombosis

[a]The efficacy of this drug for this use has been reported in controlled clinical trials.
[b]Cyclosporine is contraindicated in patients with acute meningoencephalitis or chronic progressive central nervous system lesions.
[c]This drug should be used with caution in patients with pulmonary vascular lesions.
[d]Low-dose aspirin is used as an antiplatelet agent.
Reproduced from Sakane T, et al. Behçet's Disease. *N Engl J Med.* 1999; 341:1284.

anemia, mild leukocytosis, and an elevated erythrocyte sedimentation rate, are common during attacks of active inflammation. Patients with active Behçet disease also often show elevated levels of serum IgD. Cerebrospinal fluid analysis in patients with meningoencephalitis usually reveals elevations of protein and IgG and a pleocytosis of either polymorphonuclear cells or lymphocytes.

C. IMAGING STUDIES

Patients with neurologic disease can have abnormalities evident on computed tomography or magnetic resonance imaging (MRI). The most frequent MRI abnormalities are seen with T2 weighting and consist of multiple high-intensity focal lesions that are widely distributed. Angiograms or magnetic resonance angiography can demonstrate large-artery thrombosis and aneurysm, typically seen in the chest or abdomen.

D. SPECIAL TESTS

Biopsies of mucocutaneous lesions and gastrointestinal ulcers reveal a neutrophilic vascular reaction. True vasculitis is rare. The pathergy phenomenon is uncommon in Americans.

Diagnosis & Differential Diagnosis

Since Behçet disease produces no pathognomic laboratory finding, the diagnosis rests upon clinical criteria, which have been refined by an International Study Group (Table 37–1).

The differential diagnosis of recurrent oral and genital aphthous ulceration includes recurrent aphthous stomatitis or complex aphthous, herpes simplex virus infection, Crohn disease, and Reiter syndrome. All patients with recurrent oral and genital ulcers should have cultures or polymerase chain reaction (PCR) testing for herpes simplex virus infection. Medications, especially nonsteroidal anti-inflammatory drugs, can cause recurrent oral ulcerations. Another cause of recurrent oral lesions is systemic lupus erythematosus. The oral and pharyngeal lesion of Wegener granulomatosis and histoplasmosis are not usually recurrent. Stevens-Johnson syndrome, pemphigoid, and lichen planus can involve the mouth, genitals, and eye, but do not produce aphthous lesions.

Erythema nodosa has many causes besides Behçet disease, including sarcoidosis and inflammatory bowel disease. As noted, only erythema nodosa associated with Behçet tends to ulcerate. Some of the skin lesions in Behçet can mimic those of Sweet syndrome.

Syphilis and sarcoidosis are two diseases that, like Behçet disease, can cause both anterior and posterior uveitis. Anterior uveitis can also be caused by inflammatory bowel disease, ankylosing spondylitis, and Reiter syndrome.

It can be virtually impossible to distinguish Behçet disease from Crohn disease unless the patient has bowel biopsies showing granulomatous lesions (supporting the diagnosis of Crohn disease).

Neurologic disease can sometimes mimic multiple sclerosis.

Treatment

Treatment—like the disease itself—runs the gamut in intensity and illustrates how important it is to ensure that the treatment fits the disease manifestation. Recurrent oral ulcers, although painful, can be treated with topical glucocorticoids. Vision-threatening uveitis or life-threatening meningoencephalitis requires high-dose systemic glucocorticoids and immunosuppressive agents such as chlorambucil. Other treatments and their indications are listed in Table 37–2.

Course & Prognosis

Behçet is a chronic disease characterized by recurrent attacks. Most manifestations, except for eye disease and large-vessel inflammation, tend to burn out over 1–2 decades. Disability most commonly results from uveitis (causing blindness), central nervous system disease (causing stroke and dementia), and gastrointestinal disease. Mortality results from central nervous system disease, rupture of arterial aneurysms, and infection and oncologic complications of immunosuppressive therapy.

When to Refer to a Specialist

Almost all patients will require referral to a rheumatologist for diagnosis and treatment. Early consultation with an ophthalmologist to diagnose and treat uveitis is also warranted. Depending on the patient's manifestation, the patient may also need to consult with a gynecologist, otolaryngologist, neurologist, or gastroenterologist.

REFERENCES

Kaklamani VG, et al. Behçet's Disease. *Semin Arthritis Rheum.* 1998;27:197. [PMID: 9514126]

Sakane T, et al. Behçet's disease. *N Engl J Med.* 1999;341:1284. [PMID: 10528040]

Relevant World Wide Web Site

[The Johns Hopkins Vasculitis Center]
http://vasculitis.med.jhu.edu

Henoch-Schönlein Purpura

38

John H. Stone, MD, MPH

ESSENTIALS OF DIAGNOSIS

- *Nonthrombocytopenic purpura, caused by inflammation in blood vessels of the superficial dermis, is the sine qua non of Henoch-Schönlein purpura (HSP).*
- *The pathologic hallmark of HSP is the deposition of immunoglobulin (Ig) A in the walls of involved blood vessels.*
- *The tetrad of purpura, arthritis, glomerulonephritis, and abdominal pain is often observed. However, all four elements are not required for the diagnosis.*
- *More than 90% of cases occur in children. The disease is self-limited most of the time, resolving within a few weeks. Adult cases are sometimes more recalcitrant.*
- *Renal insufficiency develops in fewer than 5% of patients with HSP.*
- *HSP can be mimicked by other forms of systemic vasculitis that are more often life-threatening. For example, Wegener granulomatosis and microscopic polyangiitis (see Chapters 31 and 32, respectively) may also present with purpura, arthritis, and renal inflammation. Both of these disorders have the potential for serious involvement of other organs (eg, the lungs and peripheral nerves) and carry more dire renal prognoses.*

General Considerations

Henoch-Schönlein purpura (HSP) is the most common form of vasculitis in children, with an annual incidence of 140 cases per million persons. The mean age of patients with HSP is 5.9 years. The disease may be misdiagnosed as another form of vasculitis—most commonly hypersensitivity vasculitis—because of the frequent failure to perform direct immunofluorescence (DIF) testing on skin biopsy specimens. In two-thirds of the cases, the disease follows an upper respiratory tract infection, with onset an average of 10 days after the start

of respiratory symptoms. Despite this association, no single microorganism or environmental exposure has been confirmed as an important cause of HSP. The American College of Rheumatology 1990 criteria for the classification of HSP are shown in Table 38–1. The Chapel Hill Consensus Conference on the nomenclature of vasculitides defined HSP as a form of vasculitis characterized by (1) IgA-dominant immune deposits within vessel walls; (2) small-vessel involvement (ie, capillaries, venules, or arterioles); and (3) skin, gut, renal, and joint manifestation.

The skin histopathology of HSP shows a leukocytoclastic vasculitis of small blood vessels within the superficial dermis. Necrosis is often present, but features of granulomatous inflammation are not. Immunofluorescent staining of biopsy specimens shows coarse, granular IgA staining in and around small blood vessels. In the kidney, the renal inflammation is indistinguishable from IgA nephropathy, with a predilection for IgA deposition within the mesangium. Most patients have increased serum IgA levels and circulating immune complexes that contain IgA, as well as IgA deposition in inflamed blood vessels.

Clinical Findings

A. SYMPTOMS AND SIGNS

The classic full presentation includes the acute onset of fever, palpable purpura on the lower extremities and buttocks (Figure 38–1), abdominal pain, arthritis, and hematuria. All components of this presentation are not required for the diagnosis, however. Conversely, classic presentations are not diagnostic of this disorder.

1. Skin—The cutaneous findings of HSP include purpura and urticarial papules and plaques. Among adults, 60% of the patients have bullous or necrotic lesions (Figure 38–2), but these are uncommon in children. Lesions are concentrated over the buttocks and lower extremities and tend to involve the small blood vessels in the superficial dermis. Medium-sized vessels are rarely involved in HSP except in the setting of HSP associated with IgA paraproteinemia.

2. Joints—Joint disease, which occurs in more than 80% of patients with HSP, manifests itself as arthralgias or arthritis in large joints, especially the knees and ankles and, to a lesser degree, the wrists and elbows.

Table 38–1. American College of Rheumatology 1990 criteria for the classification of Henoch-Schönlein purpura.[a]

Palpable purpura
Age at onset < 20 years
Bowel angina
Vessel wall granulocytes on biopsy

[a]The presence of two criteria classified Henoch-Schönlein purpura with a sensitivity of 87% and specificity of 88% in a group of persons with forms of systemic vasculitis.

Migratory patterns of joint involvement are common. Lower extremity involvement among patients with HSP and arthritis is nearly universal; up to one-third of patients have upper extremity involvement as well. The pain associated with HSP arthritis may be incapacitating. The arthritis is nondeforming in nature.

3. Gastrointestinal tract—Approximately 60% of patients with HSP have abdominal pain and 33% have evidence of gastrointestinal bleeding. Abdominal symptoms result from edema of the bowel wall as well as hemorrhage induced by mesenteric vasculitis. Abdominal pain may precede the appearance of purpura by up to 2 weeks, leading often to diagnostic confusion and occasionally to invasive testing. The abdominal pain is typically colicky and may worsen after eating (ie, intestinal angina). Some patients experience nausea, vomiting, and upper or lower gastrointestinal bleeding. Mesenteric ischemia in HSP rarely leads to gut perforation. Massive gastrointestinal hemorrhage occurs in only 2% or so of patients. Gastrointestinal involvement in children with HSP can cause intussusception, a rare

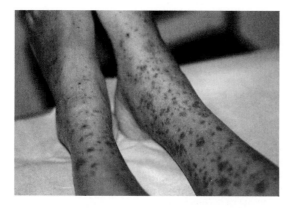

Figure 38–1. Palpable purpura with some superficial ulcerations in a patient with Henoch-Schönlein purpura. Note also the presence of right ankle swelling due to arthritis.

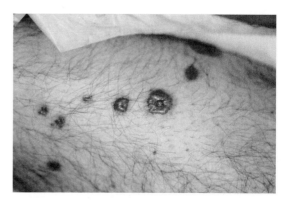

Figure 38–2. A bullous lesion with a purpuric component in a patient with Henoch-Schönlein purpura.

complication in adults. In contrast to idiopathic intussusception, which typically is ileocolic, HSP-associated intussusception is usually ileoileal.

4. Kidney—Forty percent of patients with HSP have renal disease. Unlike gastrointestinal disease and arthritis, which occasionally precede the onset of purpura, glomerulonephritis almost always appears after the development of skin manifestations. The occurrence of glomerulonephritis may be delayed by several weeks in up to 25% of all patients with this complication. The clinical hallmark of nephritis in HSP is hematuria, which is usually microscopic. Proteinuria never occurs in the absence of hematuria. Renal lesions range from minimal change disease to focal or diffuse proliferative glomerulonephritis with crescents. DIF studies characteristically demonstrate IgA deposition in the mesangium. Renal disease occurs in a higher percentage of adult patients with HSP, affecting between 50% and 80%, and is more likely to lead to renal insufficiency (13% of adult cases, compared with 1% of cases in children). Even in cases in which the renal disease resolves spontaneously, many patients have persistent urinary abnormalities (eg, proteinuria).

5. Other organs—Pulmonary and central nervous system (CNS) complications of HSP have been described, but these are very rare. When present, the usual lung manifestation of the disease is alveolar hemorrhage. Seizures are the usual CNS manifestation of HSP; the precise mechanism is obscure. Testicular involvement occurs in up to 10% of boys with this disease and may mimic torsion.

B. LABORATORY FINDINGS

The results of routine laboratory tests and more specialized assays in HSP are shown in Table 38–2. All of these tests are appropriate at the initial evaluation of a patient with possible HSP. The exclusion of other

Table 38–2. The laboratory evaluation in Henoch-Schönlein purpura.

Test	Typical Result
Complete blood cell count, with differential	Mild to moderate leukocytosis common, but otherwise the complete blood cell count is usually normal.
Electrolytes	Hyperkalemia in the setting of advanced renal dysfunction
Liver function tests	Normal
Urinalysis with microscopy	• Hematuria (ranging from mild to too numerous to count red blood cells) • Red blood cell casts • Proteinuria (nephritic range proteinuria in a small minority)
Erythrocyte sedimentation rate/ C-reactive protein	Modestly elevated acute phase reactacts may be observed. Approximately one-third of patients have abnormal erythrocyte sedimentation rates.
Serum IgA level	60% of patients have an elevated serum IgA. Although there are two subclasses of IgA, Henoch-Schönlein purpura is associated with increases only in IgA1.
ANA	Negative
Rheumatoid factor	Negative
C3, C4	Even though immune complexes containing IgA are essential to the pathophysiology of Henoch-Schönlein purpura, serum complement levels are usually normal.
ANCA	Negative (both IgG and IgA ANCA)
Cryoglobulins	Negative

ANA, antinuclear antibody; ANCA, antineutrophil cytoplasmic antibody.

forms of vasculitis that may mimic HSP in presentation is essential. Sixty percent of patients have an elevated serum IgA. Although there are two subclasses of IgA, HSP is associated with serum elevations and tissue deposits of IgA1 only. The reason for the preferential elevation of IgA1 is not clear.

C. IMAGING STUDIES

Chest radiography should be performed to rule out pulmonary lesions. The presence of pulmonary involvement, unusual in HSP, raises the possibility of other diagnoses that may require other treatment approaches (see Differential Diagnosis).

D. SPECIAL TESTS

DIF studies of skin biopsies can only be performed on fresh samples, and therefore must be planned at the time the biopsy is performed. The usual procedure is to biopsy one skin lesion for hematoxylin and eosin staining and another for DIF.

Differential Diagnosis

The differential diagnosis of HSP is shown in Table 38–3. HSP must be distinguished from other small-vessel vasculitides, from autoimmune inflammatory conditions associated with joint disease and rashes, and from infections. Other disorders may be associated occasionally with mild IgA deposition in blood vessels, but the process is rarely so florid as with HSP. IgA nephropathy is pathologically indistinguishable from the renal disease associated with HSP (including the preferential deposition of IgA1) but has a typically chronic course and is not associated with disease in other organ systems.

A particularly crucial distinction is between HSP and the antineutrophil cytoplasmic antibody (ANCA)–associated conditions, primarily Wegener granulomatosis and microscopic polyangiitis. (Churg-Strauss disease may be distinguished more readily by the presence of eosinophilia.) The ANCA-associated vasculitides often present with purpura, migratory arthritis, and renal inflammation but, in contrast to HSP, do not typically have self-limited courses. Organ manifestations that are atypical for HSP, such as pulmonary involvement, symptoms or signs compatible with vasculitic neuropathy, or inflammatory eye disease, should broaden the differential diagnosis. Misdiagnoses of HSP because of failure to perform DIF testing on tissue biopsies and ANCA assays can lead to poor outcomes.

Table 38–3. Differential diagnosis of Henoch-Schönlein purpura.

Other vasculitides
Hypersensitivity vasculitis
Microscopic polyangiitis
Churg-Strauss syndrome
Wegener granulomatosis
Mixed cryoglobulinemia
Polyarteritis nodosa
Systemic autoimmune conditions
Systemic lupus erythematosus
Rheumatoid arthritis
Renal disorders
IgA nephropathy
Infections
Acute viral or bacterial infections
Malignancies
Childhood leukemias
Miscellaneous
Acute hemorrhagic edema of infancy

Treatment

Nonsteroidal anti-inflammatory drugs may alleviate arthralgias but can aggravate gastrointestinal symptoms and should be avoided in any patient with renal disease. Dapsone (100 mg/d) may be effective in cases of HSP, perhaps through interference with the interactions of IgA and neutrophils. Although glucocorticoids have not been evaluated rigorously in HSP, they appear to ameliorate joint and gastrointestinal symptoms. Glucocorticoids do not appear to improve the rash, however, and their effectiveness in renal disease is controversial. Uncontrolled trials suggest that high-dose methylprednisolone followed by oral prednisone or high-dose prednisone combined with azathioprine or cyclophosphamide may help patients with severe nephritis (ie, nephrotic syndrome and > 50% crescents).

Complications

In most cases, HSP follows a self-limited course, resolves without substantial morbidity, and does not recur. The vast majority of cases resolve within 6–8 weeks. Recurrences, found in 33% of patients, usually develop within the first few months after resolution of the first bout. Even when associated with small ulcerations, the cutaneous lesions are usually so superficial that they heal without scarring. A small percentage of patients have progressive renal insufficiency. Chronic renal failure is rare except in adults with more than 50% crescents on renal biopsy.

When to Refer to a Specialist

Diagnosis should be made in consultation with either a dermatologist or a rheumatologist who can help determine whether a skin biopsy is necessary to confirm the diagnosis. Another form of vasculitis should be suspected if the disease fails to follow its usual pattern. The small subset of patients with progressive renal insufficiency should be managed in consultation with a nephrologist.

REFERENCES

Saulsbury FT. Henoch-Schönlein purpura in children. Report of 100 patients and review of the literature. *Medicine (Baltimore)*. 1999;78:395. [PMID: 10575422] (Well-characterized cohort of pediatric patients evaluated and followed at one center.)

Tancrede-Bohin E, et al. Schönlein-Henoch purpura in adult patients. Predictive factors for IgA glomerulonephritis in a retrospective study of 57 cases. *Arch Dermatol.* 1997;33:438. [PMID: 9126006] (Adults are more likely to have persistent disease and serious renal involvement.)

Relevant World Wide Web Sites

[The Johns Hopkins Vasculitis Center]
http://vasculitis.med.jhu.edu
[The International Network for the Study of the Systemic Vasculitides]
http://www2.ccf.org/inssys
[The Cleveland Clinic Foundation Center for Vasculitis]
http://www.clevelandclinic.org/arthritis/vasculitis/default.htm

Vasculitis of the Central Nervous System

David B. Hellmann, MD

Central nervous system (CNS) vasculitis is not a single disease but a collection of conditions that cause inflammatory damage of blood vessels in the brain and spinal cord. About half of the cases have no known cause and are, therefore, classified as *primary* vasculitis of the CNS. The other half of the cases arise in the setting of some other disorder, often a rheumatic disease such as systemic lupus erythematosus (SLE), and are classified as secondary forms of CNS vasculitis. Primary vasculitis of the CNS has been referred to by many names. Bowing to tradition, this chapter will use the term "primary angiitis of the CNS" (PACNS).

CNS vasculitis presents a two-handed clinical challenge. On the one hand, clinicians need to recognize and treat those rare patients whose strokes and other neurologic deficits result from CNS vasculitis. On the other hand, clinicians need to avoid overdiagnosis of CNS vasculitis and must realize that the angiographic and magnetic resonance image (MRI) abnormalities observed in CNS vasculitis can be mimicked by infection, tumor, and other conditions.

ESSENTIALS OF DIAGNOSIS

- *Common presentation includes headache, encephalopathy, and multiple strokes.*
- *Brain MRI sensitive but not specific.*
- *Most patients in whom PACNS is suspected have some other disorder.*
- *Angiographic abnormalities suggestive but not specific.*
- *Definitive diagnosis requires brain biopsy.*

General Considerations

PACNS is a disease of unknown cause characterized by vasculitis limited to the brain and spinal cord. PACNS is rare: At large medical centers, PACNS constitutes only about 1% of all cases of systemic vasculitis. Evidence suggests that PACNS is not one disease. Indeed, the clinical picture of PACNS that emerges from re-

viewing the literature depends a great deal on whether the analysis focuses on biopsy-proven cases (BP-PACNS) or cases defined by angiography (AD-PACNS) without biopsy proof. Some clinicians have speculated that AD-PACNS may be caused by spasm rather than by inflammation, but the evidence for spasm is largely circumstantial. The term "benign angiography of the CNS" is sometimes applied to cases of AD-PACNS. Such a name is unsatisfactory because some patients with AD-PACNS have a progressive disease, and the benignity of AD-PACNS can only be established over time. Table 39–1 outlines the clinical pictures of both BP-PACNS and AD-PACNS.

Clinical Findings

A. Symptoms and Signs

BP-PACNS chiefly affects middle-aged men. The initial presentation is typically headache and encephalopathy, and multifocal strokes develop later. BP-PACNS usually develops insidiously, unfolding with additive neurologic deficits over weeks or months before the diagnosis is suspected. Strokes in the absence of diffuse cortical dysfunction would be most unusual for BP-PACNS. However, the presentation of BP-PACNS is highly variable. Some patients may appear to have had one stroke, but PACNS is suspected after an MRI reveals multiple strokes of varying age. In other patients, headache may be the dominating feature. In some patients who have headache and what appears to be mass lesions on MRI, a brain tumor is suspected. Diffuse cortical dysfunction can manifest as either a decline in cognitive ability or an alteration in consciousness. The English teacher who can no longer spell accurately or the bank teller who cannot count change exemplifies how cognitive changes from diffuse cortical dysfunction may present. Seizure and brainstem or cranial nerve dysfunction develop in approximately one-third of patients. Spinal cord involvement occurs less commonly. Isolated dementia is a very rare presentation of BP-PACNS. It is a common misconception that BP-PACNS is associated with systemic symptoms such as fever, weight loss, or sweats. In reality, such symptoms develop in fewer than 20% of cases.

Table 39–1. Clinical and laboratory features of PACNS based on the method of diagnosis.[a]

Feature	BP-PACNS	AD-PACNS	P value
Sex, no. (%)			
Males	78 (69.0)	17 (30.8)	< .001
Females	38 (31.0)	38 (69.1)	< .001
Age, mean ± SD	46 ± 17	33 ± 14	
Headache, no. (%)			
Yes	63 (55.8)	43 (78.2)	
No	50 (44.3)	12 (21.8)	
Stroke, no. (%)			
Yes	83 (86.5)	15 (32.6)	
No	13 (13.5)	31 (67.4)	< .008
Seizure, no. (%)			
Yes	29 (30.2)	11 (23.9)	
No	67 (69.8)	35 (76.1)	
Cerebral hemorrhage, no. (%)			
Yes	13 (11.5)	5 (9.1)	
No	100 (88.5)	50 (90.9)	
Diffuse neurologic dysfunction, no. (%)			
Yes	77 (68.1)	26 (47.3)	
No	36 (31.9)	29 (52.7)	< .009
Decreased cognition, no. (%)			
Yes	64 (83.1)	20 (76.9)	
No	13 (16.9)	6 (23.1)	
Days from symptom onset to diagnosis, mean ± SD	170 ± 261	46 ± 73	< .001
Abnormal CSF/total tested (%)	90	50	< .005

[a]An abnormal cerebrospinal fluid sample had > 5 cells/μL or protein > 55 mg% or both.
PACNS, primary angiitis of the central nervous system; BP-PACNS, biopsy-proven PACNS; AD-PACNS, angiographically defined PACNS.
From Calabrese LH, Duna GF, Lie JT. Vasculitis in the central nervous system. *Arthritis Rheum.* 1997; 40: 1189. Reprinted by permission of Wiley-Liss, Inc., a subsidiary of John Wiley & Sons, Inc.

The clinical picture of AD-PACNS differs in several important ways. The typical patient is a woman in her 30s who presents suddenly with headache and stroke (Table 39–1). Diffuse cortical abnormalities develop less commonly. In AD-PACNS, as in BP-PACNS, systemic symptoms and signs are usually absent.

B. Laboratory Findings

In BP-PACNS, about one-fifth of the patients have anemia (usually mild), one-half have an elevated white blood cell count, and two-thirds have an elevated erythrocyte sedimentation rate (ESR). The hematocrit and ESR are less frequently abnormal in AD-PACNS cases. The cerebrospinal fluid (CSF) is abnormal in nearly 90% of BP-PACNS cases and in about 50% of AD-PACNS cases. The most common abnormalities are an elevated CSF protein (with a mean of 177 mg/dL and a median of 100) and a CSF lymphocytosis (with a mean of 77 cells/μL). A CSF cell count exceeding 250/μL al-

most never occurs in PACNS. In AD-PACNS, the CSF abnormalities are typically very mild. CSF protein levels are usually below 60 mg/dL and the CSF white blood cell count is usually less than 10 cells/μL.

C. Imaging Studies

MRI is the most sensitive imaging method for detecting PACNS, being abnormal in approximately 90% of cases. However, the abnormalities are not specific for vasculitis. On average, patients with PACNS have multiple lesions that are predominantly bilateral and supratentorial. The most commonly affected areas are the subcortical white matter, the deep gray matter, the deep white matter, and the cortex. The lesions appear most commonly as infarcts but can also appear as mass lesions or areas of signal change. Hemorrhagic lesions are uncommon. MRI angiograms are normal in the vast majority of cases. Even though PACNS is classified as a medium-sized-vessel vasculitis, MRI angiography lacks the resolution to detect the size of arteries usually affected by PACNS.

Computed tomography (CT) of the brain is much less sensitive in PACNS, detecting abnormalities in only about two-thirds of the cases. However, CT is more sensitive than MRI at detecting hemorrhagic lesions.

Traditional angiography is abnormal in 50–80% of patients with PACNS. The classic finding in PACNS of "beading" of the small intracranial arteries is caused by lesions of constitution or dilations interspersed with normal areas (Figure 39–1). Slow flow, thread-like thinning of arteries, and occlusion are other angiographic (albeit nonspecific) abnormalities found in PACNS. Microaneurysms occur much less commonly in PACNS than in polyarteritis nodosa. The small branches of the middle anterior arteries and the posterior cerebral arteries are the most commonly affected. Angiographic abnormalities of larger more proximal arteries are unusual. Angiographic abnormalities are usually bilateral and more widespread than the MRI lesions. None of the angiographic abnormalities are absolutely specific for PACNS. In patients in whom CNS vasculitis is suspected, angiography carries an 11.8% risk of transient neurologic deficit and a 0.8% risk of permanent stroke.

The role of positron emission tomography scanning in PACNS has not been defined.

D. Special Tests

Brain biopsy, required for definitive diagnosis of PACNS, carries a risk of serious morbidity of 0–2%, and will be falsely negative in at least one-quarter of cases. Sampling the tip of the nondominant temporal lobe can reduce the chance of neurologic deficits from

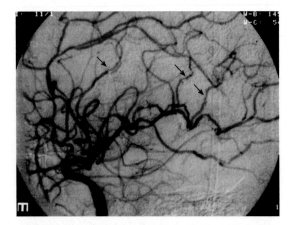

Figure 39–1. Angiogram of intracranial arteries showing segmental narrowing typical of central nervous system vasculitis.

biopsy. Biopsy should include the leptomeninges as this tissue is often involved by PACNS. Biopsies should be processed for histologic examination and cultures and should be stained for bacteria, fungi, and viruses. PACNS affects chiefly small- and medium-size arteries and arterioles of the brain and spinal cord. Affected vessels are infiltrated chiefly with lymphocytes. A minority of biopsies will show granulomatous inflammation. Thrombosis and rupture can lead to infarction and hemorrhage of the surrounding tissue.

E. Evaluation

Most patients in whom CNS vasculitis is suspected will need to undergo a battery of tests. Since MRI is the most sensitive noninvasive imaging method overall, it is preferred over CT unless hemorrhage is a concern. After MRI has excluded mass lesion, the patient should undergo lumbar puncture. The CSF analysis can help support the diagnosis of CNS vasculitis, as noted above, and can help exclude the many infections and tumors that can mimic CNS vasculitis (see below). Although angiograms are invasive and not highly specific, they do help support the diagnosis of CNS vasculitis and should usually be performed. Whether all patients in whom PACNS is suspected should undergo brain biopsy is controversial. Few centers have a large experience with either PACNS or brain biopsy. Traditionally, few patients in whom PACNS was suspected have undergone biopsy. Other laboratory evaluations will depend on the patient's presentation and differential diagnosis (see below).

Diagnostic Criteria

A definite diagnosis of PACNS requires the following:

1. Symptoms and signs of an acquired neurologic deficit consistent with the diagnosis of PACNS (eg, headache, confusion, and multiple strokes).

2. No evidence of a systemic vasculitis or another disorder that could cause the clinical picture, despite a thorough investigation.

3. A brain or spinal cord biopsy demonstrating vasculitis in the absence of infection.

The diagnosis of PACNS should be regarded as *probable* if, in the absence of a positive biopsy, the patient meets the first two criteria and has an angiogram with classic changes of vasculitis in multiple intracranial vessels.

Differential Diagnosis

Since most patients in whom CNS vasculitis is suspected have some other disorder, the differential diagnosis should be reviewed meticulously (Table 39–2). Among the rheumatic diseases, SLE, polyarteritis nodosa, and Wegener granulomatosis are the disorders that most

Table 39–2. Differential diagnosis of primary angiitis of the central nervous system.[a]

Category	Examples
Rheumatic disorders	Systemic lupus erythematosus, Wegener granulomatosis, polyarteritis nodosa, Takayasu arteritis, temporal arteritis, Behçet disease, Sjögren syndrome, Cogan syndrome
Infections	Bacteria (eg, endocarditis, bacterial meningitis, tuberculosis, syphilis, Lyme disease), fungi (eg, histoplasmosis, aspergillus), viruses (eg, herpes zoster, HIV, hepatitis C)
Drugs	Cocaine, ephedrine, amphetamine, allopurinol, phenylpropanolamine, heroin
Vasculopathies	Atherosclerosis, antiphospholipid antibody syndrome, cerebral amyloid angiopathy, moya moya, radiation-induced vasculopathy, vasospasm associated with severe hypertension or hemorrhage, arterial fibromuscular dysplasia, cardiac myxoma embolism, cholesterol embolism, pregnancy- and postpartum-associated vasculopathy, sickle cell anemia, thrombotic thrombocytopenic purpura
Malignancy	Vascular lymphoma, Hodgkin disease, small-cell lung cancer
Heritable disorders	Cerebral autosomal dominant arteriopathy with subcortical infarcts and leukoencephalopathy (CADASIL)
Other inflammatory disorders	Sarcoidosis, inflammatory bowel disease, celiac disease
Metabolic disorders	Pheochromocytoma

[a]References: (Lie, 1997; Razavi, 1999; Williamson, 1999; Younger, 1997; Calabrese, 1997; Calabrese, 1987)
Reproduced from Hellmann DB, Stone J. Vasculitis of the central nervous system. In: Asbury AK, McKhann GM, McDonald WI, Goadsby PJ, McArthur JC, eds. *Diseases of the Nervous System: Clinical Neuroscience and Therapeutic Principles.* 3rd ed. Cambridge University Press, 2002:1547. Reprinted with the permission of Cambridge University Press.

often cause secondary CNS vasculitis. Rarely, however, are these conditions confused with PACNS. Almost all patients with those conditions have other organs involved (eg, skin in SLE) and have other characteristic laboratory abnormalities (eg, positive antineutrophil cytoplasmic antibodies in Wegener granulomatosis).

Infection can be more difficult to distinguish from PACNS. HIV, herpes zoster virus (HZV), syphilis, and histoplasmosis are among the infections that can closely mimic PACNS. Most patients affected are immunosuppressed by HIV, alcoholism, or cancer chemotherapy. Many of the infections, especially fungi, preferentially affect the base of the brain. Infection should also be considered whenever the number of cells in the CSF exceeds 250/μL.

The possibility of HZV-related vasculitis should be considered in a person who is immunosuppressed or who has had shingles in a V_1 distribution in the last few weeks. Angiographic abnormalities seen with infection can perfectly mimic the changes seen with PACNS. Because of the difficulty of recognizing when infection is causing vasculitis, spinal fluid and brain biopsies should be cultured and stained for infection. Blood cultures, HIV testing, and CSF VDRL tests should also be routinely performed when evaluating a patient for PACNS. Special tests (eg, polymerase chain reaction assay) for other infections may be warranted if the patient is immunosuppressed.

Cocaine, amphetamines, and ephedrine derivatives are the drugs that most commonly produce CNS vasculopathy. There is some evidence that these drugs can produce vasculitis itself and not just a vasculopathy that imitates PACNS. Most patients with cocaine-induced vasculitis are men in their 20s. However, profiling for PACNS is an inexact science, so detailed drug histories and toxicology screens should be used routinely.

Atherosclerosis should always be considered because it is so common, especially if the patient is over the age of 50 and has hypertension, hypercholesterolemia, or diabetes. No angiogram should be interpreted as showing vasculitis if atherosclerosis is evident in the carotid siphon or other vessels. Cerebral amyloid should be considered if the patient is over the age of 65 and has cerebral hemorrhages. Other conditions that can resemble PACNS are listed in Table 39–2.

Treatment

Patients with BP-PACNS should be treated with glucocorticoids. The role of immunosuppressive drugs such as cyclophosphamide is not yet established. Patients who have declined rapidly should be started on solumedrol 1000 mg intravenously daily for 3–5 days, followed by prednisone (or equivalent) 1 mg/kg/d. Patients who have not progressed rapidly can begin treatment with prednisone. The rarity of PACNS means that no large, detailed studies are available to guide tapering. Prednisone should not be reduced until the patient has stabilized and after all manifestations of inflammation (ESR, hematocrit, CSF abnormalities) have resolved. Typically this takes a month. Thereafter, prednisone can be tapered by 10% every 1–2 weeks until 20 mg is reached, at which time the reduction schedule is slowed further. New symptoms or signs or new imaging abnormalities will require an increase in prednisone dose. Cyclophosphamide or other immunosuppressive drugs should be considered if the patient has severe deficits or if the disease progresses despite glucocorticoid therapy.

Treatment of AD-PACNS is also not well defined. However, studies suggest that some cases result more from spasm of the arteries than from true inflammation. Spasm appears to be especially likely in young women who have an abrupt onset of headache and focal deficits and who have no or minimal abnormalities of the CSF. There is growing evidence that these patients infrequently require immunosuppressive drugs. Some experts advocate treating these cases with a calcium channel blocker such as verapamil (to reduce spasm) and prednisone (1 mg/kg/d). Following resolution of the acute illness, the prednisone is tapered over 6–12 weeks. Repeat angiography is recommended after 4–6 weeks. Failure to demonstrate substantial angiographic improvement should cast doubt on spasm as a major component and should suggest true vasculitis that will require a slower tapering of prednisone. All patients with PACNS should be instructed to avoid drugs that cause vasoconstriction or thrombosis (such as birth control pills, ephedrine, nicotine, and cocaine). All patients who take prednisone for more than 2 months should be evaluated and treated to minimize the risks of osteoporosis.

When to Refer to a Specialist

Given the rarity of PACNS, it is prudent to refer each patient in whom PACNS is suspected to a rheumatologist, a neurologist, or both. A physician familiar with the side effects of immunosuppressive drugs should closely monitor patients.

Prognosis

In the absence of treatment, almost all patients with BP-PACNS die of progressive neurologic deficits. Treatment has reduced mortality in the first year to 5%. The prognosis of AD-PACNS appears to be better. More than 90% of patients in whom spasm is suspected will recover.

REFERENCES

Calabrese LH, et al. Vasculitis in the central nervous system. *Arthritis Rheum.* 1997;40:1189. [PMID: 9214418]

Hajj-Ali RA, et al. Benign angiopathy of the central nervous system: cohort of 16 patients with clinical course and long-term followup. *Arthritis Rheum.* 2002;47:662. [PMID: 12522842]

Hellmann DB, Stone J. Vasculitis of the central nervous system. In: Asbury AK, McKhann GM, McDonald WI, Goadsby PJ, McArthur JC, eds. *Diseases of the Nervous System: Clinical Neuroscience and Therapeutic Principles.* 3rd ed. Cambridge University Press, 2002:1547.

Moore PM. Diagnosis and management of isolated angiitis of the central nervous system. *Neurology.* 1989;39:167. [PMID: 2915784]

Relevant World Wide Web Site

[The Johns Hopkins Vasculitis Center]
http://vasculitis.med.jhu.edu

Buerger Disease

John H. Stone, MD, MPH

ESSENTIALS OF DIAGNOSIS

- *Active, strong history of tobacco use.*
- *The finding of severe digital ischemia without evidence of internal organ involvement.*
- *Angiography reveals segmental involvement of medium-sized arteries, with abrupt vascular cutoffs and corkscrew collaterals. The major vessel involvement occurs at the levels of the ankle and wrist.*

General Considerations

Buerger disease is also called thromboangiitis obliterans. Typically, patients are young male smokers. The mean age of onset is approximately 40 years, with a broad age range that includes both late teens and the elderly. Although the patients described initially were men, the disease may afflict women as well, probably in direct proportion to the number of women in any particular society who smoke. The precise mechanism underlying the relationship between Buerger disease and cigarette smoking is unknown; autoimmune reactions to constituents of tobacco have been postulated. Cases may present several years after the start of smoking, but Buerger disease does not occur in the absence of ongoing tobacco exposure.

The diagnosis of Buerger disease is made by delineation of the typical pattern of vascular involvement by angiography, exclusion of diseases that may mimic Buerger disease (Table 40–1), and confirmation that the major risk factor, ongoing tobacco exposure, is present. Because of difficulty in accessing medium-sized vessels for biopsy, the diagnosis is rarely confirmed histologically. The exceptions to this rule are superficial thrombophlebitis, which seldom comes to medical attention, and amputation specimens, by which time medical attention is (at least in some senses) too late. When biopsy is possible, acute Buerger disease is characterized by a highly inflammatory thrombus, composed of a variety of cell types: lymphocytes, neutrophils, giant cells, and occasional microabscesses.

Fibrinoid necrosis, a hallmark of most systemic vasculitides, is absent in Buerger disease.

Clinical Findings

A. SYMPTOMS AND SIGNS

1. Extremities—A major hallmark of Buerger disease is its confinement to the extremities. The initial symptoms may be nonspecific pains in the calf, foot, or toes. The progression of thrombosis and vasculitis can lead to horrific pain in the digits and limbs and ultimately to gangrene and tissue loss, through either autoamputation or elective amputation. For unknown reasons, however, other vascular beds (eg, the cardiac, pulmonary, renal, and mesenteric vasculature) are nearly always spared in Buerger disease. Although Buerger disease has a predilection for the feet and toes, the hands and fingers may also be affected prominently. More than 60% of patients have abnormal Allen tests, indicating compromise of circulation to the hand; many demonstrate obliterations of the radial or ulnar artery pulses on physical examination. In contrast to atherosclerosis, which is a disease of the proximal vasculature, Buerger disease is characterized by inflammation and thrombosis of medium-sized, distal blood vessels (both arteries and veins), most intense at the levels of the ankles and wrists.

2. Skin—The earliest lesion may be a superficial thrombophlebitis. This complaint is often disregarded by the patient or misdiagnosed as deep varicosities. Histologic examination of these lesions reveals an acute thrombophlebitis with marked perivascular infiltration. This herald lesion is then followed by progressive occlusion of the deeper veins and arteries, leading the patient to seek medical attention. Patients with Buerger disease may have splinter hemorrhages, arousing suspicions of infective endocarditis. Most cutaneous features of disease are those of a process involving the medium-sized vessels exclusively (purpura, for example, a manifestation of small-vessel disease, is absent). Gangrene occurs in the most distal tissues, ie, the toes and fingers, first (Figure 40–1). If the process remains undiagnosed or if the patient continues to smoke even after the diagnosis, larger portions of the extremities become compromised. In advanced cases, the major arterial supplies to the hands and feet may become occluded, leading to cool-

Table 40–1. Differential diagnosis
of Buerger disease.

Cardiovascular conditions
  Atherosclerosis
  Cardiogenic emboli (eg, infective endocarditis)
Systemic disorders associated with autoimmunity
  Systemic lupus erythematosus
  Antiphospholipid antibody syndrome
  Systemic sclerosis (particularly limited scleroderma, or
    CREST syndrome)
  Mixed connective tissue disease
Systemic vasculitides
  Rheumatoid vasculitis
  Polyarteritis nodosa
  Wegener granulomatosis
  Microscopic polyangiitis
  Churg-Strauss syndrome
  Cryoglobulinemia
Miscellaneous
  Paraproteinemia
  Ergotism

CREST, calcinosis, Raynaud phenomenon, esophageal motility,
sclerodactyly, telangiectasias.

ness and pain of the entire distal extremity, necessitating amputation (Figure 40–2).

3. Peripheral nerve—Early in the disease, nonspecific pains in the calf, foot, or toes may recall a primary neuropathic process. These sensory symptoms may result from thickening of the tissues immediately surrounding the veins and arteries, leading to connective tissue proliferation around the nerve bundles that are intimately connected with the vasculature. True vasculitic neuropathy, however, does not occur in Buerger disease.

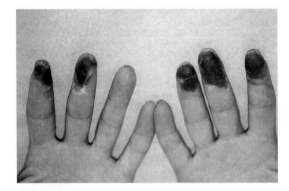

Figure 40–1. Digital ischemia with gangrene in Buerger disease.

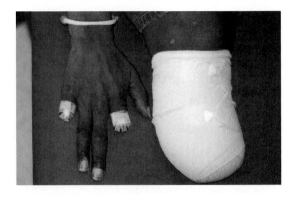

Figure 40–2. The consequence of failure to stop smoking: multiple amputations. This patient proceeded to amputations of every finger on both hands and bilateral below-the-knee amputations.

4. Gastrointestinal tract and other organs—Extremely rare cases of Buerger disease involving the gastrointestinal tract and other organs have been reported.

B. LABORATORY FINDINGS

There is no single diagnostic test for Buerger disease. The demonstration of "corkscrew collaterals" (Figure 40–3) on angiography is highly characteristic but not pathognomonic. Such vessels may also be observed in polyarteritis nodosa and other forms of medium-vessel

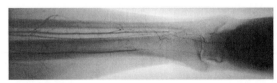

A

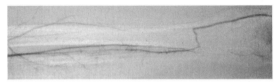

B

Figure 40–3. Angiographic findings in Buerger disease. **A:** Attenuation of the anterior tibial artery in the mid-calf. This artery forms a collateral at the site of occlusion with the peroneal artery. The posterior tibial artery is occluded superiorly. **B:** Abrupt arterial cut-offs several centimeters above the ankle, with minimal blood flow distal to the cut-offs.

vasculitis. Laboratory and radiologic investigations are important in Buerger disease, both to identify the typical vascular lesions and to exclude conditions that require other approaches to management. Table 40–2 lists the results of routine laboratory tests and specialized assays that are done to rule out disorders masquerading as Buerger disease.

The erythrocyte sedimentation rate and C-reactive protein levels are generally lower than observed in many other types of diffuse systemic vasculitis, but most patients have at least moderate elevations of these acute phase reactants. Routine hematologic, serum chemistry, and urinalysis studies are normal in Buerger disease; abnormalities in these tests suggest other diagnoses.

Table 40–2. Laboratory and radiologic evaluation in possible Buerger disease.

Test	Typical Results
Complete blood cell count	Normal. Mild elevations of the white blood cell and platelet count would not be unexpected.
Renal and hepatic function	Normal
Urinalysis with microscopy	Normal
Erythrocyte sedimentation rate (ESR)/C-reactive protein	Mild to moderate elevations in patients with severe digital ischemia. Dramatically elevated acute phase reactants (eg, an ESR > 100 mm/h) unusual.
ANA	Negative
Rheumatoid factor	Negative
C3, C4	Normal
ANCA	Negative
Hepatitis B and C serologies	Negative
Antiphospholipid antibodies	Negative rapid plasma regain and anticardiolipin antibody assays. Normal Russell viper venom time (for lupus anticoagulant).
Blood cultures	Negative
Echocardiography (or TEE)	No cardiac valvular vegetations. Normal aortic root.
Angiography	Corkscrew collaterals (see Figure 40–3). Abrupt cut-offs of medium-sized arteries at levels of the ankles and wrists, and often higher. Segmental areas of involvement, with diseased regions interspersed with normal-appearing arterial stretches

ANA, antinuclear antibody; ANCA, antineutrophil cytoplasmic antibody; TEE, transesophageal echocardiography.

Markers of hypercoagulable states that may be associated with widespread arterial thromboses, eg, antiphospholipid antibodies, should be investigated.

C. IMAGING STUDIES

Echocardiography (possibly including a transesophageal study) should examine the heart valves and aortic root. Comprehensive angiographic studies that define the vasculature of the extremities, proximal aorta, gastrointestinal tract, and renal arteries should be considered. Such studies are critical in identifying vascular involvement typical of Buerger disease and excluding atheroembolic sources as well as findings more typical of other vasculitides (eg, microaneurysms). The arterial involvement in Buerger disease is highly segmental, with abrupt vascular occlusions interspersed with regions of vessels that appear angiographically normal (Figure 40–3). In advanced cases, the thready appearance of vessels distal to the wrists and ankles may resemble a disorganized spider web. The most commonly involved vessels are the digital arteries of the fingers and toes as well as the palmar, plantar, tibial, peroneal, radial, and ulnar vessels.

Differential Diagnosis

The major conditions in the differential diagnosis of Buerger disease are cardiovascular diseases, autoimmune disorders, and systemic vasculitides (see Table 40–1). Among the cardiovascular diseases, atherosclerosis and cardiogenic emboli are the principal considerations. Echocardiography (including transesophageal echocardiography) and angiography may be helpful in distinguishing Buerger disease from cardiovascular conditions. Careful imaging of the proximal aorta is essential. In contrast to Buerger disease, atherosclerotic disease characteristically affects the proximal vessels. Sources of cardiogenic emboli must be excluded by echocardiography and blood cultures.

Among the autoimmune disorders, systemic lupus erythematosus, the antiphospholipid syndrome, and scleroderma all may present with digital ischemia. Limited scleroderma (the CREST [calcinosis, Raynaud phenomenon, esophageal dysmotility, sclerodactyly, telangiectasias] syndrome; see Chapter 22) may pose special diagnostic challenges because of its propensity to cause digital loss, particularly when associated with anticentromere antibodies. Careful examination of the vasculature in the nailbeds, where dilated capillary loops appear in scleroderma and other connective tissue disorders, may help distinguish these conditions from Buerger disease.

The systemic vasculitides commonly associated with distal ischemia and gangrene are rheumatoid vasculitis, polyarteritis nodosa, Wegener granulomatosis, microscopic polyangiitis, Churg-Strauss syndrome, and cryoglobulinemia. In general, the lack of visceral involvement in Buerger disease helps distinguish Buerger disease from other vasculitides. For example, ulcerations of the shins, calves, and malleolar regions are atypical of Buerger disease but common among other forms of vasculitis listed above. Vasculitic neuropathy, often striking in the other forms of systemic vasculitis, does not occur in Buerger disease.

Treatment

The only effective intervention in Buerger disease is complete smoking cessation. Despite the similarities of Buerger disease to systemic vasculitides that affect medium-sized blood vessels and to hypercoagulable states, there is no role for immunosuppressive interventions or anticoagulation in this condition. Moreover, because of the obliterative nature of the vascular inflammatory and thrombotic processes, the vasculature distal to the lesions generally offers no blood vessels large enough to sustain bypass grafts. Thrombolysis, which has not been studied in substantial numbers of patients, carries with it significant risks and perhaps a low likelihood of success, given the length of thromboses present in Buerger disease. Effective pain control is important during periods of intense pain from digital ischemia (without it, patients may only smoke more).

Complications

Without smoking cessation, Buerger disease progresses inexorably through an obliterative vascular process, leading to coolness of the digits, hands, and feet; paresthesias; intermittent claudication symptoms; skin ulcerations over the fingers and toes; and gangrenous infarctions of the extremities. Once established, the disease may be maintained by even small exposures to tobacco (even smokeless tobacco or second-hand smoke). Failure to stop smoking is associated with a dramatic increase in the risk of limb loss by amputation. The angiogram often looks far worse than the patient does: The extent of vascular obliteration may hold out little hope for preserving the patient's extremities, but complete abstinence from tobacco may be remarkably successful in saving limbs.

When to Refer to a Specialist

Consultation with a rheumatologist to rule out other forms of systemic vasculitis is useful. Because of the absence of vessels large enough to bypass into, vascular surgery consultation is usually not required except, unfortunately, for amputation.

REFERENCES

Buerger L. Thromboangiitis obliterans: a study of the vascular lesions leading to presenile spontaneous gangrene. *Am J Med Sci.* 1908;136:567. (Perceptive, detailed summaries of the first cases described and recognized to be a new disease.)

McKusick VA, et al. Buerger's disease: A distinct clinical and pathological entity. *JAMA.* 1962;181:93.

Olin JW. Thromboangiitis obliterans (Buerger's disease). *N Engl J Med.* 2000;343:846. [PMID: 10995867] (An up-to-date, comprehensive review.)

Relevant World Wide Web Sites

[The Johns Hopkins Vasculitis Center]
http://vasculitis.med.jhu.edu
[The International Network for the Study of the Systemic Vasculitides]
http://www2.ccf.org/inssys/
[The Cleveland Clinic Foundation Center for Vasculitis]
http://www.clevelandclinic.org/arthritis/vasculitis/default.htm

Miscellaneous Forms of Vasculitis

Philip Seo, MD, & John H. Stone, MD, MPH

RHEUMATOID VASCULITIS

ESSENTIALS OF DIAGNOSIS

- Palpable purpura, cutaneous ulcers (particularly in the malleolar region), digital infarctions, and peripheral sensory neuropathy are common manifestations.
- Tissue biopsy establishes the diagnosis of rheumatoid vasculitis. Nerve conduction studies help identify involved nerves for biopsy. Muscle biopsies should be performed simultaneously with nerve biopsies to increase the diagnostic yield of the procedure.

General Considerations

Rheumatoid vasculitis (RV) is a medium-vessel vasculitis occurring in patients with "burnt-out" but previously severe rheumatoid arthritis (RA). The typical patient has long-standing RA characterized by rheumatoid nodules, destructive joint disease, and high titers of rheumatoid factor. The diagnosis of RV should be considered in any patient with RA in whom new constitutional symptoms, skin ulcerations, serositis, digital ischemia, or symptoms of sensory or motor nerve dysfunction develop. RV resembles polyarteritis nodosa because it tends to cause cutaneous ulcerations, digital ischemia, mononeuritis multiplex, and mesenteric vasculitis (see Chapter 34).

Pathogenesis

Immune complex deposition and antibody-mediated destruction of endothelial cells both appear to contribute to RV. Certain HLA-DR4 alleles that predispose patients to severe RA may also heighten patients' susceptibility to RV. Cigarette smoking increases the risk of RV. However, the inciting events leading to the development of RV upon the substrate of previously destructive arthritis are not known. The manifestations of RV may be the result of a vasculopathy in which true vascular inflammation plays only a small part. Other factors, such as diabetes, atherosclerosis, and hypertension, likely play an important role in promoting vascular occlusion.

Clinical Findings

A. SYMPTOMS AND SIGNS

1. Skin—Dermatologic findings are the most common manifestation of RV, and may include palpable purpura, cutaneous ulcers (particularly in the malleolar region), and digital infarctions (Figure 41–1).

2. Nervous system—A peripheral sensory neuropathy is a common manifestation of RV. A mixed motor-sensory neuropathy or mononeuritis multiplex may also be seen. Central nervous system manifestations (such as strokes, seizures, and cranial nerve palsies) are considerably less common.

3. Eyes—Retinal vasculitis as a manifestation of RV is common but frequently asymptomatic. Necrotizing scleritis and peripheral ulcerative keratitis (Figure 41–2) pose threats to vision and require aggressive immunosuppressive therapy.

4. Serositis—Pericarditis and pleuritis may occur in association with RV. Other cardiopulmonary manifestations of RV are unusual.

B. LABORATORY FINDINGS

Most laboratory findings in RV, for example, elevations in the erythrocyte sedimentation rate, are nonspecific and merely reflect the presence of an inflammatory state. Hypocomplementemia, antinuclear antibodies (ANAs), atypical antineutrophil cytoplasmic antibodies (ANCAs) (by immunofluorescence testing but not enzyme immunoassay; see Chapter 31, Wegener Granulomatosis), and anti-endothelial cell antibodies are all detected more frequently in patients with RV than in those with RA alone. The usefulness of these findings for diagnosing RV, however, is not well established.

C. IMAGING STUDIES

The presence of bony erosions is a risk factor for the development of RV, but plain radiographs and other imaging studies have no consistent role in the evaluation of this disorder.

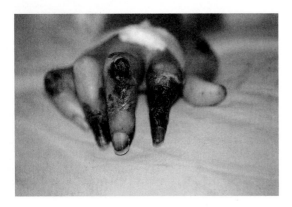

Figure 41–1. Digital infarctions in rheumatoid vasculitis.

D. Special Tests

Because the treatment implications for RV are so severe, the diagnosis must be established by tissue biopsy whenever possible. Deep skin biopsies (full-thickness biopsies that include some subcutaneous fat) taken from the edge of ulcers are very useful in detecting the presence of medium-vessel vasculitis. Nerve conduction studies help identify involved nerves for biopsy. Muscle biopsies (eg, of the gastrocnemius muscle) should be performed simultaneously with nerve biopsies.

Differential Diagnosis

Patients with erosive RA are at increased risk for infections. When patients with RA seek medical attention for the new onset of nonspecific systemic complaints, infection must be first on the differential diagnosis. Cholesterol embolization may cause digital ischemia and a host of other symptoms that mimic vasculitis. Diabetes mellitus is another major cause of mononeuritis multiplex, but multiple mononeuropathies occurring over a short period of time are unusual in that condition. Many clinical features of RV mimic those of polyarteritis nodosa and other forms of necrotizing vasculitis.

Treatment

Therapy must reflect the severity of organ involvement. Small, relatively painless infarctions around the nail bed develop in some patients with nodular RA (Figure 41–3). Such lesions do not herald the presence of a necrotizing vasculitis and require no adjustment in the patients' therapy. With other disease manifestations, however, such as cutaneous ulcers, vasculitic neuropathy, and inflammatory eye disease, glucocorticoids may be required. The role of tumor necrosis factor inhibitors in the treatment of RV is not known. Cyclophosphamide may be required in some cases of RV but should be used with extreme caution and moderate doses in this patient population, which is usually quite debilitated at baseline.

When to Refer to a Specialist

Patients in whom RV develops have a life-threatening complication of their RA and should be referred immediately to a rheumatologist. Other subspecialty consultations may also be required to confirm the diagnosis. Particular caution must be exercised when using cyclophosphamide in the elderly or in patients with renal

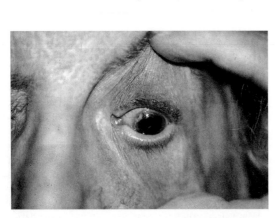

Figure 41–2. Peripheral ulcerative keratitis in a patient with nodular, destructive rheumatoid arthritis and rheumatoid vasculitis.

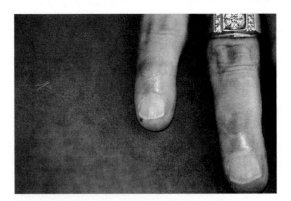

Figure 41–3. Nail bed infarctions in a patient with rheumatoid arthritis. Such lesions do not necessarily herald the onset of rheumatoid vasculitis.

dysfunction. All patients treated with cyclophosphamide benefit from management by clinicians accustomed to its use.

Prognosis

Although RV is a treatable condition, the development of this complication is a poor prognostic indicator.

COGAN SYNDROME

 ESSENTIALS OF DIAGNOSIS

- *The hallmark of Cogan syndrome is the presence of ocular inflammation and audiovestibular dysfunction in a young adult, which may be accompanied by evidence of a systemic vasculitis.*
- *Interstitial keratitis is the most common form of ocular involvement.*
- *Audiovestibular dysfunction may lead to the acute onset of vertigo, tinnitus, nausea, and vomiting.*
- *Vasculitis in Cogan syndrome may take the form of aortitis, renal artery stenosis, or occlusion of the great vessels.*

General Considerations

Cogan syndrome (CS) is an immune-mediated condition that primarily affects young adults. CS is an inflammatory disorder associated with ocular inflammation (usually interstitial keratitis) and audiovestibular dysfunction. This syndrome may be accompanied by a systemic vasculitis of large- and medium-sized arteries that may resemble Takayasu arteritis.

Pathogenesis

The onset of CS is frequently preceded by an upper respiratory tract infection. Because many features of CS can be caused by known pathogens (eg, *Treponema pallidum*), CS may be the direct consequence of an unidentified pathogen affecting the eyes, ears, and blood vessels. Alternatively, CS may be the indirect consequence of a pathogen that induces an immune response that continues to attack the host long after the pathogen has been eliminated (a phenomenon known as molecular mimicry). Neither of these theories has been proved.

Clinical Findings

A. SYMPTOMS AND SIGNS

1. Eye—Half of patients with CS will suffer from ocular involvement, most commonly the sudden onset of interstitial keratitis, which is accompanied by photophobia, lacrimation, and eye pain. Although keratitis is the classic ocular manifestation of CS, this disorder may be associated with inflammation in any part of the eye: Scleritis, episcleritis, anterior uveitis, conjunctivitis, and retinal vascular disease are all possible.

2. Ear—Patients with CS frequently suffer the acute onset of vertigo, tinnitus, nausea, and vomiting. These symptoms may be enormously disabling. The audiovestibular symptoms may occur before or after the onset of ocular disease. (These features are often separated in onset by weeks or months.) If not treated promptly and aggressively, permanent hearing loss may ensue. Recurrent attacks, which are common, may cause decremental loss of hearing. Ultimately, complete hearing loss occurs in as many as 60% of patients.

3. Large-vessel vasculitis—The most common manifestation of vasculitis in patients with CS is aortitis. Aortitis may lead to dilatation of the aorta and subsequent incompetence of the aortic valve. Involvement of aortic branches may cause claudication in the arms or legs. Renal artery stenosis or occlusion of the great vessels may also occur. These manifestations may be accompanied by nonspecific constitutional symptoms such as malaise, fever, or weight loss as well as arthralgias and frank arthritis.

B. LABORATORY FINDINGS

Laboratory findings are nondiagnostic and generally reflect the presence of inflammation. An antibody against a 68-kD antigen has been identified in cases of autoimmune sensorineural hearing loss but is not found in patients with CS. Exclusion of syphilis with fluorescent treponemal antibody testing (ie, FTA-ABS, not just the rapid plasma reagin) is essential.

C. IMAGING STUDIES

Gadolinium-enhanced T1-weighted magnetic resonance imaging (MRI) studies may demonstrate a hyperintensity in the membranous labyrinth secondary to vessel inflammation in the stria vascularis. This enhancement is not seen in patients with inactive CS and may be useful in identifying the activity of the disease.

Brainstem MRI studies are also essential to exclude tumors of the cerebellopontine angle, which may mimic the audiovestibular features of CS. Angiography may be useful to define the involvement of the great vessels (Figure 41–4). Magnetic resonance angiography is useful in evaluating vessel wall thickness and edema as well as the degree of luminal stenosis. Serial echocardiography may be used to assess and monitor aortic insufficiency.

D. Special Tests

Formal audiometric testing is important early in the evaluation to distinguish conductive hearing loss from sensorineural hearing dysfunction. In CS, audiometry demonstrates sensorineural hearing loss that preferentially affects the low- and high-range frequencies. This

may be a useful way to document response to therapy, although subsequent hearing loss is not always due to active disease.

Differential Diagnosis

The differential diagnosis of immune-mediated inner ear disease (sensorineural hearing loss with or without vestibular dysfunction) is shown in Table 41–1. Inflammatory eye disease may be caused by a variety of pathogens, including bacterial (eg, *Chlamydiae, Neisseriae*), spirochetal (eg, *Borrelia burgdorferi*), viral (eg, herpes simplex, varicella zoster), and mycobacterial (eg, *Mycobacterium tuberculosis, M leprae*).

Treatment

Some manifestations of CS respond well to symptomatic therapy. In general, the ocular manifestations are more amenable to therapy than the auricular complications. Interstitial keratitis may be treated with topical

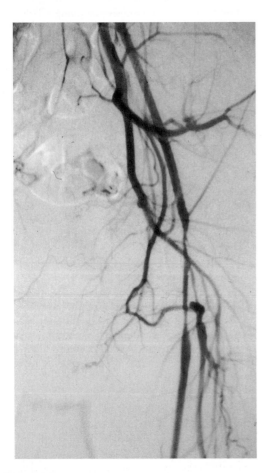

Figure 41–4. Large-vessel vasculitis in Cogan syndrome. Femoral artery disease led to lower extremity claudication.

Table 41–1. Differential diagnosis of the audiovestibular complications of Cogan syndrome.

Alternate Diagnoses	Comments
Immune-mediated inner ear disease	Sensorineural hearing loss and vestibular dysfunction in the absence of eye inflammation.
Syphilis	Latent and tertiary forms of this disease. Ordering both rapid plasma reagin and FTA-ABS essential.
Other infections	Lyme disease, mumps
Acoustic neuroma	Performance of brainstem magnetic resonance imaging essential to exclude this tumor.
Meniere syndrome	Inner ear disturbances in Meniere are generally more intermittent, with a waxing/waning character.
Systemic vasculitides	Wegener granulomatosis, giant cell arteritis
Collagen vascular diseases	Sjögren syndrome
Other inflammatory conditions	Sarcoidosis, Susac syndrome
Barotrauma	Other etiologies of perilymph fistula formation
Medications	Aminoglycosides, loop diuretics, antimalarials

atropine or glucocorticoids. Sensorineural hearing loss in CS is analogous to rapidly progressive glomerulonephritis in other forms of systemic vasculitis: Prompt treatment with cyclophosphamide and glucocorticoids is indicated. For patients with advanced, irreversible hearing loss, hearing aids and cochlear implants are feasible. Vestibular retraining may be required for some patients with significant cochlear damage.

Complications

The prevention of complications depends directly on the rapid recognition of this diagnosis, and the equally swift institution of therapy. Permanent damage may result early in the course of immune-mediated inner ear disease, and hearing deficits will not respond to therapy if initiated too late. Therefore, a high index of suspicion for this diagnosis must be maintained when evaluating patients with compatible complaints.

When to Refer to a Specialist

A patient who has a red eye (potentially related to a variety of ocular complications in CS) will require referral to an ophthalmologist for definitive diagnosis. Similarly, the involvement of an otolaryngologist will be essential to diagnose the nature of the hearing loss, to document its degree, and to monitor patients over time. Immunosuppressive medications should be managed by a rheumatologist.

Prognosis

Even if the initial event is recognized and responds the therapy, recurrent bouts of sensorineural hearing loss may cause the gradual loss of hearing. Up to 60% of patients experience some degree of permanent hearing loss. Some patients become completely deaf.

URTICARIAL VASCULITIS

ESSENTIALS OF DIAGNOSIS

- *The lesions of urticarial vasculitis are frequently associated with burning or pain rather than pruritus and require more than 24 hours to resolve.*
- *Immunofluorescence on skin biopsy specimen is the critical test. Intense staining for immunoreactants (ie, IgG, IgM, C3, C4, C1q) not only in and around small blood vessel walls but also in a ribbon along the dermal/epidermal junction is*

pathognomonic of hypocomplementemic urticarial vasculitis.

General Considerations

Urticarial vasculitis (UV) is a leukocytoclastic vasculitis that presents as hives (often associated with pain or discomfort) that last longer than 24 hours. Although UV is occasionally seen in isolation, it most often appears in association with connective tissue disorders such as serum sickness, cryoglobulinemia, and systemic lupus erythematosus (SLE).

UV targets the capillaries and postcapillary venules in the skin, leading to the appearance of hive-like lesions. In approaching patients with this problem, it is critical to distinguish cases associated with hypocomplementia from those in which the serum complement levels are normal.

Hypocomplementemic UV is associated with depressed serum levels of C3 and C4. Such cases often overlap with known connective tissue disorders, particularly SLE. At the severe end of the spectrum of this disorder are patients with a distinct disorder known as the **hypocomplementemic urticarial vasculitis syndrome** (HUVS).

The normocomplementemic form is a subset of cutaneous leukocytoclastic angiitis (see Chapter 36) in which the leukocytoclastic vasculitis manifests clinically as urticaria. In general, these cases are secondary to "hypersensitivity" reactions (usually caused by a medication) and respond to discontinuation of the offending agent. This form of UV is not discussed further in this chapter.

Pathogenesis

Hypocomplementemic UV is mediated at least in part by immune complex deposition. In one model, following an unknown inciting event, the deposition of IgG and C3 leads to further complement activation. The complement cascade activates mast cells and eosinophils, both of which act to form the typical urticarial wheal. The eosinophils are gradually replaced by neutrophils, leading to the leukocytoclastic destruction of capillary walls.

Clinical Findings

A. SYMPTOMS AND SIGNS

The lesions of UV, typically between 0.5 and 2.0 cm in diameter (Figure 41–5), are frequently associated with burning or pain rather than pruritus. In contrast to

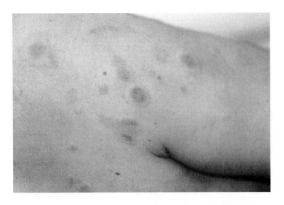

Figure 41–5. Lesions of hypocomplementemic urticarial vasculitis.

common urticaria, UV lesions usually require more than 24 hours to resolve, and typically leave small amounts of hyperpigmentation in the skin, caused by red blood cell extravasation.

Like SLE, hypocomplementemic UV may also be associated with malaise, arthralgias, fever, and glomerulonephritis. Unlike SLE, HUVS is characterized not only by recurrent or chronic UV, but also by angioedema. Moreover, severe chronic obstructive pulmonary disease (COPD) and uveitis—manifestations that are atypical of SLE—often complicate this condition. Jaccoud arthropathy has been noted in some patients with HUVS and possibly correlates with the presence of cardiac valvular lesions.

B. LABORATORY FINDINGS

Serum C3, C4, and CH50 levels are depressed. Hypocomplementemic UV is generally accompanied by the presence of anti-C1q autoantibodies. The presence of these antibodies is not pathognomonic, since they also may be found in patients with SLE who do not have UV. Patients with hypocomplementemic UV have antinuclear antibodies and, if significant overlap with SLE is present, may also have other autoantibodies (eg, anti-dsDNA, anti-Ro/SS-A, anti-La/SS-B, anti-Sm, and anti-RNP).

C. SPECIAL TESTS

Hematoxylin and eosin staining of skin biopsy specimens reveal a leukocytoclastic vasculitis in the superficial dermis. Older lesions may have a predominantly lymphocytic infiltrate. The critical test is the performance of immunofluorescence on the skin biopsy specimen, which reveals intense staining for immunoreactants (ie, IgG, IgM, C3, C4, C1q) not only in and around small blood vessel walls, but also in a ribbon

along the dermal/epidermal junction. These findings are pathognomonic of hypocomplementemic UV.

Differential Diagnosis

The skin lesions of hypocomplementemic UV must be distinguished from common urticaria (lesions are always pruritic and resolve completely over 2–8 hours, leaving no traces of the original lesion), neutrophilic urticaria (a persistent, treatment-refractory form of urticaria not associated with vasculitis), and normocomplementic UV (see above).

Treatment

UV may respond to therapies commonly used in SLE, such as low-dose prednisone, hydroxychloroquine, dapsone, or other immunomodulatory agents. There is anecdotal evidence that antihistamines, calcium channel antagonists, doxepin, methotrexate, indomethacin, colchicine, and pentoxifylline are effective in some cases.

HUVS is frequently a therapeutic challenge. Serious cases, particularly those presenting with glomerulonephritis or other organ involvement, may require treatment with high doses of glucocorticoids, cyclophosphamide, or cyclosporine. Angioedema, COPD, and cardiac valvular abnormalities may all necessitate other specific interventions.

When to Refer to a Specialist

Hypocomplementemic UV should always be managed with a subspecialist and may require a team of subspecialists depending on the specific organs involved. Accurate diagnosis through consultation with dermatologists and rheumatologists is the essential first step.

Prognosis

Hypocomplementemic UV frequently reflects the presence of an underlying disorder, which may influence the prognosis substantially. HUVS may be associated with multiple complications (eg, severe COPD) that affect prognosis adversely.

ERYTHEMA ELEVATUM DIUTINUM

ESSENTIALS OF DIAGNOSIS

- *New lesions come in the form of tender papules, associated with pruritus or a burning sensation.*
- *Lesions develop into red, reddish brown, or purple papules or nodules.*

- *Lesions may coalesce to form large plaques, usually over the extensor surfaces of joints.*

General Considerations

Erythema elevatum diutinum (EED) is a chronic, recurring cutaneous vasculitis in which tender papules appear on the extensor surfaces of the extremities. The onset of these lesions is usually heralded by the presence of pruritus or stinging, followed by the development of tender papules or nodules that coalesce with others to form plaques. The skin findings are frequently located near joints, such as on the extensor surfaces of the hands and fingers.

Pathogenesis

The pathogenesis of EED is unknown but may involve recurrent immune complex deposition, followed by incomplete attempts at healing. Persistence of an antigen, with a subsequent increase in dendrocyte activity, may also play a role in its pathogenesis. There is an association between EED and multiple infections (including HIV, hepatitis B and C, tuberculosis, and streptococcal infections), autoimmune diseases (such as RA, relapsing polychondritis, and type 1 diabetes mellitus), and the paraproteinemias (such as multiple myeloma).

Clinical Findings

A. Symptoms and Signs

A new lesion is heralded by the presence of pruritus or a burning sensation in the skin, which then leads to the development of a red, reddish brown, or purple papule or nodule. These lesions may coalesce to form large plaques, usually over the extensor surfaces of joints. With healing, the lesions often assume a yellowish or brown color, resembling xanthomata.

B. Laboratory Findings

Patients in whom EED is suspected should be screened for possible causes, including HIV infection, viral hepatitis, syphilis, cryoglobulinemia, and monoclonal gammopathy. When appropriate, patients may benefit from screening for associated autoimmune diseases as well.

C. Special Tests

Skin biopsy specimens usually show a nonspecific leukocytoclastic vasculitis with C3 deposition and are important for excluding nonvasculitis mimickers. In older lesions, the neutrophils are replaced by histiocytes, and there is marked granulation tissue and fibrosis.

Differential Diagnosis

Biopsy of lesions at various stages of development may demonstrate findings that are also consistent with a wide variety of diagnoses, including Sweet syndrome, pyoderma gangrenosum, drug reaction, erythema multiforme, fibrous histiocytoma, Kaposi sarcoma, xanthoma, and necrobiotic xanthogranuloma. The diagnosis can be established only by clinical judgement, supplemented by supportive findings on pathology.

Treatment

When a cause can be established, EED may respond to treatment of the underlying disorder. It is well established, for instance, that patients with EED as a consequence of HIV infection experience a regression of the cutaneous lesions with institution of highly active antiretroviral therapy. Nonspecific therapies are less successful. Lesions may be suppressed by dapsone but tend to recur when the drug is stopped. Lesions may also respond to tetracycline, colchicine, chloroquine, and glucocorticoids (either topical or systemic).

Complications

Although recurrent and frequently unresponsive to therapy, EED is limited to the skin and does not lead to significant morbidity.

When to Refer to a Specialist

Patients who have an underlying disorder, such as HIV, multiple myeloma, or an autoimmune condition, may benefit from evaluation by a specialist.

Prognosis

The prognosis associated with EED itself, even when unresponsive to therapy, is generally quite good. The overall prognosis for the patient, however, largely depends on the underlying disease process.

DRUG-INDUCED ANCA-ASSOCIATED VASCULITIS

 ESSENTIALS OF DIAGNOSIS

- *Cutaneous eruptions, such as palpable purpura or a maculopapular rash limited to the lower extremities, are the most common manifestation of the drug-induced AAV.*

- *Frequently associated with very high titers of anti-myeloperoxidase ANCA.*
- *Tissue biopsy provides a definitive diagnosis.*

General Considerations

Drug-induced, ANCA-associated vasculitis (AAV) is a form of vasculitis induced by certain medications in some patients. The majority of cases are associated with ANCA directed against myeloperoxidase, often in very high titers. Drug-induced AAV may resolve following discontinuation of the offending agent. Other cases, however, are indistinguishable from idiopathic AAV and require intensive therapy with glucocorticoids and cytotoxic agents.

Many cases of drug-induced AAV are associated with relatively minor symptoms (eg, constitutional symptoms, arthralgias or arthritis, and purpura). Propylthiouracil is a well-documented cause of drug-induced AAV. Other drugs implicated thus far include hydralazine, sulfasalazine, minocycline, D-penicillamine, ciprofloxacin, phenytoin, clozapine, and allopurinol. Leukotriene inhibitors have been linked to the occurrence of the Churg-Strauss syndrome, but the true direct relationship (if any) between these medications and that condition remains unclear (see Chapter 33).

Pathogenesis

All of the events in the pathogenesis of drug-induced AAV remain undefined. Propylthiouracil is known to accumulate within neutrophil granules and alter myeloperoxidase, an event that may trigger the production of antimyeloperoxidase ANCA. The presence of this human model of ANCA-associated disease forms one of the strongest arguments for a direct contribution of ANCA to the pathophysiology of other human disorders. Recent mouse models also strongly support the concept that ANCA may be pathogenic in humans.

Clinical Findings

A. SYMPTOMS AND SIGNS

Cutaneous eruptions are the most common manifestation of drug-induced AAV. These often present as palpable purpura or a maculopapular rash limited to the lower extremities. Unlike other AAV, the skin lesions in the drug-induced form frequently appear in "crops" (ie, simultaneously). Arthralgias and myalgias are common. The kidneys and upper respiratory tract may also be involved, as with the classic forms of AAV.

B. LABORATORY FINDINGS

In drug-induced AAV, very high titers of anti-myeloperoxidase antibodies are characteristic. Reports of cases associated with anti-proteinase 3 antibodies are rare. Even when the vasculitis resolves after discontinuation of the causative agent and initiation of immunosuppression, ANCA titers often remain elevated.

C. SPECIAL TESTS

Tissue biopsy is usually necessary to provide a definitive diagnosis.

Differential Diagnosis

Drug-induced AAV is frequently slow to resolve after cessation of the offending agent and may be difficult to distinguish from the primary ANCA vasculitides. In general, the manifestations of drug-induced AAV are mild and responsive to short courses of immunosuppression, although this is not always the case.

Treatment

The first step in treatment is the identification of the potential offending agents. Clinicians should take into account all exposures during the 6 months before the onset of symptoms, including nonprescription medications, herbal and dietary supplements, and illicit substances. Withdrawal of the offending agent may result in the resolution of the symptoms, although this may take months and may require the withdrawal of numerous agents simultaneously.

Patients with severe organ involvement may require aggressive immunosuppression with glucocorticoids and cytotoxic agents such as cyclophosphamide. The required length of therapy in drug-induced AAV may be shorter than that recommended for primary AAV.

When to Refer to a Specialist

Drug-induced, ANCA-associated vasculitides may require the institution of cytotoxic agents for prolonged periods of time. Therefore, patients with evidence of severe organ involvement may benefit from referral to a specialist who is accustomed to the treatment of systemic vasculitis.

Prognosis

Overall, the prognosis associated with drug-induced AAV is quite good. Organ involvement is frequently limited to the skin, and even systemic involvement frequently responds to lower doses of immunosuppressive agents administered for shorter periods of time than that required for primary AAV.

REFERENCES

Choi HK, et al. Drug-associated antineutrophil cytoplasmic antibody-positive vasculitis: prevalence among patients with high titers of antimyeloperoxidase antibodies. *Arthritis Rheum.* 2000;43:405. [PMID: 10693882]

Garcia Berrocal JR, et al. Cogan's syndrome: an oculo-audio-vestibular disease. *Postgrad Med J.* 1999;75:262. [PMID: 10533627]

Gibson LE, el-Azhary RA. Erythema elevatum diutinum. *Clin Dermatol.* 2000;18:295. [PMID:10856661]

Goronzy JJ, Weyand CM. Vasculitis in rheumatoid arthritis. *Curr Opin Rheumatol.* 1994;6:290. [PMID: 8060764] (Focuses on some of the predisposing factors to this complication of rheumatoid arthritis, particularly on potential genetic risk factors.)

Gunton JE, et al. Prevalence of positive anti-neutrophil cytoplasmic antibody (ANCA) in patients receiving anti-thyroid medication. *Eur J Endocrinol.* 2000;142:587. [PMID: 10822221]

Stone JH, Francis HW. Immune-mediated inner ear disease. *Curr Opin Rheumatol.* 2000;12:32. [PMID: 10647952] (A basic review that quantifies many of the unknowns about this condition.)

Stone JH, Nousari HC. 'Essential' cutaneous vasculitis: what every rheumatologist should know about vasculitis of the skin. *Curr Opin Rheumatol.* 2001;13:23. [PMID: 11148712] (A logically ordered review of the approach to cutaneous vasculitis, with an emphasis on diagnosis.)

Vollertsen RS, Conn DL. Vasculitis associated with rheumatoid arthritis. *Rheum Dis Clin North Am.* 1990;16:445. [PMID: 2189161] (Comprehensive description of this disease complication.)

Wisnieski JJ. Urticarial vasculitis. *Curr Opin Rheumatol.* 2000;12:24. [PMID: 10647951] (Thoughtful synthesis of the different clinical forms of this disorder.)

SECTION V

Degenerative Joint Disease & Crystal-Induced Arthritis

Osteoarthritis

42

Allan C. Gelber, MD, MPH, PhD

ESSENTIALS OF DIAGNOSIS

- *Joint pain brought on and exacerbated by activity and relieved with rest.*
- *Stiffness that is self-limited upon awakening in the morning or when rising from a seated position after an extended period of inactivity.*
- *Absence of prominent constitutional symptoms.*
- *Examination notable for increased bony prominence at the joint margins, crepitance or a grating sensation upon joint manipulation, and little if any associated joint effusion.*
- *Diagnosis supported by radiographic features of joint space narrowing and spur (or osteophyte) formation.*

General Considerations

Osteoarthritis is the leading cause of arthritis in the adult American population and affects an estimated 20 million people in the United States. Joint pain is a frequent symptom that often prompts a patient to seek medical attention, for which osteoarthritis figures prominently in the differential diagnosis. The challenge for clinicians is to correctly identify the cause of the patient's pain and to initiate appropriate therapy, both medicinal and nonmedicinal. Synonymous with degenerative joint disease, osteoarthritis is characterized by joint pain related to use, the absence of pain at rest, self-limited morning stiffness, an audible grating sound

or crepitus on palpation, reduction in joint range of motion, and minimal to no associated joint swelling or warmth.

Characteristic sites of involvement in the peripheral skeleton include the hand (distal interphalangeal joint, proximal interphalangeal [PIP] joint, and first carpometacarpal joint), knee, and hip. Common axial sites with a predilection for osteoarthritis are the lumbar and cervical spine. Constitutional symptoms are characteristically absent. Other than pain or discomfort in the involved joint, the patient with osteoarthritis most often feels well and reports good health.

The diagnosis of osteoarthritis can usually be made relatively easily and confidently based on the history and examination alone. The bedside diagnosis of osteoarthritis can be supported by plain radiography.

Epidemiology

At the population level, osteoarthritis results in substantial morbidity and disability, particularly among the elderly. It is the leading indication for several hundred thousand knee and hip replacement surgeries performed each year in the United States. Therefore, much effort has been invested in improving the understanding of the epidemiology of this disorder, including identifying the factors that predispose persons to osteoarthritis, especially those risk factors that are reversible or modifiable.

Several factors heighten the risk of incident osteoarthritis, including age, gender, and joint injury. While the clinical expression of osteoarthritis begins to manifest during the fourth and fifth decades of life, the incidence of osteoarthritis continues to increase with each decade of aging. Moreover, women in their 50s, 60s, and 70s have a greater prevalence of osteoarthritis in the hand, knee, and hip than do men. There is evidence to suggest that racial differences exist in osteoarthritis prevalence, with greater frequency of knee osteoarthritis in African Americans than in white Americans. Also, prior trauma to a previously pristine joint, such as a ruptured anterior cruciate ligament or torn medial meniscus, increases the risk of later osteoarthritis at that joint site.

Pathogenesis

The pathophysiology of this disorder is related to excessive degradation of cartilage within the involved joint. Elevated production of degradative metalloproteinases, including collagenases, results in tissue breakdown and disruption in assembly of the extracellular matrix. This disruption to the structural integrity of articular cartilage in turn leads to functional compromise of the patient.

Prevention

At present, there are no definitive data available from randomized controlled trials regarding what preventive measures can be taken to reduce a patient's risk of developing osteoarthritis. While certain factors, such as age, gender and race, cannot be altered, others such as body weight are more amenable to modification. Moreover, findings from observational studies suggest that weight loss and a change in dietary patterns may reduce a patient's risk of developing osteoarthritis at the knee or diminish the probability of osteoarthritis progression.

Among women who participated in the Framingham Osteoarthritis Study, those who experienced a 5-kg or more weight reduction over 10 years had half the risk of developing symptomatic knee osteoarthritis. Such data support the claim that weight reduction can alter the risk of developing osteoarthritis. Moreover, higher levels of vitamin D in serum and in the diet and greater intake of vitamin C were associated with a reduced risk of disease progression. Dietary consumption of these nutrients was not, however, related to the risk of developing new, or incident, osteoarthritis.

Clinical Findings

A. SYMPTOMS AND SIGNS

The patient with osteoarthritis affecting a joint in the peripheral skeleton, such as the finger, knee, or hip, may initially experience relatively minor pain or discomfort with use of the involved joint (Table 42–1). For example, at the outset of osteoarthritis involving the hip joint, patients may have some difficulty crossing their legs to put on a pair of shoes or pants; however, once they are dressed and upright, bearing weight and

Table 42–1. Signs, symptoms, and diagnostic features of osteoarthritis.

Joint pain that increases with activity
Morning stiffness that is relatively brief and self-limited
Crepitus (a grating sensation with motion)
Bony enlargement at the joint margin
Tenderness to palpation
Minimal to no joint warmth
Minimal to no joint effusion
Noninflammatory synovial fluid (< 2000 WBC/µL)
ESR normal for age
Radiographic evidence of osteoarthritis (nonuniform joint space narrowing, osteophyte [spur] formation, subchondral cysts, and eburnation [bony sclerosis])
Negative serologic tests for antinuclear antibody and rheumatoid factor

WBC, white blood cell; ESR, erythrocyte sedimentation rate.

ambulation are still well tolerated. As osteoarthritis progresses, a patient will gradually experience progressively severe joint discomfort and increasing difficulty with related activities of daily living.

With further disease progression, such as at an osteoarthritic hand or finger, increasing difficulty with previously routine activities often follows. Thus, even gripping, holding, or writing with a pen or pencil can be a painful feat to accomplish. Putting car keys in and turning the ignition switch, lifting a gallon of milk out of the refrigerator, or removing a pot of water from the stove can become quite difficult tasks to accomplish. At this stage, the signs of osteoarthritis joint involvement include bony enlargement of the involved joint and possibly joint misalignment. At the extreme end of the disease spectrum, marked impairment in activity follows. Even walking from room to room in one's home may be unbearably painful when advanced or end-stage osteoarthritis affects the hip or knee joint.

B. LABORATORY FINDINGS

There is no specific laboratory test that is used in clinical practice to confirm a diagnosis of osteoarthritis. Instead, routine laboratory blood testing, including complete blood cell counts, acute phase reactants (erythrocyte sedimentation rate and C-reactive protein), and screening autoantibodies (rheumatoid factor and antinuclear antibody) are of value in their negativity. These parameters may be of key diagnostic value when determining whether particular signs and symptoms in the hand represent underlying osteoarthritis or rheumatoid arthritis. Thus, normal white blood cell and platelet counts, the absence of anemia, normalcy of acute phase reactants, and seronegativity for rheumatoid factor are each expected in the patient whose PIP joint changes are the result of bony remodeling and joint space narrowing from osteoarthritis (termed "Bouchard nodes") rather than the result of active rheumatoid synovitis, which may affect this same joint group.

C. IMAGING STUDIES

Radiographic imaging can confirm the diagnosis of osteoarthritis. More than 4 decades ago, Kellgren and Lawrence described characteristic radiographic features of osteoarthritis—joint space narrowing, osteophytes, subchondral cysts, and bony sclerosis (eburnation). To the present, these parameters remain the radiographic hallmarks of osteoarthritis. While scintigraphy (bone scan) may reveal increased radionuclide uptake at osteoarthritic joints and computed tomography and magnetic resonance imaging may demonstrate characteristic radiographic features of osteoarthritis, these imaging modalities are not routinely used to confirm the diagnosis of osteoarthritis.

D. SPECIAL TESTS

Pursuit of a histologic diagnosis via synovial or bone biopsy is not a conventional strategy in the evaluation of a patient with suspected osteoarthritis. However, in the appropriate setting, a joint tap is a valuable test when encountering a patient with presumptive osteoarthritis. When there is subtle—if not moderate evidence—of a mild joint effusion, diagnostic arthrocentesis may be a key aid to confirm the clinical impression. This is because a synovial fluid cell count of 200–2000 cells/μL is characteristic of an osteoarthritic effusion; this synovial fluid white blood cell count is intermediate between the upper bound of normal and the lower bound of an inflammatory arthritis.

Differential Diagnosis

The challenge when evaluating a patient with joint pain is to effectively use the history, examination, and available tests to arrive at the correct diagnosis. The presence of pain at the symptomatic joint, brought on by activity and relieved with rest, is quite suggestive of a degenerative arthropathy. Moreover, the absence of constitutional signs and symptoms and the presence of bony enlargement at the joint margin, with little if any evidence of joint inflammation, serve to reinforce this clinical impression. Finally, the pattern of joint involvement is meaningful because primary osteoarthritis has a predilection for particular joint sites in the peripheral skeleton, predominantly the hands (distal interphalangeal joints, PIP joints, first carpometacarpal joint), knees, and hips. The cervical and lumbar spine are preferentially involved sites of involvement in the axial

skeleton. These features serve to distinguish osteoarthritis from inflammatory arthropathies (such as rheumatoid arthritis and gout) that have overlapping sites of involvement.

It is also worth noting that a variety of secondary disorders represent identifiable causes of osteoarthritis. Several such disorders, including those resulting from inborn errors of metabolism and metabolic derangements, are listed in Table 42–2. Recognition of their distinct features, such as predilection for involvement of the second and third metacarpophalangeal joints in hemochromatosis-associated arthropathy, may serve to identify the true underlying cause of the joint pain and may impact upon therapeutic decision making. Finally, one need also bear in mind that the presence of known osteoarthritis does not negate consideration of an alternate explanation, such as an occult malignancy, when a meaningful change in the pattern of joint pain occurs.

Treatment

Notwithstanding the substantial population burden and the deleterious impact on quality of life for affected persons, there is no known curative therapy for osteoarthritis. Nevertheless, conventional treatment has been demonstrated to reduce symptoms and improve function and quality of life in randomized clinical trials. Goals of therapy are to control pain, improve function, minimize disability, and enhance health-related quality of life. It is a priority to furnish the patient and his or

Table 42–2. Identifiable causes of osteoarthritis.

Inherited genetic predisposition
Type II procollagen gene (COL2A1)
Congenital disorder
Legg-Calvé-Perthes disease
Acetabular dysplasia
Inborn error of connective tissue
Ehlers-Danlos syndrome
Marfan syndrome
Post-traumatic
Anterior cruciate ligament tear
Meniscus tear with or without prior meniscectomy surgery
Metabolic disorders
Hemochromatosis
Wilson disease
Ochronosis (alkaptonuria)
Postinflammatory
Underlying rheumatoid arthritis
Generalized osteoarthritis
Predilection for first CMC, DIP, PIP, knee, and hip joints

CMC, carpometacarpal; DIP, distal interphalangeal; PIP; proximal interphalangeal.

her family with appropriate education and understanding on this disorder as well as reasonable expectations regarding the course and hazards of therapy. A further therapeutic priority is to minimize, if not avoid altogether, drug-associated toxicity, particularly that which may result from nonsteroidal anti-inflammatory drug (NSAID) therapy.

A specific set of guidelines regarding the medical management of osteoarthritis at the knee and hip joints has been published by the American College of Rheumatology. The major goals of therapy are the alleviation of pain and improvement in function. In patients with mild to moderate osteoarthritis, therapeutic benefit can often be achieved without resorting immediately to the use of prescription medication. For example, an assistive device, such as a cane or walker, can be substantially beneficial. Similarly, quadriceps strengthening and aerobic exercise have been shown to be effective in the management of osteoarthritis at the knee. In terms of nonprescription therapy, it is also pertinent to inquire about what other forms of therapy the patient may be taking. For example, many persons resort to alternative medicine modalities, including ingestion of shark tooth cartilage, application of magnets to osteoarthritic joints, or standing in front of an electromagnetic field.

A front-line approach to medicinal therapy for osteoarthritis includes use of acetaminophen. This drug has been demonstrated to be effective in improving pain and function and has a safer toxicity profile, particularly with regard to the gastrointestinal tract, than other NSAIDs. For many years, the NSAIDs have been widely used in the management of osteoarthritis. Via their inhibition of cyclooxygenase (COX), particularly the inducible isoform at sites of joint damage, symptomatic benefit is achieved.

However, the toxicity profile of NSAID therapy remains a major concern, at both the individual and population aggregate level. An estimated 10,000 Americans die each year of gastrointestinal complications resulting from NSAID therapy. The following factors increase the risk of such toxicity:

- Persons with prior peptic ulcer disease.
- Persons older than 65 years.
- Concomitant tobacco and alcohol use.
- Coadministration of glucocorticoids or anticoagulation therapy.
- Comorbid *Helicobacter pylori* infection.

In 1999, a new category of NSAID agents, the selective COX-2 antagonists, that selectively and preferentially inhibit the inducible isoform at the site of joint injury (but not the constitutive form of the enzyme that has gastroprotective properties) was introduced into the marketplace. Their use has exploded in just the last 4 years, on the strength of furnishing a safer gastrointestinal profile. However, this improved safety profile has been questioned, including concern of an enhanced cardiovascular toxicity profile that may offset the improved gastrointestinal benefits.

Increasing evidence now exists to support use of glucosamine sulfate, a component of human articular cartilage, in the medical management of osteoarthritis. In particular, two recent European reports have furnished evidence from randomized, placebo-controlled trials that demonstrated improvement in joint pain and functionality in patients with knee osteoarthritis managed with oral glucosamine at a dose of 1500 mg/d compared with placebo. Moreover, in both trials glucosamine was also shown to halt radiographic progression of joint space narrowing. The concept that a therapeutic intervention may actually arrest or reverse structural compromise to an osteoarthritic joint is a novel and highly noteworthy development in the management of osteoarthritis. Whether similar benefit may be accrued with use of chondroitin sulfate (also commercially available)—or whether additive benefit can be obtained from concomitant administration of both glucosamine and chondroitin—remains to be determined.

Complications

After a diagnosis of osteoarthritis has been firmly established, subsequent change in symptoms or course will not necessarily be directly attributable to the known osteoarthritis. Such a change ought to command the clinician's attention to search for, or at least entertain, the possibility of an alternate consideration (Table 42–3). For example, the abrupt onset of heat, redness, and swelling in a known yet previously stable osteoarthritic knee may herald the onset of a superimposed microcrystalline arthritis or of a ruptured Baker (or popliteal) cyst. Alternately, new-onset joint locking or giving way

Table 42–3. Acute complications of osteoarthritis.

Microcrystalline arthropathy
  Gout
  Pseudogout
Spontaneous osteonecrosis of the knee
Ruptured Baker cyst (pseudothrombophlebitis syndrome)
Bursitis
  Supraspinatus tendinitis
  Trochanteric bursitis
Radiculoneuritis
  Sciatica
  Femoral

may suggest the presence of a loose body that warrants arthroscopic intervention before a catastrophic fall were to occur. Similarly, nerve entrapment from a spinal osteophyte encroaching upon an exiting nerve root in the foraminal space may lead to new or rapidly progressive burning or electrical pain in the affected extremity. Not to be forgotten is that a change in symptoms in the region of an osteoarthritic join may also be attributable to active inflammation of adjacent nonarticular tissues, including regional tendons and bursae.

When to Refer to a Specialist

An important consideration when weighing the merit of referral to a specialist is whether there exists a lack of diagnostic clarity. This is particularly germane when the clinician's judgement suggests that a given patient's symptoms are poorly explained by invoking osteoarthritis as the underlying cause. This concern often arises because of the high background prevalence of osteoarthritis in the general population. For example, even though clinical and radiographic evidence of osteoarthritis may be present, ongoing symptoms may be attributable to an unrelated superimposed process.

A second opinion is also advisable when a patient's pain and functional decline appear refractory to treatment. Finally, evaluation by an orthopedic surgeon is in order when the persistence of symptoms and functional decline necessitate consideration of joint replacement surgery.

Future Directions

Ongoing research in this field is largely directed at identification of factors that predispose some but not all aging adults to the development of osteoarthritis. In addition, there is an intense effort underway to identify biomarkers—of bone and cartilage turnover—that may identify those at risk for osteoarthritis and those at risk for disease progression. In the future, availability of drug therapy that may inhibit the adverse effects of degradative enzymes or promote the growth of deficient cartilaginous structures will be critical to realizing therapies that may effectively control, if not cure, osteoarthritis.

REFERENCES

Ettinger WH Jr, et al. A randomized trial comparing aerobic exercise and resistance exercise with a health education program in older adults with knee osteoarthritis. The Fitness Arthritis and Seniors Trial (FAST). *JAMA.* 1997;277:25. [PMID: 8980206] (A substantive randomized clinical trial that demonstrated the benefit of exercise in the management of osteoarthritis.)

Mukherjee D, et al. Risk of cardiovascular events associated with selective COX-2 inhibitors. *JAMA.* 2001;286:954. [PMID: 11509060] (A thought-provoking report that raised the possibility of unintended adverse cardiovascular events associated with use of selective COX-2 inhibitors.)

Pavelka K, et al. Glucosamine sulfate use and delay of progression of knee osteoarthritis: a 3-year, randomized, placebo-controlled, double-blind study. *Arch Intern Med.* 2002;162:2113. [PMID:12374520]

Recommendations for the medical management of osteoarthritis of the hip and knee: 2000 update. American College of Rheumatology Subcommittee on Osteoarthritis Guidelines. *Arthritis Rheum.* 2000;43:1905. [PMID: 11014340]

Reginster JY, et al. Long-term effects of glucosamine sulphate on osteoarthritis progression: a randomised, placebo-controlled clinical trial. *Lancet.* 2001;357:251. [PMID: 11214126] (A landmark trial demonstrating therapeutic benefit from use of glucosamine in the management of osteoarthritis.)

Relevant World Wide Web Sites

[OsteoArthritis Research Society International]
http://www.oarsi.org
[Arthritis Foundation]
http://www.arthritis.org

Gout

43

Sherri Sanders, MD, & Robert L. Wortmann, MD

ESSENTIALS OF DIAGNOSIS

- *Caused by deposition of uric acid crystals and usually associated with hyperuricemia.*
- *Usually begins as an intermittent, acute monoarthritis, especially of the first metatarsophalangeal joint.*
- *Over time, attacks become more frequent, less intense, and involve more joints.*
- *Diagnosed by demonstrating uric acid crystals in joint fluid.*
- *Extra-articular manifestations include tophi and renal stones.*
- *Arthritis responds to nonsteroidal anti-inflammatory drugs or colchicine.*

General Considerations

The underlying basis for gout is an increased total body urate pool. This is generally manifested as hyperuricemia, which is defined as a serum urate concentration more than 7.0 mg/dL. The concentration of 7.0 mg/dL is important because fluids with urate content greater than that are supersaturated with urate, a condition that favors urate crystal precipitation.

At least 5% of asymptomatic Americans manifest hyperuricemia on at least one occasion during adulthood. Hyperuricemia may be even more common in Europe and in countries in the Far East.

The likelihood of developing symptomatic gout and the age at which that occurs correlates with the duration and magnitude of hyperuricemia. In one study, persons with urate levels between 7.0 and 8.0 mL/dL had a cumulative incidence of gouty arthritis of 3% while those with urate levels greater than 9.0 mL/dL had a 5-year cumulative incidence of 22%. Hyperuricemia alone is not sufficient for the diagnosis of gout, however, and asymptomatic hyperuricemia in the absence of gout is not a disease. It appears that clinical gout will develop in fewer than one in four hyperuricemic persons at any point.

Gout presents predominantly in men with a peak age of onset in the fifth decade. The incidence of gout in women approaches that of men only after they have reached age 60 years. The onset of disease in men prior to adulthood or in women before menopause is quite rare and is almost always due to an inborn error of metabolism or congenital condition. The prevalence of self-reported gout is estimated to be 13.6 per 1000 men and 6.4 per 1000 women.

Hyperuricemia can result from increased urate production, decreased uric acid excretion by the kidneys, or a combination of the two mechanisms. Fewer than 5% of patients with gout are hyperuricemic because of urate overproduction. These persons can be recognized because they excrete more than 800 mg of uric acid in their urine during a 24-hour period. Those who excrete less uric acid than 800 mg are hyperuricemic because of impaired renal excretion. Defining individuals as "overproducers" or "underexcreters" is helpful in predicting whether the hyperuricemia is associated with a variety of acquired or genetic disorders (Table 43–1) and may be useful in some cases in determining the most appropriate treatment.

Clinical Findings

A. SYMPTOMS AND SIGNS

The natural history of gout can be divided into three distinct stages (Figure 43–1):

1. Asymptomatic hyperuricemia.
2. Acute and intermittent (or intercritical) gout.
3. Chronic tophaceous gout.

Although most untreated patients with gout will progress to chronic tophaceous gout, the course varies considerably from one patient to another. Some patients experience only one or two attacks of acute gouty arthritis during their lifetime. It is quite unusual for tophi to develop in a patient with no history of acute gouty arthritis.

The initial episode of acute gouty arthritis usually follows 10 to 30 years of asymptomatic hyperuricemia, and there is no evidence that damage occurs to any organ system during that time. Just why and when the first attack of gout occurs in susceptible persons remains a mystery. Although some patients experience

Table 43–1. Classification of hyperuricemia.

Urate overproduction
    Primary hyperuricemia
        Idiopathic
        Complete or partial deficiency of HGPRT
        Superactivity of PRPP synthetase
    Secondary hyperuricemia
        Excessive purine consumption
        Myeloproliferative or lymphoproliferative disorders
        Hemolytic diseases
        Psoriasis
        Glycogen storage diseases: types 1, 3, 5, and 7
Uric acid underexcretion
    Primary hyperuricemia
        Idiopathic
    Secondary hyperuricemia
        Decreased renal function
        Metabolic acidosis (ketoacidosis or lactic acidosis)
        Dehydration
        Diuretics
        Hypertension
        Hyperparathyroidism
        Drugs including cyclosporine, pyrazinamide, ethambutol
          and low-dose salicylates
        Lead nephropathy
Overproduction and underexcretion
    Alcohol use
    Glucose-6-phosphatase deficiency
    Fructose-1-phosphate-aldolase deficiency

HGPRT, hypoxanthine-guanine phosphoribosyltransferase; PRPP, 5′-phosphoribosyl-1-pyrophosphate.

prodromal episodes of mild discomfort, the onset of a gouty attack is usually heralded by the rapid onset of exquisite pain associated with warmth, swelling, and erythema of the affected joint (Figure 43–2). The pain escalates from the faintest twinges to its most intense level over an 8- to 12-hour period. Initial attacks usually affect only one joint and, in half the patients, the first attack involves the first metatarsophalangeal joint. Other joints frequently involved in the early stage of gout include the midfoot, ankle, heel, and knee. Wrist, fingers, and elbows are more typical sites of attacks later in the course of the disease. The intensity of the pain is such that patients cannot stand even the weight of a bed sheet on the affected part and most find it difficult or impossible to walk when the lower extremities are involved in an acute attack. The acute attack may be accompanied by fever, chills, and malaise. Cutaneous erythema associated with the attack may extend beyond the involved joint and resemble cellulitis. Desquamation of the skin may occur as the attack resolves.

Symptoms resolve quickly with appropriate treatment, but even untreated, an acute attack resolves spontaneously over 1 to 2 weeks. With resolution of the attack, patients enter an interval termed the "intercritical period" when they are again completely asymptomatic. The rare patient will not experience a second attack of gout but most will. Early in the intermittent stage, episodes of arthritis are infrequent and the intervals between the attacks vary from months to years. Over time, the attacks become more frequent, less acute in onset, longer in duration, and tend to involve more joints.

During the intercritical periods of acute intermittent gout, the previously involved joints are virtually free of symptoms. Despite this, monosodium urate crystal de-

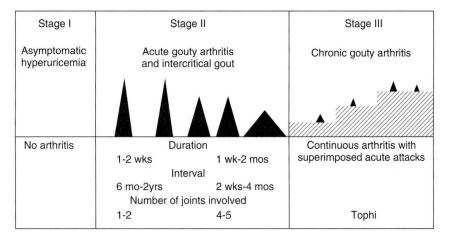

Figure 43–1. The natural history of gout progress through three stages.

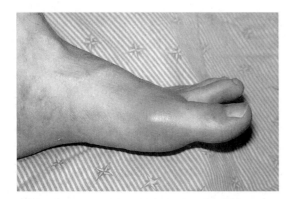

Figure 43–2. Acute gouty attack of the first metatarsophalangeal joint.

position continues. Urate crystals often can be identified in the synovial fluid despite the absence of symptoms and erosive changes indicative of bony tophi begin to appear on radiographs.

Although the reasons why acute gout develops when it does are not clear, attacks tend to be associated with rapid increases, and more often, decreases in the concentration of urate in synovial fluid. These concentrations mirror the fluctuations seen in the serum. Accordingly, a person may experience a sudden drop in the serum urate level, leading to an acute attack and, therefore, is found to be normouricemic when blood is tested at that time. Trauma, alcohol ingestion, and the use of certain drugs are known to trigger gout attacks as well. Gouty attacks not infrequently occur as a person is recovering from an alcoholic binge. Drugs known to precipitate attacks do so by rapidly raising or lowering serum urate levels. Candidate agents include diuretics, salicylates, and the urate-lowering drugs allopurinol and radiographic contrast agents. It is believed that these fluctuations in urate levels destabilize tophi in the gouty synovium. The sudden addition of urate to them may render them unstable, or the sudden lowering of the urate concentration may cause partial dissolution and instability. As the microtophi break apart, crystals are shed into the synovial fluid and the gouty attack is initiated by the ingestion of these crystals by polymorphonuclear leukocytes.

As gout continues to progress, the patient gradually enters the stage of chronic gouty arthritis. This usually develops after 10 or more years of acute intermittent gout. The transition to chronic gout is complete when the intercritical periods are no longer pain free. The involved joints are now persistently uncomfortable and may be swollen. Patients report stiffness or gelling sensations as well. Visible or palpable tophi may be detected on physical examination during this stage of

gout, even though they may have been recognized by radiographs prior to entry into this stage (Figure 43–3). The development of tophaceous deposits in individual patients varies; in general, they are a function of the duration and severity of the hyperuricemia, with a mean occurrence approximately 12 years after the onset of the first attack of gout in those not treated with urate-lowering drugs.

B. LABORATORY FINDINGS

Hyperuricemia remains the cardinal feature of gout. The usefulness of this laboratory finding in establishing the diagnosis of gout is limited. Whereas most patients with gout will have an elevated serum urate (greater than 7.0 mg/dL), levels may fall within the normal range on occasion; in fact, levels in the normal range are not uncommon during acute attacks, as described above. In addition, during the acute attack, the complete blood cell count may show a leukocytosis with increased polymorphonuclear leukocytes on the differential and elevations of the erythrocyte sedimentation rate and C-reactive protein. The greatest utility of measuring serum urate is in monitoring the effects of urate-lowering therapy.

During an acute attack, the synovial fluid findings are consistent with moderate to severe inflammation (see Chapter 2). The leukocyte count usually ranges between 5 and 80,000 cells/µL with an average between

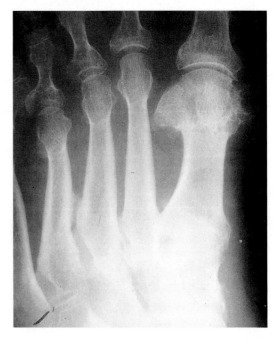

Figure 43–3. Radiographic changes of gout.

15,000 and 20,000 cells/μL. The cells are predominately polymorphonuclear leukocytes.

The definitive diagnosis of gout is made by examination of synovial fluid or tophaceous material with compensated polarized light microscopy and identifying the characteristic monosodium urate crystals. These crystals appear as bright yellow needle-shaped objects when parallel to the access of slow vibration on the first-order compensator. When these crystals are perpendicular to that axis, they are blue. Crystals are usually intracellular and needle-shaped during acute attacks but may be small, blunted, and extracellular as the attack subsides or during intercritical periods.

The 24-hour urine uric acid measurement is not required in all patients with gout but is useful for determining potential causes of hyperuricemia (see above) as well as determining whether uricosuric therapy can be effective, since this form of therapy is effective only in underexcretors.

C. IMAGING STUDIES

No radiographic abnormalities are present early in the disease course. In acute gouty arthritis, the only finding may be soft tissue swelling in the involved joint. Bony abnormalities indicative of deposition of urate crystals (microtophi) develop only after years of disease. These abnormalities are most frequently asymmetric and confined to previously symptomatic joints. The advanced bony erosions of advanced gout are often radiographically distinct. Typically, they are slightly removed from the joint space, have a rounded or oval shape, and are characterized by a hypertrophic calcified "overhanging edge." The joint space may be preserved or show osteoarthritic type narrowing.

D. SPECIAL TESTS

Patients with gout often suffer from hyperlipidemia, glucose intolerance, hypertension, coronary artery disease, and obesity. Accordingly, it is appropriate to measure serum lipids and fasting blood sugars in patients with gout. Because renal dysfunction develops in many patients with hypertension and gout, it is appropriate to monitor serum creatinine levels as well.

Diagnosis & Differential Diagnosis

The definitive diagnosis of gout is made by identifying monosodium urate crystals in polymorphonuclear leukocytes in synovial fluid or from aspirates of tophi (Figure 43–4). The presumptive diagnosis of gout can be made by the presence of the characteristic triad of (1) hyperuricemia, (2) acute monarticular arthritis, and (3) a gratifying clinical response to therapy with colchicine, defined as complete resolution of symptoms within 48 hours and no recurrence for 1 week. Finally, clinicians may also use the criteria proposed by American

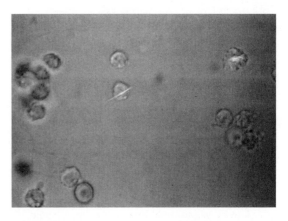

Figure 43–4. Urate crystal ingested by a polymorphonuclear leukocyte in synovial fluid. This finding is pathognomonic for acute gouty arthritis.

College of Rheumatology for the diagnosis of gout (Table 43–2).

Because gouty arthritis often occurs in association with other diseases, those conditions in Table 43–1 should be considered as possible in any person with gout. A variety of conditions can mimic or be confused with gouty arthritis. These include other crystal-induced diseases such as those related to the deposition of calcium pyrophosphate dihydrate crystals (pseudogout) or basic calcium phosphate crystals. The latter

Table 43–2. Criteria for the diagnosis of acute gouty arthritis.

- Presence of characteristic urate crystals in joint fluid, or
- A tophus proved to contain urate crystals by chemical means or polarized light microscopy, or
- The presence of 6 of the following 12 clinical, laboratory, and x-ray phenomena listed below:
    1. More than one attack of acute arthritis
    2. Maximal inflammation developed within 1 day
    3. Attack of monarticular arthritis
    4. Joint redness observed
    5. First metatarsophalangeal joint painful or swollen
    6. Unilateral attack involving first metatarsophalangeal joint
    7. Unilateral attack involving tarsal joint
    8. Suspected tophus
    9. Hyperuricemia
    10. A symptomatic swelling within a joint (radiograph)
    11. Subcortical cysts without erosions (radiograph)
    12. Negative culture of joint fluids for microorganisms during attack of joint inflammation

may cause a calcific tendinitis that is similar in presentation to gout. Septic arthritis can also mimic gout, although a gouty attack may coexist with an infected joint. The more common causes of septic arthritis are gonococcal, staphylococcal, or streptococcal infections. However, infections with fungi or mycobacteria may also be seen. A hemarthrosis or fracture in the joint line may be confused with a gouty attack. Finally, some conditions that are usually considered oligoarticular or polyarticular in presentation may involve only one joint early in the course and be confused with gout. This is particularly true with the peripheral arthritis associated with ankylosing spondylitis, Reiter syndrome, psoriatic arthritis, and the arthritis of inflammatory bowel disease. Rarely, palindromic rheumatism may herald the onset of rheumatoid arthritis and begins with monarticular arthritis.

Occasionally, chronic gouty arthritis and tophi are misdiagnosed as rheumatoid arthritis. The chronic symptoms are polyarticular and symmetric, and the tophaceous deposits mimic rheumatoid nodules. This problem is compounded by the fact that up to 25% of patients with gout have positive tests for rheumatoid factor although these are usually of low titer.

Treatment

The management of gout includes the following:

1. Providing rapid and safe pain relief
2. Preventing further attacks
3. Preventing formation of tophi and destructive arthritis
4. Addressing associated medical conditions

The goal of treating the acute gout attack is to eliminate the pain and other symptoms caused by the intense inflammation as rapidly as possible. The choices in this situation include nonsteroidal anti-inflammatory drugs (NSAIDs), colchicine, and glucocorticoids. Effective management of the acute attack is not so much determined by which agent is used but, rather, by how quickly that agent is initiated after the onset of the attack. If a single dose is given in the first minutes of an attack, it may eradicate the symptoms and terminate the attack. If, however, medication is not taken during the first 48 hours of symptoms, it will probably take at least 2 days before control is gained. Once symptoms have resolved, the particular agent used should be continued at a reduced dose for another 48–72 hours.

NSAIDs have become the most frequently used agents to treat gout because they are so well tolerated. Indomethacin is historically the NSAID of choice for acute gout, but other NSAIDs may be just as effective. The selected NSAID should be started at its recommended maximal dose. The dose may be lowered as symptoms resolve. NSAIDs should be avoided in patients with active or recent peptic ulcer disease and should be used in caution in patients with renal insufficiency or conditions associated with impaired renal blood flow (see Chapter 56).

Colchicine is effective but less well-tolerated than NSAIDs. Colchicine is taken in 0.5- or 0.6-mg doses hourly until one of three end points is reached: (1) significant clinical improvement, (2) onset of severe gastrointestinal side effects, or (3) 10 doses are taken without relief (in which case the diagnosis of gout should be questioned). Gastrointestinal side effects include gas, nausea, vomiting, diarrhea, and severe cramping abdominal pain. Gastrointestinal symptoms eventually develop (at a particular dose) in everyone who takes colchicine. However, there is much individual variation in the tolerance to this medication. Often, the development of these side effects coincides with the control of the gouty attack, but they may develop before symptomatic relief.

Intravenous colchicine may be used, particularly in persons who are recovering from surgery or for those where oral intake is not possible. Intravenous use of colchicine has the advantages of a rapid onset and no gastrointestinal toxicity, provided oral colchicine is not being used simultaneously. When used, the drug should be diluted in 20–50 mL of normal saline administered over 15 to 20 minutes through a secured intravenous line. Extravasation of colchicine into soft tissues results in a severe reaction. A single intravenous dose of colchicine should not exceed 2 mg and the total cumulative dose for an attack should not exceed 3 mg in a 24-hour period. Patients should not receive additional colchicine through any route for 7 days after receiving an intravenous dose. Usage of colchicine by the intravenous route is not recommended in the presence of renal or hepatic disease. Absolute contraindications to intravenous colchicine include combined renal and hepatic disease, a glomerular filtration rate less than 25 mL/min, and extrahepatic biliary obstruction. Relative contraindications include significant intercurrent infection, preexisting bone marrow suppression, or the concomitant use of oral colchicine. The improper use of colchicine has led to serious toxicities and even death. All reported cases of death and severe toxicity have involved unusually high doses, or recurrent dosage in patients with renal insufficiency.

Glucocorticoids are usually reserved for patients in whom colchicine or NSAIDs are contraindicated or ineffective. Anecdotal reports suggest early recurrence of gout after treating acute attacks with glucocorticoids, but recent studies have not confirmed that observation. The response time for glucocorticoids is comparable to that for NSAIDs and colchicine. Doses of prednisone of 20–40 mg/d have been used. The dosage is usually tapered over 1 to 2 weeks after symptoms resolve. Intramuscular or intravenous glucocorticoids provide alternatives for use in the hospitalized patient who can take nothing by mouth. Finally, intra-articular injections with 10–40 mg of prednisone or 10 mg of triamcinolone can also be used.

Most often the gout attack will resolve with the use of one of these agents. However, when this does not occur or in the extremely severe case of gout, these agents may be used in combination. Potent analgesics, including narcotics, may also be added to the regimen.

Once a patient has had an acute gouty attack, the likelihood of further attacks can be reduced by prophylactic therapy with low-dose colchicine or an NSAID on a daily basis. Prophylactic therapy, however, should not be prescribed unless a urate-lowering agent is added to the regimen. The use of prophylactic colchicine without controlling the hyperuricemia only allows tophi and destructive arthritis to continue to develop without the usual warning signs of recurrent acute gouty attacks. The prophylactic use of colchicine in doses of 0.5–0.6 mg 1 to 3 times a day reduces the frequencies of attacks by 75–85%. These small doses of colchicine rarely cause gastrointestinal side effects and appear to be relatively safe. Long-term colchicine use can cause neuromuscular complications in patients with decreased renal function, especially older patients. It is prudent to avoid using more than 0.6 mg of colchicine daily in a patient with a serum creatinine above 1.5 mg/dL. This toxicity manifests with proximal muscle weakness, painful paresthesias, elevated creatine phosphokinase levels, and abnormalities on electromyograms. This axonal neuromyopathy resolves completely over several weeks after discontinuing the colchicine. Ultimately, specific urate-lowering drugs must be used to eliminate acute attacks and to prevent tophi from forming or cause them to disappear. Although dietary manipulation is essential for control of the comorbid conditions often found with gout, diet cannot reduce serum urate levels sufficiently.

The goal of treatment is to maintain the serum urate level at 5.0 mg/dL or less. Maintaining the serum level at this target allows precipitated crystals to dissolve and be cleared. If the urate level remains above 7.0 mg/dL, supersaturated conditions will persist and urate deposition will continue. In other words, lowering the serum urate from 10.0 mg/dL to 8.0 mg/dL will not reverse the disease; it will only allow it to continue to progress at a slower rate.

The xanthine oxidase inhibitor allopurinol is the agent of choice for most patients with gout. It can effectively lower serum urate levels in those patients with hyperuricemia due to underexcretion and is specifically indicated for those who overproduce urate. Patients with tophi, those with nephrolithiasis, and those who are intolerant of uricosuric therapy are also candidates for xanthine oxidase inhibition. Allopurinol may be used in the presence of renal insufficiency, but its dosage must be reduced to prevent toxicity. Allopurinol at a dose of 300 mg/d adequately controls the serum urate in most patients with normal renal function. If the patient is already taking prophylactic colchicine (which is recommended), then allopurinol can be started at a dose of 300 mg/d. Otherwise, it is recommended that patients start with 100 mg/d for a week and gradually increase the dose until the lowest level of medication that keeps the serum urate level in the target range is reached. Most patients will achieve the desired serum urate level of 5 mg/dL or less while taking 300–400 mg of allopurinol daily. The maximum recommended daily dose is 800 mg. Allopurinol must be used cautiously when the patient is also taking azathioprine or 6-mercaptopurine. Allopurinol reduces the catabolism of these agents, thereby greatly increasing their effective doses.

Side effects and toxicity of allopurinol include fever, headaches, diarrhea, dyspepsia, pleuritis, skin rashes, granulomatous hepatitis, and toxic epidermal necrolysis. The syndrome of allopurinol hypersensitivity is rare but serious with a mortality rate of 20–30%. Allopurinol hypersensitivity reactions are more common in older patients with impaired renal function taking diuretics. The development of a rash in patients with allopurinol is an indication to stop the medicine. After the rash is cleared, allopurinol may be cautiously reinstituted if the rash was not deemed to be severe. With more severe reactions, hypersensitivity may be overcome through desensitization protocols.

Uricosuric agents are also effective in lowering serum urate levels. The patients in whom they are most effective are those who have good renal function (glomerular or filtration rate above 60 mL/min), those who have no history of nephrolithiasis, those who can avoid all salicylate ingestions, and those under 65 years of age. Salicylate use in doses in excess of 81 mg/d will interfere with the effectiveness of uricosuric agents. These agents should be avoided in patients with a history of nephrolithiasis because stone formation is more likely due to the flooding of urine with uric acid. Finally, uricosuric agents require good renal function to be effective. Probenecid is started at a dosage of 500 mg twice a day and advanced slowly up to a maximum dosage of 1 gram twice a day or until the target urate level is reached. The most common side effects of this agent are rash and gastrointestinal upset. Sulfinpyrazone is the other uricosuric agent available in the

United States. This drug is slowly advanced from 100 mg to approximately 800 mg/d in two or three divided doses until the desired level of serum urate is reached. Benzbromarone, an agent available in Europe, is more potent and may be effective in the face of moderate renal insufficiency.

Unfortunately, the treatment of gout is complicated by poor compliance. This is probably related to the difficulty people have in remembering how to take three different medicines on three different schedules. Frequently, they become confused in which medicines to take in what situations. An analogy has been developed that may help patients understand and better remember how to take their medications (Box, Gout is Like Matches).

Hyperuricemia alone is rarely an indication for treatment with specific urate-lowering drugs. Therefore, use of a xanthine oxidase inhibitor or uricosuric agent is not recommended in the treatment of asymptomatic hyperuricemia. On the other hand, the identification of asymptomatic hyperuricemia should not be ignored. First, the cause should be determined (Table 43–1), and any associated problems, such as hypertension, obesity, alcoholism, diabetes, or hyperlipidemia, should be addressed rigorously.

GOUT IS LIKE MATCHES

The following paragraph is an analogy that can be used to explain gout to patients.

Gout is caused by uric acid. Everyone has uric acid in their blood but some people have too much of it, and some of those get gout. In those who get gout, the uric acid accumulates around the joints and acts like matches. When you get gout attack, one of the matches strikes and catches the joint on fire. When that happens, you should take your indomethacin (or nonsteroidal anti-inflammatory drug of choice). It is important to take it right away. If not, more matches will catch fire and the attack will worsen. Taking indomethacin does not cure the gout because it only puts out the fire. The matches are still there and can light again. A urate-lowering drug will remove the matches. If there are no matches, you cannot get gout. But until the urate-lowering drug has time to work, you can still get gout. Therefore, you should take colchicine, one pill twice a day. Colchicine is very good at preventing gout attacks. You can think of colchicine as something that makes the matches damp and harder to strike.

From Wortmann RL. *Am J Med.* 1998;105:513.

Complications

As described above, untreated and severe gout leads to visible and palpable tophaceous deposits and a destructive arthropathy. However, these complications are preventable with accurate diagnosis and appropriate therapy.

Nephrolithiasis develops in 10–25% of patients with gout at some time during the disease course. In 40% of these patients, the first episode of renal colic precedes the first attack of acute gouty arthritis. Most of these calculi are composed of uric acid; however, calcium-containing stones are 10 times more common in patients with gout than in the general population. The incidence of nephrolithiasis correlates with the serum urate level, but more strongly with the amount of uric acid excreted in the urine. The likelihood of developing a stone reaches 50% with either a serum urate level above 13.0 mg/dL or a 24-hour urinary uric acid excretion in excess of 1100 mg.

In the past, progressive renal failure has been common in the gouty population with up to 25% of patients with gout dying of renal disease. Today, this frequency is much less. Hypertension, diabetes, chronic lead exposure, and chronic atherosclerosis are the most important contributing factors to this complication. In fact, if blood pressure is rigorously controlled, it is very unusual for renal failure to develop in a patient with gout. Chronic urate nephropathy has been described and is a distinct condition caused by the deposition of monosodium urate crystals in the renal parenchyma and pyramids. Although chronic hyperuricemia is thought to be the cause of this urate nephropathy, this form of kidney disease is never seen in the absence of gouty arthritis. Furthermore, with appropriate management, urate nephropathy should be easily prevented.

Hyperuricemia and gout are frequently accompanied by obesity, alcoholism, glucose intolerance related to insulin resistance, and hyperlipidemia. In addition, a very high percentage of patients with gout have hypertension. These associated conditions should be managed aggressively.

When to Refer to a Specialist

Primary care physicians should easily and appropriately manage the majority of patients with gouty arthritis. A rheumatologist should be consulted if there are questions about the diagnosis or if a patient is difficult to manage, either in controlling the number of acute attacks or in maintaining his or her serum urate level below the target of 5.0 mg/dL.

Patients requiring therapy with allopurinol in whom an allergic reaction develops can be referred to an allergist for attempts at desensitization.

REFERENCES

Agudelo CA, Wise CM. Gout: diagnosis, pathogenesis, and clinical manifestations. *Curr Opin Rheumatol.* 2001;13:234. [PMID: 11333355]

Emmerson BT. The management of gout. *N Engl J Med.* 1996; 334:445. [PMID: 8552158]

Wortmann RL. Gout and hyperuricemia. *Curr Opin Rheumatol.* 2002;14:281. [PMID: 11981327]

Wortmann RL, Kelley WN. Gout and hyperuricemia. In: Ruddy S, Harris ED Jr, Sledge CB, eds. *Kelley's Textbook of Rheumatology.* 6th ed. WB Saunders and Company, 2001: 1339–1376.

Pseudogout: Calcium Pyrophosphate Dihydrate Crystal Deposition Disease

44

Jeffrey S. Alderman, MD, & Robert L. Wortmann, MD

ESSENTIALS OF DIAGNOSIS

- *Calcium pyrophosphate dihydrate (CPPD) crystal deposition disease can mimic gout, rheumatoid arthritis, or osteoarthritis.*
- *Pseudogout causes an intermittent monoarthritis, often of the knee or wrist.*
- *Diagnosis of pseudogout established by demonstrating CPPD crystals in joint fluid.*
- *CPPD crystal deposition disease is associated with other diseases, especially hemochromatosis and hyperparathyroidism.*

General Considerations

Calcium pyrophosphate dihydrate (CPPD) deposition disease may be asymptomatic or may result in a variety of clinical presentations (Table 44–1). Although the term "pseudogout" is often used to represent the entire spectrum of CPPD, it more accurately is used to describe the acute gout-like attacks of inflammation that occur in some patients with CPPD crystal deposition disease. In fact, the name pseudogout was coined when it was discovered that a subset of patients believed to have gout had CPPD crystals in their synovial fluids rather than uric crystals. CPPD deposition may give rise to clinical presentations that mimic septic arthritis, polyarticular inflammatory arthritis, or osteoarthritis (Table 44–1). In addition, CPPD crystals can coexist with urate or basic calcium phosphate crystals in inflammatory and osteoarthritic-like diseases and in Charcot joints.

Although the cause of CPPD crystal deposition is unknown, several contributory factors have been identified. Perhaps the most important factor is aging. CPPD deposition will probably develop in everyone if they live long enough. Genetic factors are probably also at play,

given that numerous familial cases of CPPD deposition have been described in many nationalities. Interestingly, the pattern of clinical manifestation differs from family to family. For example, in some families, disease onset occurs at an early age and mimics a spondyloarthropathy. In others, presentation is in later years with sporadic joint distribution. The prevalence of CPPD deposition is greater in joints that have been traumatized, even when there have also been attempts to surgically repair these joints. Finally, several metabolic conditions including hyperparathyroidism, hemochromatosis, hypothyroidism, amyloidosis, hypomagnesemia, and hypophosphatasia have been associated with an increased frequency of CPPD disease.

Clinical Findings

A. SYMPTOMS AND SIGNS

Approximately 25% of patients with CPPD deposition disease exhibit the pseudogout pattern of disease. Signs and symptoms are characterized by acute, typically monarticular inflammatory arthritis lasting for several days to 2 weeks. These self-limited attacks may vary in intensity but can occur as abruptly—or feel as severe—as an acute gout attack. Patients are usually asymptomatic between episodes. Almost half of all attacks involve the knees, although attacks can affect nearly all other joints, including the first metatarsophalangeal joint (the site most common in gout). Pseudogout attacks can occur spontaneously or be provoked by trauma, surgery, or severe medical illness. Differentiation from gout or joint infection may be difficult and requires arthrocentesis examination of synovial fluid for crystals and culture. A subset of patients with pseudogout may have fever. Without appropriate analysis of synovial fluid, it is impossible to differentiate this presentation from that of septic arthritis.

Nearly 5% of patients with CPPD deposition manifest symptoms that mimic rheumatoid arthritis. These patients have symmetric distribution and low-grade inflammation in multiple joints. This arthritis is fre-

Table 44–1. CPPD crystal deposition can be asymptomatic or cause clinical presentations that mimic several conditions.

Gout
Septic Arthritis
Rheumatoid Arthritis
Osteoarthritis
Spondyloarthritis
Meningitis

CPPD, calcium pyrophosphate dihydrate.

quently accompanied by morning stiffness, fatigue, synovial thickening, joint contractures, and an elevated erythrocyte sedimentation rate. Because of these findings, this presentation is often misdiagnosed as rheumatoid arthritis. A small percentage of patients with CPPD deposits have low titers of rheumatoid factor, a finding that leads to further diagnostic confusion.

Nearly half of patients with CPPD deposits have a progressive, degenerative disease termed "pseudoosteoarthritis." Although there is some overlap with the pattern of joint involvement in primary osteoarthritis, the distribution of joint degeneration with CPPD deposition may differ. The knees are most commonly affected, followed by the wrists, metacarpophalangeal joints, hips, shoulders, elbows, and ankles. Symmetric involvement is typical. Deformities and flexion contractures of affected joints are not uncommon. Severe derangement and destruction like that seen in a Charcot joint has been reported. Valgus deformity of the knees is especially suggestive of underlying CPPD crystal deposition, as is disease localized to the patellofemoral joint. Patients with this pseudoosteoarthritic pattern may have intermittent episodes of acute joint inflammation of varying severity, superimposed upon their baseline disease state.

Rarely, CPPD crystal deposition occurs in the axial skeleton but can be a cause of acute neck pain. The ligamentum flavum has been the most regularly reported site of CPPD crystal deposition in the spine. At times, neck pain may be accompanied by stiffness and fever and can mimic meningitis. Crystal deposits, ligament hypertrophy, and cartilage metaplasia contribute to encroachment of the spinal cord. Infrequently, lumbar spine involvement causes an acute radiculopathy or neurogenic claudication from spinal stenosis. Long tract neurologic signs and symptoms develop in some patients as a result of CPPD deposition and related changes.

Many patients with CPPD crystal deposits have no joint symptoms. Even patients who have symptoms in some joints have other joints with crystal deposition that are completely asymptomatic and clinically normal.

B. Laboratory Findings

The critical laboratory feature of any form of CPPD crystal deposition disease is the demonstration of CPPD crystals. They are most commonly recognized in synovial fluid (Figure 44–1). Their identification requires the use of compensated polarized light microscopy. CPPD crystals are generally rhomboid-shaped and positively birefringent. They appear blue when parallel to the long axis of the compensator and yellow when perpendicular.

Findings on routine synovial fluid analysis are representative of the individual clinical presentation. The pseudogout and pseudorheumatoid presentations generally result in cloudy fluid with low viscosity and a white blood cell count between 5000 and 25,000 cells/μL. However, white blood cell counts over 100,000 cells/μL, a finding that is typically associated with septic arthritis, can be observed. The white blood cells in the synovial fluid in the pseudogout or pseudoseptic presentation are mostly polymorphonuclear leukocytes. In contrast, the fluid from the pseudoosteoarthritic form is clear, viscous, and has a very low white blood cell count (generally less than 300 cells/μL). Inflammatory presentation of CPPD crystal deposition disease may be accompanied by a peripheral blood leukocytosis with a left shift on the differential and an elevated erythrocyte sedimentation rate and C-reactive protein.

C. Imaging Studies

The radiographic findings of punctate and linear densities in hyaline articular cartilage or fibrocartilaginous tissues are diagnostic of CPPD crystal deposition (Figure 44–2). Other radiographic features include degen-

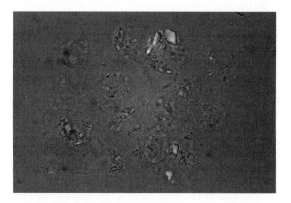

Figure 44–1. Positive birefringent calcium pyrophosphate dihydrate crystals.

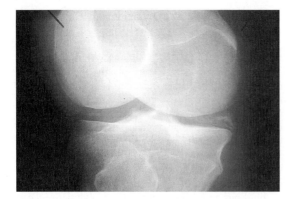

Figure 44–2. Chondrocalcinosis of the knees.

erative changes in an uncommon site along with sub-chondral cyst formation. The most characteristic sites of CPPD crystal deposition include the wrist (triangular cartilage of the radiocarpal joint) (Figure 44–3), the synthesis pubis, and the knees. The finding of isolated patellofemoral joint space narrowing or degenerative change in the wrist may provide helpful clinical clues to the presence of CPPD deposition-related arthropathy.

When the deposits are typical or unequivocal, the radiographic appearance can be viewed as specific. However, the interpretation of atypical or calcific deposits is often difficult largely because degenerative change is often already present. These changes can be extremely severe with subchondral collapse, bone fragmentation, and intra-articular radiodense bodies.

Changes in the metacarpophalangeal joints such as squaring of the bone ends, subchondral cysts, and hook-like osteophytes are characteristic features of the arthritis associated with hemochromatosis. However, these can also be observed in patients with CPPD crystal deposition alone or related to another metabolic disorder, such as Wilson disease.

A patient can be screened for CPPD crystal deposition with four radiographs. These include an anterior-posterior view of the knees, anterior-posterior view of the pelvis, and a posterior-anterior view of both hands to include the wrists. If these views show no evidence of crystal deposits, it is unlikely that further study will be fruitful. Tomographic views may be required to identify CPPD deposits surrounding the odontoid process.

D. SPECIFIC TESTS

Because of the recognized association between CPPD deposition and various metabolic diseases, the evaluation of a patient with newly diagnosed CPPD deposition should include tests for a serum calcium, phosphorus, magnesium, alkaline phosphatase, and thyroid-stimulating

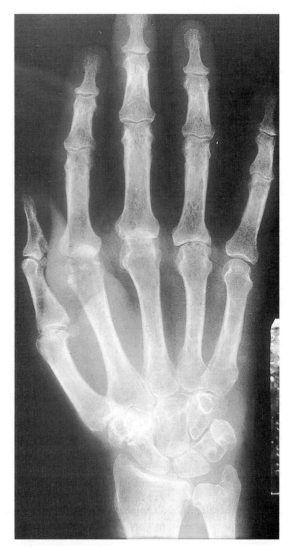

Figure 44–3. Chondrocalcinosis of the radiocarpal triangular cartilage.

hormone levels. The serum ceruloplasmin levels should also be assessed if Wilson disease is suspected. Hypophosphatasia and Wilson disease need not be considered in patients who become symptomatic after the age of 60 years.

Diagnosis & Differential Diagnosis

The diagnosis of CPPD crystal deposition disease is made through the identification of CPPD crystals in tissue or synovial fluid by definitive means of polarized light microscopy or x-ray defraction. The radiographic finding of chondrocalcinosis (calcium-containing radio-densities) in articular cartilage is also an indication of CPPD deposition. A criteria scheme for the diagnosis of these diseases has been provided and is outlined in Table 44–2.

Because CPPD crystal deposition disease can be associated with so many presentations, the differential diagnosis is quite extensive. Acute monarticular attacks (pseudogout) can be misdiagnosed as gout, acute basic calcium phosphatecrystal arthritis or periarthritis, or septic arthritis. Polyarticular or oligoarticular inflammatory presentations mirror rheumatoid arthritis and other inflammatory joint diseases. The polyarticular presentation may be difficult to distinguish from primary or post-traumatic osteoarthritis. Uncommonly, an acute inflammatory response to CPPD involvement

Table 44–2. Diagnostic criteria for CPPD crystal deposition disease.

Criteria
1. Demonstration of CPPD crystals and tissue or synovial fluid by definitive means (for example, characteristic x-ray defraction or chemical analysis)
2A. Identification of monoclinic or triclinic crystals showing no or weekly positive birefringence by compensated polarized light microscopy
2B. Presence of typical radiographic calcifications
3A. Acute arthritis, especially of the knees or other large joints
3B. Chronic arthritis, especially of the knee, hip, wrist, carpus, elbow, shoulder, or metacarpophalangeal joint, especially if accompanied by acute exacerbations. The chronic arthritis shows the following features helpful in differentiating it from osteoarthritis:
   Uncommon site—wrist metacarpophalangeal, elbow, or shoulder joint
   Radiographic appearance—radiocarpal or patellofemoral joint space narrowing, especially if isolated (patella "wrapped around" the femur)
   Subchondral cyst formation for severity of degeneration—progressive, with subchondral bony collapse and fragmentation with formation of intra-articular radiodense bodies.
   Osteophyte formation—variable and inconstant
   Tendon calcifications—especially triceps, Achilles, obturators

Categories
Definite disease: Criteria 1 or 2A must be fulfilled
Probable disease: Criteria 2A or 2B must be fulfilled
Possible disease: Criteria 3A or B should alert the clinician of the possibility of underlying CPPD deposition

---

CPPD, calcium pyrophosphate dihydrate.

of the ligament flavum or cervical spine can mimic meningitis.

Treatment of CPPD Crystal Deposition

The recommendations for the management of acute attacks of pseudogout are exactly those that are recommended for the treatment for acute gouty arthritis (see Chapter 43). Therefore, the choices include non-steroidal anti-inflammatory drugs (NSAIDs), colchicine orally, intravenous colchicine, and intravenous or intra-articular glucocorticoids in the patients who cannot take medication by mouth.

Oral colchicine at a dose of 0.5–0.6 mg one to three times per day is useful in the patient who has frequent bouts of pseudogout. The efficacy of this prophylactic therapy is not quite as successful as it is for gout. Nevertheless, it can prove helpful in some patients. The management of the pseudoosteoarthritic type of disease uncomplicated by acute attacks is similar to that for the management of other forms of osteoarthritis. Activity planning and pacing, assistive devices, analgesic medication (eg, NSAIDs and intra-articular glucocorticoid injections), and eventually surgery are all effective tools.

Unfortunately, there is no equivalent to allopurinol or a uricosuric agent for the treatment of CPPD deposition disease. Until the cause of this condition is determined, there will likely not be a specific medicine that removes the crystals from joints. However, in patients with an associated metabolic condition, such as hyperparathyroidism, hemochromatosis, or hypothyroidism, treatment of the associated disease may decrease the number of attacks but does not result in resorption of crystals.

Complications

The development of CPPD crystal deposition disease leads to progressive degenerative damage of the joint. This may be severe with joint collapse and a Charcot-like picture. Fortunately, an abnormality this severe is unusual.

Flares of pseudogout can follow general anesthesia and surgery. This can be quite dramatic after parathyroidectomy. The sudden decline in calcium may precipitate a flare of polyarticular inflammation with fever and mental confusion.

When to Refer to a Specialist

Most cases of CPPD crystal deposition disease can be managed by primary care physicians if they are confident of the diagnosis. Patients with confusing clinical pictures should be referred to a rheumatologist. For example, a polyarticular inflammatory presentation in a patient with chondrocalcinosis can be confusing. Such a presentation could be caused by the inflammatory response to the crystals, or the patient has both rheumatoid arthritis and CPPD deposition. Patients with intractable pain from the degenerative forms of CPPD deposition should be referred to an orthopedic surgeon for possible joint replacement surgery.

REFERENCES

Canhao H, et al. Cross-sectional study of 50 patients with calcium pyrophosphate dihydrate crystal arthropathy. *Clin Rheumatol.* 2001;20:L119. [PMID: 11346223]

Reginato AJ, et al. Familial and clinical aspects of calcium pyrophosphate deposition disease. *Curr Rheumatol Rep.* 1999;1: 112. [PMID: 11123024]

Reuge L, et al. Local deposition of calcium pyrophosphate crystals in evolution of knee osteoarthritis. *Clin Rheumatol.* 2001;20: 428. [PMID: 11771528]

Rosenthal AK, Mandel N. Identification of crystals in synovial fluids and joint tissues. *Curr Rheumatol Rep.* 2001;3:11. [PMID: 11177766]

SECTION VI

Infection

<table>
<tr><td>

Septic Arthritis & Disseminated Gonococcal Infection

</td><td>

45

</td></tr>
</table>

Monica Gandhi, MD, MPH, & Richard Jacobs, MD, PhD

ESSENTIALS OF DIAGNOSIS

Septic Arthritis

- *Classic presentation is abrupt onset of hot, painful, and swollen joint, usually monarticular and affecting large weight-bearing joints.*
- *Staphylococcus aureus is the most common cause of septic arthritis in native joints.*
- *White blood cell counts > 50,000 cells/μL with over 80% neutrophils are typical findings in synovial fluid analysis in bacterial arthritis.*

Disseminated Gonococcal Infection (DGI)

- *Typical presentation is triad of polyarthritis, tenosynovitis, and dermatitis.*
- *Although synovial fluid Gram stain and culture are less often positive in DGI than other forms of bacterial arthritis, urethral or cervical swabs significantly increase the yield of diagnosis.*

General Considerations

The reported incidence of septic arthritis varies from 2–10 per 100,000 per year in the general population, with significantly higher rates in patients with rheumatoid arthritis (RA) or joint prostheses (both ~30–70 cases per 100,000 per year). The incidence of bacterial arthritis is significantly higher among children than adults. Disseminated gonococcal infection (DGI) remains the most common cause of acute septic arthritis

in young sexually active persons in the United States; dissemination of *Neisseria gonorrhoeae* occurs in 1–3% of cases of untreated infections. Women are affected with DGI 2–3 times more commonly than men, with dissemination of *N gonorrhoeae* observed most frequently within 7 days of menses, during pregnancy, or in the postpartum period. Inherited deficiencies in either the terminal complement components (C5–C9) or in properdin synthesis result in inefficient outer membrane attack of *Neisseria* species and predispose patients to dissemination of *N gonorrhoeae* from localized sites of infection.

Septic (bacterial) arthritis is a medical emergency, and delay in diagnosis and treatment can lead to irreversible joint destruction and an increase in mortality. Even with the advent of better antimicrobial agents and techniques of joint incision and drainage, the rate of permanent joint damage from septic arthritis is 25–50%. The case fatality rate for bacterial arthritis also remains high at 5–15%, with increased mortality rates seen in the setting of polyarticular arthritis and underlying RA or in immunocompromised states. The prognosis of arthritis in DGI is much more favorable, with virtually all patients completely recovering after the institution of appropriate antibiotic therapy.

Risk factors and underlying mechanisms for the development of bacterial arthritis (Table 45–1) include chronic arthritic syndromes, prosthetic joints, parenteral drug use, extremes of age, diabetes mellitus, and immunocompromised conditions. DGI tends to cause acute septic arthritis in young, sexually active persons without prior joint disease.

Septic arthritis in **prosthetic joints** has some unique characteristics in terms of incidence, risk factors, and management. The rate of prosthetic joint infection fell

Table 45–1. Risk factors and mechanisms of infection in bacterial arthritis.

Risk Factor	Mechanism of Infection	Comments
Rheumatoid arthritis (RA)	Local and systemic factors play role. Damaged joint from RA serves as a nidus for infection, and patient with RA has compromised defenses from chronic illness and immunosuppressive medications.	RA complicated by septic arthritis in 0.3–4% of patients, usually following the administration of oral or intra-articular glucocorticoids. Patients with RA and a poly-articular septic arthritis have > 50% mortality rate. Most likely organism is *S aureus*.
Prosthetic joint	Foreign body in joint serves as nidus for infection, especially for pathogens that lay down a glycocalyx layer (ie, *S epidermidis*).	Rates of infection in prosthetic joints have decreased over the past 30 years. The incidence of prosthetic joint infection is much higher in revision arthroplasty. See text for details.
Parental drug use, recurrent injections, chronic skin infections	Recurrent bacteremia with subsequent hematogenous seeding of joints can result from repeated injections. Patients on chronic hemodialysis, with chronic indwelling lines, with repeated skin injections (eg, insulin), or with chronic skin infections, are also susceptible to joint infections through this process of recurrent bacteremia.	The knee is still the most commonly infected joint in parenteral drug use-associated septic arthritis, but axial joint infections, including the sternoclavicular and sacroiliac joints, also occur. *S aureus* (often methicillin-resistant) is the most common cause of infection in parenteral drug use, although *Pseudomonas aeruginosa* is seen in ~10% of cases.
Crystal-induced arthritis (gout, pseudogout)	Local factors. Joint damage from crystals. Synovial fluid acidosis in crystal-induced synovitis may also promote cartilage damage.	Crystal-induced arthritis can lead to high WBC counts in synovial fluid without the additional component of infection. However, the presence of crystals does not rule out infection. Infection-mediated destruction of articular cartilage can rarely lead to a high crystal count within the synovial space.
Severe osteoarthritis, Charcot joint, hemarthroses	Joint disorganization, chronic synovitis, and blood within the synovial space can all provide a nidus for infection.	Always send a bloody synovial effusion for culture to exclude infection.
Chronic, systemic disease (eg, lupus, cancer, diabetes mellitus, other immunosuppressive conditions, including extremes of age—children < 5 or adults > 65)	Impaired host defenses from chronic illness, including phagocytic deficiencies. Medications for these conditions (eg, glucocorticoids) can also predispose to infection.	*S aureus* and gram-negative bacilli are the most common organisms implicated. In systemic lupus, a selective functional hyposplenism may occur, which leads to susceptibility to encapsulated organisms, eg, *N gonorrhoeae, Salmonella, Proteus*.
Intra-articular injection (or arthrocentesis)	Mechanism of infection is direct inoculation of the offending organism.	Most common agents are skin flora, including *S epidermidis* and *S aureus*.
HIV infection	Immunosuppression and an increased tendency to develop bacteremia with localized infections lead to a higher rate of septic arthritis in HIV-positive persons.	Even when HIV-positive patients are relatively immunocompetent, underlying risk factors for the acquisition of HIV, such as parenteral drug use or hemophilia, can predispose to septic arthritis.
Sexual activity	Predisposes to localized gonococcal infection, which may disseminate to cause joint and skin disease.	DGI 2–3 times more common in women than men, especially after menses or in postpartum period. Terminal complement deficiencies also predispose to DGI.

WBC, white blood cell; DGI, disseminated gonococcal infection.

from 10% in the 1960s to < 1% by 1990 due to improvements in surgical technique, equipment, and preoperative antibiotics. The rate of prosthetic joint infection is 5–10 times more likely with a revision arthroplasty, however. Prosthetic joint infections can be divided into the categories of "early" or "late," depending on the temporal relationship to the surgical joint replacement (Table 45–2). Early postoperative infections reflect contamination of the wound in the perioperative period from skin flora, contaminated equipment, operating room personnel, or airborne bacteria. Risk factors for early postoperative infections include prolonged duration of surgery, an inexperienced primary surgeon, and patient factors such as advanced age, underlying chronic illnesses, RA, or a perioperative nonarticular infection. Late infections, which occur more than 1 month after the joint replacement, are the result of hematogenous seeding of the foreign body and damaged native tissue within the prosthetic joints.

Pathogenesis

A. Nongonococcal Arthritis

Bacterial pathogens reach the joint spaces by hematogenous spread (> 50% of cases), by direct inoculation, or by direct spread from bony or soft tissue infections. Although skin infections are the most common predisposing infections to joint infections, transient bacteremia from respiratory, gastrointestinal, or genitourinary infections can also lead to septic arthritis. Bacteria enter the closed joint space and, within hours, the synovium becomes infected, leading to synovial membrane proliferation and infiltration by polymorphonuclear (PMN)

and other inflammatory cells. This inflammatory response in turn leads to enzymatic and cytokine-mediated degradation of the articular cartilage, neovascularization, and the eventual development of granulation tissue. Without appropriate treatment, irreversible subchondral bone loss and cartilage destruction occur within a few days of the initial infection.

B. Disseminated Gonococcal Infection

The joint and skin manifestations of DGI are mediated by both circulating immune complexes and the direct effects of microbial proliferation. Mucosal infection with *N gonorrhoeae* always precedes the development of DGI, although this herald infection may be asymptomatic.

Clinical Findings

A. Symptoms and Signs

1. Nongonococcal arthritis—The classic presentation of bacterial arthritis is the abrupt onset of a hot, painful, and swollen joint. More indolent presentations are seen in patients with preexisting rheumatic illnesses, immunocompromised states, or in "late" prosthetic joint infections. An obvious joint effusion, moderate to severe joint tenderness to palpation, and marked restriction of both passive and active motion are common signs of septic arthritis.

A patient with an acute monarticular arthritis should be considered to have septic arthritis until proven otherwise. Nongonococcal bacterial arthritis is monarticular in 80–90% of cases, with polyarticular involvement

Table 45–2. Timing and characteristics of prosthetic joint infections.

Classification of Joint Infection	Timing from Joint Replacement Surgery	Signs and Symptoms	Microorganisms Involved	Treatment
Early	≤ 4 weeks	Pain, fever, erythema, edema	*S aureus*, then coagulase-negative staphylococci	"Prostheses salvage" with debridement and appropriate antibiotics
Late	≥ 4 weeks	Insidious onset, pain, occasionally drainage from joint	Coagulase-negative staphylococci, *Propionibacterium acnes* and diptheroids, *S aureus*	Joint debridement and prolonged courses of antibiotics (including rifampin, if staphylococcal infection) if feasible
Hematogenous	>2 years	Typical symptoms of septic arthritis, but occurring after patient has done initially well	*S aureus*, streptococci, gram-negative rods	Usually requires two-stage removal of joint with antibiotics for cure

(10–20%) carrying a poorer chance of survival. Poly-articular septic arthritis is more likely to occur in patients with RA or other systemic connective tissue diseases or in the syndrome of overwhelming sepsis. Infectious monoarthritis typically involves the knee (40–50%), hip (13–20%), shoulder (10–15%), wrist (5–8%), ankle (6–8%), elbow (3–7%), and the small joints of the hand or foot (5%). Bursitis, especially olecranon and prepatellar, may be the first manifestation of septic arthritis in patients with RA.

Septic arthritis manifests with fever in 60–80% of cases, although the temperature elevation is not usually pronounced. Twenty percent of patients with fever have shaking chills that usually correspond to waves of bacteremia. Cough, gastrointestinal symptoms, or dysuria may represent symptoms of the precedent infection. Indeed, a preceding source of infection, such as pneumonia, otitis, bronchitis, pharyngitis, or cutaneous, gastrointestinal, or genitourinary infection, can be identified in 50% of septic arthritis cases.

Prosthetic joint infections have varying clinical presentations depending on the duration since orthopedic implant (Table 45–2). Such infections can present early (≤ 4 weeks after joint replacement) or late (≥ 1 month after surgery). Furthermore, prosthetic joints are more susceptible to infection from hematogenous spread than normal joints throughout their lifetime because of the presence of a foreign body. Early prosthetic joint infections typically present with the classic symptoms of acute bacterial arthritis with fever, erythema, edema, and pain persisting beyond the postoperative period. Late infections usually present with a more indolent course of increasing joint pain, sometimes accompanied by joint drainage, but usually without concurrent fever or peripheral leukocytosis.

2. DGI—The duration from sexual contact to the onset of DGI varies from 1 day to 2 months, although the average duration of symptoms prior to presentation is 5 days. Twenty-five percent of patients with DGI will have the genitourinary or pharyngeal symptoms of the precedent mucosal infection.

DGI usually presents with the clinical triad of polyarthritis, tenosynovitis, and dermatitis. The initial symptoms include fevers; chills; and migratory symptoms of polyarthralgias, which usually progress to frank monoarthritis or polyarthritis in the knees, ankles, or wrists. Migratory symptoms of tenosynovitis occur in two-thirds of patients and are most often present over the dorsum of the hand, the wrist, the ankle, or the knee. Dermatitis is seen in approximately two-thirds of patients with DGI, usually presenting as maculopapular, vesicular, or pustular lesions on an erythematous base, often with a necrotic center (Figure 45–1). The rash is typically found on the trunk and distal extremities (including digits) in a relatively sparse distribution (10–25 lesions usually found in total). Hemorrhagic bullae, erythema multiforme, and vasculitic lesions have also been reported. The skin lesions of DGI are usually asymptomatic and require careful inspection for their detection. Biopsy of these skin lesions demonstrates perivascular inflammation, leukocytoclastic vasculitis, intra-epidermal neutrophilic infiltration, and microthrombi; *N gonorrhoeae* can be cultured from biopsy specimens of the skin lesions approximately 10% of the time.

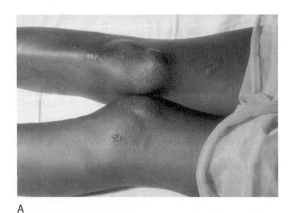

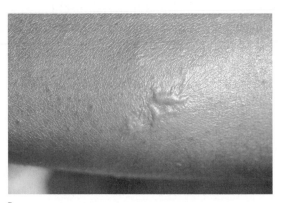

A   B

Figure 45–1. **A:** Skin lesions and joint involvement in disseminated gonococcal infection (DGI). **B:** Close-up view of a pustular DGI lesion on the skin of a patient's arm. (Images contributed by Dr. Thomas F. Sellers and are in the public domain; Centers for Disease Control Public Health Image Library [phil.cdc.gov].)

Unusual clinical manifestations of DGI include pericarditis, meningitis, aortitis, endocarditis, myocarditis, pyomyositis, and osteomyelitis.

B. PHYSICAL EXAMINATION

The initial physical examination for septic arthritis should determine whether the source of inflammation and pain is articular or periarticular (specifically, localized to skin, bursae, or tendons). Septic arthritis produces warmth, swelling, and tenderness of the involved joint, and attempts at passive and active motion of the joint usually produce considerable discomfort. Similar findings occur in noninfectious forms of severe inflammatory arthritis, such as acute gout. In contrast, cellulitis and inflammation of bursae and tendons do not cause joint effusions, and passive motion of the adjacent joint usually does not elicit severe pain unless there is stretching of an inflamed tendon. Because septic arthritis can involve more than one joint, all joints should be examined for warmth, swelling, deformity, range of motion, pain on motion, and tenderness.

Septic arthritis of the sacroiliac (SI) joint is often difficult to distinguish from infection in the hip because both present with fever and pain upon ambulation and because examination of the SI joints is difficult (see Chapter 1). Moreover, findings of SI septic arthritis can be subtle and can be mistaken for the syndrome of a protruded disk or a paraspinous muscular strain.

Infection of the shoulder joint is often difficult to identify given the usual lack of a visible effusion. Adults with shoulder infections tend to be elderly, with multiple risk factors for the development of septic arthritis. Infections of the sternoclavicular joint most often occur in injecting drug users. Furthermore, an abscess of the chest wall or in the intrathoracic extrapleural space will develop in 20% of patients with septic arthritis of the sternoclavicular joint.

Septic olecranon bursitis is distinguished from infection of the elbow joint by the presence of swelling and erythema overlying the olecranon process and the absence of joint pain with passive extension of the elbow. Infection of the olecranon bursa often follows minor trauma to the region, which leads to inoculation of organisms (usually *S aureus*) into the bursal space.

C. LABORATORY FINDINGS

1. Peripheral markers of inflammation—Peripheral white blood cell (WBC) counts are elevated in bacterial arthritis approximately two-thirds of the time. The erythrocyte sedimentation rate and C-reactive protein are usually elevated in the setting of septic arthritis and may be useful to monitor during treatment, especially in children with septic hip infections.

2. Blood and extra-articular cultures—Blood cultures are positive approximately 50–60% of the time in nongonococcal septic arthritis, with lower rates observed in prosthetic joint infections. Blood cultures for *N gonorrhoeae* in DGI, however, are rarely positive. Targeted cultures from extra-articular sites, such as respiratory, cutaneous, gastrointestinal, or genitourinary, should be collected after a careful history and physical examination. If DGI is suspected, urethral, cervical, pharyngeal, and rectal cultures should be collected. Genitourinary cultures are positive in 70–90% of patients with DGI.

3. Synovial fluid analysis—Synovial fluid analysis is critical for the definitive diagnosis of septic arthritis. Synovial fluid is usually obtained by emergent arthrocentesis, with fluoroscopic or computed tomographic guidance if necessary (see Chapter 2). An open surgical procedure may be required to obtain synovial fluid and biopsies for the diagnosis of bacterial arthritis, especially in suspected sternoclavicular, hip, or shoulder infections or in the presence of prosthetic joints. Of note, arthrocentesis is contraindicated if the needle must pass through an area of cellulitis, heavily colonized skin lesions (eg, psoriatic plaques), or infection of any kind because of the risk of introducing bacteria into the joint space. Bacteremia is also a relative contraindication for the performance of arthrocentesis.

Once synovial fluid has been collected, the following analyses should be performed (see Chapter 2):

- Appearance: Look for color and clarity of the fluid, since purulence or turbidity or both suggest a septic process.

- Cell count and differential: The joint fluid in nongonococcal septic arthritis has more than 50,000 WBC/μL in 50–70% of cases. Low synovial fluid cell counts may be seen early in the process of infectious arthritis and in the setting of partially treated infections. The majority of WBCs in infected synovial fluid are neutrophils (usually > 80% PMNs). The synovial fluid in gonococcal septic arthritis generally has lower WBC counts than in nongonococcal infections, with a typical range of 30,000–60,000 WBC/μL.

- Gram stain for organisms: A positive Gram stain is diagnostic for septic arthritis (highly specific), but a Gram stain that is negative for bacteria does not rule out an infected joint. The Gram stain is positive 50–75% of the time in nongonococcal bacterial arthritis (depending on the organism) and should be used to guide presumptive therapy. The Gram stain for gonococcal organisms in synovial fluid is positive < 25% of the time in the DGI syndrome (Figure 45–2).

- Culture: Bacterial culture of the synovial fluid is positive in 70–90% of cases of nongonococcal arthritis,

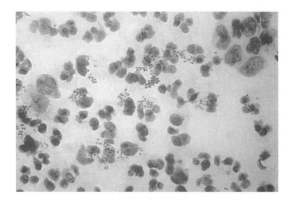

Figure 45–2. Gram stain of purulent fluid sample showing the small intracellular gram-negative diplococci of *Neisseria gonorrhoeae* with surrounding polymorphonuclear cells. (Image is in the public domain; Centers for Disease Control Public Health Image Library [phil.cdc.gov].)

depending on the organism. In contrast, the culture for *N gonorrhoeae* in synovial fluid is positive in only 20–50%. Reasons for this low yield of positive synovial cultures in DGI include its pathogenesis, which often involves circulating immune complexes rather than direct infection, and the fastidious growth requirements of the *N gonorrhoeae*.

Optimal growth conditions for the gonococcus involve the immediate plating of synovial fluid at the bedside on chocolate or Thayer-Martin media with incubation at 5–10% CO_2 concentration. *N gonorrhoeae* organisms may take more than 48 hours of incubation to grow, so the laboratory should be alerted to hold these cultures if DGI is suspected. As these stringent procedures of collection and incubation are not always followed, the yield of recovering *N gonorrhoeae* from any culture site is usually lower than could be optimally achieved. Synovial fluid in DGI is more likely to be positive for gonococcus when the fluid has a high WBC count.

• Microbiology: Table 45–3 shows the typical pathogens of nongonococcal bacterial arthritis and risk factors for their acquisition. *S aureus* is the most common cause of septic monoarthritis in native joints (60–70%) (Figure 45–3). The remaining causes of septic arthritis include streptococcal species, gram-negative rods, and anaerobes in relatively constant proportions. *N gonorrhoeae* accounts for only 20% of cases of monarticular septic arthritis in young adults, since the most common presentation of DGI involves an oligoarthritis or polyarthritis.

In prosthetic joint infections, the microbiology of early postoperative infections involves mainly *S aureus* and the coagulase-negative staphylococci introduced at the time of surgical repair (Table 45–2). Late prosthetic joint infections that present at least a month after surgery usually evolve from a pathogen of low virulence or of low inoculum introduced at the time of the procedure. These pathogens include skin flora such as *Staphylococcus epidermidis, Propionibacterium acnes,* or diptheroids, although anaerobes and *S aureus* can also be involved. Hematogenous infection in a prosthetic joint, as in a normal joint, can result from transient bacteremia secondary to a remote infection or a surgical procedure, including dental work or respiratory, gastrointestinal, or genitourinary manipulations. Group A streptococci are often isolated from the infected joint after procedures in the oral cavity, whereas gastrointestinal, procedures can lead to bacteremia with non–group A streptococcal species, gram-negative bacilli, or anaerobes, all of which can seed the prosthetic joint.

D. IMAGING STUDIES

1. Plain radiographs—Plain radiographs are of little diagnostic usefulness in acute septic arthritis but are often obtained as a baseline and to exclude contiguous osteomyelitis. Radiographs will usually reveal only soft tissue swelling; in cases of infection with *Escherichia coli* or anaerobic organisms, however, radiographs may demonstrate gas formation within an untapped joint. In late septic arthritis (at least 8–10 days after infection), films may show subchondral bone destruction, periosteal new bone formation, joint space narrowing, or osteoporosis. Radiographs of a suspected septic prosthetic joint may show zones of radiolucency at the bone-cement interface to suggest joint loosening, although infection-mediated loosening is difficult to distinguish from aseptic mechanical loosening.

2. Computed tomography—Because the hip, shoulder, sternoclavicular, and SI joints are difficult to palpate and to aspirate, evaluation of these joints usually requires computed tomography (CT) or magnetic resonance imaging (MRI). CT is preferred for the sternoclavicular joint. CT scans may demonstrate early bone erosions, reveal soft tissue extension, detect effusions, and facilitate arthrocentesis of the hip, shoulder, sternoclavicular, and SI joints. Prosthetic joints often have distorted joint architecture and may require CT image guidance for fluid aspiration.

3. MRI—MRI scans demonstrate adjacent soft tissue edema or abscesses and may be especially helpful in detecting septic sacroiliitis. MRI can also detect the early bone erosions of incipient contiguous osteomyelitis.

Table 45–3. Major bacterial organisms implicated in nongonococcal septic arthritis in adults.

Organism	% Adult Infections	Comments
Staphylococcus aureus	60–70%	*S aureus* is the most common pathogen implicated in native joint septic arthritis and late prosthetic joint infections. Increasing rates of methicillin-resistant *S aureus* (MRSA) seen in injection drug users and in the community.
Streptococcal species	15–20%	Group A streptococcus is the most common streptococcal agent implicated in septic arthritis and usually results from a primary skin or soft tissue infection. Increasing reports of non–group A β-hemolytic streptococcal species (eg, groups B, C, G streptococci) in infectious arthritis, especially in the immunocompromised patient or following gastrointestinal or genitourinary infections. *Streptococcus pneumoniae* infectious arthritis is uncommon.
Gram-negative bacilli	5–25%	Gram-negative rods cause septic arthritis more commonly in neonates, infants younger than 2 months, the elderly, injection drug users, and the chronically ill (diabetes mellitus, cancer, sickle cell anemia, connective tissue disorders, renal transplant recipients, and other immunosuppressed conditions). Most infections begin as urinary tract or skin infections, with subsequent hematogenous spread to a single joint. Septic arthritis from *Hemophilus influenzae* type E has decreased markedly since routine childhood vaccination for this organism.
Anaerobes	1–5%	Common anaerobes recovered from joints include *Bacteroides* species, *Propionibacterium acnes* (skin flora), and various anaerobic gram-positive cocci. 50% of anaerobic arthritis syndromes are polymicrobial. Predisposing factors include diabetes mellitus, immunocompromised state, or postoperative wound infections, especially following total joint replacement or joint arthroplasty. Higher suspicion if synovial fluid is foul-smelling or if gas is present in the joint space radiologically. Cultures must be collected under anaerobic conditions and incubated for at least 2 weeks.
Staphylococcus epidermidis	Rare in native joints	Most common agent in late postoperative prosthetic joint infections (≥4 weeks after surgery). *S epidermidis* forms a glycocalyx layer over foreign surfaces, which makes the organism difficult to eradicate without joint removal.
Brucella species (*Brucella melitensis* is most common *Brucella* species implicated in septic arthritis)	Rare	Not common in the United States, but prevalent in many parts of the world. Risk factors include ingestion of unpasteurized milk or cheese or occupational exposures (farmers, meat packers, etc). *Brucella* causes a monoarthritis or an asymmetric peripheral oligoarthritis. Sacroiliitis and spondylitis also common. Diagnose with scintigraphy, CT scan, PCR, and/or positive blood or joint cultures. Treatment courses are lengthy and usually involve antimicrobial combinations.
Mycoplasma	Rare	More common in children than adults. Occurs more frequently in immunocompromised patients, particularly those with agammaglobulinemia.

CT, computed tomography; PCR, polymerase chain reaction.

4. Scintigraphy—Scintigraphy makes use of various agents, such as labeled WBCs, technetium colloid, or immunoglobulin, to highlight areas of infection. The drawback of this imaging technique in the diagnosis of septic arthritis is the rate of false positives with contiguous soft tissue infections; scintigraphy cannot reliably differentiate septic from aseptic joint inflammation. False-positive scans can also result from underlying fracture or a recent operation. Given this low sensitivity, scintigraphy is rarely used as the imaging study of choice for the diagnosis of septic arthritis.

5. Gallium scan—Gallium accumulates where there is a extravasation of serum proteins and leukocytes and has a much higher sensitivity than scintigraphy in distinguishing infection from mechanical damage. Gallium scans have shown an increasing utility in the diagnosis of septic arthritis and the identification of concurrent osteomyelitis.

E. Special Tests

Various nonculture techniques have been developed for the detection of *N gonorrhoeae*. Particularly promising

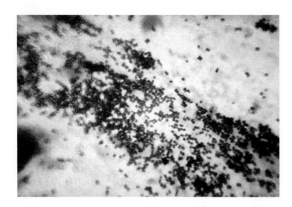

Figure 45–3. Gram stain of an inflammatory exudate showing the clustered gram-positive cocci of *Staphylococcus aureus*. (Image contributed by Dr. Thomas F. Sellers and is in the public domain; Centers for Disease Control Public Health Image Library [phil.cdc.gov].)

are nucleic acid amplification tests, which given their excellent sensitivity and specificity, may be useful for the diagnosis of patients with clinically typical but culture-negative gonococcal arthritis. Polymerase chain reaction techniques to identify nongonococcal bacteria in septic joints are not as well developed.

Differential Diagnosis

Septic arthritis usually presents as acute monoarthritis, occasionally as an acute oligoarthritis or a polyarthritis. The differential diagnoses of these syndromes are reviewed in Chapter 4, but several points warrant emphasis here. The diagnosis of acute monoarthritis is infection unless proved otherwise. Differentiating infection from crystal-induced arthritis can be particularly difficult, since acute flares of pseudogout or gout can also cause fever, peripheral leukocytosis, and markedly elevated synovial cell counts. Bacterial superinfection can complicate crystal-induced arthritis, although this is rare. A history of recurrent monoarthritis, typical podagra, or radiologic evidence of chondrocalcinosis are suggestive of crystal-induced arthritis. However, only arthrocentesis with culture of the synovial fluid and analysis for crystals can definitively distinguish septic arthritis from crystal-induced arthritis.

The differential diagnosis for DGI includes nongonococcal polyarticular septic arthritis, bacterial endocarditis, viral arthritis, and meningococcemia. Up to 40% of cases of meningococcemia have articular symptoms; meningococcus-associated arthritides are almost always sterile and present either as monarticular or polyarticular disease. Postinfectious forms of arthritis (acute rheumatic fever and reactive arthritis) also can be diffi-

cult to differentiate from DGI early in their course. Both can begin abruptly and be associated with fever; tenosynovitis is often prominent in reactive arthritis, as it is in DGI.

Treatment

Early diagnosis is the key to successful treatment of septic arthritis; delay in instituting appropriate antibiotic therapy and debridement measures leads to poor outcomes. The two mainstays of treatment are drainage and intravenous antibiotic therapy. Progressive joint mobilization will also help prevent some of the long-term complications of septic arthritis.

A. Drainage

The management of septic nongonococcal arthritis usually mandates hospitalization for drainage of the infected joint. The joint must be thoroughly drained to decrease the number of inflammatory cells, which produce cytokines and proteolytic enzymes that cause permanent joint damage. Early arthroscopic lavage, debridement, and drain insertion have largely replaced the standard procedure of performing daily aspirations of the joint. Response to therapy can be gauged by following the synovial fluid cell counts and culture results over the subsequent days of hospitalization.

Open surgical drainage and debridement (arthrotomy) may be required for the following indications:

- Failure to respond to more conservative therapy in 5–7 days.
- Coexistent osteomyelitis that needs surgical intervention.
- Involvement of joints that are difficult to drain using more conservative approaches: hips, shoulders, or SI joints.
- Involvement of a prosthetic joint.
- Difficulty in performing adequate drainage of the joint with needle aspiration or arthroscopic manipulations.
- Refusal of the patient to accept repeated needle aspirations or catheter drainage (eg, young children).
- Open drainage is the initial procedure of choice in children with septic arthritis of the hip.

B. Antibiotics

1. Nongonococcal arthritis—After the initial diagnostic joint aspiration, intravenous antibiotics should be immediately administered. Empiric antibiotic therapy is based on either the initial Gram stain result or the clinical situation (Table 45–4) in suspected nongonococcal bacterial arthritis. Antibiotics are usually administered for a total of 6 weeks, with longer dura-

Table 45–4. Initial antibiotic therapy for septic arthritis based on synovial Gram stain or clinical situation.

Synovial Fluid Gram Stain/Clinical Situation	Antibiotic Therapy
Gram-positive cocci	Use intravenous vancomycin as initial therapy given increasing rate of methicillin-resistant *Stapholococcus aureus* (MRSA) in the community. Switch to high-dose ceftriaxone, ceftizoxime, or the appropriate penicillin class if the culture reveals methicillin-sensitive *S aureus* or streptococcal growth. Oral options include ciprofloxacin plus rifampin for sensitive stapholococcal strains, which achieve bactericidal intra-articular concentrations in combination. Initial reports suggest linezolid may have good efficacy in MRSA gram-positive infections of the joint and may therefore provide another oral treatment option.
Gram-negative bacilli	Initial intravenous therapy usually includes an aminoglycoside in synergistic combination with an antipseudomonal penicillin or high-dose third-generation cephalosporin.
Injection drug use	Initial therapy should include vancomycin for MRSA coverage as well as either single-agent or combination therapy for pseudomonal infections. Tailor subsequent therapy based on culture results.
Immunocompetent normal patient	Initial therapy can be intravenous vancomycin alone given the high rate of resistant *S aureus* infections in the normal patient. Tailor subsequent therapy based on culture results.
Chronically ill, immunocompromised patient	Initial therapy should include broad coverage for gram-positive organisms (eg, vancomycin), gram-negative organisms, and anaerobes if clinically suspected. Tailor subsequent therapy based on culture results.
Young adults with negative smear	As gonococcal infection is the most likely diagnosis in this clinical situation, empiric ceftriaxone should be instituted.
Neonates and children < 2 months	Broad-spectrum initial antibiotic coverage for *H influenzae* (assume ampicillin resistance), *S aureus*, group B streptococcus, and gram-negative bacilli. A combination of vancomycin, an extended-spectrum penicillin, and an aminoglycoside may be used as initial therapy with subsequent tailoring based on culture results.

tions of therapy (up to 3–6 months) required in the presence of retained prosthetic material (see below). Intra-articular antibiotic distillation has not been shown to be beneficial and may lead to a chemical synovitis.

2. DGI—Penicillin can no longer be used as initial therapy for gonococcal arthritis given increasing rates of penicillinase production or chromosomally mediated resistance to penicillin. Table 45–5 lists the options for initial intravenous or oral therapy for DGI. (DGI can be treated primarily or exclusively with oral therapy in mild disease.) The initiation of antibiotics for DGI usually results in very rapid improvement (over 24–48 hours) in signs and symptoms, which can be a clue to the diagnosis. Indeed, the management of gonococcal arthritis rarely requires repeat arthrocentesis given the brisk response to antibiotics alone. Unless complicated by systemic manifestations such as carditis, meningitis, endo-

carditis, or osteomyelitis, the duration of treatment for DGI is only 10–14 days. Intravenous therapy is usually given for 2–4 days, followed by 7–10 days of oral therapy. Uncomplicated cases of DGI are increasingly being treated in the outpatient setting with oral therapy alone. Given the high prevalence of concurrent chlamydial infections in patients with *N gonorrhoeae* infections, management of DGI usually requires additional treatment for *Chlamydia trachomatis* (eg, azithromycin or doxycycline).

3. Prosthetic joint infections—Therapy of **prosthetic joint infections** varies by the temporal relationship of the infection to the surgical procedure. Infections occurring in the acute postoperative period (≤ 4 weeks after surgery) may be able to be managed with surgical debridement and prolonged antibiotic therapy alone, without subsequent prostheses removal. This treatment course has been labeled "prostheses salvage" and has

Table 45–5. Recommended antibiotic therapy
for treatment of gonococcal arthritis.

Antibiotic	Comments
Parenteral third-generation cephalosporin	Ceftriaxone 1 g IV/IM daily is the most common third-generation cephalosporin used in DGI; ceftizoxime or cefotaxime can also be used.
Spectinomycin	Usually reserved for patients with β-lactam allergies. Dose is 2 g IM every 12 h.
Fluoroquinolones	Increasing resistance of *Neisseria gonorrhoeae* to fluoroquinolones reported, mainly in Thailand and other Asian countries, Hawaii, the western Pacific countries, and some regions of California. The dose of ciprofloxacin is 500 mg orally twice daily, the dose of ofloxacin is 400 mg orally twice daily, and the dose of levofloxacin is 500 mg orally once daily. IV formulations can be used initially, but fluoroquinolones have excellent oral bioavailability.
Cefixime	Dose is 400 mg orally twice daily. Of note, the MMWR recently reported that Wyeth Pharmaceuticals (the only company manufacturing cefixime tablets) has discontinued the manufacturing of cefixime in the US (*MMWR Morb Mortal Wkly Rep.* 2002 Nov 22; 51 (46): 1052), although the drug is still being manufactured in Europe.
Penicillin or ampicillin	If *N gonorrhoeae* is identified as penicillin-susceptible, switch to one of the following agents: ampicillin 1 g IV every 6 h, penicillin G 10 million units IV once daily (divided), or amoxicillin 1 g orally every 8 h.

demonstrated up to a 70% success rate for early infections. Infections occurring in the late postoperative period and through hematogenous spread usually require removal of the prostheses for successful cure, although factors that predict success with debridement and antibiotics alone are being identified. A recent randomized controlled trial looked at patients with culture-proven staphylococcal infection associated with stable orthopedic implants who had short durations of infectious symptoms (0–3 weeks). These patients all underwent surgical debridement of the joint without prosthetic material removal followed by prolonged oral antibiotic therapy (3–6 months) with either oral ciprofloxacin alone or a combination of oral ciprofloxacin and rifampin. The group treated with the oral antibiotic combination had a higher cure rate (100%) than the group treated with ciprofloxacin alone (58%), presumably because of rifampin's superior ability to penetrate tissues and biofilms. Factors associated with the achievement of cure with antibiotics and debridement alone in later prosthetic joint infections caused by staphylococcal species include stable orthopedic implants, a short duration of infections prior to debridement, immediate surgical debridement, and the addition of rifampin to the antibiotic regimen.

If surgical removal of the device is necessary, two-stage procedures may be more successful than one-stage exchange, although this has not been extensively studied. One-stage exchange combines removal of the infected implant, debridement, and replacement of the joint, followed by prolonged courses of antibiotics. However, management most often involves a two-stage procedure: (1) removal of the infected joint prostheses (with concomitant debridement and collection of appropriate diagnostic cultures), (2) administration of appropriate antibiotics for at least 6 weeks, and (3) revision arthroplasty.

C. MOBILIZATION

Management of septic arthritis also includes passive motion exercises to prevent formation of adhesions and to enhance the clearance of purulent exudates after the acute inflammatory response has subsided. Passive mobilization is gradually followed by active strengthening of periarticular structures to help prevent joint contractures.

Complications

The major complications of septic arthritis include osteomyelitis, persistent or recurrent infection, a marked decrease in joint mobility, ankylosis, or persistent pain.

Prognosis

The clinical outcome of septic arthritis is determined by the duration of symptoms before the initiation of effective treatment, the number of infected joints, the age and immune status of the patient, preceding joint disease, the virulence and susceptibilities of the organism, and the particular joint infected. Virtually all patients with gonococcal arthritis recover completely. Seventy to eight-five percent of patients with group-A streptococcal infections recover without residual symptoms. Up to 50% of patients with septic arthritis secondary to *S aureus* or gram-negative rods, however, have residual joint damage. Patients with RA in whom polyarticular infection develops carry a very poor prognosis, with less than a 50% survival rate.

REFERENCES

Gillespie WJ. Prevention and management of infection after total joint replacement. *Clin Infect Dis.* 1997;25:1310. [PMID: 9431369] (A thorough review of the risk factors and management in prosthetic joint infections.)

Goldenberg DL. Septic arthritis. *Lancet.* 1998;351:197. [PMID: 9449882] (An excellent and thorough review of nongonococcal and gonococcal septic arthritis.)

Kaandorp CJ, et al. Risk factors for septic arthritis in patients with joint disease: a prospective study. *Arthritis Rheum.* 1995;38: 1819. [PMID: 8849354] (One of a series of prospective community-based trials (all with CJ Kaandorp as the first author) looking at the incidence, risk factors, and outcomes of septic arthritis.)

Liebling MR et al. Identification of *Neisseria gonorrhoeae* in synovial fluid using the polymerase chain reaction. *Arthritis Rheum.* 1994;37:702. [PMID: 8185697] (A case control study of the utility of PCR in the detection of *N gonorrhoeae* in synovial fluid samples.)

Stengel D, et al. Systematic review and meta-analysis of antibiotic therapy for bone and joint infections. *Lancet Infect Dis.* 2001; 1:175. [PMID: 11871494] (A meta-analysis that describes the paucity of high-quality data regarding the appropriate use and administration of antibiotics for septic arthritis. Consultation with an infectious diseases specialist may aid in the selection of appropriate antimicrobial therapy for this condition.)

Zimmerli W, et al. Role of rifampin for treatment of orthopedic implant-related staphylococcal infections: a randomized controlled trial. Foreign-Body Infection (FBI) Study Group. *JAMA.* 1998;279:1537. [PMID: 9605897]. (The results of this important study are reviewed in the text.)

Lyme Disease

Linda K. Bockenstedt, MD

The multisystem disorder of Lyme disease is due to a tick-transmitted infection with the spirochete *Borrelia burgdorferi*. The diagnosis should be considered in persons who have a reasonable risk of exposure to infected ticks, such as those who live or vacation in areas endemic for the disorder, and in persons who have the characteristic complex of signs and symptoms. Classic clinical features occur in stages: **early localized disease** (3–30 days after tick bite), **early disseminated disease** (weeks to months after tick bite), and **late disease** (several months to years after tick bite). Supporting serologic evidence of exposure to *B burgdorferi* is present in most cases but can be absent in persons with early infection.

ESSENTIALS OF DIAGNOSIS

- *A single hallmark skin lesion, erythema migrans, occasionally associated with fever, malaise, arthralgias, and myalgias, is seen in early disease.*
- *Multiple erythema migrans lesions and associated fever, migratory arthralgias, and myalgias; acute pauciarticular arthritis; and carditis manifested primarily as atrioventricular nodal block; neurologic features, including cranial nerve (especially facial nerve) palsies, lymphocytic meningitis, and radiculoneuropathies are manifestations of early disseminated disease.*
- *Primarily neurologic features, especially peripheral neuropathies and chronic mild encephalopathy, and arthritis, including monarticular and migratory pauciarticular arthritis, may be present in late disease.*

General Considerations

Lyme disease is a multisystem disorder caused by infection with spirochetes of the genus *B burgdorferi sensu lato: B burgdorferi sensu stricto, Borrelia garinii,* and *Borrelia afzelii.* Hard-shelled ticks of the *Ixodes* family, primarily *Ixodes scapularis* and *Ixodes pacificus* in the United States and *Ixodes ricinus* in Europe, serve as vectors for infection. In the United States, the disease first came to medical attention in 1975, with the evaluation of a clustering of children with presumed juvenile rheumatoid arthritis around the area of Lyme, Connecticut. Lyme arthritis, as it was initially termed, was soon found to be one manifestation of systemic infection with *B burgdorferi.* Beginning with a characteristic skin lesion, erythema migrans (EM), early infection was either localized to the skin or disseminated to other sites, with disease most commonly found in the skin, heart, joints, and nervous system. Lyme disease is not a new condition; in Europe, EM had been associated with *I ricinus* tick bites since the early twentieth century, and the skin disease was treated successfully with penicillin after spirochetes were visualized in biopsy specimens in the mid-1900s. Other systemic manifestations were occasionally present, especially neurologic disease (Bannwarth syndrome), but the broad clinical spectrum was not fully appreciated until the late 1970s.

Since its emergence in the United States more than a quarter century ago, Lyme disease has become the most common vector-borne infection in this country. In 1999, 16,273 cases from 49 states were reported to the Centers for Disease Control and Prevention (CDC), with 93% originating from only 9 states: Connecticut, Rhode Island, New York, Pennsylvania, New Jersey, Maryland, Massachusetts, Minnesota, and Wisconsin. Cases of Lyme disease also occur in other areas of North America as well as in Europe and Asia. In the latter two continents, other *B burgdorferi sensu lato* members—*B garinii* and *B afzelii*—are the main causative agents.

Lyme disease begins when humans serve as incidental bloodmeal hosts for *B burgdorferi*–infected ticks. Although all three forms of ticks—larvae, nymphs, and adults—can harbor *B burgdorferi,* nymphs are more likely to transmit infection to humans because of their promiscuous feeding patterns and small size (see CDC web site for description of vector life cycle and image of ticks). *Ixodes* ticks feed only once per developmental stage, so that the incidence of Lyme disease follows the seasonal feeding patterns of nymphs (late spring, summer, and early fall). Larvae are rarely, if ever, vectors for the disease because they must first acquire infection by feeding on a reservoir host. Nymphs feed for 3–8 days, during which time spirochetes migrate from their residence in the tick midgut to the salivary gland and egress into the host through salivary secretions. Transmission of infection generally requires 24–48 hours of tick feeding, so that tick surveillance and early removal of embedded ticks is a primary preventive strategy in areas endemic for Lyme disease. Spirochetes first establish infection in the skin, where local immune responses give rise to EM, a hallmark of early, localized infection. This rash is present in up to 80% of cases and typically appears within the first month after tick bite. Thereafter, spirochetes can disseminate hematogenously to all areas of the body, but disease primarily manifests in other areas of the skin, the heart, the joints, and the nervous system.

The diagnosis of Lyme disease relies on a characteristic clinical presentation and can be supported by serologic tests showing the presence of antibodies to *B burgdorferi*. Patients early in the course of their treatment or, rarely, those treated early with antibiotics may test negative. The majority of patients with Lyme disease can be treated successfully with antibiotics, with little in the way of long-term sequelae. Misdiagnosis of other conditions as Lyme disease remains the most common reason that patients do not respond to conventional therapy. Oral antibiotics for 2–4 weeks are appropriate initial therapy for all patients except those with severe cardiac or neurologic involvement who should receive intravenous therapy. One exception may be patients with isolated Bell palsy because they respond equally well to oral antibiotics. Patients with chronic residual signs and symptoms after treatment for Lyme disease may have irreversible tissue damage, a post-Lyme fibromyalgia syndrome, or infection-induced autoimmunity. Extended courses of oral or intravenous antibiotics, or both, have not been shown to provide benefit over placebo for this patient population and should be avoided unless clear objective evidence of active infection is present.

Pathogenesis

B burgdorferi survives in nature through alternating infection with ticks and reservoir hosts, including mammals and birds. Ticks feed only once per developmental stage and can lay dormant for years. Thus, spirochetes require that their vertebrate hosts survive in order to increase the probability of transmission back to ticks. In mammals, spirochetes cause disease as they initially infect and disseminate within the host, but inflammation generally resolves even if the organism is not cleared. In animal models, few spirochetes can be seen in infected tissues, yet an exuberant inflammatory response can be transiently present. Spirochete lipoproteins, which are expressed on internal and surface-exposed pathogen membranes, are highly inflammatory and some lipoproteins are the targets of borreliacidal antibodies. Downregulation of surface exposure of lipoproteins may be one way that spirochetes avoid host immunity. Lysis of spirochetes with antibiotic therapy may cause release of internally sequestered lipoproteins and contribute to the Jarisch-Herxheimer reaction, a febrile response and transient exacerbation of symptoms noted by up to 15% of Lyme disease patients with initiation of antibiotic therapy. Delayed clearance of spirochete inflammatory products may also contribute to lingering symptoms after antibiotic treatment for Lyme disease.

Prevention

The best way to prevent Lyme disease is to reduce the risk of exposure to *B burgdorferi*–infected ticks through personal preventive behavior and environmental controls. Avoiding physical contact with common tick habitats, such as wooded areas, stone fences, woodpiles, and tall grass and brush, helps limit exposure risk in areas endemic for Lyme disease. Environmental controls such as the removal of tall grass and brush, clearance of woodpiles, and the application of area insecticides, can reduce the risk of human contact with infected ticks. If entry into tick habitats is anticipated, wearing protective, light-colored clothing such as long-sleeved shirts and long pants tucked into socks allows for ticks to be readily seen and reduces their access to exposed skin. Insect repellants containing diethyltoluamide (DEET) applied to the clothing and exposed skin surfaces provide added protection. Permethrin can also be sprayed on clothing and kills ticks directly.

Daily tick checks are essential for persons with exposure risk to ticks. Prompt removal of ticks embedded in the skin can effectively reduce the incidence of Lyme disease in endemic communities. Attached ticks should be removed by grasping the mouthparts with tweezers and pulling steadily up. Use of alcohol, heat, or vaso-occlusive substances will not promote tick detachment. A single 200-mg dose of doxycycline administered within 72 hours of tick bite has been shown to prevent Lyme disease. However, the risk of infection after tick-bite is low (~ 1.4% even in endemic areas), making the routine use of prophylactic antibiotics in persons bitten by ticks unwarranted. Such persons should be observed for 30 days for the development of a rash at the site of tick bite or for unexplained fever, which may be indicative not only of Lyme disease but of other tick-borne infections as well.

One effective method for prevention of Lyme disease is vaccination. Two vaccines using the spirochete lipoprotein Osp A were developed and tested in humans for safety and efficacy. Although immune responses to

Osp A that arise after natural infection have been associated with chronic arthritis (see below), the incidence of arthritis in patients undergoing Osp A vaccination did not differ from those receiving placebo. One of the two Osp A vaccines, LYMErix, was approved by the Food and Drug Administration; 76% of adults (aged 18–75) who received three doses of LYMErix were protected from symptomatic Lyme disease. However, limited demand for the vaccine led to its discontinuation by the manufacturer.

Clinical Findings

Lyme disease typically occurs in stages that reflect the in vivo biology of the spirochete. After establishing infection in the skin at the site of tick feeding, spirochetes that escape initial immune destruction disseminate through the blood and lymphatics to infect virtually any organ system. The clinical manifestations of Lyme disease thus depend on the stage of the illness—early localized infection, early disseminated disease, or late disease.

A. Symptoms and Signs

1. Early localized infection—The most common early manifestation of Lyme disease is the skin rash EM, present in up to 80% of patients. EM appears within 1 month after exposure to *B burgdorferi,* with a median of 7–10 days, and first appears at the site of tick bite. Ticks may initially bind to clothing or exposed skin, but typically choose skin folds or creases and areas where clothes are particularly confining (eg, near elastic bands). In adults, the most common sites for EM are the popliteal fossa, gluteal fold, trunk, and axilla; in children, EM often arises near the hairline.

The most characteristic feature of EM is its morphology (Figure 46–1A): a flat, macular erythematous lesion that expands rapidly, 2–3 cm/d, and can enlarge to more than 70 cm in diameter. The lesion should be > 5 cm in diameter to fulfill diagnostic criteria. Although central clearing to produce a target or bull's-eye rash can occur in up to 40% of cases, especially when the lesion is large, more often it presents with uniform erythema. Occasionally, the center can be intensely erythematous, vesicular, or even necrotic (Figure 46–1B). Despite its appearance, EM itself rarely produces much in the way of local symptoms other than tingling. Rarely, the lesion is intensely pruritic or painful. Systemic symptoms may be present, including low-grade fever, malaise, neck pain or stiffness, arthralgias, and myalgias. Lyme disease can also manifest with these same nonspecific systemic symptoms in the absence of EM, but this presentation is uncommon.

2. Early disseminated disease—Within weeks to months of initial infection, spirochetes can disseminate

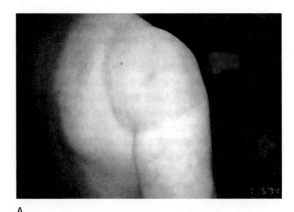

A

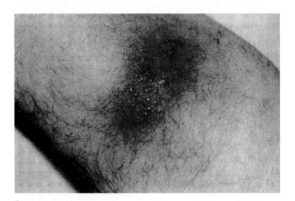

B

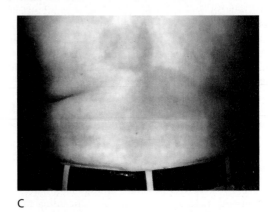

C

Figure 46–1. **A:** Erythema migrans rash with central clearing on the shoulder of a patient. Note the central hyperpigmentation at prior tick bite site (punctum). *Borrelia burgdorferi* was isolated from a biopsy culture performed at the periphery of the lesion. **B:** Vesicular erythema migrans lesion. **C:** Multiple erythema migrans lesions on the back of a patient whose primary lesion is depicted in **A.** Note absence of central papule or postinflammatory skin change.

widely throughout the patient. At this stage, infection can be present in multiple tissues, but disease most commonly arises in four organ systems: the skin, the heart, and the musculoskeletal and nervous systems. Patients are generally ill-appearing and complain of debilitating fatigue and malaise. While specific localizing signs and symptoms may be intermittent, persistent fatigue is a hallmark of untreated disseminated Lyme disease.

a. Skin—Multiple EM lesions are a sign of dissemination and arise in about 50% of patients with untreated early, localized infection (Figure 46–1C). Secondary lesions have a random distribution, are smaller than the primary lesion, and are less often necrotic or vesicular, although they may exhibit central clearing.

b. Musculoskeletal—A variety of musculoskeletal signs and symptoms may be present in disseminated Lyme disease. Migratory pains in muscles, joints, and periarticular structures, especially tendons and ligaments, that last only hours to days are seen in early localized infection as well as in acute disseminated disease. True inflammatory arthritis usually involves a single joint, particularly the knee, and presents with a large effusion (> 50–100 mL) accompanied by stiffness and only mild pain. Other joints involved in order of frequency include the shoulder, ankle, elbow, temporomandibular joint, and wrist. It is rare for Lyme arthritis to involve more than five joints at any time. Acute Lyme arthritis is usually episodic, with attacks of monarticular or oligoarticular arthritis lasting only weeks and decreasing in frequency with time. In a minority of patients, arthritis can become chronic (see below).

c. Nervous system—Central or peripheral nervous system disease, or both, occurs in about 15% of patients with early, disseminated Lyme disease. The classic triad consists of aseptic meningitis with cranial neuropathy, especially involving the seventh nerve, and painful peripheral radiculoneuropathy. Central nervous system (CNS) involvement most commonly presents as aseptic meningitis, although meningoencephalitis with subtle cognitive deficits can occur. In comparison to other forms of meningitis, headache may be waxing and waning and neck stiffness is generally mild, so that a high index of suspicion may be required to make the diagnosis. Cranial neuropathy occurs in about 50% of patients with early neuroborreliosis and most often affects the facial nerve. Cerebrospinal fluid (CSF) abnormalities may be present in cases of facial palsy and reflect asymptomatic CNS involvement. Although usually unilateral, bilateral facial nerve palsies occur in nearly 30% of patients with facial nerve involvement. Peripheral radiculoneuropathy is a mixed motor and sensory neuropathy that presents with sharp, lancinating pain in the distribution of the affected nerves and, later, hyporeflexia. Often, multiple nerves and nerve roots are involved in an asymmetric fashion. Acute radiculoneuritis is rarely seen in the United States but is common in Europe, where it is also known as Bannwarth syndrome. In untreated patients, neurologic signs and symptoms can have a relapsing, remitting course over many months. Rarely, Lyme disease can be a cause of transverse myelitis.

d. Heart—Lyme carditis is relatively rare, occurring in fewer than 10% of patients with disseminated Lyme disease. Conduction system abnormalities with varying degrees of atrioventricular (AV) block are the most common cardiac manifestation, with symptomatic third-degree AV block occurring in about 50% of such patients. Occasionally, myocarditis with heart muscle dysfunction and pericarditis can also occur, but valvular disease is not found. Because Lyme carditis is usually self-limited, cardiac involvement in disseminated Lyme disease may be overlooked, especially if it remains clinically asymptomatic in comparison to other features.

e. Other organ system involvement—A variety of other organs can exhibit disease with disseminated *B burgdorferi* infection. These include the eye (keratitis), the ear (sensorineural hearing loss), the liver (hepatitis), the spleen (necrosis), skeletal muscle (myositis), and subcutaneous tissue (panniculitis). In general, other more classic manifestations of Lyme disease are present concurrently or have been present in the recent past to suggest the diagnosis.

3. Late persistent disease—Chronic manifestations of the disorder, most often in the skin, joints, and nervous system, develop in fewer than 10% of patients with acute Lyme disease. In Europe, infection with *B afzelii* is associated with the late skin lesion acrodermatitis chronic atrophicans. It first appears as an erythematous, hyperpigmented lesion that evolves to a chronic stage of hypopigmentation and atrophic, cellophane-like skin. Antibiotic treatment during the inflammatory phase of this lesion can lead to resolution. Lyme disease can also be the cause of chronic cardiomyopathy in Europe, but this late manifestation has not been documented within the United States.

Late neurologic manifestations include subtle cognitive dysfunction, meningoencephalitis, sensorimotor neuropathies, and rarely, leukoencephalitis. Chronic encephalomyelitis is more commonly found in Europe and is best documented by CSF examination and neuropsychology testing.

A small percentage of patients with acute intermittent Lyme arthritis (fewer than 10%) may subsequently evolve a pattern of chronic arthritis, usually involving a single joint and often the knee. These patients may not respond to antibiotics, particularly if polymerase chain reaction (PCR) of synovial fluid is negative for *B burgdorferi* DNA. Such "treatment-resistant" Lyme arthritis occurs primarily in patients who possess the HLA-DR4 allele and who have T-lymphocyte and antibody responses to the spirochete lipoprotein Osp A. It has been postulated that synovitis can be perpetuated by immune responses to Osp A that cross-react with a human protein (LFA-1), which is expressed in inflamed joints, even though the spirochete itself has been eliminated. Chronic arthritis may also be due to the immune response to poorly degraded spirochete debris or to persistent infection with multiple antigenic variants transmitted by the tick.

B. LABORATORY FINDINGS

1. Routine studies—Results of laboratory studies of patients with Lyme disease depend on the stage and organ system involved. Routine laboratory tests are nonspecific, with some patients exhibiting a mild elevation in the white blood cell (neutrophil) count, erythrocyte sedimentation rate, and modest abnormalities of liver function tests (Table 46–1). The synovial fluid from patients with acute arthritis is inflammatory. Cell counts range from 2000 to 100,000/μL with a predominance of neutrophils. The synovial fluid protein and glucose levels are usually normal. Serum antinuclear antibody and rheumatoid factor tests should be negative. Patients with neurologic Lyme disease, including isolated facial palsy, may have abnormalities within the CSF. It is debated whether all patients with isolated facial palsy should have a lumbar puncture to exclude

Table 46–1. Laboratory tests in Lyme disease.

Test	Result
Complete blood cell count	White blood cell count normal or slightly elevated (neutrophil predominance)
Erythrocyte sedimentation rate	Elevated in 50% of cases
Liver function tests	Mild elevation in GGT and ALT
ANA, rheumatoid factor	Negative
Synovial fluid	Inflammatory, cell counts ranging from 2000 to 100,000 (neutrophil predominance); normal or elevated protein; normal glucose
Cerebrospinal fluid	Lymphocytic pleocytosis; elevated protein; normal glucose; negative oligoclonal bands

GGT, gamma-glutamyl transpeptidase; ALT, alanine transaminase; ANA, antinuclear antibody.

CNS involvement, since these patients appear to respond well to oral antibiotics. A lymphocytic pleocytosis accompanied by elevated protein and normal glucose is consistent with CNS infection but not specific for Lyme neuroborreliosis.

2. *B burgdorferi*–specific tests—

a. Culture—In contrast to other infectious diseases for which isolation of the causative organism is a viable tool for diagnosis, it is rare to culture *B burgdorferi* from tissues and body fluids of patients with Lyme disease. EM provides an exception, with spirochetes readily cultivated from biopsies of the leading margin of the lesion. The morphologic features of EM, however, are sufficiently distinct to make this skin manifestation virtually diagnostic for Lyme disease so that biopsy and culture are rarely performed.

b. Serologic tests—Serologic tests that measure antibodies to *B burgdorferi* provide evidence of exposure to the pathogen and can be used to support a clinical diagnosis of Lyme disease. A two-tiered approach to serologic testing uses an enzyme-linked immunosorbent assay (ELISA) with *B burgdorferi* antigens as a screening tool for IgM and IgG reactivity to *B burgdorferi*. IgM responses appear within the first 2–3 weeks of infection, whereas IgG responses can usually be detected after 1 month. IgM responses should be used to support a diagnosis of Lyme disease only in patients who have had suggestive signs and symptoms for 1–2 months. For persons with a clinical history of longer duration, IgG responses alone should be considered. A persistently positive IgM ELISA over many months without an IgG response suggests a false-positive test. An immunoblot (Western blot), in which individual proteins of *B burgdorferi* are separated by molecular weight, should be used to confirm specificity of antibodies for all positive or equivocal ELISA tests but should not be routinely performed on negative ELISA samples. Criteria for positive IgM and IgG immunoblots are listed in Table 46–2. The most commonly detected antigen, the 41-kDa protein, flagellin, is not unique to *B burgdorferi*, and patients may have detectable antibodies because of past exposure to other bacteria. Patients with early Lyme disease may initially be seronegative, but the majority will seroconvert after 1 month despite the use of antibiotics. Rarely, patients who received inadequate antibiotic treatment for early Lyme disease may remain seronegative. False-positive test results are far more frequent than false-negative test results, especially among patients whose pretest probability of having the disorder is low. A history of previous vaccination for Lyme disease, including participation in vaccine trials, should be obtained from patients before testing because standard Lyme ELISA and immunoblot tests will be posi-

Table 46–2. Criteria for Western blot interpretation in the serologic confirmation of Lyme disease.

Isotype Tested	Criteria for Positive Test
IgM	two of the following three bands are present: 24 kDa (OspC), 39 kDa (BmpA), and 41 kDa (Fla)
IgG	five of 10 bands are present: 18 kDA, 21 kDa (OspC), 28 kDa, 30 kDa, 39 kDa, 41 kDa, 45 kDa, 58 kDa (not GroEL), 66 kDa, and 93 kDa

Adapted from Centers for Disease Control and Prevention. Recommendations for Test Performance and Interpretation from the Second National Conference on Serologic Diagnosis of Lyme Disease. *MMWR.* 1995; 44 : 590.

tive in such persons. Some laboratories offer modified Lyme ELISA and immunoblot tests that have eliminated the vaccine antigen Osp A from the assays so that infection-induced antibodies can be distinguished from those related to vaccination.

In patients with suspected neuroborreliosis, *B burgdorferi*–specific antibody testing of paired serum and CSF samples can demonstrate the production of intrathecal antibodies. If present, intrathecal *B burgdorferi*–specific antibody production is highly suggestive of CNS involvement in Lyme disease.

Recently, a synthetic C6 peptide ELISA has been developed that measures antibodies to a conserved region of the VlsE protein of *B burgdorferi*. This assay has a high specificity (99%) and sensitivity (ranging from 74% in acute Lyme disease to 100% in late Lyme disease) and can be used to distinguish infection-induced antibodies in patients who have received Lyme vaccination.

Once present, antibodies to *B burgdorferi* can persist indefinitely, and serologic titers should not be used to assess efficacy of antibiotic therapy. In this regard, it should be emphasized that serologic tests at best confirm exposure to the pathogen at some time in the past and are not by themselves indicative of active infection with *B burgdorferi*.

c. DNA tests—The PCR has widespread use in the diagnosis of many infectious diseases, especially for pathogens that are difficult to culture or when rapid diagnosis is critical for management. This technique has been used to detect *B burgdorferi* DNA in synovial fluid and CSF specimens from patients with Lyme disease with variable success. Up to 85% of synovial fluid samples may test positive, whereas fewer than 40% of CSF

samples from patients with Lyme meningitis yield positive results. The lower sensitivity is believed to be due, in part, to the preference of spirochetes for connective tissue rather than body fluids.

d. Other laboratory tests—A Lyme urine antigen test has been purported to detect *B burgdorferi* proteins in the urine of patients with chronic symptoms after Lyme disease, and some physicians have used this test to monitor response to treatment. This test, however, has been discredited because of its inconsistent results and marked inter-laboratory variability. Currently, there is no *B burgdorferi*–specific test that can be used to monitor efficacy of treatment.

C. IMAGING STUDIES

Radiographic studies have limited use in establishing the diagnosis of Lyme disease and are used primarily to eliminate other diagnoses. Plain radiographs of inflamed joints may be normal or show only soft tissue swelling and effusion. In contrast to septic arthritis due to other bacterial pathogens in which radiographic evidence of infection can be present early, overt changes with periarticular osteoporosis, cartilage loss, and bony erosions are relatively late findings in Lyme arthritis.

Magnetic resonance imaging (MRI) of the brains of patients with CNS Lyme disease are generally normal, but 25% of patients with encephalopathy will have white matter lesions that may or may not enhance with gadolinium. The majority of patients with Lyme encephalopathy have multifocal abnormalities in cerebral blood flow on single photon emission computed tomography (SPECT) scans. These findings are not specific for Lyme encephalopathy, however, and can be seen in normal persons. Abnormalities on SPECT scans alone should not be used as evidence of Lyme disease in the absence of suggestive clinical history and laboratories tests.

D. SPECIAL TESTS

Specialized tests for Lyme disease are primarily used to evaluate the extent of cardiac and nervous system involvement. The electrocardiogram can show evidence of conduction system disease (especially varying degrees of AV block and escape rhythms) or, less commonly, more diffuse myocardial involvement with changes consistent with myocardial dysfunction and pericarditis. Electrophysiologic studies reveal a predilection for the AV node, but any part of the conduction system can be affected.

Patients with radicular symptoms should have nerve conduction testing and electromyography to document changes consistent with axonal polyradiculopathy. For patients with cognitive complaints, neuropsychological tests are useful to evaluate for depression and to provide objective evidence of memory loss.

Differential Diagnosis

The protean manifestations of Lyme disease have led to its nickname, "the new great mimicker." Despite this label, Lyme disease typically follows a characteristic presentation and clinical course. Accurate diagnosis requires that the patient have an appropriate clinical history and a reasonable risk of exposure to *B burgdorferi*–infected ticks. The hallmark skin lesion EM is a diagnostic criterion for early Lyme disease, but other more common skin disorders can be mistaken for EM (Table 46–3). The seasonal occurrence of EM in late spring and summer months, the size and number of lesions, and the paucity of associated cutaneous symptoms such as itch or pain are useful distinguishing features. Although early Lyme disease can less commonly present as a summer "flu-like" illness, headache, myalgia, and arthralgia are nonspecific symptoms of a variety of viral pathogens. Presence of upper respiratory symptoms or gastrointestinal complaints is unusual in Lyme disease. Patients with fibromyalgia and chronic fatigue syndrome often have debilitating fatigue and musculoskeletal complaints in the absence of objective findings or laboratory abnormalities. These syndromes are more insidious in onset than Lyme disease and patients may be symptomatic for many months before diagnosis. History of a sleep disturbance and the presence of trigger points on physical examination should suggest a diagnosis of fibromyalgia. Acute Lyme arthritis can mimic other causes of monarticular or pauciarticular arthritis, including reactive arthritis and other seronegative spondyloarthropathies, juvenile rheumatoid arthritis, and systemic lupus erythematosus. Low back pain and spine involvement are commonly seen in the seronegative spondyloarthropathies but are rare in patients with Lyme disease. Patients with Lyme arthritis generally have strong antibody responses to *B burgdorferi* and negative tests for rheumatoid factor and antinuclear antibodies. Presence of high-titer rheumatoid factor and antinuclear antibodies can lead to false-positive ELISA tests for *B burgdorferi,* emphasizing the need to confirm ELISA results by immunoblot analysis. Other causes of acute monoarthritis, such as septic arthritis and crystal-induced disease, can usually be distinguished by the severity of pain and by examination of joint fluid for infectious microorganisms and crystals.

Even in areas endemic for Lyme disease, isolated facial palsy is more often found to be idiopathic in origin than due to *B burgdorferi* infection. Only a few conditions are common causes of bilateral facial palsy—Guillain-Barré syndrome, HIV infection, sarcoidosis and other causes of chronic meningitis—and these are readily distinguished from Lyme disease. Acute meningitis due to *B burgdorferi* infection resembles viral meningitis, but most patients should have positive serologic tests at this stage of Lyme disease. The radiculoneuropathy of Lyme disease must be distinguished from neuropathy associated with disc disease or diabetes, or other infections, such as herpes zoster. Chronic encephalopathy can be confused with multiple sclerosis when the MRI scan of the brain shows evidence of white matter disease. Oligoclonal bands are generally not found in CSF of patients with Lyme disease, and multiple sclerosis patients have negative serologic tests for Lyme disease. Subtle neurocognitive deficits due to chronic fatigue syndrome, fibromyalgia, or aging are often incorrectly attributed to chronic Lyme encephalopathy. As for any chronic encephalopathy, toxic-metabolic causes should be excluded.

Cardiac manifestations of Lyme disease can resemble those of acute rheumatic fever, except that valvular heart disease is absent. Coronary atherosclerotic disease, structural defects within the heart, and certain medications (especially β blockers, calcium channel blockers, and digoxin) can lead to conduction system abnormalities characteristic of Lyme carditis. When patients have myocardial dysfunction, other infectious causes should be considered, such as infection with coxsackievirus A and B, echovirus, *Yersinia enterocolitica,* and *Rickettsia rickettsii* (the pathogen that causes Rocky Mountain spotted fever).

Treatment

Practice guidelines for the treatment of Lyme disease have been established by the Infectious Disease Society of America (Tables 46–4 and 46–5). Because many of the manifestations of Lyme disease can resolve without specific therapy, the goal of antibiotic treatment is to hasten resolution of signs and symptoms and to prevent later clinical manifestations due to ongoing infection. This is particularly true for facial palsy, in which the rate of recovery is the same as for untreated patients, and for cardiac involvement. Patients with localized or early disseminated disease without neurologic involvement or third-degree AV block can be treated with oral antibiotics. Although the ideal duration of antibiotics has not been firmly established, administration of oral doxycycline or amoxicillin for 14–28 days is effective therapy for EM, isolated facial palsy, first- or second-degree heart block, and acute arthritis. Doxycycline has the advantage of also being effective against *Anaplasma phagocytophila,* the pathogen that causes human granulocytic ehrlichiosis (see below). Parenteral antibiotics should be reserved for patients with other forms of neurologic involvement (central or peripheral), recurrent

Table 46–3. Differential diagnosis of erythema migrans.

Differential Diagnosis	Seasonal Occurrence	Associated Symptoms	Location	Size	Evolution	Morphology
Erythema migrans	Yes	Mild systemic symptoms Paucity of pain or itch	Skin folds, central	Large	2–3 cm per day	See text
Tinea corporis	No	Itch	Variable	Variable	Slow progression	Ring-like; may have satellite lesion; scaling much more common
Cellulitis	No	Systemic symptoms Painful	Typically acral	Variable but rarely large except on legs	Grows more in typical cases	Usually a homogeneous erythema; tender to touch
Hypersentivity to insect or tick bite	Yes	No	Variable	Small	Variable	Can be uniform erythema, often with tick still attached
Contact dermatitis	No	Itchy	Variable	Variable	Slow progression	Often linear (rhus) or in an area that suggests the diagnosis
Spider bite	Yes	Painful bite	Acral	Variable	Can develop dependent edema but spreads centrifugally	Often necrotic with eschar
Urticaria	No	Itch	Variable	Individual lesions vary	Individual lesions wax and wane over hours	Raised, multiple, often serpiginous around edges
Pityriasis rosea	More in spring and fall	Mild to moderate itch	Diffuse; usually not on face	Herald patch may be confused with erythema migrans	Tends to stay same day to day when it is expressed	Oval lesions, slightly scaly, with long axis oriented with skin cleavage lines
Fixed drug eruption	No	Variable, but often a burning sensation; recent drug ingestion	Fixed, often in genitals, hands, feet, and face	Variable	Tends to stay fixed	Plaque with deep violaceous hue and well-demarcated borders
Granuloma annulare	No	No	Acral	Several centimeters	Fixed over weeks to months	Tend to skin peripherally; can have central clearing
Erythema multiforme	No	Variable (may be associated with viral syndrome or medication)	Usually diffuse; often palms, soles, mucosae	Most lesions small without a single large one	Slow enlargement or stagnant over days	Target lesion is classic, but these lesions are usually much smaller than erythema migrans; often there is an obvious precipitant

Reprinted from *Medical Clinics of North America,* Vol. 86, Edlow, J.A.: "Erythema Migrans", pp 252–253, 2002, with permission from Elsevier Science.

Table 46–4. Recommended antimicrobial regimens for treatment of patients with Lyme disease.

Recommendation, Drug	Dosage for Adults	Dosage for Children
Preferred oral		
Amoxicillin	500 mg 3 times a day	50 mg/kg/d divided into 3 doses (maximum, 500 mg/dose)
Doxycycline	100 mg twice daily[a]	Age < 8 y: not recommended; age > 8 y: 1–2 bid (maximum, 100 mg/dose)
Alternative oral		
Cefuroxime axetil	500 mg twice daily	30 mg/kg/d divided into 2 doses (maximum, 500 mg/dose)
Preferred parenteral		
Ceftriaxone	2 g IV once daily	75–100 kg/kg IV per day in a single dose (maximum, 2 g)
Alternative parenteral		
Cefotaxime	2 g IV 3 times a day	150–200 mg/kg/d IV divided into 3 or 4 doses (maximum, 6 g/d)
Penicillin G	18–24 million units IV/d divided into doses given every 4 hours[b]	200,000–400,000 units/kg/d, divided into doses given every 4 hours (maximum, 18–24 million units/d)

[a]Tetracyclines are relatively contraindicated for pregnant or lactating women.
[b]The penicillin dosage should be reduced for patients with impaired renal function.
Reprinted from *Clin. Infect. Dis.*, Vol. 31, Suppl. 1, Wormser, G.P., Nadelman, R.B., Dattwyler, R.J., et al: "Practice guidelines for the treatment of Lyme disease: The Infectious Disease Society of America", pp 1–14, 2000, with permission from The University of Chicago Press.

arthritis after oral antibiotic therapy, or third-degree heart block. This latter group of patients should be hospitalized and monitored by telemetry for the need for temporary pacemaker insertion. The rationale for intravenous therapy for high-degree heart block is based on the concern that intense or prolonged inflammation may lead to irreversible cardiac damage. However, no study has directly addressed whether parenteral therapy is more effective than oral therapy in this setting, or whether other means for suppressing inflammation provide added benefit. In this regard, the use of glucocorticoids to limit cardiac inflammation may be considered for patients with severe disease who do not respond rapidly to antibiotic therapy.

Pregnant patients and children younger than 8 years can be treated in similar fashion to adult patients except that tetracyclines should be avoided.

A puzzling feature of Lyme disease is that patients may experience a delay in resolution of symptoms after antibiotic treatment. This is particularly true for disseminated disease with neurologic abnormalities or arthritis, which may take several months to resolve. For patients with persistent arthritis, a second course of oral antibiotics (generally of 4 weeks duration) or a single 2–4-week course of parenteral therapy is reasonable after several months of observation. Repeat treatment is not recommended for chronic neurologic abnormalities unless objective signs of relapse are present.

Complications

Ixodes ticks can carry multiple pathogens simultaneously, some of which are also infectious for humans. These include *Babesia microti,* a protozoan, and *A phagocytophila,* the pathogen that causes human granulocytic ehrlichiosis. *B microti* infection presents as a malaria-like illness with fever, drenching sweats, and severe constitutional symptoms, especially myalgias, along with hemolytic anemia. Examining the peripheral blood smear for the characteristic ring-like organisms within red blood cells can make the diagnosis. *A phagocytophila* infects granulocytes and leads to leukopenia and thrombocytopenia. The presence of morulae within granulocytes can establish a diagnosis, but PCR of peripheral blood for *A phagocytophila* DNA or antibody testing is more sensitive. Coinfection with these pathogens should be suspected in patients who have Lyme disease who live in endemic areas and have severe constitutional symptoms and hematologic abnormalities. In one study of patients with *B microti* infection, 20% also tested positive by serologic tests for exposure to *B burgdorferi*. Coinfection can increase the morbidity associated with Lyme disease; a fatality associated with Lyme carditis was reported in a patient with concomitant *Babesia* infection.

Maternal-fetal transmission of *B burgdorferi* has been reported, but earlier concerns that Lyme disease can cause congenital abnormalities appear unwarranted. Several prospective studies have failed to document an increased prevalence in adverse fetal outcomes (spontaneous abortion, premature delivery, or congenital abnormalities) among pregnant women who were treated with standard therapy for Lyme disease.

Table 46–5. Recommended therapy for patients with Lyme disease.

Indication	Treatment	Duration, d
Tick bite	None recommended; observe	
Erythema migrans	Oral regimen[a,b]	14–21
Acute neurologic disease		
Meningitis or radiculopathy	Parental regime[a,c]	14–28
Cranial-nerve palsy	Oral regimen[a]	14–21
Cardiac disease		
First- or second-degree heart block	Oral regimen[a]	14–21
Third-degree heart block	Parenteral regimen[a,d]	14–21
Late disease		
Arthritis without neurologic disease	Oral regimen[a]	28
Recurrent arthritis after oral regimen	Oral regimen[b] or	28
	parenteral regimen[a]	14–28
Persistent arthritis after two courses of antibiotics	Symptomatic therapy	
CNS or peripheral nervous system disease	Parenteral regimen[a]	14–28
Chronic Lyme disease or post–Lyme disease syndrome	Symptomatic therapy[e]	

[a]See Table 46–4.
[b]For adult patients who are intolerant of amoxicillin, doxycycline, and cefuroxime axetil, alternatives are azithromycin (500 mg orally daily for 7–10 days), erythromycin (500 mg orally 4 times per day for 14–21 days), or clarithromycin (500 mg orally twice daily for 14–21 days [except during pregnancy]). The recommended dosages of these agents for children are as follows: azithromycin, 10 mg/kg daily (maximum, 500 mg/d), erythromycin, 12.5 mg/kg 4 times daily (maximum, 500 mg/dose); clarithromycin, 7.5 mg/kg twice daily (maximum, 500 mg/dose). Patients treated with macrolides should be closely followed.
[c]For nonpregnant adult patients intolerant of both penicillin and cephalosporins, doxycycline (200–400 mg/d orally [or IV if oral medications cannot be taken], divided into two doses) may be adequate.
[d]A temporary pacemaker may be required.
[e]See the discussion of chronic lyme disease or post–lyme disease syndrome in the text.
Reprinted from *Clin. Infect. Dis.,* Vol. 31, Suppl. 1, Wormser, G.P., Nadelman, R.B., Dattwyler, R.J., et al: "Practice guidelines for the treatment of Lyme disease: The Infectious Disease Society of America", pp 1–14, 2000, with permission from The University of Chicago Press.

Adverse reactions from antibiotic usage occur at a frequency comparable to that seen in other infectious diseases. Cholestasis has been reported with intravenous ceftriaxone therapy, so its use should be limited to patients with disseminated disease. About 15% of patients with Lyme disease may experience a Jarisch-Herxheimer reaction, a sudden worsening of clinical symptoms (especially fever and musculoskeletal complaints) within 24–48 hours of initiation of antibiotic therapy for Lyme disease. This condition is self-limited and believed to be due to a sudden release of inflammatory products by dead spirochetes. Supportive care with reassurance and nonsteroidal anti-inflammatory drugs helps relieve symptoms.

When to Refer to a Specialist

Primary care physicians who are knowledgeable about the disorder and who follow the recommended evaluation and treatment guidelines can care for the majority of cases of early Lyme disease. Referral to a specialist is appropriate when the diagnosis is uncertain, when other tick-transmitted pathogens or pregnancy complicate *B burgdorferi* infection, or if patients do not respond to a standard course of antibiotics for presumed Lyme disease. Patients who have disseminated infection should be monitored jointly by relevant subspecialists for optimum management and to exclude other disorders that have features in common with Lyme disease.

Prognosis

Overall, the majority of patients with Lyme disease respond to antibiotic therapy with little in the way of adverse sequelae. Complete resolution of clinical signs and symptoms may take several months, however, especially in persons with arthritis or nervous system involvement. In some cases, permanent damage may result in residual deficits that do not improve with antibiotic therapy. A chronic arthritis that is unresponsive to antibiotic therapy may develop in a small percentage of patients, especially those with HLA-DR4 genotype or Osp A antibodies (or both). These patients are believed to be genetically predisposed to an autoimmune arthritis triggered by the immune response to *B burgdorferi* infection. As for other forms of chronic arthritis, treatment regimens directed toward suppression of the inflammatory response are effective. Arthroscopic synovectomy can achieve clinical remission in 80% of patients.

Patients who receive recommended treatment for Lyme disease can have persistent subjective complaints such as fatigue, memory loss, myalgias, and arthralgias. In such cases, evaluation to exclude conditions other than persistent *B burgdorferi* infection should be considered. Rarely, coinfection with *B microti* or *A phagocytophila* may explain unresolved symptoms of patients who acquired Lyme disease from areas in which ticks harbor multiple pathogens. More commonly, fibromyalgia can be seen as a consequence of Lyme disease. A clinical trial evaluating the efficacy of extended courses of antibiotics for patients with chronic unexplained symptoms after standard treatment for Lyme disease failed to show benefit over placebo. Alternative therapeutic approaches should be considered.

REFERENCES

Klempner MS, et al. Two controlled trials of antibiotic treatment in patients with persistent symptoms and a history of Lyme disease. *N Engl J Med.* 2001;345:85. [PMID: 11450676] (Results of the NIH-sponsored multicenter, randomized, placebo-controlled trial of extended antibiotic treatment (IV and oral) for chronic symptoms after Lyme disease. The study was terminated early because of lack of efficacy based on interim analysis of the first 64 patients who received antibiotics versus 65 patients who received placebo.)

Logician EL, et al. Successful treatment of Lyme encephalopathy with intravenous ceftriaxone. *J Infect Dis.* 1999;180:377. [PMID: 10395852] (Results of treatment of patients with Lyme encephalopathy with intravenous ceftriaxone. Includes an excellent description of the various manifestations of chronic neuroborreliosis along with objective clinical measures and reference to previous studies.)

Nadelman RB, Wormser GP. Lyme borreliosis. *Lancet.* 1998;352: 557. [PMID: 9716075] (Informative review of the epidemiology, clinical manifestations, and treatment of Lyme borreliosis in the United States and Europe.)

Reed KD. Laboratory testing for Lyme disease: possibilities and practicalities. *J Clin Microbiol.* 2002;40:319. [PMID: 11825936] (This article provides a comprehensive review of laboratory tests for Lyme disease and discusses interpretation of ELISA and immunoblot analyses.)

Steere AC, et al. The early clinical manifestations of Lyme disease. *Ann Intern Med.* 1983;99:76. [PMID: 6859726] (Description of clinical manifestations seen in 314 patients in whom Lyme disease was diagnosed based on the presence of erythema migrans. Includes some patients in whom antibiotic treatment was delayed because the spirochetal etiology of Lyme disease had not yet been determined at the time of initial presentation.)

Wormser GP, et al. Practice guidelines for the treatment of Lyme disease. *Clin Infect Dis.* 2000;31(Suppl 1):S1. [PMID: 10982743] (Guidelines from the Infectious Disease Societies of America on the treatment of all stages of Lyme disease in adults, children, and pregnant patients. Includes rationale behind recommendations based on quality of evidence and cost considerations.)

Relevant World Wide Web Sites

[The American Lyme Disease Foundation]
http://www.aldf.com
[ACP-ASIM Online—Initiative on Lyme Disease]
http://www.acponline.org/lyme/
[MEDLINEplus: Lyme Disease]
http://www.nlm.nih.gov/medlineplus/lymedisease.html
[Centers for Disease Control and Prevention: Lyme disease]
http://www.cdc.gov/ncidod/dvbid/lyme/index.htm

Mycobacterial & Fungal Infections of Bone & Joints

47

John B. Imboden, MD

■ INFECTIONS WITH *MYCOBACTERIUM TUBERCULOSIS*

Musculoskeletal infection with *M tuberculosis* accounts for 1–5% of cases of tuberculosis (TB) and can produce spondylitis (Pott disease), arthritis, osteomyelitis, tenosynovitis, bursitis, and pyomyositis. In developing countries, where the prevalence of TB is high, musculoskeletal TB remains an important source of morbidity and mortality, particularly among children. In the developed world, musculoskeletal TB is uncommon and largely affects adults. Immigrants from countries where TB is prevalent account for a substantial proportion of musculoskeletal TB in the United States and Europe. Musculoskeletal infection has been reported in HIV-infected persons and in patients whose TB reactivated in the setting of anti-tumor necrosis factor therapy.

SPINAL TUBERCULOSIS (POTT DISEASE)

ESSENTIALS OF DIAGNOSIS

- Back pain.
- Radiographic evidence of spondylitis or spondylodisciitis.
- Identification of M tuberculosis in aspirates or biopsy specimens of skeletal lesions.

General Considerations

Tuberculous infection of the spine accounts for approximately 50% of musculoskeletal TB. The thoracic and lumbar vertebrae are most often affected; the cervical spine is involved in fewer than 10% of cases. Organisms reach the vertebrae either by hematogenous spread (at the time of initial infection or during reactivation) or through lymphatic spread from renal, pleural, or other foci of disease. Most patients do not have active TB at sites outside the skeleton. Pulmonary TB, which is the most common form of concomitant extraskeletal disease, occurs in fewer than 20% cases.

Infection usually begins within the body of a vertebra and then extends to involve adjacent vertebrae and discs; however, "skipping" to noncontiguous vertebrae is not rare. Soft tissue involvement is common, and paravertebral cold abscesses develop in about 75% of cases. Isolated involvement of the posterior elements is unusual (5% in one large series).

Clinical Findings

A. SYMPTOMS AND SIGNS

The most common presenting complaint is pain localized to the spine. The pain typically is not relieved by rest and may be present for months or longer before the patient seeks medical attention. In contrast to pulmonary TB, constitutional symptoms (weight loss, fever, and night sweats) occur in only 50% of cases.

Radicular pain is common. Approximately 50% of patients have lower extremity weakness at presentation; these figures are higher in case series from the developing world. Compression of either the cauda equina or the spinal cord by an inflammatory mass or abscess is the leading cause of neurologic compromise. Meningitis and menigomyelitis are less common. Severe spinal instability can lead to compression or ischemia of the cord.

Destruction of the anterior vertebral body can result in severe angular kyphosis: the gibbus deformity of Pott disease. Paravertebral cold abscesses can track from the lumbar vertebrae along the psoas muscle and present as inguinal masses or can extend from the thoracic spine into the pleural space. Fistulae occur in a small number of patients and can become superinfected with pyogenic organisms.

B. Laboratory Findings

Routine laboratory investigations are of little diagnostic help. Patients may or may not manifest a peripheral leukocytosis. There usually is a moderate elevation in the erythrocyte sedimentation rate (ESR), but in 10% of cases the ESR is < 20 mm/h.

C. Imaging Studies

Plain radiographs can be normal early in the course of disease but then demonstrate evidence of spondylitis including osteolysis, a combination of lytic and sclerotic lesions, and bony destruction. Initially, there may be relative preservation of the intervertebral disc, but disc narrowing is common later in the disease course. Computed tomography (CT) and magnetic resonance imaging (MRI) reveal changes earlier than plain radiography, provide greater detail of the extent of bony involvement, and can reveal paraspinal abscesses not suspected on clinical grounds. MRI permits prompt detection of compression of the spinal cord or cauda equina and is the preferred imaging technique in cases with signs or symptoms of neurologic compromise.

D. Special Tests

Most patients (90–95%) have a positive reaction to purified protein derivative (PPD). Cultures of material obtained by percutaneous needle aspiration of paraspinal abscesses, percutaneous needle biopsy of spinal lesions, and open surgical biopsy are positive for *M tuberculosis* in 70–90% of reported cases. Smears of biopsy material reveal acid-fast bacilli in a lower percentage (20–25%) than do smears of aspirates of paraspinal abscesses (60%). Biopsies reveal characteristic caseating granulomas in 70%. These percentages on the yields of culture, staining, and histopathology may be inflated by the relatively strict case definitions of the studies. The bacillary burden in spinal TB is low, and some writers with extensive clinical experience in endemic areas estimate that the false-negative rates of aspirates and biopsies approach 50%. DNA amplification techniques may facilitate earlier diagnosis but have only been studied in small numbers of patients with spinal TB. In patients with extraspinal disease, identification of *M tuberculosis* in the extraspinal foci may be sufficient to establish the diagnosis of spinal TB.

Differential Diagnosis

Infections by organisms other than *M tuberculosis* and neoplastic disease can cause diagnostic difficulty. Vertebral osteomyelitis due to pyogenic organisms generally has a more acute presentation and is more often associated with fever and clinical toxicity than spinal TB. Imaging studies cannot reliably differentiate pyogenic and tuberculous spondylitis. Noncaseating granulomas, which occasionally are the only histologic evidence of spinal TB, also may be seen on biopsy specimens of vertebral osteomyelitis due to *Brucella* or fungi (either of which can mimic spinal TB clinically). Certain imaging features, such as the presence of paravertebral abscesses, can help distinguish spinal TB from neoplastic disease, but these are not always present.

Treatment

Antimicrobial therapy is the cornerstone of treatment for spinal TB. Unless there is strong suspicion of resistance to first-line drugs, the Centers for Disease Control and Prevention, the American Thoracic Society, and the Infectious Diseases Society of America recommend 6- to 9-month regimens of isoniazid, rifampin, pyrazinamide, and ethambutol for 2 months followed by isoniazid and rifampin for 4–7 months (see http://www.thoracic.org/statements/).

The role for surgical intervention remains controversial. Uncomplicated cases generally respond well to antituberculous therapy alone. A randomized trial conducted by the Medical Research Council found no additional benefit of surgery over medical therapy alone, but critics of these studies point out that there was a trend toward greater spinal instability in the medically treated groups and that patients with extensive disease were excluded. Most clinicians agree that surgery is indicated for patients with persistent neurologic deficits and spinal cord compression, with severe spinal instability, or with ongoing infection despite appropriate antibacterial therapy.

Complications

Complications of spinal TB include destruction of vertebral bodies and discs with consequent spinal deformities and instability; paraparesis or paraplegia; and tracking of paravertebral cold abscesses to distant sites in the chest, abdomen, groin, and neck.

When to Refer to a Specialist

A neurosurgeon or orthopedist should evaluate patients with signs or symptoms of neurologic compromise or with spinal instability or deformity. The diagnosis often depends on CT-guided aspiration or biopsy by an interventional radiologist.

TUBERCULOUS ARTHRITIS

ESSENTIALS OF DIAGNOSIS

- *Usually monarticular with predilection for hip or knee.*
- *Periarticular abscesses and sinus tracts in late stages of disease.*
- *Culture of M tuberculosis from synovial fluid or biopsy.*
- *Demonstration of caseating granulomas on synovial biopsy.*

General Considerations

Tuberculous arthritis is the second most common form (after spinal TB) of musculoskeletal TB. Tuberculous arthritis is seen mostly in children and young adults who live in developing countries. In nonendemic regions, tuberculous arthritis tends to affect older persons. The hip is most often involved, followed by the knee. Any joint may be infected, however, and infection of non-weight-bearing joints and the sacroiliac joints were prominent in a recent European series. The great majority of cases (85%) of tuberculous arthritis are monarticular; oligoarticular TB is an uncommon but well-recognized condition.

Tuberculous arthritis usually develops from adjacent TB osteomyelitis but also can be initiated by hematogenous spread directly to the synovium. Because *M tuberculosis* does not produce collagenases, joint destruction is more insidious than in septic arthritis due to pyogenic organisms.

Clinical Findings

A. SYMPTOMS AND SIGNS

The classic presentation is that of a monoarthritis with pain, stiffness, and gradual loss of function over weeks to months. Some patients seek medical attention after years of symptoms. Approximately 15%, however, have an acute presentation that mimics septic arthritis or microcrystalline disease.

Constitutional symptoms such as fever, night sweats, and weight loss are present in only 50% of patients. Most patients do not have active TB elsewhere, and the chest radiograph may be normal.

On examination there is swelling with or without warmth of the affected joint. Pain limits motion, par-

ticularly when the hip is involved. Cold abscesses and draining sinus tracts may be present in those with longstanding disease.

B. LABORATORY FINDINGS

A mild anemia is common. Peripheral leukocytosis is variable. Most patients have an elevated ESR.

C. IMAGING STUDIES

The classic radiographic changes of tuberculous arthritis are juxta-articular osteopenia, bony erosions at the periphery of the joint, and gradual narrowing of the joint space (Phemister triad). CT and MRI detect changes earlier than plain radiography and can better visualize the extent of bony destruction. MRI is superior to CT for the detection of para-articular abscesses, sinus tract formation, and other soft tissue abnormalities.

D. SPECIAL TESTS

The great majority (> 90%) of patients have a positive reaction to PPD, but false-negative tests can occur in immunocompromised patients. Synovial fluid analysis reveals inflammatory fluid; cell counts vary but usually are in the range of 10,000–20,000 cells/μL with a predominance of neutrophils. Smears of synovial fluid reveal acid-fast bacilli in only 20% of cases, but 80% of cultures of synovial fluid grow *M tuberculosis*. Synovial biopsies yield positive cultures (> 90%) and compatible histopathology (> 90%) and are the test of choice when there is clinical suspicion of tuberculous arthritis and smears of synovial fluid are unrevealing. The sensitivity and specificity of DNA amplification techniques are not yet known for tuberculous arthritis.

Differential Diagnosis

Infection with *M tuberculosis* should be suspected in any patient with an unexplained, chronic inflammatory monoarthritis. Fungal infections can have a similarly indolent course. The chronic nature of the infection may cause confusion with the spondyloarthropathies, particularly when there is sacroiliac joint involvement or in the unusual patient with oligoarticular involvement. Conversely, acute presentations of tuberculous arthritis can lead to a misdiagnosis of septic arthritis or crystal-induced arthritis. Noncaseating granulomas can be observed in synovial biopsy specimens from patients with sarcoidosis, Crohn disease, foreign body reactions, gout (rarely), brucellosis, and infections due to fungi or atypical mycobacteria.

Treatment

Antimicrobial therapy is the primary treatment. Six- to 9-month regimens of isoniazid, rifampin, pyrazinamide, and ethambutol for 2 months followed by isoniazid and rifampin for 4–7 months are recommended (see http://www.thoracic.org/statements/). Drainage or joint lavage is necessary if there is thick purulent material in the joint. Occasionally, surgical intervention is required for debridement of extensive foci of osseous infection or for drainage of cold abscesses. Arthroplasty has been successful for patients with joint destruction.

Complications

Untreated infection leads to pannus formation that erodes cartilage and subchondral bone, eventually destroying the joint. Para-articular cold abscesses and draining sinus tracts develop in long-standing disease; the latter can be superinfected with pyogenic organisms.

OTHER FORMS OF MUSCULOSKELETAL TB

Spinal TB and tuberculous arthritis account for the great majority of cases of musculoskeletal TB. Although TB can cause tenosynovitis of the hand and wrist, olecranon bursitis, and trochanteric bursitis, infections of tenosynovium and bursae are more common with atypical mycobacteria than with *M tuberculosis*. Tuberculous osteomyelitis of the phalanges can produce dactylitis, particularly in children. Poncet disease is a polyarthritis seen with extra-articular TB. The failure to isolate *M tuberculosis* from involved joints led to the concept that Poncet disease is a reactive arthritis, but this hypothesis has been questioned. Primary tuberculous myositis is rare and typically affects the psoas muscle. Muscle also can be infected secondarily by sites in joints or bone.

◼ FUNGAL INFECTIONS

Fungal infections of bones and joints are uncommon in the United States. Histoplasmosis, coccidioidomycosis, blastomycosis, and cryptococcosis are acquired through inhalation. The primary infection is usually asymptomatic but may be associated with transient arthralgias or arthritis, probably on the basis of a hypersensitivity reaction to the pulmonary infection. Osteomyelitis and joint infection are the sequelae of disseminated infection; the clinical presentation is usually that of an indolent process and may mimic skeletal TB. Diagnosis is based on histologic demonstration of organisms on biopsy specimens of affected synovium or bone or on smears and cultures of synovial fluid and biopsy material.

HISTOPLASMOSIS

Primary infection with *Histoplasma capsulatum,* a soil fungus endemic in the midwestern and southeastern United States, can produce a self-limited syndrome of erythema nodosum or erythema multiforme with polyarthralgias or polyarthritis. Disseminated disease is uncommon, and infection of bone and joints is rare. In contrast, African histoplasmosis, due to *H capsulatum* var *duboisii,* frequently leads to osteomyelitis.

COCCIDIOIDOMYCOSIS

Coccidioides immitis is endemic in the southwestern United States. Primary infection is usually asymptomatic but, in a minority of cases, results in self-limited arthralgias or arthritis, often in association with erythema nodosum or erythema multiforme. Disseminated disease, which can occur in otherwise healthy persons, commonly produces osteomyelitis and arthritis, due either to direct seeding of synovium or to extension from adjacent infected bone.

BLASTOMYCOSIS

Blastomyces dermatitidis is endemic in the central and southeastern United States. Polyarthralgias may accompany the primary lung infection. Osteomyelitis develops in most patients with disseminated disease and can lead to cold abscesses and sinus tracts. Vertebral involvement can mimic spinal TB. Arthritis is uncommon and usually due to extension of infection from adjacent osteomyelitis.

CRYPTOCOCCOSIS

Cryptococcus neoformans is ubiquitous. Disseminated disease occurs in immunocompromised persons and leads to osteomyelitis, particularly of the vertebra, in 5–10% of cases. Cryptococcal arthritis is rare.

REFERENCES

Five-year assessment of controlled trials of short-course chemotherapy regimens of 6, 9, or 18 months' duration for spinal tuberculosis in patients ambulatory from the start or undergoing radical surgery. Fourteenth report of the Medical Research Council Working Party on Tuberculosis of the Spine. *Int Orthop.* 1999;23:73. [PMID: 10422019]

Luk KD. Tuberculosis of the spine in the new millennium. *Eur Spine J.* 1999;8:338. [PMID: 10552315] (Critique of the Medical Research Council report favoring conservative treatment over surgical intervention for spinal tuberculosis.)

Malaviya AN, Kotwal PP. Arthritis associated with tuberculosis. *Best Pract Res Clin Rheumatol.* 2003;17:319. [PMID: 12787528] (Detailed review of peripheral arthritis due to tuberculosis.)

McGill PE. Geographically specific infections and arthritis, including rheumatic syndromes associated with certain fungi and parasites, *Brucella* species and *Mycobacterium leprae. Best Pract Res Clin Rheumatol.* 2003;17:289. [PMID: 12787526]

Pertuiset E, et al. Spinal tuberculosis in adults. A study of 103 cases in a developed country, 1980–1994. *Medicine (Baltimore).* 1999;78:309. [PMID: 10499072] (Detailed clinical description of spinal tuberculosis.)

Wallace R, Cohen AS. Tuberculous arthritis: a report of two cases with review of biopsy and synovial fluid findings. *Am J Med.* 1976;61:277. [PMID: 952297] (This classic review of the literature is the basis for the recommendation that synovial biopsy is the diagnostic procedure of choice for tuberculous arthritis.)

RELEVANT WORLD WIDE WEB SITE

[Joint statement by the Centers for Disease Control and Prevention, the American Thoracic Society, and the Infectious Diseases Society of America on the treatment of tuberculosis.]

http://www.thoracic.org/statements/

Rheumatic Manifestations of Acute & Chronic Viral Arthritis

48

Sharon E. Banks, DO, & Stanley J. Naides, MD

PARVOVIRUS B19 ARTHRITIS

 ESSENTIALS OF DIAGNOSIS

- Polyarthritis in a rheumatoid-like distribution that is symmetric with an acute onset.
- Serum anti-B19 IgM antibody positivity.

General Considerations

Parvovirus B19 is a single-stranded DNA virus that does not possess a lipid membrane envelope. It replicates in erythroid precursors. B19 infection is common and widespread geographically. Approximately 50% of all adults have acquired anti-B19 IgG serum antibodies as a result of prior childhood or adolescent infection. Approximately 70% of childhood infections are asymptomatic.

While sporadic cases occur, outbreaks account for the larger number of infections. Outbreaks occur in 5- to 7-year cycles in a given community, reflecting the time required to acquire a school age cohort without immunity. Outbreaks typically occur in the late winter and the spring, although outbreaks in the summer and fall have been recorded.

School teachers, school or pediatric nurses, and day-care workers are at increased risk for infection because of the exposure to multiple children. Risk of infection is as high as 50% among school teachers who have five children in a classroom with the bright red "slapped cheeks" of fifth disease. Transmission is by nasopharyngeal secretions, presumably transmitted as respiratory droplets. Incubation from infection to symptoms is 7–18 days.

Pathogenesis

In experimental infections, illness was biphasic with a flu-like illness characterized by malaise and myalgia occurring at day 7 and associated with viremia. During this phase, B19 growth in erythroid precursors results in maturation arrest at the giant pronormoblast stage of erythroid maturation. At this junction, nuclear inclusions may be seen in bone marrow cells, representing replicated viral particles. Areticulocytosis occurs as does intense viremia, with up to 10^{15} B19 particles per milliliter of serum. By day 11 postinfection, the nascent anti-IgM antibody response begins to clear the viremia. Temporally correlated with anti-B19 IgM antibody is the onset of the second clinical phase of illness characterized by rash, myalgia, arthralgia, and arthritis. Anti-B19 IgG antibody may be measurable soon after anti-B19 IgM, often detectable when rash or joint symptoms present. In natural infections, the two phases of the illness may not be clearly separated.

Anti-B19 IgG antibodies are required to clear B19 infection. Failure to make neutralizing antibodies to the minor capsid protein VP1 allows persistence. This occurs in the setting of immune compromise, such as inherited immunodeficiency, previous therapy for lymphoma or leukemia, or AIDS. Persistence of detectable B19 in bone marrow may cause chronic or recurrent anemia, leukopenia, or thrombocytopenia.

Prevention

Good hand washing and avoiding coughing or sneezing into the face of others is helpful in preventing transmission. This may be difficult in interactions with children. Avoidance of work exposures for teachers and workers by work furlough is often impractical because both child and adult household contacts may be the source of infection in a community outbreak.

Clinical Findings

Typically, sudden-onset pain and swelling in the small, medium, and large joints develops in a rheumatoid distribution. Involvement of the metacarpophalangeal, proximal interphalangeal, wrist, knee, and ankle joints is prominent. Pain is more prominent than swelling. Swelling is more prominent than erythema or heat. The joint symptoms are often severe. Fever, malaise, chills, and myalgias may precede joint symptoms. Rarely, patients experience brief nausea, vomiting, or diarrhea.

The joint symptoms may begin in the hands or knees but spread to include the wrists, elbows, shoulders, feet, and ankles within 48 hours. The spine is usually spared. Morning stiffness is prominent.

Joint symptoms improve within 2 weeks. Up to 12% of patients may experience prolonged joint symptoms. The mean duration is 6 months, but prolonged symptoms may occur up to 8 years. Those with chronic joint symptoms fall into one of two patterns: Two-thirds have continuous arthralgias and morning stiffness with intermittent flares while one-third are symptom free between flares.

B19 infection is associated with a number of nonarticular presentations, and features of these may be present in persons seeking medical attention for arthritis. B19 causes the childhood rash illness of erythema infectiosum or fifth disease. Fifth disease is the most common manifestation of B19 infection in children. Facial rash is common with spread to the torso and then to extremities. The rash is usually macular or maculopapular but may be vesicular or pustular, at least in limited areas. The rash may resolve over a few days but recrudesce, especially after sun exposure, a hot shower, or physical exertion. In adults, the rash is often subtle, and the patient may be unaware of its presence. Children usually have milder joint symptoms when they are present. Adults tend to have more severe flu-like symptoms but lack the classic "slapped cheeks" seen in children. B19 may also cause an unusual "gloves and socks" rash characterized by acral erythema of the hands distal from the wrists and the feet distal from the ankles. Several other viruses have been reported to precipitate this type of rash.

Persons with chronic hemolytic anemia are at risk for developing a transient aplastic crisis. B19-induced maturation arrest of erythroid precursors and subsequent areticulocytosis during viremia leads to severe anemia in those who require a brisk ongoing production of erythrocytes to offset peripheral destruction. B19 may be transmitted to the fetus when pregnant women are infected. The fetus may develop an "aplastic crisis," leading to high-output cardiac failure and hydrops fetalis with death and spontaneous abortion.

Laboratory Findings

B19 may induce isolated anemia, thrombocytopenia or leukopenia, or pancytopenia. The erythrocyte sedimentation rate may be normal or moderately elevated. Rheumatoid factors may be present in low to moderate titers, which confounds the diagnosis given the pattern of joint involvement. Anti-DNA, antinuclear, antilymphocyte, or antiphospholipid antibodies may also be present, which suggests a diagnosis of systemic lupus erythematosus in the setting of arthralgia, arthritis, rash, cytopenias, and fever. Autoantibodies, when present, are usually transient.

The diagnosis is confirmed by detection of anti-B19 IgM antibody in the serum. Anti-B19 IgM is usually present at the time of presentation of arthritis and may wane by 2 months but may last up to 6 months. Anti-B19 IgG antibody is usually present at the time of anti-B19 IgM detection. Identification of anti-B19 IgG alone is not diagnostic because the prevalence of anti-B19 IgG antibody in the adult population is approximately 50%. Detection of B19 virus or B19 DNA in the serum is diagnostic of acute B19 infection, but viremia is usually cleared by the time of presentation for arthritis. Certainly, prolonged viremia would suggest immune dysfunction or deficiency. Testing for B19 virus by DNA-based detection methods in bone marrow or synovial tissue is usually not diagnostic of an acute infection because B19 may be found in the synovial tissue of normal, healthy persons, suggesting that B19 can persist normally.

Differential Diagnosis

Rheumatoid arthritis is in the differential diagnosis. Patients infected with B19 do not have rheumatoid nodules or erosions on roentgenograms. Women with an antecedent history to suggest psoriasis may manifest the psoriatic arthritis after a B19 infection. The initial presentation may be typical for B19 infection, but the chronic disease appears to be psoriatic arthritis in its joint distribution, although psoriatic arthritis may manifest a rheumatoid pattern of joint distribution, making the diagnosis all the more difficult. Persons with fever, rash, cytopenias, arthralgia, or arthritis may appear to have systemic lupus erythematosus. Other viral arthritides, including rubella arthritis in young adults, should be considered.

Treatment

Treatment of B19 arthritis is symptomatic. Nonsteroidal anti-inflammatory drugs are helpful. In those patients with chronic joint pain, tricyclic antidepressants in low doses, eg, 10 mg of oral amitriptyline at bedtime, may be useful adjuncts. Glucocorticoids have not been shown to be beneficial and theoretically may delay viral clearance or promote persistence. In persons who are immunocompromised with persistent or recurrent viremia, especially with chronic or recurrent anemia or other cytopenias, intravenous immunoglobulin may be used. The doses required are 0.4 g/kg/d for 5 consecutive days. Patients may be retreated should the viremia not be cleared. Intravenous immunoglobulin has not been shown to be effective in the absence of viremia. Therefore, intravenous immunoglobulin is *not* indicated for patients with arthralgias or arthritis without persistent viremia.

Complications

Arthritis usually resolves without complications although resolution may require months to years.

When to Refer to a Specialist

Referral may be helpful in delineating the differential diagnosis when serologic diagnosis is delayed and the window of opportunity to identify an anti-B19 IgM antibody is missed and symptoms persist. Atypical symptoms should also prompt a referral because B19 infection may occur in the setting of nonviral disease.

Prognosis

Prognosis is good. B19 arthritis is not associated with joint destruction. Development of joint erosions or deformities should prompt reconsideration of the diagnosis.

Anderson MJ, et al. Experimental parvoviral infection in humans. *J Infect Dis*. 1985;152:257. [PMID: 2993431] (The classic experiment defining the clinical presentation of B19 infection.)

Gillespie SM, et al. Occupational risk of human parvovirus B19 infection for school and day-care personnel during an outbreak of erythema infectiosum. *JAMA*. 1990;263:2061. [PMID: 2157074] (The epidemiologic study defining occupational risk of B19 infection.)

Naides SJ, et al. Rheumatologic manifestations of human parvovirus B19 infection in adults. Initial two-year clinical experience. *Arthritis Rheum*. 1990;33:1297. [PMID: 2169746] (A description of B19 arthritis presentation in a rheumatology practice with demonstration of molecular diagnostics.)

Söderlund-Venermo M, et al. Persistence of human parvovirus B19 in human tissues. *Pathol Biol* (Paris). 2002;50:307. [PMID: 12116849]

RUBELLA VIRUS

ESSENTIALS OF DIAGNOSIS

- *Polyarthralgia or polyarthritis.*
- *Anti-rubella IgM antibody or anti-rubella IgG antibody conversion.*

General Considerations

Rubella is a member of the Togaviridae family of enveloped RNA viruses. Rubella is the sole member of the genus *Rubivirus*. The Togaviridae include arthritogenic viruses in the *Alphavirus* genus found outside the United States.

Rubella is transmitted by nasopharyngeal secretions. In the prevaccination era, rubella occurred among children in outbreaks during the late winter and spring, occurring in 6–9-year cycles. With widespread vaccination of children, the demography has shifted to young adults whose risk of infection is 10–20% of that in the prevaccination era. Outbreaks have occurred among college students.

The incubation time from infection to rash is 14–21 days. Viremia begins 6–7 days before the rash appears and peaks immediately before the onset of rash. Viremia clears within 48 hours of the appearance of the rash. Virus is shed in nasopharyngeal secretions from 7 days before until 14 days after rash, but maximal shedding occurs from just before rash onset until 5–6 days after.

Prevention

Rubella vaccination is required in most jurisdictions in the United States. However, rubella vaccination is not universal in many countries. Rubella vaccination uses live, attenuated virus. The currently used vaccine strain is RA27/3.

Clinical Findings

Rubella infection may be asymptomatic. The classic presentation includes low-grade fever, coryza, malaise, rash, and prominent posterior cervical, postauricular, and occipital lymphadenopathy. Constitutional symptoms may precede the rash by 5 days. The rash can vary over a 2–3-day period, first appearing morbilliform on the face before spreading to the torso, and upper then lower extremities. The facial rash may coalesce and clear as the extremities become involved. Alternatively, the rash is limited to a transient blush.

Joint involvement is common in adult infection, especially in women. Arthralgia or arthritis may occur 1 week before or after onset of rash. The joint involvement is usually symmetric but may be migratory. Metacarpophalangeal, proximal interphalangeal, hand, knee, wrist, ankle, and elbow joints are commonly involved. Arthralgia is more frequent than frank arthritis. Stiffness is prominent. Tenosynovitis, periarthritis, and carpal tunnel syndrome may be seen. Symptoms may persist for months to years.

Rubella vaccination may be associated with joint symptoms, usually occurring 2 weeks postvaccination.

As many as 15% of RA27/3 vaccine recipients experience joint symptoms. These are usually transient, but they persist in a minority of recipients. Postvaccination rubella arthritis mirrors clinical findings in wild-type rubella infections. In children, two unusual syndromes may occur 2 months after vaccination. In the "arm syndrome," brachial radiculoneuropathy causes arm pain, hand pain, and dysesthesias that are worse at night. In the "catcher's crouch syndrome," a lumbar radiculoneuropathy causes popliteal pain on arising in the morning; pain decreases through the day. In both pain syndromes, the initial episode may last 2 months, but recurrences become less severe and less frequent over the subsequent year.

Laboratory Findings

Rubella virus may be cultured from body fluids and tissues, including throat swabs. Detection of anti-rubella IgM antibody or seroconversion of anti-rubella IgG is diagnostic. Anti-rubella IgM and IgG are usually present at the time of onset of joint symptoms. Anti-rubella IgM peaks 8–21 days after onset of symptoms and then wanes over the next 4–5 weeks. Ordering "rubella titer" is inadequate as typically only the IgG antibody is reported. The presence of anti-rubella IgG only documents immunity. Anti-rubella IgM documents a recent rubella infection, usually within the proceeding 1–2 months.

Differential Diagnosis

The differential diagnosis includes other viral arthritides. Rubella and parvovirus B19 arthritides may be indistinguishable on clinical grounds. The setting, exposure history, and vaccination history may help differentiate the two conditions. When an infection with one is suspected but the serologic tests are negative, testing for the other virus should be performed.

Treatment

Treatment is supportive.

Complications

Infection in pregnant women may cause fetal anomalies.

When to Refer to a Specialist

Referral to a rheumatologist may be helpful in discerning the diagnosis and eliminating inflammatory autoimmune arthritis from consideration.

Prognosis

While symptoms may be prolonged in a small number of persons, permanent sequelae of the arthritis do not occur.

Chantler JK, et al. Persistent rubella virus infection associated with chronic arthritis in children. *N Engl J Med.* 1985;313:1117. [PMID: 4047116] (Classic study of rubella in children suggesting persistence.)

Howson CP, Fineberg HV. Adverse events following pertussis and rubella vaccines. Summary of a report to the Institute of Medicine. *JAMA.* 1992;267:392. [PMID: 1727962] (Summary of the Institute of Medicine study showing the rate and nature of rubella vaccination complications.)

Mitchell LA, et al. Chronic rubella vaccine-associated arthropathy. *Arch Intern Med.* 1993;153:2268. [PMID: 8215730] (Follow-up of vaccine outcome.)

HEPATITIS C VIRUS

ESSENTIALS OF DIAGNOSIS

- *Anti-hepatitis C virus (HCV) antibody or HCV reverse transcriptase-polymerase chain reaction (RT-PCR).*

General Considerations

HCV is a linear single-stranded RNA virus that shares similarities with the genomes of the flaviviruses and pestiviruses. The term "hepatitis C virus" was accepted in 1989 after the viral genome was identified. Previously, cases of post-transfusion hepatitis not due to hepatitis A or B virus infection, the majority of which were due to HCV, were simply labeled "non-A, non-B hepatitis." Early studies on non-A, non-B hepatitis described a blood-borne pathogen that could be transmitted to chimpanzees and cause alterations in the structure of infected hepatocytes. In 1989, an RNA viral genome was identified from a cDNA library derived from a virally infected human sample. The complete HCV virus genome has been identified.

Approximately 3.9 million residents of the United States are infected with HCV, and the prevalence is estimated to be 1.8%. Only 20% of persons who are acutely infected show signs and symptoms of acute hepatitis. Thus, chronic infection will develop in 80%, most of whom have subclinical disease despite histologic evidence of inflammation. Hepatitis C is the most common blood-borne infection and the leading cause of liver transplantation in the United States. There are two forms: **acute symptomatic,** which accounts for about 20% of cases, and **chronic disease,** which accounts for the other 70–80%. Many persons with chronic infection are not aware they carry the virus.

The majority of cases of acute infection can be attributed to injection drug use and needle-stick exposure. As many as 43% can be attributed to injection drug use. Transmission through sexual contact is somewhat controversial but appears to contribute in only a minority of cases. Fewer than 10% of cases in more recent years are attributed to blood transfusion or household exposures. The incubation period ranges from 2 to 12 weeks. Infected persons usually express HCV RNA positivity within 2 weeks of exposure. Jaundice, dark urine, and HCV antibody positivity occur in those showing acute symptoms. The symptoms will usually abate within 2 weeks. The return of appetite usually marks the start of the convalescent phase and the disappearance of jaundice, but mild symptoms may continue for months. Chronic infection will develop in 60–90% of patients.

Chronic hepatitis C affects approximately 2 million people in the United States. Chronic hepatitis C tends to remain subclinical. The possibility of hepatitis C is raised by detecting elevated liver enzymes—often inadvertently—over a 6-month period and the exclusion of other causes of transaminitis. Cirrhosis usually develops after an average of 20 years of infection, but the time course can be shorter. Histologically, liver biopsy typically shows varying degrees of fibrosis, ultimately leading to cirrhosis should viral activity continue unaltered by therapy. Risk factors implicated in the development of chronic disease include male sex, age less than 40 years, and a history of heavy alcohol ingestion.

Musculoskeletal dysfunction in HCV infection is becoming increasingly recognized. Often, patients will complain of musculoskeletal pain prior to the diagnosis of significant detectable viral titers. Therefore, this diagnosis is important to recognize when evaluating a person with various musculoskeletal complaints.

Prevention

Blood-borne pathogen precautions contribute to decreased transmission. Newly adopted solvent detergent methods of decontamination of pooled blood products remove enveloped viruses including HCV.

Clinical Findings

Extrahepatic manifestations of HCV infection are increasingly recognized. Musculoskeletal symptoms are common. Presentation is variable, and a wide variety of symptoms are seen, which may be easily confused with other forms of arthritis. The best association between musculoskeletal dysfunction and hepatitis C is in those patients with mixed essential cryoglobulinemia, which usually presents with Raynaud phenomenon, membranoproliferative glomerulonephritis, arthritis (which is nondestructive), arthralgias, and leukocytoclastic vasculitis. Sialadenitis and sicca symptoms of dry mouth and dry eyes can be seen as well as a pseudorheumatoid picture of symmetric synovitis. Nonspecific myalgias as well as fibromyalgia have been identified in 16% of patients in hepatitis C cohorts. Screening for hepatitis C is recommended for patients who have subacute rheumatic complaints.

Laboratory Findings

Detectable levels of autoantibodies are often found in the serum of patients with hepatitis C. During an initial patient encounter, these positive antibodies are frequently confused as being indicative of other forms of arthritic disease. The clinical significance of these antibodies is not clear. There is no known association between the extent and severity of the liver disease and the types and titers of the antibodies seen. Serologic diagnosis uses an array of antigens in an enzyme immunoassay. A recombinant strip immunoblot assay (RIBA) is confirmatory. HCV RNA may be detectable by RT-PCR. A minority of patients may have HCV RNA detectable by PCR amplification methods in the absence of a positive serologic test.

Differential Diagnosis

The joint symptoms and signs may suggest rheumatoid arthritis. The presence of rheumatoid factor may further confound the diagnosis. The presence of lower extremity palpable purpura, Raynaud phenomenon, livedo reticularis, or digital gangrene should prompt screening for HCV. The presence of tattoos or a history of illicit drug use or transfusion should likewise prompt screening. The use of nasal cocaine should be considered as parenteral because shared cocaine straws allow transmission via blood from nasal trauma, ulcers, and bleeding. The presence of autoantibodies may confound the diagnosis (Table 48–1).

Treatment

The management of the musculoskeletal manifestations of hepatitis C is controversial. In general, especially in cases of superimposed cryoglobulinemic vasculitis, treatment of the underlying hepatitis C with interferon-α and ribavarin has resulted in improvement of the

Table 48–1. Auto antibodies detected in hepatitis C virus infection.

Frequently associated
 Rheumatoid factor (most common, especially with cryoglobulinemia)
 Antinuclear antibodies
 Anticardiolipin antibodies (not usually associated with hypercoagulable state)
Less frequently associated
 Thyroid autoantibodies
 Anti-smooth muscle antibodies
 Antineutrophil cytoplasmic antibodies
 Anti-liver, kidney microsomal antibodies
 Anti-SS-A, anti-SS-B antibodies

renal manifestations, but the response to the musculoskeletal manifestations is less impressive. Glucocorticoids and cyclophosphamide are required at times to control the neurologic and renal effects of cryoglobulinemia, but the concern over worsening infection remains. There is also a concern that interferon-α may exacerbate underlying autoimmune processes, such as autoimmune thyroiditis, or rheumatoid arthritis. The myalgias, arthralgias, and arthritis that occur as part of hepatitis C are at times difficult to manage. A conservative approach with low-dose acetaminophen (≤ 2 g/d) has generally been accepted. Nonsteroidal anti-inflammatory medications have been discouraged because of past case reports of reversible liver toxicity with moderate doses. However, no clinical trials to address this question have been performed. The benefit or toxicity of antimalarials has not been reported and is yet to be shown. Disease-modifying antirheumatic drugs with the potential for hepatic toxicity are generally not recommended.

Complications

Cirrhosis and cryoglobulinemia are complications of hepatitis C. Cryoglobulinemia may be associated with severe vasculitis presenting as cutaneous ulcers, digital gangrene, severe Raynaud phenomenon, and major organ dysfunction. Malaise, fatigue, depression, thyroiditis, and exacerbation of other underlying autoimmune disease complicate treatment with interferon-α.

When to Refer to a Specialist

A diagnosis of HCV infection warrants a nonurgent referral to a hepatologist. Cryoglobulinemia warrants a referral to a rheumatologist.

Prognosis

The long-term prognosis of HCV infection is guarded. While a minority of infected patients clear the virus with antiviral treatment, the majority can achieve control of viremia at best. Cryoglobulinemia is a serious prognostic sign requiring control of both viremia and inflammation. Use of glucocorticoids and cyclophosphamide in the setting of viral infection is apparently paradoxical, but the clinical picture often demands simultaneous treatment of viremia, cryglobulinemia, and vasculitis.

Barkhuizen A, et al. Musculoskeletal pain and fatigue are associated with chronic hepatitis C: a report of 239 hepatology clinic patients. *Am J Gastroenterol.* 1999;94:1355. [PMID: 10235218]

Laurer GM, Walker BD. Hepatitis C virus infection. *N Engl J Med.* 2001;345:41. [PMID: 11439948] (A more manageable review than Liang for short sitting.)

Liang TJ, Hoofnagle JH. *Hepatitis C.* Academic Press, 2000: 1–313. A major review of the field.

Munoz-Fernandez S, et al. Evidence of hepatitis C virus antibodies in the cryoprecipitate of patients with mixed cryoglobulinemia. [Review]. *J Rheumatol.* 1994;21:229. [PMID: 7514225] (An early demonstration of HCV in the cryoglobulins of patients with essential mixed cryoglobulinemia.)

Ompad DC, et al. Lack of behavior change after disclosure of hepatitis C virus infection among young injection drug users in Baltimore, Maryland. *Clin Infect Dis.* 2002;35:783. [PMID: 12228813] (A reminder of the challenge to public health management of HCV.)

Riley TR 3rd, Smith JP. Ibuprofen-induced hepatotoxicity in patients with chronic hepatitis C: a case series. *Am J Gastroenterol.* 1998;93:1563. [PMID: 9732947] (A cautionary note to monitor dosing of over-the-counter drugs in HCV patients.)

HEPATITIS B VIRUS

 ESSENTIALS OF DIAGNOSIS

- *Transaminasemia.*
- *Serum hepatitis B surface antigen (HB$_s$Ag), anti-hepatitis B surface antigen antibody (HB$_s$Ab), or serum hepatitis B virus DNA.*
- *Arthritis, urticaria.*

General Considerations

Hepatitis B virus (HBV) is an enveloped, icosahedral double-stranded DNA virus measuring 42 nm in diameter. HBV is transmitted both parenterally and sexually.

HBV occurs worldwide, but the prevalence has been reduced in industrialized nations through vaccination and screening of blood products. Prevalence in the United States is 0.01% compared with 10% in China. Prevalence is likewise high in the Middle East and the rest of Asia. In endemic regions, infection occurs in early childhood, acquired during delivery from infected mothers. Such childhood infections are usually asymptomatic. The incidence of HBV infection in children may be as high as 5% annually, with gradual decline of carriage rates and specific antibody with advancing age. In contrast, in the West, most infections are acquired during sexual or needle exposures in adulthood. Acute hepatitis follows infection more often in adults. Of those with acute hepatitis, persistent infection develops in 5–10%. HBV is a common cause of chronic liver disease and a leading cause of hepatocellular carcinoma in endemic regions.

HBV may cause an immunecomplex–mediated arthritis. It is generally more sudden and explosive when compared with hepatitis C because of the significant viremia early in infection when circulating anti-HBsAb formed. The musculoskeletal manifestations are usually present during the acute phase of infectivity, and present with a symmetric and migratory arthritis. There is a subset of patients in whom chronic viremia and intermittent arthritis and arthralgias develop in the chronic form of HBV infection. One general consideration is the identification of polyarteritis nodosa associated with HBV infection.

Prevention

Blood-borne pathogen precautions contribute to decreased transmission. HBV vaccine using recombinant HBsAg is well tolerated.

Clinical Findings

Following an incubation period of 45–120 days, a pre-icteric prodrome lasting several days to a month occurs. The prodrome may be associated with fever, malaise, anorexia, nausea, vomiting, and myalgia. HBV infection may cause an immune complex–mediated arthritis during this period. Significant viremia occurs early in infection. As anti-hepatitis B surface antigen antibodies (HBsAb) are produced, soluble immune complexes form with circulating HBsAg. Arthritis onset is usually sudden and often severe. Joint involvement is usually symmetric with simultaneous involvement of several joints at onset, but arthritis may be migratory or additive. Hand and knee joints are most often affected. Fusiform swelling may be seen in the small joints of the hand. Wrists, ankles, elbows, shoulders, and other large joints may also be involved. Morning stiffness is common. Arthritis and urticaria may precede jaundice by days to weeks and may persist several weeks after jaundice. However, patients usually have elevated liver transaminases and bilirubin at the time of presentation with arthritis or rash, classically urticaria. Urticaria with polyarthritis should raise the possibility of HBV infection. Arthritis and rash usually subside soon after onset of clinical jaundice. Persons with chronic active hepatitis or chronic HBV viremia may have recurrent arthralgias or arthritis. Polyarteritis nodosa is frequently associated with chronic hepatitis B viremia.

Laboratory Findings

At the time of arthritis onset, peak serum HBsAg titers are high. Virions, viral DNA, polymerase, and hepatitis B e antigen may be detectable in serum. The presence of anti-hepatitis B core antigen IgM antibodies indicates acute HBV infection. Decreases in complement components indicate immune complex–mediated inflammation.

Differential Diagnosis

Differential diagnosis includes serum sickness and other causes of urticaria. Urticaria is unusual with other hepatitis viruses and should alert the physician to consider HBV infection.

Treatment

Treatment is supportive. Hepatotoxic agents should be avoided. Nonsteroidal anti-inflammatory drugs may be used to control symptoms, but liver function should be monitored.

Complications

The arthritis-urticaria syndrome of HBV infection resolves without musculoskeletal sequelae. Attention should be paid to the impact on hepatic health and function.

When to Refer to a Specialist

Patients in whom chronic HBsAg positivity or chronic transaminasemia develops should be referred to a hepatologist.

Prognosis

The arthritis-urticaria syndrome usually resolves with development of jaundice. Rarely, chronic active hepatitis and persistent viremia are associated with chronic arthritis.

Guillevin L, et al. Polyarteritis nodosa related to hepatitis B virus. A prospective study with long-term observation of 41 patients.

Medicine (Baltimore). 1995;74:238. [PMID: 7565065] (A classic description of polyarteritis nodosa associated with HBV.)

Segool RA, et al. Articular and cutaneous prodromal manifestations of viral hepatitis. *J Pediatr*. 1975;87:709. [PMID: 1185334] (A classic description of the arthritis-urticaria syndrome.)

HIV

 ESSENTIALS OF DIAGNOSIS

- *HIV serologic tests positive with confirming RT-PCR.*
- *Musculoskeletal symptoms.*
- *Exclusion of opportunistic infections and coinfections.*
- *CD4 lymphocyte count < 200 cells/μL.*

General Considerations

Management of HIV infection focuses on the induced immunodeficiency, opportunistic infections, and wasting disease. The current discussion will focus on several defined musculoskeletal syndromes associated with HIV infection without known coinfections. Reactive arthritides (including psoriatic arthritis) are more prevalent in some HIV populations, likely reflecting differences in the racial and ethnic composition of the population, geography, local microbial flora, risk behaviors, modes of HIV transmission, and patient ascertainment.

Prevention

Avoidance of risk behaviors, including illicit drug abuse, multiple sexual partners, unprotected sex, and folk practices that lead to blood or tissue exposure, reduces infection rates. Universal precautions in the health care workplace have contributed to reduced occupational acquisition.

Clinical Findings

Acute HIV infection may be associated with a flu-like illness. Several acute pain syndromes have been described in established HIV infection. Several cases of acute symmetric polyarthritis involving the small bones of the hands have been associated with periarticular periosteal new bone formation. In another presentation, subacute oligoarthritis of the knees and ankles may be extremely painful and debilitating; fortunately, it peaks in 1–6 weeks and is responsive to nonsteroidal anti-inflammatory drugs. As many as 10% of HIV-infected patients may experience a third syndrome, "painful articular syndrome," characterized by severe but intermittent arthralgia of the elbows, shoulders, and knees. While each episode of painful articular syndrome lasts only 1 day, it often requires narcotic analgesia.

A high prevalence of fibromyalgia has been reported, up to 29%, in HIV-infected patients. The cause remains unclear.

A CD8 lymphocytic infiltrative disease of the salivary glands called DILS, or diffuse infiltrative interstitial lymphocytosis syndrome, may develop in patients with HIV infection.

Laboratory Findings

There are no laboratory findings specific to the musculoskeletal manifestations of HIV infection.

Differential Diagnosis

The differential diagnosis of HIV infection includes the array of similarly presenting arthritides. DILS needs to be differentiated from Sjögren syndrome, sarcoidosis, sialoadenitis, and lymphoma.

Treatment

Treatment is supportive.

When to Refer to a Specialist

Referral to a specialist is warranted when there is doubt that the presenting syndrome is self-limited or explained.

Prognosis

The articular syndromes attributable to HIV are self-limited. The overall prognosis for the underlying HIV infection determines patient prognosis.

Cuellar ML, Espinoza LR. Rheumatic manifestations of HIV-AIDS. *Baillieres Best Pract Res Clin Rheumatol*. 2000;14:579. [PMID: 10985987] (An excellent review, along with Reveille below, of the rheumatic manifestations of HIV infection.)

Reveille JD. The changing spectrum of rheumatic disease in human immunodeficiency virus infection. *Semin Arthritis Rheum*. 2000;30:147. [PMID: 11124280] (An excellent review, along with Cuellar and Espinoza above, of the rheumatic manifestations of HIV infection.)

HUMAN T-LYMPHOCYTE LEUKEMIA VIRUS 1

This virus is endemic in Japan, especially those areas with a history of early contact with Portuguese sailors who sojourned in Africa. Human T-lymphocyte leukemia virus 1 (HTLV1) infection is associated with oligoarthritis and a nodular rash. The patients have positive serologic tests for anti-HTLV antibodies. Skin nodules contain type C retroviral particles. Atypical synovial cells with lobulated nuclei and T-cell synovial infiltrates are seen in synovial tissue. Sicca symptoms may occur.

Nishioka K, et al. Rheumatic manifestation of human leukemia virus infection. *Rheum Dis Clin North Am.* 1993;19:489. [PMID: 8502784] (A rare review of the rheumatic manifestations of HTLV infection.)

ALPHAVIRUSES

ESSENTIALS OF DIAGNOSIS

- *Fever.*
- *Rash.*
- *Arthritis.*
- *Correct geography.*

General Considerations

The *Alphavirus* genus of the Togaviridae family includes a number of mosquito-transmitted viruses capable of causing febrile episodes of rash and arthritis in humans. Chikungunya virus (chikungunya, "that which twists or bends up") causes sporadic cases and outbreaks of febrile arthritis in Africa and Asia. O'nyong-nyong ("joint breaker") virus is closely related to chikungunya and has been responsible for outbreaks centered in Uganda. Igbo-ora virus, isolated in the Ivory Coast, is serologically related to chikungunya and o'nyong-nyong viruses. Ross River virus (epidemic polyarthritis) causes annual outbreaks of an illness characterized by fever, rash, and polyarthritis in Australia, New Zealand, and the islands of Micronesia. Ross River virus outbreaks occur during the winter wet season when mosquito populations rise. Barmah Forest virus shares clinical features and geographic range with Ross River virus. Sindbis virus infection occurs in Sweden, Finland, and the neighboring Karelian isthmus of Russia, where it is known locally as Okelbo disease,

Pogosta disease, or Karelian fever, respectively. Mayaro virus infection occurs in the tropical rain forest in the trinational area defined by the confluence of Brazil, Bolivia, and Peru. Several cases have been imported to the United States by travelers to the endemic areas.

The reinfestation of previously eradicated mosquitoes, eg, *Aedes aegypti,* the introduction of others, eg, *Aedes albopictus,* and the example of the emergence of West Nile virus in the United States underscore the potential for alphaviruses to spread to new geographic ranges. Mayaro virus has been isolated from a bird in Louisiana.

Prevention

Care to avoid mosquito bites in endemic areas reduces the risk of infection. Insect repellant and bed netting help. Avoiding outdoor activities during the time of day when the host mosquito vector feeds is prudent.

Clinical Findings

Alphaviruses have an explosive onset of fever, rash, and arthritis accompanied by constitutional symptoms. Chikungunya fever reaches 40 °C. Myalgia and back and shoulder pain are common. Macular or maculopapular eruption is typical. Petechiae and mucosal bleeding may be noted. Recrudescence of fever is common following apparent resolution. In Ross River virus, the arthralgia is incapacitating. Fever in Sindbis virus infection is usually not high. Constitutional symptoms are usually not severe. A macular rash typically begins on the torso and spreads to the arms, legs, palms, soles, and occasionally head. The macules evolve to papules that may vesiculate, particularly on the palms and soles. Vesicles on the palms and soles may become hemorrhagic. Mayaro virus causes abrupt onset of fever, headache, dizziness, rigors, and arthralgias in the wrists, fingers, ankles, and toes.

Laboratory Findings

Specific serologic tests for alphaviruses are available through public health reference laboratories.

Differential Diagnosis

Differential diagnosis includes systemic lupus erythematosus, parvovirus B19 infection, rubella, HBV infection, HCV infection, dengue, Henoch-Schönlein purpura, and drug hypersensitivities.

Treatment

Treatment is supportive. In chikungunya fever, 250 mg/d of oral chloroquine phosphate has been used when nonsteroidal anti-inflammatory drugs have failed.

When to Refer to a Specialist

Referral to an infectious disease specialist is warranted when the diagnosis of alphavirus infection is suspected. Public health officials should be advised.

Prognosis

Prognosis is good, although full recovery may be delayed over months. A minority of patients will have residual joint symptoms for an extended period.

Calisher CH, et al. Isolation of Mayaro virus from a migrating bird captured in Louisiana in 1967. *Bull Pan Am Health Organ.* 1974;8:243. [PMID: 4418030] (A cautionary note.)

Doggett SL, et al. Barmah Forest virus epidemic on the south coast of New South Wales, Australia, 1994-1995: viruses, vectors, human cases, and environmental factors. *J Med Entomol.* 1999;36:861. [PMID: 10593092] (A description of an emerging virus.)

Fraser JR. Epidemic polyarthritis and Ross River virus disease. *Clin Rheum Dis.* 1986;12:369. [PMID: 3026719] (A review of the rheumatic manifestations of the annually occurring febrile arthritis.)

Kelly-Hope LA, et al. The risk of Ross River and Barmah Forest virus disease in Queensland: implications for New Zealand. *Aust N Z J Public Health.* 2002;26:69. [PMID: 11895031] (Further analysis of an emerging virus.)

Laine M, et al. Prolonged arthritis associated with sindbis-related (Pogosta) virus infection. *Rheumatology (Oxford).* 2000;39: 1272. [PMID: 11085809] (A description underscoring the minority of patients with prolonged symptoms following alphavirus infection.)

Lam SK, et al. Chikungunya infection—an emerging disease in Malaysia. *Southeast Asian J Trop Med Public Health.* 2001;32: 447. [PMID: 11944696] (A description of how the global village encourages emerging viral infections.)

Lanciotti RS, et al. Emergence of epidemic O'nyong-nyong fever in Uganda after a 35-year absence: genetic characterization of the virus. *Virology.* 1998;252:258. [PMID: 9875334] (After a nearly 40-year absence, a virus returns.)

Tesh RB, et al. Mayaro virus disease: an emerging mosquito-borne zoonosis in tropical South America. *Clin Infect Dis.* 1999;28: 67. [PMID: 10028074] (A description of the clinical presentation and epidemiology of the danger lurking next door.)

Woodruff RE, et al. Predicting Ross River virus epidemics from regional weather data. *Epidemiology.* 2002;13:384. [PMID: 12094092] (Confirmation for avid weather watchers that our environment impacts our health.)

OTHER VIRUSES

On occasion, arthritis has been described as part of the presentation of a number of other commonly encountered viral infections. Varicella rarely causes brief monarticular or pauciarticular arthritis. Small- or large-joint synovitis occasionally develops in adults with mumps. Adenovirus and coxsackievirus A9, B2, B3, B4, and B6 infections have been associated with recurrent episodes of polyarthritis, pleuritis, myalgia, rash, pharyngitis, myocarditis, and leukocytosis. Polyarthralgia frequently occurs in mononucleosis associated with Epstein-Barr virus; occasionally, monarticular knee arthritis occurs. Echovirus 9 infection has been associated with polyarthritis, fever, and myalgias in a few cases. Herpes simplex virus arthritis is rare. A severe cytomegalovirus polyarthritis may occur after bone marrow transplantation. "Herpes gladiatorum" is a herpes hominis knee arthritis occasionally seen in wrestlers. Vaccinia virus has been associated with postvaccination knee arthritis in two cases.

Evaluation of Rheumatic Complaints in Patients with HIV

49

Jeff Critchfield, MD, & Meg Newman, MD

ESSENTIAL FEATURES

- *Potential causes of rheumatic complaints among patients infected with HIV include the underlying retroviral infection itself, inflammatory conditions that are heightened (paradoxically) by the presence of HIV, opportunistic infections, and the effects of medications.*

- *Arthralgias are the most common rheumatic complication encountered by patients who are not receiving highly active antiretroviral therapy (HAART).*

- *Myalgias with minimal laboratory evidence of muscle damage are consistent with several conditions, including fibromyalgia and the HIV wasting syndrome.*

- *Elevation of serum muscle enzymes with pain or weakness raises the specter of myositis secondary to pyomyositis, polymyositis, or the myopathies that sometimes accompany treatment with antiretroviral drugs.*

- *HIV may cause abnormal B-cell activation and a polyclonal hypergammaglobulinemia. The high frequency of false-positive autoantibody assays may complicate the serologic evaluation of HIV patients with rheumatic complaints.*

- *Painless parotid enlargement may herald the development of diffuse infiltrative lymphocytosis syndrome.*

- *In the pre-HAART era, patients with HIV often suffered from profound neutropenia and thrombocytopenia and were not appropriate candidates for the most immunosuppressive therapies used to treat inflammatory disease. With HAART, sup-*

pression of viral load in plasma and the bone marrow have reversed these problems, permitting the use of these therapies in selected HIV patients.

GENERAL CONSIDERATIONS

The approach to any rheumatic complaint in a patient with HIV must begin with the recognition that the complaint could stem directly or indirectly from the underlying immunodeficiency, from a secondary infection, or from a complication of medications used to treat HIV. The clinical spectrum of rheumatologic complaints in HIV ranges from arthralgias (very common) to multiorgan system illnesses such as systemic vasculitis (unusual). Nearly every rheumatic condition has been reported in HIV-infected patients, although several are found only in this patient population (Table 49–1). Serologic evaluations of complaints in these patients are complicated by disturbances of both the cellular and humoral arms of the immune system.

JOINT COMPLAINTS: ARTHRALGIAS & ARTHRITIS

Initial Clinical Evaluation

The principles of evaluating patients with arthritis (discussed in Chapter 4) are thoroughly relevant to patients with HIV. Thus, the presence of synovitis, the pattern and number of joints involved, and the patient's demographic features all help refine the differential diagnosis. The diagnostic algorithm changes according to whether the joint syndrome is one of arthralgias or whether frank arthritis is present. Through the history and physical examination, the clinician must localize the pain to the precise articular structure involved. Patients frequently describe pain arising from bursae, ligaments,

Table 49–1. HIV-specific rheumatic syndromes.

HIV painful articular syndrome
HIV-associated arthritis
Immune reconstitution syndrome
Nucleoside analogue mitochondrial toxicity
Diffuse infiltrative leukocytosis syndrome
Abacavir hypersensitivity

and even the skin as "joint pain." Persons using injection drugs are at higher risk for septic arthritis (see Chapter 45), especially with *Staphylococcus aureus*. Patients who engage in high-risk sexual behaviors may contract gonococcal infections (see Chapter 45). Arthrocentesis is essential for all cases of undiagnosed arthritis whenever joint effusions are present.

Differential Diagnosis

A. HIV PAINFUL ARTICULAR SYNDROME

This dramatic syndrome is characterized by debilitating arthralgias that are often sufficiently severe to precipitate evaluations in the emergency department. This syndrome resolves spontaneously, nearly always within 24 hours. The joint complaints are usually oligoarticular and asymmetric. The affected joints—most commonly the knees, elbows, and shoulders—are free of any sign of inflammation on examination. Hospital admission may be required until other conditions can be excluded. Symptomatic relief requiring narcotics and reassurance that symptoms should resolve quickly should suffice. If symptoms do not improve within 1–2 days, reevaluation is essential.

B. HIV-ASSOCIATED ARTHRITIS

An asymmetric oligoarthritis may affect the large joints of patients with HIV. This form of arthritis usually has a self-limited course, with a mean duration of 6–12 weeks. The prevalence has been reported as 3–25% of HIV-positive cohorts, the higher prevalence coming from a cohort in Zambia. The arthritis is thought to be secondary to HIV itself; viral particles have been recovered from synovia. Treatment has centered on nonsteroidal anti-inflammatory drugs, with some reports of benefit from low-dose glucocorticoids and hydroxychloroquine. The impact of HAART on the course of this complication is not clear.

C. THE IMMUNE RECONSTITUTION INFLAMMATORY SYNDROME

Another diagnosis to consider in the patient who has initiated HAART within the past 1–2 months is the immune reconstitution inflammatory syndrome (IRIS). This syndrome is a paradoxical worsening in clinical status that is caused by an improved capacity of the patient to mount an inflammatory response against persistent microbial antigens or self-antigens. IRIS is usually associated with a response to organisms that were present before the initiation of HAART, eg, mycobacterial infections. The manifestations of IRIS are diverse and depend largely on the particular infectious agent involved. In addition to responses to microorganisms, cases of autoimmunity (eg, of the occurrence of Graves disease) have also been reported in patients with IRIS.

Following the institution of HAART, suppression of the viral load permits the expansion of memory CD4+ cells within 1–2 weeks. Cytokine production shifts from a T_{H-2} profile to a T_{H-1} profile with increases in interferon-gamma and interleukin-2. When mycobacterial organisms have been identified previously and even sterilized in the bone, joint spaces, or soft tissue, aggressive immune responses have been reported to occur at those specific tissue sites. Bone biopsies should include smears and cultures for fungi and acid-fast bacilli in addition to bacterial pathogens, which will be negative if IRIS is the underlying cause. Cessation of HAART is rarely necessary. Short courses of glucocorticoids will mitigate symptoms and may be necessary.

D. OSTEOMYELITIS

Injection drug use is a risk factor common to both HIV and osteomyelitis. Even in HIV-negative persons, the presentation of osteomyelitis can be subtle, with persistent low-grade fevers and malaise initially attributed to other causes. Despite its low incidence among patients with HIV (fewer than 1% of patients suffer this complication), the onset of persistent discomfort that localizes to the skeleton should raise the specter of this disease. As with any infection, the pathogen will greatly influence the presentation and course of the illness. The most commonly involved organism is *S aureus*. Other bacterial pathogens include *Salmonella, Pseudomonas,* and *Streptococcus* species. In the pre-HAART era, *Bartonella* species were found in erosive bone lesions. As the CD4 count declines to < 100/μL, the clinician must consider bone infections with atypical mycobacterial organisms, *Candida*, and *Sporothrix,* which rarely cause such problems in normal patients. Interestingly, it is not clear that *Mycobacterium tuberculosis* osteomyelitis is more prevalent in HIV-positive patients.

E. OSTEONECROSIS

The importance of osteonecrosis as a complication in patients with HIV has been appreciated in both the pre-HAART and the post-HAART eras. One recent report of 118 asymptomatic HIV-positive patients showed a prevalence of hip osteonecrosis in 4.4% of patients. The femoral head is the most common site of involvement, but studies from the pre- and post-HAART eras have also demonstrated involvement of knees, shoulders, and elbows. Among persons with AIDS, osteonecrosis is frequently bilateral. Studies conflict on the number of involved sites present concurrently as well as the correlation of disease with stage of AIDS. Initially, protease inhibitors were thought to be causative. More recent evidence suggests that traditional risk factors for osteonecrosis—trauma, smoking, alcohol abuse, glucocorticoid use, and pancreatitis—are also important in HIV-associated osteonecrosis. Evaluation with magnetic resonance imaging (MRI) is essential for patients with strongly suggestive clinical histories and physical examination findings (eg, pain with internal rotation) but normal plain films. Prompt diagnosis at an early stage may allow successful core decompression. Late-stage disease is treated most effectively with hip replacement.

F. SEPTIC ARTHRITIS

Infected joints are relatively uncommon among HIV-positive patients, with series suggesting fewer than 1% of patients. As in osteomyelitis, more than 70% of affected persons are injection drug users. As the CD4+ T-cell count drops below 200 cells/μL, the risk of musculoskeletal infections rises. *S aureus* is the most common pathogen described.

Gonococcal infection, either isolated arthritis or in its disseminated form presenting with oligoarthritis, small papules, pustules, and enthesitis, must be considered in patients engaging in high-risk sexual behaviors. The cell counts and microbiologic data from the synovial fluid will guide diagnosis and treatment of these conditions that do not differ from non-HIV-positive patients (see Chapter 4).

G. SPONDYLOARTHROPATHIES

1. Reactive arthritis—Studies from the late 1980s suggested an increased risk of reactive arthritis in HIV-positive patients. Data from several subsequent cohorts found no change in prevalence of reactive arthritis between seronegative or seropositive populations. This suggested the observation of reactive arthritis was not due to HIV per se but due to the prevalence of high-risk sexual behavior leading to postvenereal reactive arthritis. Recent literature derived from sub-Saharan African patients, however, suggests a more complicated relationship. The prevalence of spondyloarthropathies has clearly risen with the increase in HIV infections, with no apparent change in triggers for reactive arthritis. In contrast to seronegative patients, these HIV-positive patients are predominantly HLA-B27 negative and seem to have a more aggressive course of arthritis. The classic presentation of reactive arthritis—an asymmetric oligoarthritis involving the lower limbs, with prominent involvement of periarticular soft tissues (eg, enthesitis)—does not differ appreciably in HIV-positive patients. Extra-articular manifestations include conjunctivitis/uveitis, mucocutaneous ulcers, and a scaling plaque termed "keratoderma blennorrhagicum."

2. Psoriatic arthritis—Literature from the late 1980s clearly described an increased prevalence of psoriasis in seropositive patients, with a tendency for appearance or exacerbation in more advanced stages of the infection. Arthritis developed in as many as 30% of patients with cutaneous psoriasis. The pattern of psoriatic arthritis—polyarticular, asymmetric involvement with dactylitis and enthesopathy—differed from seronegative individuals in that sacroiliac and axial skeleton involvement initially seemed less common. As the natural history of HIV has been altered by new treatments, the axial bony changes commonly seen in seronegative patients are now developing in patients living longer than 5 years with psoriatic arthritis. These include unilateral sacroiliitis and bulky spondylitis that skips adjacent vertebral bodies. Therapy is the same as that described for seronegative patients and may require the aggressive use of immunosuppressive agents (see Chapter 18).

Laboratory Evaluation

The white blood cell count may provide clues to the presence of infection. However, patients in the later stages of HIV infection (eg, full-blown AIDS) may not be able to mount a leukocytosis. The presence of a relative leukocytosis, eg, an increase from a baseline of $1.5–3.0 \times 10^3/\mu L$ to $3.0–6.0 \times 10^3/\mu L$, may be significant. Synovial fluid should be sent for culture (ie, bacterial, mycobacterial, and fungal), WBC count, and Gram stain, and be examined for crystals by polarized light microscopy. Basic laboratory studies (eg, complete blood cell count, serum electrolytes and creatinine, and urinalysis) can also provide helpful information.

Patients with HIV have heightened activation of the B-cell compartment and a high prevalence of polyclonal hypergammaglobulinemia. Partly as a consequence of this, the frequency with which autoantibody production is detected in patients with HIV is increased compared with healthy persons. The interpretation of positive autoantibody assays (eg, for antinuclear antibodies, rheumatoid factor, and antineutrophil cytoplasmic antibodies) may be complicated in patients with HIV. The types of tests affected by this phenomenon include serologic titers, enzyme-linked immunoassays, and pattern-based fluorescent microscopy studies.

Imaging Studies

Plain radiographs have low sensitivities for lesions associated with acute clinical syndromes. Infectious arthritides, for example, require 7–10 days to produce bony pathology detectable by plain radiography. Osteomyelitis usually requires at least 10 days before bony changes are detectable. In contrast, disease due to osteonecrosis may be clear radiographically with only recently appreciated symptoms. MRI studies are quite valuable in the characterization of lesions detected by plain radiography.

MUSCLE COMPLAINTS

Initial Clinical Considerations

The distinction between muscle pain and muscle weakness is an important initial step in the evaluation of patients with muscle complaints. Among HIV-negative persons who have been infected with HIV recently, systemic symptoms of fever, arthralgias, and myalgia may correspond with acute HIV seroconversion. In the current era of HAART, chronically infected patients who have terminated their HAART medications are at risk for the development of second acute HIV seroconversion syndromes. The rate at which viral load increases after cessation of therapy is extremely variable; it appears that patients with nadir CD4 counts < 100/μL reaccumulate viral loads more quickly. Cases of acute HIV syndrome in chronically infected patients have been documented as early as 1 week after cessation of HAART. While the long-standing HIV-positive patient may have symptoms secondary to autoimmune phenomenon, infection or adverse drug effects must always be considered. The use of statins to control hyperlipidemia induced by protease inhibitors is extremely common in patients receiving HAART. Symptoms in the setting of elevated levels of serum muscle enzymes direct the clinician to consider HIV medications as causes of myositis.

Differential Diagnosis

A. MYALGIAS

Complaints of muscle pains of varying duration have been reported in as many as 30% of HIV-positive patients in several cohorts. The pathophysiology is unclear with explanations including fibromyalgia, particularly in patients with a history of depression. At times, these myalgias can be localized. Analgesics often are quite useful. Some clinicians recommend strategies similar to those for patients without HIV who have fibromyalgia.

B. MUSCLE WEAKNESS

Seropositive patients experiencing muscle weakness or evidence of muscle damage identified by elevated serum creatinine kinase are subject to several myopathic conditions. Biopsy of affected muscles is an important part of evaluation. The myopathies may be divided into those with biopsy-proven inflammation and those with tissue necrosis mediated by minimal inflammatory infiltrate.

1. Noninflammatory myopathies—The best-characterized myopathy associated with an HIV medication is zidovudine-induced myopathy. This is observed commonly after prolonged therapy (> 1 year). In addition to weakness, patients may first complain of muscle discomfort or pain. Histopathologic studies indicate the drug disrupts skeletal muscle mitochondrial function, yielding characteristic "ragged-red" fibers on biopsy. The quantity of ragged fibers present correlates loosely with clinically observed weakness.

All nucleoside analogues preferentially inhibit reverse transcriptase. Some of these medications also inhibit other DNA polymerases, including mitochondrial DNA polymerases. This type of mitochondrial toxicity can be the cause of myopathy, as well as other drug-induced complications such as a demyelinating polyneuropathy (similar to the Guillain-Barré syndrome) and hepatic steatosis. When zidovudine myopathy is diagnosed, cessation of therapy leads to normalization of serum creatinine kinase levels within several weeks, presaging return of power to affected muscles in subsequent months.

A clinical condition termed "HIV-associated myopathy" describes weakness in the setting of a biopsy showing nonspecific type 2 muscle fiber atrophy with evidence of denervation and abnormal oxidation. Although the presentation and biopsy results are quite similar to zidovudine myopathy, it is usually the diagnosis in patients not taking zidovudine. Some clinicians have posited a causative role of malnutrition, with HIV simply exacerbating the dietary deficiency. A similar biopsy pattern has been described in patients experiencing clinical signs of HIV-associated wasting syndrome. Several case studies have demonstrated therapeutic benefit from glucocorticoids. Finally, the rare condition nemaline rod myopathy has been observed in HIV-positive patients, although it also occurs in seronegative patients in both a congenital and acquired form. The diagnosis is made on biopsy with characteristic type 1 muscle fiber atrophy with myocytes containing small, punctate rods and vacuoles. A clear therapeutic strategy for this condition has not been defined.

2. Inflammatory myopathies—An inflammatory muscle disease clinically indistinguishable from polymyositis in HIV-negative persons has been described clearly in HIV-infected persons. Thus, the picture of progressive proximal muscle weakness, either subtle or dramatic, with minimal myalgia should prompt consideration of polymyositis. Inflammation-induced necrosis yields elevated muscle enzymes in the serum. Electromyographic (EMG) evaluations demonstrate the identical disruption patterns as described in seronegative patients (see Chapter 25). Confirmation of the diagnosis by muscle biopsy is important because therapy will involve pharmacologic immunosuppression. The EMG can direct the clinician to biopsy muscle groups most affected, thus lowering risk of false-negative results due to sampling bias. On biopsy, myositis will manifest as predominantly CD8+ lymphocytic infiltrate among myofibrils of variable states of destruction and regeneration.

Regardless of the person's state of HIV-induced immunosuppression, immunotherapy with glucocorticoids is a cornerstone of therapy. Patients with CD4 counts < 300/μL should receive prophylaxis against *Pneumocystis jiroveci* and *Candida* infections when using any immunosuppressive agent. Some patients may require adjunctive therapy either to control symptoms or facilitate glucocorticoid taper. In these cases, methotrexate or azathioprine is the agent used most often. Patients with HIV infection are susceptible to bone marrow suppression and may require growth factors (eg, erythropoietin) while undergoing chemotherapy.

An infectious myositis, pyomyositis, is also observed presenting as a deep muscle abscess. Patients complain of focal myalgia, localizing to the region of the affected muscle, frequently associated with fevers. Muscle enzymes may not be elevated depending on the volume of muscle involved. Persistence of localizing symptoms merits further evaluation with ultrasonography, although MRI also is quite sensitive for muscle abscesses. The pathogen most commonly encountered is *S aureus*, although other bacteria such as *Salmonella*, *Streptococcus pyogenes*, *M tuberculosis*, and *Nocardia asteroides* have also been described. Surgical incision and drainage or drainage by percutaneous interventional radiology often is necessary as an adjunct to parenteral antibiotics.

Laboratory Evaluation

Assessment of serum levels of creatinine kinase and aldolase are necessary to determine muscular disease. Muscle enzymes levels provide indications of treatment response, but clinical symptoms serve as the primary guide to the duration and intensity of treatment. A leukocytosis is typical of pyomyositis.

Imaging Studies

When considering pyomyositis, ultrasonographic evaluation of localizing muscular symptoms can reveal an abscess. MRI is also valuable for assessing infectious causes of muscular symptoms and for evaluating idiopathic inflammatory myopathies.

SICCA SYNDROME

Initial Clinical Considerations

A significant number of patients with HIV complain of dry eyes and dry mouth. These are often assumed to be HAART-related symptoms, yet only indinavir (5% of patients who take the drug) and efavirenz, ritonavir, saquinavir, and didanosine (all < 2%) are associated with xerostomia. Mycobacterial infections should also be considered but are usually not subtle in presentation. Concurrent symptoms with evidence of systemic process (eg, arthritis and shortness of breath) should indicate Sjögren syndrome or diffuse infiltrative lymphocytosis syndrome (DILS), a condition that occurs exclusively in HIV (see below).

Differential Diagnosis

A. GRANULOMATOUS PROCESSES

Chronic granulomatous processes such as mycobacterial infections or sarcoidosis should be considered. Systemic symptoms are expected to accompany mycobacterial infections, but the presentation may be complicated in the setting of HIV. Sarcoidosis, although rare in HIV, has been reported in patients experiencing immune reconstitution. Medication changes may be considered after other conditions have been excluded.

B. DIFFUSE INFILTRATIVE LYMPHOCYTOSIS SYNDROME

First described in the late 1980s, the prevalence of DILS has been reported as 3–7% of outpatient HIV cohorts. Characterized by painless parotid gland swelling with concurrent asymmetric salivary gland enlargement, 60% of patients will also experience sicca symptoms. Tissue biopsy of the minor salivary gland reveals prominent infiltrate of CD8+ lymphocytes, distinctly different from the inflammatory process of Sjögren syndrome. Extraglandular infiltrates also cause visceral organ disease with up to 50% of affected patients experiencing lymphocytic interstitial pneumonitis. Neurologic deficits can include cranial nerve VII palsies, likely secondary to parotid gland compression, and occasionally peripheral neuropathies. Treatments for both glandular and extraglandular manifestations range from moderate doses of prednisone to the use of HAART.

Laboratory Evaluation

A biopsy of the minor salivary gland has a very low risk of morbidity and may contribute significantly to the work-up.

Imaging Studies

Gallium scintigraphy reveals significant signal enhancement in the affected salivary glands. This finding, however, is nonspecific.

VASCULITIS SYNDROMES

Initial Clinical Considerations

Despite the immunodeficiency that often accompanies HIV infection, there have been many reports of tissue-confirmed polyarteritis nodosa, Henoch-Schönlein purpura, Behçet disease, and cutaneous vasculitis secondary to drug-induced hypersensitivity. It is unclear whether HIV alters the patient so he or she is predisposed to these conditions or simply is a marker for coinfection or an exposure that initiates the cascade resulting in vasculitis.

Differential Diagnosis

Among the true systemic vasculitides, the most commonly described in HIV patients is drug-induced small-vessel hypersensitivity vasculitis. Palpable purpura is the most common manifestation, with skin biopsy yielding the nonspecific description of leukocytoclastic vasculitis. These lesions may be accompanied by arthritis of wrists, fingers, knees, or ankles as well as low-grade fevers. The typical symptomatic HIV patient is taking multiple drugs, but abacavir, β-lactam agents, and sulfa-based medications are the most common offenders.

Abacavir hypersensitivity is observed in 3–5% of patients and most often presents with a combination of fever, rash (usually urticarial or maculopapular), fatigue, and gastrointestinal symptoms. Symptoms worsen progressively during continued therapy and notably improve substantially within 24–48 hours of discontinuation. A patient with a presumed abacavir hypersensitivity reaction should never be rechallenged with abacavir. Ordinarily, cessation of the drug is sufficient for improvement, which occurs over the ensuing several weeks. An identical clinical condition can occur in the weeks following streptococcal infections or subacute bacterial endocarditis, with the sensitizing antigen being a bacterial epitope rather than a medication.

Several groups have described clear examples of tissue, confirmed polyarteritis nodosa. The prevalence of the disease is quite low but has been described in patients at any stage of disease and at any level of CD4 cell number. Clinical pathology seems to be muscular, neurologic, and cutaneous, although examples of gut and kidney ischemia have been described. Cases of cryoglobulinemia with cutaneous, neurologic, and renal pathology suggestive of a vasculitis are well documented. For both of these diseases, it is likely that HIV patients are predisposed to these conditions because of high coinfection rates with hepatitis B and C, respectively.

Finally, when the diagnosis of vasculitis is entertained in the HIV patient, the numerous potential mimickers of vasculitis must also be considered. Case reports describe examples of cutaneous and neurologic pathology from infectious pathogens, including the herpesviruses (herpes simplex, varicella-zoster, and cytomegalovirus) and parasites such as *Toxoplasma gondii* and *P carinii*. Similarly, hypercoagulable states such as the antiphospholipid antibody syndrome can mimic vasculitis by causing multiorgan system dysfunction. Antiphospholipid antibodies such as the lupus anticoagulant occur with increased frequency in patients with HIV, but their clinical significance is not always clear.

Laboratory Evaluation

The evaluation should include urinalysis with careful attention to the presence of protein, blood, and red blood cell casts. Serum complement levels are often depressed in the setting of immune complex–mediated processes, such as the cryoglobulinemic vasculitis associated with hepatitis C. The status of patients' exposure to hepatitis B and C is important. An elevation in the partial thromboplastin time may hint at an underlying hypercoaguable state, which can then be further studied by Russell viper venom time and a mixing study.

Imaging Studies

Plain films may clarify underlying pathology of skeletal complaints to build a picture of a vasculitis associated with a systemic rheumatic disease; however, these are rarely sufficient to reliably make the diagnosis of vasculitis. In the patient with chronic active hepatitis B, complaints of abdominal pain may ultimately require selective mesenteric artery angiography to confirm polyarteritis nodosa (see Chapter 34).

REFERENCES

Biviji AA, et al. Musculoskeletal manifestations of human immunodeficiency virus infection. *J Am Acad Orthop Surg.* 2002;10: 312. [PMID: 12374482]

Casado E, et al. Musculoskeletal manifestations in patients positive of human immunodeficiency virus: correlation with CD4 count. *J Rheumatol.* 2001;28:802. [PMID: 11327254]

Kolson DL, Gonzalez-Scarano F. HIV-associated neuropathies: role of HIV-1, CMV, and other viruses. *J Peripher Nerv Syst.* 2001;6:2. [PMID: 11293803]

Miller KD, et al: High prevalence of osteonecrosis of the femoral head in HIV-infected adults. *Ann Intern Med.* 2002;137:17. [PMID: 12093803]

Reveille JD. The changing spectrum of rheumatic disease in human immunodeficiency virus infection. *Semin Arthritis Rheum.* 2000;30:147. [PMID: 11124280] (Outstanding review of 494 HIV-positive patients referred to academic rheumatology practice between 1994 and 2000.)

Shelburne SA 3rd, et al. Immune reconstitution inflammatory syndrome, emergence of a unique syndrome during highly active antiretroviral therapy. *Medicine (Baltimore).* 2002;81:213. [PMID: 11997718]

SECTION VII

Rheumatic Manifestations of Systemic Disease

Sarcoidosis

50

Irina Petrache, MD, & David R. Moller, MD

ESSENTIALS OF DIAGNOSIS

- *Multisystem disease due to noncaseating epithelioid granulomatous inflammation in affected organs.*
- *Most frequently affected organs are lung, lymph nodes, eye, skin, joints, brain, and heart.*
- *More common and severe in African Americans.*
- *Diagnosis requires a consistent clinical picture and a biopsy with typical compact noncaseating granulomas after excluding diseases that can cause similar granulomatous reactions.*

General Considerations

Sarcoidosis is found worldwide with a prevalence ranging from 10 to 60 cases per 100,000 in North America and Europe. In the United States, there is a higher frequency among African Americans. Worldwide, there is a slight female predominance. Although all ages can be affected, more than 80% of patients are between the ages of 20 and 50 years.

The cause of sarcoidosis remains unknown. A genetic predisposition to sarcoidosis is supported by familial clustering in approximately 5–10% of cases of sarcoidosis and linkage to the MHC locus on chromosome 6. The genetic pattern of inheritance suggests that susceptibility to sarcoidosis is polygenic and interacts importantly with environmental factors. A recent multicenter study on the etiology of sarcoidosis in the United States (ACCESS) found little evidence for dominant or common environmental or occupational exposures associated with an increased risk of developing sarcoidosis. Speculation continues to focus on a potential microbial cause of sarcoidosis with mycobacterial and propionibacterial organisms most frequently implicated in laboratory-based studies of sarcoidosis.

While the etiology of sarcoidosis remains to be elucidated, there is consensus that the pathogenesis of the disease is the result of activated mononuclear phagocytes and oligoclonal CD4+ T cells driving a polarized T_H1 immune response to yet unknown tissue antigens. This immune response is characterized by increased production of interferon (IFN) γ, interleukin (IL) 12, IL18, and tumor necrosis factor (TNF) α at sites of disease.

Clinically, sarcoidosis may present acutely or in a subacute or chronic fashion. Distinct presentations of sarcoidosis are associated with different clinical courses, with approximately 50% of patients undergoing remission, usually within 2–3 years. The other 50% of patients have persistent, generally progressive disease requiring treatment to mitigate the consequences of unremitting inflammation and subsequent fibrosis. There are no biomarkers that have been found to be useful in predicting outcomes or to assist in treatment decisions.

Standard therapies include glucocorticoids, antimalarial drugs, and immunosuppressive agents. Since these therapies are associated with substantial potential toxicities, newer drugs and biologics are under study.

Clinical Findings

A. SYMPTOMS AND SIGNS

1. Pulmonary sarcoidosis—The most common symptoms are progressive shortness of breath, nonproductive cough, and chest discomfort (Table 50–1).

Table 50–1. Clinical features of systemic sarcoidosis.

Organ System (% involvement)	Major Clinical Features
Pulmonary (90%)	Bilateral hilar adenopathy, restrictive and obstructive disease, fibrocystic disease, bronchiectasis, mycetomas
Ocular (25%)	Anterior and posterior uveitis, chorioretinitis, conjunctivitis, optic neuritis, glaucoma, lacrimal gland enlargement
Hematologic (30–50%)	Lymphadenopathy, splenomegaly, hypersplenism, anemia, lymphopenia, thrombocytopenia
Skin (20%)	Erythema nodosum, chronic nodules and plaques, lupus pernio, alopecia
Joints/musculoskeletal (10–20%)	Polyarthritis, bone cysts, Achilles tendinitis, heel pain, myopathy
Hepatic (10%)	Hepatomegaly, pruritus, jaundice, cirrhosis
Cardiac (5–10%)	Arrhythmias, heart block, cardiomyopathy, sudden death
Central nervous system (5–10%)	Cranial neuropathy (eg, Bell palsy, aseptic meningitis, brain mass, seizures, obstructing hydrocephalus, myelopathy, polyneuropathy, mononeuritis multiplex)
Salivary and parotid gland (10%)	Salivary and parotid gland enlargement, sicca syndrome
Endocrine (< 10%)	Hypercalciuria (more common), hypercalcemia, hypopituitarism, diabetes insipidus
Renal (< 5%)	Renal calculi, nephrocalcinosis, renal failure, epididymitis, testicular mass
Upper airway (5–10%)	Hoarseness, laryngeal or tracheal obstruction, nasal congestion, sinusitis, saddle-nose deformity

Chronic sputum production and hemoptysis are more frequent in advanced fibrocystic disease. Typically, there are few physical findings of pulmonary sarcoidosis, with lung crackles heard in fewer than 20% of patients. Clubbing is rare. Findings of pulmonary hypertension or cor pulmonale are seen in 1–4% of patients, usually from severe fibrocystic sarcoidosis or, rarely, a granulomatous pulmonary vasculitis.

2. Löfgren syndrome—This syndrome is a well-defined presentation of acute sarcoidosis characterized by erythema nodosum, bilateral hilar adenopathy, polyarthritis, and often uveitis. Löfgren syndrome is common among Scandinavians and Irish women but occurs in fewer than 5% of African American patients with sarcoidosis.

3. Musculoskeletal sarcoidosis—Systemic constitutional symptoms such as fever, malaise, and weight loss are seen in over 20% of patients and may be disabling.

Arthralgias are common in active multisystem sarcoidosis, although joint radiographs are usually normal. Acute, often incapacitating polyarthritis involving the ankles, feet, knees, and wrists is commonly seen in patients with Löfgren syndrome; usually the polyarthritis regresses within weeks to several months with or without therapy. Persistent joint disease is found in fewer than 5% of patients with chronic sarcoidosis. Pain, swelling, and tenderness of the phalanges of the hands and feet are most common.

Although random muscle biopsies in autopsy series often demonstrate muscle granulomas in patients with sarcoidosis, symptomatic myopathy with weakness and tenderness is uncommon. Rarely, sarcoidosis can present as a polymyositis with profound weakness and elevated serum creatine kinase and aldolase levels.

4. Sarcoidosis of the upper respiratory tract (SURT)—This manifestation occurs in 5–10% of patients, usually in those with long-standing disease. Severe nasal congestion and chronic sinusitis usually are unresponsive to decongestants and nasal glucocorticoids. Chronic disease or surgical intervention may result in destruction of the nasal septum and a "saddle-nose" deformity. Laryngeal sarcoidosis may present with severe hoarseness, stridor, and acute respiratory failure secondary to upper airway obstruction. Often, SURT is associated with chronic skin lesions, particularly lupus pernio.

5. Ocular manifestations—**Uveitis** is the most common eye lesion in sarcoidosis and may be the initial presenting manifestation. The uveitis is more commonly anterior, may be unilateral or bilateral, and is frequently associated with bilateral hilar adenopathy. Severe chorioretinitis occurs uncommonly. Chronic uveitis occurs in as many as 20% of patients with chronic sarcoidosis and is more common in the African American population. **Granulomatous conjunctivitis** appears as a granular or cobblestone-like appearance of the conjunctivae. **Optic neuritis** or **retinitis** may present dramatically with blindness.

6. Chronic cutaneous sarcoidosis—This form of sarcoidosis is common and may be severe, especially in patients of African descent. Plaques and subcutaneous nodules, typically located around the hairline, eyelids, ears, nose, mouth, and extensor surfaces of the arms and legs, are common. Lupus pernio is a particularly disfiguring form of cutaneous sarcoidosis of the face with violaceous plaques and nodules covering the nose, nasal alae, malar areas, and around the eyes.

7. Gastrointestinal sarcoidosis—The liver is frequently involved in sarcoidosis but is rarely the sole manifestation of the disease. Active hepatic inflammation may be associated with fever, tender hepatomegaly, and pruritus. Characteristically, the serum alkaline phosphatase and γ-glutamyltransferase are elevated disproportionately higher than the transaminases or bilirubin. Elevated serum liver function tests frequently revert to normal spontaneously or after treatment with glucocorticoids. Progressive cirrhosis may occur if severe, persistent granulomatous hepatitis is not treated.

Symptomatic gastrointestinal involvement in sarcoidosis is rare, and therefore, other causes such as Crohn disease or ulcerative colitis must be excluded.

8. Cardiac sarcoidosis—Although myocardial sarcoidosis is clinically apparent in fewer than 5% of patients in the United States and Europe, this problem remains a major cause of mortality, particularly in young adults. Arrhythmia, heart block, dilated cardiomyopathy, or sudden death can be the presenting clinical manifestations. Endomyocardial biopsy is usually nondiagnostic because of sampling inefficiencies in the setting of a patchy inflammatory involvement. The diagnosis is usually established by a consistent clinical presentation in a patient with sarcoidosis confirmed by a noncardiac biopsy.

9. Salivary, parotid and lacrimal gland sarcoidosis—Parotid or lacrimal gland enlargement or sicca syndrome can occasionally be the dominant clinical manifestations of sarcoidosis. Heerfordt syndrome, or uveoparotid fever, is an uncommon acute presentation of sarcoidosis manifesting as fever, parotid and lacrimal gland enlargement, uveitis, bilateral hilar adenopathy, and often cranial neuropathies.

10. Neurosarcoidosis—This manifestation occurs in approximately 5% of patients with sarcoidosis. The most common manifestation is cranial neuropathy with bilateral or unilateral seventh nerve (Bell) palsy or less commonly, glossopharyngeal, auditory, oculomotor, or trigeminal palsies. The palsies may resolve spontaneously or with glucocorticoid therapy but may recur years later. Optic neuritis can result in blurred vision, field defects, and blindness. Other manifestations include mass lesions, aseptic meningitis, obstructive hydrocephalus, and hypothalamic-pituitary dysfunction. Seizures, headache, change in mental status, confusion, and diabetes insipidus may be presenting symptoms. Spinal cord involvement is rare, but paraparesis, hemiparesis, and back and leg pains may occur. Peripheral neuropathies account for about 15% of cases of neurosarcoidosis, often presenting as mononeuritis multiplex or a primary sensory neuropathy. Recently, small fiber neuropathy was implicated as a cause of chronic pain in sarcoidosis.

11. Hematologic sarcoidosis—Peripheral lymph node enlargement occurs in 20–30% of patients as an early manifestation of sarcoidosis but then typically undergoes spontaneous remission. Persistent, bulky lymphadenopathy occurs less than 10% of the time. Splenomegaly, occasionally massive, occurs in fewer than 5% of cases and is often associated with hepatomegaly and hypercalcemia. Nonclonal hypergammaglobulinemia is present in 25% or more of patients.

12. Hypercalcemia, hypercalciuria, and renal disease—Hypercalcemia and hypercalciuria are thought to be due to an increased conversion of 1-OH vitamin D_3 to the active $1,25(OH)_2$ vitamin D_3 by macrophages and epithelioid cells from granulomas. Manifestations include kidney stones, nephrocalcinosis, and occasionally, renal failure. Direct granulomatous involvement of the kidneys is rare and usually not a cause of renal failure.

B. Laboratory Findings

An initial diagnostic evaluation should consist of tests to evaluate the presence and extent of pulmonary involvement and screen for extrathoracic disease (Table 50–2). Specialized testing is indicated when symptoms or signs suggest extrapulmonary involvement.

The complete blood cell count is usually either normal or demonstrates peripheral lymphopenia. Pancytopenia may be caused by hypersplenism or bone marrow infiltration with granulomas.

Serum angiotensin-converting enzyme (SACE) is elevated in 30–80% of patients with clinically active disease. This protein is likely produced from activated epithelioid cells and macrophages at sites of granulomatous inflammation. The test has positive and negative predictive values of less than 70–80% for diagnostic purposes. SACE levels do not predict clinical course.

Table 50–2. Recommended tests for an initial evaluation of sarcoidosis.

Chest radiograph
Pulmonary function tests
    Spirometry
    Diffusing capacity
    Lung volumes
    Flow-volume loop (if suspected upper airway obstruction)
Ophthalmologic examination (to exclude subclinical uveitis)
Liver and renal function tests
Calcium level
Complete blood cell count
Electrocardiogram
Purified protein derivative

Thus, most clinicians agree this test is of limited usefulness in the management of sarcoidosis.

C. Imaging Studies

Chest radiographs are abnormal in 90% or more of patients with sarcoidosis. By international convention, the chest radiograph is divided into the following stages:

0: Normal chest radiograph (in extrapulmonary sarcoidosis)

I: Bilateral hilar adenopathy

II: Bilateral hilar adenopathy plus interstitial infiltrates

III: Interstitial infiltrates only (nonfibrotic)

IV: Fibrocystic lung disease

More unusual patterns of pulmonary sarcoidosis include large, well-defined nodular infiltrates, miliary disease, or a pattern of patchy air space consolidation with air bronchograms, termed "alveolar sarcoidosis," or the presence of mycetomas. Differential diagnoses often include mycobacterial or fungal infection, malignancy, or Wegener granulomatosis. Pleural effusions and pneumothorax are unusual in sarcoidosis.

Chest computed tomography (CT) typically demonstrates nodular infiltrates that follow central bronchovascular structures.

The gallium scan often shows uptake in the bilateral hilar and right paratracheal lymph node region ("lambda" sign) of the lungs. Uptake in the parotids or lacrimal and salivary glands lead to a "panda" sign. The combination of signs (lambda-panda) is highly suggestive of sarcoidosis, but the lack of specificity, cost, and considerable radiation exposure from this test have led most clinicians to abandon its use.

Positron emission tomography is replacing the gallium scan as a method to detect active inflammatory sites in sarcoidosis, potentially aiding in choosing sites for biopsy. The test has much less radiation exposure than gallium scanning but has a similar lack of specificity.

Joint radiographs may demonstrate "punched out" lesions with cystic changes and marked loss of trabeculae but without evidence of erosive chrondritis. Cystic lesions of the long bones, pelvis, sternum, skull, and vertebrae rarely occur.

Evaluation for central nervous system (CNS) sarcoidosis should include magnetic resonance imaging with gadolinium enhancement, which is now considered the optimal test to detect characteristic inflammatory lesions that have a propensity for periventricular and leptomeningeal areas. The images are nonspecific and can be produced by infectious (tuberculosis, fungal disease) or malignant (lymphoma, carcinomatosis) disease. A normal scan does not exclude neurosarcoidosis, particularly for cranial neuropathies or in the presence of glucocorticoid therapy.

D. Special Tests

Pulmonary function tests may show restrictive, obstructive, or combined impairment with reduction in diffusing capacity for carbon monoxide (DLCO). Gas exchange is usually preserved until extensive fibrocystic changes are evident.

Bronchoalveolar lavage (BAL) fluid in sarcoidosis is typically characterized by increased proportions and numbers of activated CD4+ alveolar lymphocytes reflective of enhanced cell-mediated immune processes at sites of granuloma formation. These findings are not specific for sarcoidosis and do not predict clinical outcome.

An electrocardiogram is routinely performed to screen for conduction abnormalities, which may signal the presence of early cardiac sarcoidosis.

A well-recognized feature of sarcoidosis is the impaired cutaneous response to common antigens that elicit delayed-type hypersensitivity reactions, seen in 30-70% of patients. Since anergy to purified protein derivative (PPD) testing is common in sarcoidosis, active tuberculosis must be strongly considered in any patient in whom a positive tuberculin skin test develops.

E. Special Examinations

Biopsy of the easiest, most accessible abnormal tissue site is used for confirmation of the diagnosis. Biopsy of a skin nodule, superficial lymph node, nasal mucosae, conjunctivae, or salivary gland (lip biopsy) sometimes can establish a diagnosis. Biopsy by fiberoptic bronchoscopy is frequently used to diagnose pulmonary sarcoidosis because of its relative safety and high yield. Endobronchial or transbronchial needle aspiration biopsies may increase the yield further. Biopsy of the liver or bone marrow is nonspecific and should be used to support a diagnosis of sarcoidosis only after malignancy, infectious granulomatous diseases, or other organ-specific diagnoses are excluded. Mediastinoscopy or thoracoscopic or open-lung biopsy should be considered in cases where lymphoma or other intrathoracic malignancy cannot be reasonably excluded. Biopsy confirmation of sarcoidosis is usually not necessary in Löfgren syndrome except in regions where histoplasmosis is endemic, and fungal infection must be excluded before initiating glucocorticoid therapy.

When cardiac sarcoidosis is suspected on the basis of symptoms or electrocardiographic abnormalities, Holter monitoring, two-dimensional echocardiography, and radionuclide imaging with gated 201-thallium scanning are indicated to detect myocardial or conduction abnormalities. If the suspicion for cardiac involvement is high, electrophysiologic testing may be indicated to exclude arrhythmias undetected by routine studies.

In patients with suspected neurosarcoidosis, magnetic resonance imaging with gadolinium enhancement of the brain or spine and examination of the cerebrospinal fluid are usually indicated. In neurosarcoidosis, the cerebrospinal fluid may demonstrate lymphocytic pleocytosis or elevated protein levels. A diagnosis of neurosarcoidosis is usually confirmed by biopsy of a non-CNS site, generally by bronchoscopic or lymph node biopsy. Rarely, brain biopsy is needed to exclude infectious or malignant disease. In suspected cases of peripheral neuropathy or myopathy, electromyography or nerve conduction studies should be considered.

Differential Diagnosis

A diagnosis of sarcoidosis is based on a compatible clinical picture, histologic evidence of noncaseating granulomas, and the absence of other known causes of this pathologic response (such as tuberculosis, fungal diseases, lymphoma, chronic beryllium disease, hypersensitivity pneumonitis, collagen vascular disease, or vasculitis such as Wegener granulomatosis).

Treatment

Indications for treatment follow:

- Persistent, symptomatic, or progressive pulmonary disease.
- Threatened organ failure, such as severe ocular, CNS, or cardiac disease.
- Persistent hypercalcemia or renal or hepatic dysfunction.
- Posterior uveitis or anterior uveitis not responding to localized glucocorticoid therapy.
- Pituitary disease.
- Myopathy.
- Significant splenomegaly or evidence of hypersplenism such as thrombocytopenia.
- Severe fatigue and weight loss.
- Disfiguring skin disease or lymphadenopathy.

A. MEDICAL

1. Glucocorticoids—These drugs are the cornerstone of therapy for serious progressive pulmonary or extrapulmonary sarcoidosis (Table 50–3). Guidelines for when to initiate therapy with glucocorticoids and proper dosing have, in general, been formulated from extensive clinical experience without being subjected to well-controlled prospective clinical trials. Controversy exists regarding their overall effectiveness in altering the long-term course of the disease. However, clinical experience indicates that glucocorticoids provide prompt symptomatic relief and reverse organ dysfunction in most patients with active inflammation. The optimal dose and duration of glucocorticoid treatment have not been established by rigorous clinical studies.

2. Antimalarial drugs—Hydroxychloroquine and chloroquine have been used as first-line drugs for dominant skin, nasal mucosal, and sinus sarcoidosis but have not been consistently effective for pulmonary or systemic disease. Hypercalcemia and laryngeal, bone, and joint involvement have been reported to respond to either hydroxychloroquine or chloroquine. Ocular toxicity is a major concern for chloroquine but is rare when low doses are used with periods of drug-free use. Ocular toxicity has also rarely been reported for hydroxychloroquine. Serial ophthalmologic evaluations should be performed during therapy.

3. Immunosuppressive drugs—Methotrexate or azathioprine have been most commonly used to treat severe extrapulmonary sarcoidosis and pulmonary sarcoidosis that is unresponsive to small doses of glucocorticoids or when there are unacceptable glucocorticoid side effects. Benefits of these drugs have not been established by rigorous clinical trials.

4. Other immunomodulatory drugs—Pentoxifylline, thalidomide, and the TNF-α inhibitors are emerging as alternative or glucocorticoid-sparing therapies from results of small case series. Further studies are needed to assess their efficacy in different clinical presentations before they can be routinely recommended.

Table 50–3. Treatment of sarcoidosis.

Drug	Typical Dose	Major Adverse Effects
Glucocorticoids	Prednisone 30–40 mg/d for 2 weeks; decrease by 5 mg/d every 2 wks until 10–15 mg/d; maintain for 8–12 mo, then taper 2.5 mg/d every 2–4 wks; reinstitute for relapse	Weight gain Hypertension Hyperglycemia Osteoporosis Cataracts
Antimalarial drugs Hydroxychloroquine	200 mg once or twice daily	Ocular toxicity (rare) Gastrointestinal upset Rashes
Chloroquine	250 mg qd (500 mg q2d) for 6 mo followed by 6-mo drug holiday	Ocular toxicity (retinopathy)
Azathioprine	100–200 mg/d	Hematologic suppression Hepatic toxicity ? Oncogenic potential
Methotrexate	10–20 mg/wk	Hepatic, pulmonary, bone marrow toxicity
Pentoxifylline	400 mg 3 or 4 times daily	Gastrointestinal upset Headache
Thalidomide	100–200 mg qhs	Teratogenicity Peripheral neuropathy Sedation

B. SURGICAL

Successful lung, heart-lung, and liver transplantations have been performed in a small number of patients with advanced organ insufficiency. Noncaseating granulomas may develop in the transplanted organs in some lung and heart transplant patients. In lung transplant patients, the recurrent granulomas seem to respond to higher doses of glucocorticoids and do not change overall survival. Heart transplantation for end-stage sarcoidosis cardiomyopathy has also been successful in a small number of patients, although experience remains limited.

Complications

Major causes of death from sarcoidosis include respiratory insufficiency and cor pulmonale, massive hemoptysis, cardiac arrest from cardiac sarcoidosis, and uremia from chronic renal failure. Several centers in the United States and Great Britain suggest that race is an important prognostic indicator, with African American and West Indian patients more likely to have chronic persistent disease and suffer from increased morbidity and mortality. Hospital statistics suggest that sarcoidosis is the direct cause of death in 1–5% of persons admitted with this disease.

Prognosis

It is estimated from various studies that approximately 50% of all patients with sarcoidosis have remission of their disease. The other 50% have chronic disease that usually persists for long periods of time, often indefinitely. The determinants of remitting versus chronic sarcoidosis are not understood, although there is evidence for a genetic basis for different clinical outcomes. The type of clinical presentation also carries prognostic information. Patients presenting with Löfgren syndrome undergo remission 80–90% of the time. Patients with fibrocystic pulmonary sarcoidosis, lupus pernio, or nasal or sinus sarcoidosis or who have multisystem disease for greater than 2 years usually will have unremitting, progressive disease if not treated.

When to Refer to a Specialist

A patient should be referred to a specialist in sarcoidosis under the following the circumstances:

- Uncertain of the diagnosis.
- Uncomfortable with a decision of whether to treat or not.
- Disease that is not responding as expected.

- Severe extrapulmonary involvement such as cardiac, neurologic, skin, or sinus involvement.
- Unsure about the use of glucocorticoid-sparing or alternative medications.

REFERENCES

Baughman RP, et al. Clinical characteristics of patients in a case control study of sarcoidosis. *Am J Respir Crit Care Med.* 2001; 164:1885. [PMID: 11734441] (Clinical characteristics of over 720 patients with sarcoidosis enrolled in the ACCESS study. A manuscript of the results from the case control study for etiologic causes is under review.)

Johns CJ, Michele TM. The clinical management of sarcoidosis. A 50-year experience at the Johns Hopkins Hospital. *Medicine (Baltimore).* 1999;78:65. [PMID: 10195091] (Insights into the clinical management of sarcoidosis from an internationally recognized expert on sarcoidosis.)

Moller DR. Treatment of sarcoidosis—from a basic science point of view. *J Intern Med.* 2003;253:31. [PMID: 12588536] (A review of the scientific foundations for our current treatment strategies in sarcoidosis.)

Sharma OP. Cardiac and neurologic dysfunction in sarcoidosis. *Clin Chest Med.* 1997;18:813. [PMID: 9413660] (The clinical experience on the challenging clinical problems of cardiac and neurologic sarcoidosis by an internationally recognized expert on sarcoidosis.)

Statement on Sarcoidosis. Joint Statement of the American Thoracic Society (ATS), the European Respiratory Society (ERS), and the World Association of Sarcoidosis and Other Granulomatous Disorders (WASOG) adopted by the ATS Board of Directors and by the ERS Executive Committee, February 1999. *Am J Respir Crit Care Med.* 1999;160:736. [PMID: 10430755] (Consensus statement of the state of the art of the understanding of the pathogenesis, diagnosis, and treatment of sarcoidosis from the American Thoracic Society, European Respiratory Society, and the World Association of Sarcoidosis and Other Granulomatous Diseases.)

Relevant World Wide Web Sites

[National Heart, Lung, and Blood Institute (NHLBI): Sarcoidosis]
http://www.nhlbi.nih.gov/health/public/lung.other/sarcoidosis/index.html
[World Association of Sarcoidosis and Other Granulomatous Disorders (WASOG)]
http://www.pinali.unipd.it/sarcoid/
[Sarcoidosis Internet Resources]
http://www.blueflamingo.net.sarcoid/sos.html

Endocrine & Metabolic Disorders   51

Jonathan Graf, MD, & Dolores Shoback, MD

Many links exist between endocrine and rheumatic diseases. Several major endocrinologic diseases, such as type 1 diabetes mellitus and Graves disease, are known to be associated with autoimmunity. Moreover, many autoimmune diseases appear to target endocrine organs secondarily. Perhaps the best example of this phenomenon is the frequent cooccurrence of connective tissue diseases and thyroid disorders associated with antithyroid antibodies. Many patients with well-established endocrine disorders seek treatment for musculoskeletal symptoms related to their primary underlying condition (Table 51–1). Finally, many endocrine disorders present with rheumatic manifestations before the nature of their underlying endocrinopathy becomes apparent. Thus, in the interest of timely diagnosis and the institution of appropriate therapies, practitioners must become familiar with these overlapping clinical features.

■ DIABETES MELLITUS

Patients with both types 1 and 2 diabetes mellitus frequently have musculoskeletal complaints. However, establishing precise cause and effect relationships between hyperglycemia and diseases of the musculoskeletal system has proved more elusive in most cases. First, the prevalence of both diabetes and soft tissue rheumatic complaints is quite high, complicating the recognition of causal relationships between the two entities. Second, as with many other clinical endocrine disorders, few well-designed studies have addressed the possible relationships between diabetes and rheumatic diseases. Finally, until recently, little has been understood about the pathophysiologic effects of hyperglycemia on bones, joints, tendons, muscles, and fascia. Theories abound about the effects of hyperglycemia on fibrous tissue proliferation, neuropathy, and small-vessel vasculopathy, but many of these hypotheses still do not explain convincingly the reasons for rheumatic complications. This section details the recognized associations of glucose intolerance and abnormalities of bones and joints (Table 51–2).

DISORDERS OF THE BONES & JOINTS

Charcot Arthropathy

Several types of arthropathy have been well characterized in patients with diabetes. In the nineteenth century, Jean Martin Charcot first described a destructive arthropathy seen in patients with tabes dorsalis. In a similar manner, many diabetic patients with longstanding hyperglycemia eventually develop progressive sensory neuropathy, with degradation in sensation occurring earliest along the axons with the greatest length, particularly those innervating the extremities. In addition to causing the classic "stocking and glove" distribution of paresthesias and numbness, this sensory neuropathy frequently progresses insidiously to inhibit normal protection of the regional joints, particularly those of the foot and ankle. The most commonly involved joints include the metatarsophalangeal, tarsal, and talar joints; however, involvement of the knees, spine, and shoulders may also occur. The deformities of the affected joints frequently occur with little or no pain or even recognition of what is actually taking place. Initially, the lack of proprioceptive protection leads to progressive microfractures and subsequent destruction of the joint. This destruction and associated reactive sclerosis can be so dramatic as to cause concern about osteomyelitis or a septic joint, especially if an ulcer is also present (Figure 51–1).

A. CLINICAL PRESENTATION

Patients usually present with a single, painless, swollen, or deformed joint. Bilateral disease may also occur. Classic radiographic findings reveal subluxations, fractures, exuberant sclerosis as well as osteolysis, and destruction of the joint. Destruction of the joint is typically out of proportion to the pain reported by the patient, owing to the existence of concomitant neuropathy. Degenerative disease affecting certain joints, including the tibiotalar, subtalar, and glenohumeral joints, is quite uncommon in the absence of other precipitating factors. In particular, the combination of unusually exuberant destructive disease in a location not usually affected by degenerative joint disease should raise the suspicion of a Charcot joint.

Table 51–1. Rheumatic manifestations associated with endocrine disorders.

Rheumatic Disorder	Endocrinopathy
Carpal tunnel syndrome	Diabetes
	Hypothyroidism
	Acromegaly
Flexor tenosynovitis	Diabetes
	Hypothyroidism
Chondrocalcinosis/ pseudogout	Diabetes
	Hypothyroidism
	Hyperparathyroidism
	Acromegaly
Osteopenia/osteoporosis	Diabetes
	Hyperthyroidism
	Hyperparathyroidism
	Hypoparathyroidism
Destructive arthropathy	Diabetes
	Hypothyroidism
	Hyperparathyroidism
Premature/unusual osteoarthritis	Chondrocalcinosis
	Charcot arthropathy
	Acromegaly
DISH	Diabetes
Myopathy	Diabetes
	Hypothyroidism
	Hyperthyroidism
	Hyperparathyroidism
	Acromegaly

DISH, diffuse idiopathic skeletal hyperostosis.

Table 51–2. Rheumatic manifestations of diabetes.

Articular
  Charcot arthropathy
  DISH
  Chondrocalcinosis
Bone
  Osteopenia
Soft tissue
  Carpal tunnel
  Flexor tendon nodule
  Dupuytren contracture
  Cheiropathy
  Adhesive capsulitis

DISH, diffuse idiopathic skeletal hyperostosis.

B. Treatment

Unfortunately, the treatment of Charcot joints, particularly those below the knee, remains suboptimal—especially once the destructive process becomes advanced. If caught early, the progress of disease can be somewhat retarded through the institution of various protective measures, including the limitation of weight bearing on the affected joint and the use of specially crafted orthotic supports for the surrounding joint structures.

Diffuse Idiopathic Skeletal Hyperostosis

Diffuse idiopathic skeletal hyperostosis (DISH) is best described as a disorder of excess calcification and bone formation along various tendinous and ligamentous insertion sites. Although seen with some degree of regularity in the general population, this condition is found with a far higher prevalence among patients with diabetes, particularly those with type 2 diabetes mellitus. This condition most commonly affects the spine, although involvement can also occur in extraspinal sites, particularly at ligamentous and tendinous insertions in the pelvis, greater trochanters, patellae, calcaneal bones, and other locations. When affecting the spine, DISH most frequently involves dramatic ossification and calcification of the anterior longitudinal spinous ligament. DISH affects the midthoracic spine most often. Although DISH can coexist with preexisting degenerative joint disease and spondylosis, in its pure form the disorder involves none of the degenerative findings found in osteoarthritis. Despite the presence of large, osteophyte-like projections, patients with DISH are rarely symptomatic. However, in advanced cases, the large bony overgrowths can cause spinal rigidity and impingement of nearby structures and nerves, particularly in the neck leading to dysphagia.

A. Clinical Presentation

As classically and radiographically defined, DISH is diagnosed when three essential criteria are met: (1) flowing calcifications involving at least four contiguous vertebral levels (Figure 51–2), (2) minimal loss of disk space, and (3) no sacroiliitis. Although DISH can be confused with both exuberant degenerative disk disease and ankylosing spondylitis, several features of the disorder distinguish it from both of those conditions. First, patients with DISH do not usually suffer pain, particularly the inflammatory types of symptoms (ie, morning pain and stiffness) characteristic of spondyloarthropathies. Second, unlike degenerative disk disease, patients with pure DISH do not suffer from loss of disk height, end plate sclerosis, or other changes commonly associated with degenerative joint disease. Finally, patients with DISH do not show characteristic changes seen with inflammatory spondyloarthropathies (Table 51–3), in-

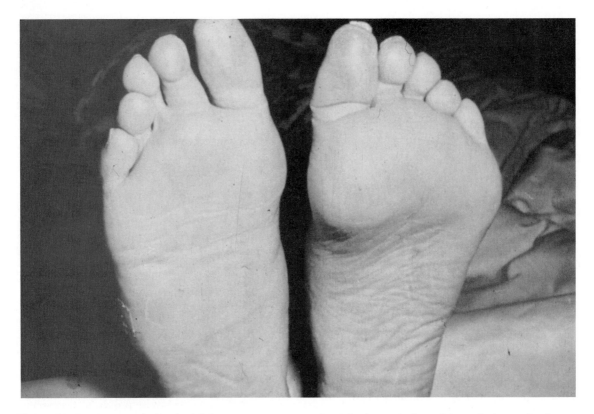

Figure 51–1. Charcot joint. **A:** The left foot in comparison to the right shows the loss of the arch due to the destruction of the first and second metatarsal joints.

cluding the lack of sacroiliac erosions or sclerosis, dactylitis, or other extra-articular features.

B. TREATMENT

The treatment of DISH is symptom-based and generally limited to analgesia as needed. Rarely, surgical removal of impinging bone bridges is undertaken when critical functions, such as swallowing, are compromised.

Osteopenia

Unlike DISH, the predisposition of diabetic patients to the development of osteopenia is not as clearly defined. To the extent that it does exist, osteopenia is thought to affect persons with type 1 diabetes more commonly than those with type 2 diabetes, and it is reported to involve those patients with poorer control of their disease. Most often, the degree of osteopenia in diabetic patients is subclinical, and treatment is based on the standard guidelines for managing patients with reduced bone mineral density. However, in the presence of destructive arthropathies, such as Charcot joints, dramatic osteolysis of the bones of the feet can be observed, with

involvement ranging from areas of patchy osteopenia to those of marked distal bone resorption.

DISORDERS OF THE LIGAMENTS, TENDONS, & SOFT TISSUES

Diabetic patients are susceptible to disorders of soft tissue rheumatism, varying from minor nuisances such as palmar flexor tendon nodules (trigger finger) to major debilitating changes such as adhesive capsulitis (frozen shoulder).

Carpal Tunnel Syndrome

The prevalences of both diabetes and carpal tunnel syndrome are high in Western societies. Even in light of this fact, the frequent coexistence of these disorders has led many to believe that the two are more than circumstantially related. The underlying mechanism by which crowding of the carpal tunnel and compression of the median nerve occur is not well defined, although it is generally accepted that proliferation of fibrous tissue may result in nerve entrapment.

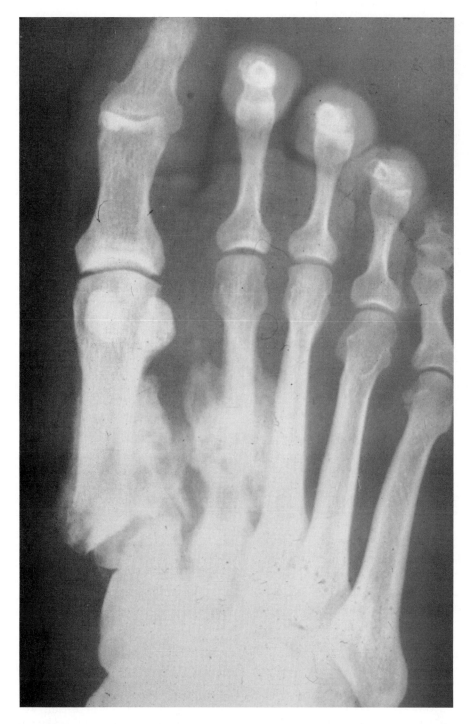

Figure 51–1. (Continued) **B:** Destruction of the first and second metatarsal joints in the foot of a patient with chronic diabetes mellitus and long-standing peripheral neuropathy. (Courtesy of Dr. Carl Grunfeld, San Francisco Department of Veterans Affairs Medical Center, University of California, San Francisco.)

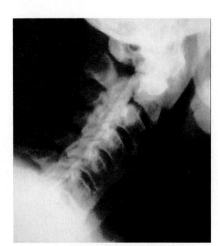

Figure 51–2. Diffuse idiopathic skeletal hyperostosis (DISH).

A. CLINICAL PRESENTATION

Patients with carpal tunnel syndrome frequently complain of numbness or paresthesias in a distribution consistent with denervation of the median nerve. These symptoms are often exacerbated at night and may even awaken a patient from sleep. The disease, if left untreated, can progress from an irritating sensory neuropathy to weakness and wasting of the intrinsic muscles (thenar) of the hand. Provocation of paresthesias in a median nerve distribution by either a Phalen maneuver or Tinel sign can help augment the physical examination. Nerve conduction studies can be used to localize the site of the nerve block and differentiate carpal tunnel syndrome from other types of neuropathy.

Table 51–3. Manifestations of endocrine disorders that can mimic other diseases.

Manifestation	Confused with
DISH	Ankylosing spondylitis
Cheiropathy	Scleroderma
Proximal myopathy	Polymyositis
Thyroid acropachy/ periosteitis/soft tissue swelling	Hypertrophic osteoarthropathy Inflammatory synovitis Scleredema
Charcot arthropathy	Osteomyelitis
Autoantobodies (RF, ANA, etc)	Other rheumatic diseases

DISH, diffuse idiopathic skeletal hyperostosis; RF, rheumatoid factor; ANA, antinuclear antibody.

B. TREATMENT

Initial treatment focuses on conservative measures. Patients are asked to wear wrist splints, particularly at night, and refrain from various activities that may exacerbate the condition. However, if symptoms persist or worsen, local glucocorticoid injection into the carpal tunnel itself or even surgical decompression can be used to treat the condition.

Flexor Tenosynovitis

Another common soft tissue ailment encountered in diabetic patients involves a flexor tenosynovitis of the hand. This condition may involve as many as 12–15% of patients with diabetes. Early in the course of this condition, patients may present with an isolated nodule on one of the flexor tendons of the hand, most commonly on the third or fourth finger. These nodules become symptomatic when they grow large enough to catch neighboring tendons as the finger is flexed, creating a symptom of locking or popping in that finger. The nodules can usually be palpated just distal to the palmar crease of the affected finger. Some patients may benefit from local glucocorticoid injections into the tendon sheath that are intended to shrink the size of the nodule. Those patients who remain symptomatic usually find relief through surgical intervention.

Chronic tenosynovitis of these flexor tendons can eventually progress to fibrosis and contracture. These Dupuytren contractures most commonly involve the fourth finger, resulting in significant disability as the affected fingers become locked in flexion. The fibrotic tendon can usually be palpated as it courses through the palm proximal to the palmar crease. Unlike flexor tendon nodules, glucocorticoid injection provides little sustained relief.

Diabetic Cheiropathy

A. CLINICAL PRESENTATION

An intriguing complication of long-standing hyperglycemia and fibrous tissue proliferation is the syndrome of limited joint mobility. Although most frequently recognized and encountered in the hands, this condition can involve joints as diverse as the shoulders, knees, and feet. Unlike Dupuytren contractures, the limited mobility encountered in this condition involves a more generalized palmar fasciitis with progressive thickening and tightening of the skin, not solely of the tendons themselves. In many instances, the skin becomes progressively puffy, shiny, and waxy in appearance, often mimicking the hands of patients with scleroderma and sclerodactyly (Table 51–3).

A simple diagnostic maneuver, referred to as the **prayer sign,** involves having the patient place his or her hands together, as if in prayer. Patients with limited mobility syndrome are unable to maintain complete contact between the palmar surfaces of their fingers.

B. TREATMENT

Improved glycemic control as well as physical and occupational therapy may help slow the progression of diabetic cheiropathy.

Adhesive Capsulitis of the Shoulder

Adhesive capsulitis, commonly referred to as "frozen shoulder," is encountered in both diabetic patients and the general population. As many as 12% of patients with diabetes may suffer this complication. Afflicted patients can suffer from a fairly rapid and significant loss of the range of motion of the shoulder. Some patients present with calcific tendinitis, peritendinitis, or bursitis of the affected shoulder, conditions that (presumably) predispose them to the development of frozen shoulder. Plain radiographs reveal few abnormalities of the glenohumeral joint, despite the degree of immobility. Early and aggressive physical therapy must be used to preserve range of motion and minimize the time in which the joint is immobile.

■ HYPERTHYROIDISM

Hyperthyroidism is associated with many classic symptoms (eg, proptosis, pretibial myxedema) that may alert physicians to the underlying diagnosis. However, conditions associated with hyperthyroidism may also present in more subtle fashions. Musculoskeletal complaints comprise a significant proportion of these symptoms, ranging from nonspecific fatigue, arthralgias, and myalgias to more florid syndromes such as thyroid acropachy (Table 51–4).

Table 51–4. Rheumatic manifestations of hyperthyroidism.

Articular
Arthralgias
Periarthritis
Thyroid acropachy
Bone
Osteopenia/osteoporosis
Muscular
Proximal myopathy

DISORDERS OF MUSCLE

Hyperthyroidism can cause a generalized musculoskeletal pain syndrome. Patients may experience fatigue, proximal muscle weakness, and joint pains that frequently involve the shoulders. The spectrum of muscular involvement can vary greatly, ranging from minor aches and pains to a profound and usually painless proximal myopathy that resembles polymyositis.

With milder muscular involvement, the patient may complain of weakness or easy fatigability but generally demonstrates minimal atrophy on physical examination. In its most extreme presentation, the myopathy can cause debilitating proximal muscle weakness with marked muscle wasting. However, hyperthyroid-induced myopathy, unlike inflammatory myopathies, causes minimal elevations of muscle enzymes. This form of myopathy usually responds to restoration of the euthyroid state.

DISORDERS OF THE BONES & JOINTS

Hyperthyroidism is frequently associated with arthralgias. For reasons that are not clear, one of the more classically involved joints includes the shoulder, where periarthritic conditions have been reported. In both overt and subclinical hyperthyroid states, increased bone turnover and reductions in bone mineral density progressing to osteopenia and frank osteoporosis are observed. Subclinical hyperthyroidism is regarded as a potentially treatable risk factor for development of osteoporosis, one that is screened for in patients with reductions in bone mineral density. As with other rheumatic features of hyperthyroidism, most bone and joint manifestations are believed to improve with correction of the underlying thyroid disorder.

THYROID ACROPACHY

Thyroid acropachy is an impressive but uncommon complication afflicting patients with Graves disease, particularly those with ophthalmic involvement and pretibial myxedema. Patients with thyroid acropachy demonstrate distal soft tissue swelling, clubbing, and periostitis, commonly of the metacarpal bones (Figure 51–3). The pathophysiologic basis of these findings, while not completely understood, is thought to be due to effects of circulating thyroid-stimulating immunoglobulin, the autoantibody responsible for many of the pathologic abnormalities observed in Graves disease. The symptoms of thyroid acropachy may continue into the euthyroid state or even present at this time because of the persistence of thyroid-stimulating immunoglobulin. However, in some cases, removal of the target antigen via thyroid ablation may diminish the levels of the circulating, offending antibody. Occasionally, treatment with nonsteroidal anti-inflammatory medications or even glucocorticoids can be used to help treat musculoskeletal symptoms associated with this disorder.

■ HYPOTHYROIDISM

General Considerations

One of the most common causes of hypothyroidism is an immune-mediated inflammatory destruction of the gland. This autoimmune process, although centered against the thyroid gland, frequently involves other organs as well. As a result, autoimmune thyroiditis can frequently mimic several common rheumatic diseases. Moreover, many rheumatic diseases, from rheumatoid arthritis and Sjögren syndrome to systemic lupus erythematosus, can coexist with thyroid disease, complicating the underlying diagnosis. Finally, the metabolic disturbances created by an underfunctioning thyroid can cause their own unique spectrum of rheumatic complaints. The diverse nature of rheumatic manifestations associated with hypothyroidism is shown in Table 51–5.

Hashimoto Thyroiditis

Hashimoto thyroiditis, also known as autoimmune or chronic lymphocytic thyroiditis, is the most common cause of hypothyroidism in the United States. Patients with autoimmune thyroid disease frequently complain of concomitant rheumatic symptoms. However, identifying patients with autoimmune thyroiditis and rheumatic complaints is rarely straightforward because many patients, depending on the stage of their disease, may not suffer from thyroid hormone deficiency.

Table 51–5. Rheumatic manifestations of hypothyroidism.

Articular
   Inflammatory synovitis associated with thyroiditis
   Noninflammatory joint effusions
   Arthralgias
   Fibromyalgia
   Chondrocalcinosis
   Erosive osteoarthritis
   Charcot-type arthropathy
Bone
   Avascular necrosis
   Epiphyseal dysplasia
Muscular
   Myopathy
Soft tissue
   Carpal tunnel syndrome
   Flexor tenosynovitis

The articular manifestations of autoimmune thyroiditis can vary in severity from nonspecific arthralgias and fibromyalgia-type complaints to overt synovitis. The synovitis associated with thyroiditis is nonerosive. The pattern of joint involvement is classically a small-joint, symmetric, polyarticular process; however, larger-joint oligoarthropathies are also frequently encountered.

Depending on the stage of disease, patients with Hashimoto thyroiditis may be clinically and serologically hyperthyroid, hypothyroid, or euthyroid while suffering from articular complications. Usually, these patients are antithyroid antibody positive (including antibodies directed against the antigen, thyroperoxidase) and are also antinuclear antibody positive. Interestingly, when patients with various rheumatic complaints who are antinuclear antibody positive were examined, approximately one-sixth were found to have antithyroperoxidase antibodies, indolent chronic lymphocytic thyroiditis, and no other eventual diagnosis. Unfortunately, thyroid replacement alone is often not enough to treat the rheumatic symptoms of these patients, and other medications such as nonsteroidal anti-inflammatory drugs, antimalarials, glucocorticoids, methotrexate, and other antirheumatic therapies must be used.

A. Other Rheumatic Diseases

Hashimoto thyroiditis has long been recognized as an associated complication of well-defined rheumatic diseases. Ten percent to 15% of patients with rheumatoid arthritis, for example, suffer from autoimmune thyroid disease. In addition, there is an association between hypothyroidism and specific HLA alleles, particularly HLA-DR3 and HLA-B8. As previously mentioned, autoimmune thyroid disease is also commonly seen in persons with Sjögren syndrome and SLE; interestingly, several case series have demonstrated a high prevalence of antithyroid antibodies and thyroid disease in family members who are otherwise apparently unaffected by autoimmunity.

B. Complications of Diminished Thyroid Function

1. Bones and joints—As with other manifestations of thyroid disease, the osseous and articular manifestations of hypothyroidism are broad. In general, patients with hypothyroidism can suffer from a generalized musculoskeletal pain syndrome resembling fibromyalgia. Frank myxedematous arthropathy can also exist, classically involving the larger, peripheral joints including the knees. However, case series examining such patients also reveal frequent involvement of the hands and wrists, with many cases demonstrating bilateral disease. Involvement of the elbows and metacarpophalangeal joints as well as flexor tenosynovitis of the hands have also been reported. Joint effusions are quite common and are characterized by generous quantities of viscous, noninflammatory synovial fluid. In many instances, calcium pyrophosphate crystals and chondrocalcinosis can be identified in the joints of patients with hypothyroidism, although the exact nature of the relationship between calcium pyrophosphate deposition disease, pseudogout, and hypothyroidism is not entirely understood.

Many studies suggest more than a casual relationship between the development of osteonecrosis and hypothyroidism, with a peculiar predilection of this occurrence for the tibial plateau. However, avascular necrosis has been reported to involve bones ranging in size from the femoral heads to the carpal lunate bones. Other reported bony abnormalities in hypothyroid patients include a Charcot-like destructive process and epiphyseal dysplasia. Correction of the underlying thyroid abnormality has been shown to be helpful in resolving many of these symptoms, although transition to a euthyroid state can be associated with nonspecific musculoskeletal complaints.

2. Muscular symptoms—Patients who are hypothyroid frequently suffer associated muscular symptoms. These include a myopathy that can vary dramatically in its clinical presentation. In actuality, elevations of muscle enzymes are very common in hypothyroid patients, with most demonstrating mild elevations in creatine kinase but few showing any clinical weakness. However, profound muscular pain and weakness can occur in other patients. In contrast to the myopathy of hyperthyroidism, elevations in creatine kinase can be dramatic in these cases.

3. Soft tissue manifestations—In thyroid hormone–deficient states, both the diminished T3 and T4 levels and the elevated levels of thyroid-stimulating hormone are involved in the deposition of mucopolysaccharides in connective tissue. This process may explain many of the soft tissue manifestations of hypothyroidism. Carpal tunnel syndrome is encountered regularly. In fact, patients with bilateral carpal tunnel syndrome, particularly those with no other known risk factors, should be tested for thyroid dysfunction. Flexor tenosynovitis of the hand and generalized sensory neuropathy, both associated with hypothyroidism, can mimic this diagnosis as well.

■ HYPERPARATHYROIDISM

Overproduction of parathyroid hormone is frequently encountered in medical practice. Primary hyperparathyroidism, the most common cause of asymptomatic hypercalcemia, is usually a result of an autonomously functioning parathyroid adenoma. Chronic renal insufficiency induces secondary and, on occasion, even tertiary parathyroid gland hyperplasia and hormone oversecretion. Both primary and secondary hyperparathyroidism are commonly complicated by rheumatic complaints affecting bones, muscles, and joints.

DISORDERS OF BONE & JOINTS

Primary hyperparathyroidism is one of the most frequently cited precipitants of acute and chronic chondrocalcinosis and pseudogout. Discovery of chondrocalcinosis, particularly in an individual not believed to be at risk, should prompt a metabolic evaluation, including a determination of serum calcium. Patients with hyperparathyroidism often complain of nonspecific bone and joint pains. These complaints can often be confused with other causes of arthritis, especially when erosive disease is detected on radiographic examination.

The pathogenesis of this erosive arthritis, in contrast to other arthritides, is primarily related to parathyroid hormone's effect on bone resorption. Thus, the bony erosions may occur anywhere, including the interphalangeal, metacarpophalangeal, carpal, and acromioclavicular joints. Moreover, bone resorption is not limited to the joints. Excess parathyroid hormone can precipitate osteoporosis, pathologic fractures, subperiosteal bone resorption, and osteolysis. In advanced stages, these processes, if undetected, can result in osteitis fibrosa cystica (Figure 51–4).

MUSCULAR COMPLICATIONS

Fatigue, muscular pain, and weakness are complaints frequently encountered in hyperparathyroid patients. Specifically, patients may complain of proximal muscle weakness, with a curious predilection for the lower extremities, and little or no elevation of muscle enzymes. Advanced renal disease and associated secondary hyperparathyroidism can lead to metastatic calcification of soft tissues and muscles, a process which, by itself or through the induction of inflammation, can produce various degrees of muscular symptoms. Calciphylaxis, usually accompanying end-stage renal failure and severe secondary hyperparathyroidism, can result in diffuse calcification of skin and subcutaneous and other soft tissues. Although not usually a subtle diagnosis, the resulting painful skin erythema and ulcerations, vascular thromboses, and digital infarctions can resemble vasculitis.

A. CLINICAL PRESENTATION

The discovery of chondrocalcinosis or pseudogout, particularly in a person not originally believed to be predisposed, should prompt an evaluation for hyperparathyroidism. Commonly, serum calcium levels are elevated

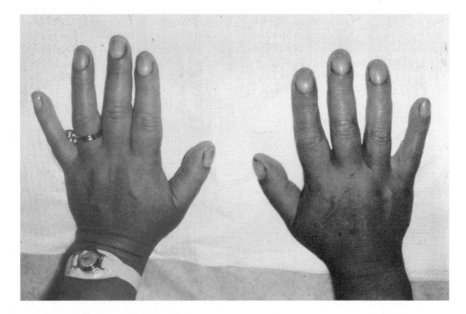

Figure 51–3. Thyroid acropachy. Hand of patient with Graves hyperthyroidism. Note swelling of digits and marked clubbing.

and phosphorous levels are depressed, while parathyroid hormone levels are inappropriately high for the level of hypercalcemia. Excessive urinary calcium excretion can help confirm this diagnosis as well. Patients with pseudogout may demonstrate calcification of articular cartilage. Radiographs from other patients with arthralgias may reveal subperiosteal, erosive, or osteolytic changes in their joints and metacarpal bones. Patients with long-bone pain may demonstrate cystic areas of demineralization (referred to as "brown tumors") or evidence of pathologic fractures. Radiographs from patients with back pain might reveal vertebral compression fractures, while those from patients with osteitis fibrosa cystica may demonstrate intense sclerosis of the vertebral endplates alternating with marked osteopenia of the vertebral bodies, a finding referred to as a "rugger jersey spine."

B. Treatment

Treatment of symptomatic primary hyperparathyroidism is usually accomplished by removing the hyperfunctioning adenomatous tissue. Most of the rheumatic symptoms associated with hyperparathyroidism improve with normalization of parathyroid hormone levels, although further therapy may be required to correct significant underlying osteoporosis.

Secondary hyperparathyroidism is a well-recognized and treatable complication of end-stage renal disease. As a result of effective vitamin D supplementation, phosphorus chelation, and dialysis, complications such as osteitis fibrosa cystica are rare.

■ HYPOPARATHYROIDISM

Hypoparathyroidism with resulting hypocalcemia is usually encountered in the context of surgical damage to or removal of the parathyroid glands; however, immune-mediated or ischemic destruction may also occur.

Muscle fatigue and weakness frequently parallel the degree of hypocalcemia. Neuromuscular irritability and tetany can result from severely low levels of calcium. Interestingly, patients sometimes demonstrate ectopic soft tissue and basal ganglia calcifications. Rarely, this process can cause calcification of the paraspinous ligaments and result in a restrictive process resembling a spondyloarthropathy.

Pseudohypoparathyroidism, caused by a tissue insensitivity to parathyroid hormone, is a disorder that also results in diminished serum calcium levels but with appropriately high serum levels of parathyroid hormone. Pseudohypoparathyroidism can be associated with distinct skeletal deformities, particularly shortening of the fourth metacarpals bilaterally (Figure 51–5). Examination of the clenched fist reveals a characteristic depression where the knuckle of the fourth metacarpal should be located.

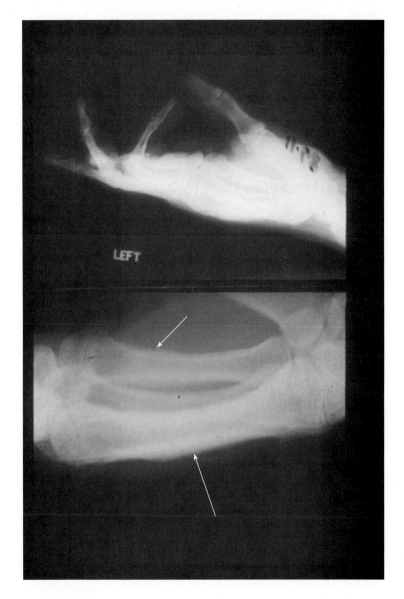

Figure 51–4. Arrows indicate periosteal reaction and periostitis. (Courtesy of Dr. Francis Greenspan, University of California, San Francisco.)

■ ACROMEGALY

Pituitary adenomas that cause excess secretion of growth hormone can be responsible for many bone and soft tissue abnormalities. In particular, the anabolic effects of excess growth hormone can cause a marked proliferation of bone, cartilage, synovium, and other soft tissues. As a result, rheumatic complaints are quite common in this condition, frequently predating the actual recognition and diagnosis of the underlying disorder. The pro-

gression of disease may be quite insidious in nature, and therefore attention to some of the finer details of these rheumatic complaints may help uncover the diagnosis before advanced disease becomes evident.

BONE & JOINT MANIFESTATIONS

Many patients with acromegaly complain of pain in various joints associated with progressive degenerative changes. This process can be both monarticular and polyarticular, affecting a large variety of joints. Early in the course of disease, cartilage overgrowth can lead to

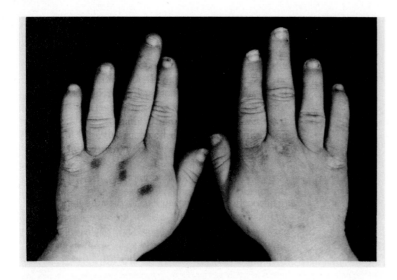

Figure 51–5. Pseudohypoparathyroidism. Shortening of the fourth and fifth metacarpals (brachydactyl) in two patients. (Courtesy of Dr. Michael Levine, The Cleveland Clinic.)

joint space widening, but this overgrowth commonly involves haphazard deposition of matrix, resulting in its fissuring and degeneration. In addition, overgrowth and hypertrophy of joint capsules can encourage progressive ligamentous laxity and hypermobility. As a result, premature osteoarthritis can ensue, particularly involving the weight-bearing joints, and invariably results in marked joint space narrowing and osteophytosis characteristic of all forms of exuberant degenerative joint disease.

Another common complaint of patients with acromegaly is back pain, which affects as many as 50%. The pattern of spinal involvement, not surprisingly, resembles that of the peripheral joints, with patients noted to have widened disk spaces, large osteophytes, and ligamentous laxity of the spine. In addition, acromegaly has been implicated in precipitating calcium pyrophosphate dihydrate deposition disease, a process that can further exacerbate any ongoing degenerative changes.

NEUROMUSCULAR INVOLVEMENT

Acromegalic patients often will manifest coarsely enlarged fingers and hands characteristic of the soft tissue, bone, and fibrous proliferation associated with excess growth hormone secretion. As a result of this tissue overgrowth, crowding of the carpal tunnel and resultant carpal tunnel syndrome can occur. This condition can often be bilateral and serve as an initial clue to the underlying diagnosis. Other neuropathies may result from the degenerative and hypermobile changes encountered in the spine, and bony overgrowth can occasionally impinge on the spinal canal. A painless, proximal myopathy has also been reported in patients with

acromegaly. Serum muscle enzyme levels are usually normal in this disorder.

A. CLINICAL PRESENTATION

Acromegaly should be suspected when precocious degenerative joint disease presents in patients. Particular attention should be paid to those patients who demonstrate excessive hypermobility or laxity of their joints or spine, a finding that would appear to be in contradiction to the degree of degenerative disease encountered. Often, a carefully taken history will reveal insidious increases in hat, glove, ring, or shoe sizes in the affected patient. Physical examination might also reveal the presence of a prognathic jaw, coarsened facial features, and increased, thickened fleshy soft tissue of the fingers and hands. Early in disease, radiographic evaluation demonstrates increased soft tissue of the hands, joint space widening, and spade-like deformities of the distal phalangeal tufts. Later, the changes observed radiologically resemble those seen in most forms of advanced osteoarthritis. The diagnosis of acromegaly can be confirmed by the serum measurement of insulin-like growth factor-1, which is usually elevated in patients with acromegaly. If these results are equivocal, serum growth hormone concentration can be measured dynamically after an oral glucose challenge.

B. TREATMENT

If treated early enough, most of the rheumatic manifestations of acromegaly will respond to removal of the pituitary adenoma or pharmacologic suppression of growth hormone secretion. However, once advanced degenerative changes have taken place, symptomatic relief is usually provided through conservative measures, including nonsteroidal anti-inflammatory medications.

Severe disease may be amenable to surgical correction once the underlying metabolic abnormality has been successfully corrected.

REFERENCES

Cagliero E, et al. Musculoskeletal disorders of the hand and shoulder in patients with diabetes mellitus. *Am J Med.* 2002;112: 487. [PMID: 11959060] (Recent study looking at hand and shoulder complications in diabetic patients and controls.)

Kloppenburg M, et al. Effect of therapy for thyroid dysfunction on musculoskeletal symptoms. *Clin Rheumatol.* 1993;12:341. [PMID: 8258232]

Lacks S, Jacobs RP. Acromegalic arthropathy: a reversible rheumatic disease. *J Rheumatol.* 1986;13:634. [PMID: 2942687] (Case report and general review.)

Lockshin M. Endocrine origins of rheumatic disease. Diagnostic clues to interrelated syndromes. *Postgrad Med.* 2002;111:87. [PMID: 11985136] (Overview for primary care clinicians.)

McGuire JL. The endocrine system and connective tissue disorders. *Bull Rheum Dis.* 1990;39:1. [PMID: 268759] (A somewhat dated, but more detailed review of the subject published by the Arthritis Foundation.)

McLean RM, Podell DN. Bone and joint manifestations of hypothyroidism. *Semin Arthritis Rheum.* 1995;24:282. [PMID: 7740308] (Case report and good general review.)

Punzi L, et al. Clinical, laboratory, and immunogenetic aspects of arthritis associated with chronic lymphocytic thyroiditis. *Clin Exp Rheumatol.* 1997;15:373. [PMID: 9272297]

Ramos-Remus C, et al. Endocrine disorders and musculoskeletal diseases. *Curr Opin Rheumatol.* 1996;8:77. [PMID: 8867544] (More of an update in selected aspects than a generalized review.)

Rheumatic Manifestations of Malignancy

52

Fiona A. Donald, MD, FRCP(C)

GENERAL CONSIDERATIONS

Rarely, tumor-like lesions, benign tumors, and malignancy involve joints directly, usually producing a monoarthritis. More commonly, paraneoplastic syndromes can have rheumatic manifestations. Certain paraneoplastic syndromes have clinical presentations that are distinctive and, therefore, warrant investigation of an underlying malignancy when recognized. Other paraneoplastic syndromes can mimic idiopathic rheumatic diseases, such as rheumatoid arthritis, and can be a source of diagnostic error.

MONOARTHRITIS DUE TO BENIGN TUMORS & TUMOR-LIKE LESIONS

ESSENTIALS OF DIAGNOSIS

- *Pain, swelling, limited motion of the affected joint.*
- *Bloody synovial fluid.*
- *Eccentric mass in or near the joint.*
- *Characteristic histologic findings.*

Benign tumors and tumor-like lesions such as synovial chondromatosis, pigmented villonodular synovitis (PVNS), and synovial hemangiomas are rare causes of monoarthritis. These disorders typically involve large joints, especially the knee, and present with chronic pain, swelling, and limited range of motion. Giant cell tumors of tendon sheaths present as painless finger nodules that can mimic ganglia.

PVNS and synovial hemangiomas produce bloody synovial effusions. Radiographs reveal numerous calcified loose bodies in cases of synovial chondromatosis. For other conditions, magnetic resonance imaging (MRI) is the imaging procedure of choice and may help guide the surgical approach, but definitive diagnosis requires histologic examination of involved tissue. The treatment for most conditions is surgical excision.

MONOARTHRITIS DUE TO MALIGNANCY

ESSENTIALS OF DIAGNOSIS

- *Pain, swelling, limited motion of the affected joint.*
- *Rapidly growing, eccentric mass in or near the joint.*
- *Characteristic histologic findings.*

Synovial sarcomas are malignant intra-articular tumors. Secondary tumors of the synovium may result from the contiguous spread of malignant bone tumors or by direct invasion from carcinoma, leukemia, or lymphoma. Leukemic infiltration of synovium also can produce an oligoarthritis or a polyarthritis.

Synovial sarcomas typically present as a rapidly growing mass in association with tendon, tendon sheath, or joint capsule in the extremities. MRI helps reveal the extent of the lesion. Treatment consists of wide surgical excision; 5-year survival rates range from 25% to 60%.

PARANEOPLASTIC SYNDROMES

The palmar fasciitis-polyarthritis syndrome, remitting seronegative symmetric synovitis with pitting edema (RS3PE), hypertrophic pulmonary osteoarthropathy, panniculitis-arthritis syndrome, and the inflammatory myopathies have known associations with malignancy. The appearance of these clinical conditions should prompt a search for an underlying cancer.

PALMAR FASCIITIS-POLYARTHRITIS SYNDROME

The development of polyarthritis (usually of the metacarpophalangeal and proximal interphalangeal joints) and rapid progression of palmar fasciitis with flexion contractures of the hands is clearly linked with ovarian cancer but also has been described in patients with gastric, lung, colon, and pancreatic cancer. The syndrome is refractory to treatment, and the prognosis is poor.

REMITTING SERONEGATIVE SYMMETRIC SYNOVITIS WITH PITTING EDEMA

RS3PE is characterized by the presence of a symmetric synovitis of the small joints of the hands in association with pitting edema of the hands and feet. Serum rheumatoid factor is negative. Treatment with low-dose systemic glucocorticoids is usually effective. Although there are idiopathic forms of the syndrome, RS3PE can herald the development of hematologic malignancies or a variety of solid tumors. Treatment of the underlying neoplasm with surgery or chemotherapy can lead to resolution of RS3PE.

HYPERTROPHIC PULMONARY OSTEOARTHROPATHY

Hypertrophic pulmonary osteoarthropathy (HPO) is a syndrome characterized by polyarthritis associated with clubbing of the fingers and periostosis of the long bones. The syndrome may exist in a primary form or in a secondary form associated with infectious diseases or malignancy. Rapidly progressive symptoms characterize paraneoplastic HPO; pain in the long bones of the legs is common. HPO is associated most commonly with intrathoracic malignancies (eg, adenocarcinoma of the lung, mesotheliomas, lymphomas) but has also been described in association with other cancers. Treatment of the underlying neoplasm often leads to remission of the syndrome.

PANNICULITIS-ARTHRITIS SYNDROME

Patients with pancreatitis or with pancreatic cancer can present with the combination of arthritis and panniculitis. The arthritis is inflammatory and ranges from a monoarthritis to a polyarthritis. The panniculitis begins as tender red subcutaneous nodules, usually on the lower extremities, that initially mimic erythema nodosum but that later liquify and may drain a yellowish material. Release of pancreatic lipase likely plays a role in the pathogenesis of the syndrome.

DERMATOMYOSITIS & POLYMYOSITIS (see Chapter 25)

Compared with the general population, the incidence ratio of malignancy has been reported to be as high as 6.2 for dermatomyositis and 2.4 for polymyositis at the time of diagnosis. Although the incidence of malignancy appears to be highest at the time of diagnosis, an

increased risk of malignancy may be present for 2–5 years postdiagnosis. A number of clinical features correlate with the presence of malignancy in association with inflammatory myositis. These include older age, fever, substantial weight loss (greater than 5%), and rapid onset of disease (defined as diagnosis within 2 months of symptoms). Dermatomyositis with cutaneous necrosis of the trunk is also associated with malignancy.

Although the distribution of malignancies seen with the inflammatory myopathies is similar to the general population, there are several specific associations with dermatomyositis and polymyositis. Cancer of the ovaries, lungs, and the gastrointestinal tract is reported most frequently in association with dermatomyositis. Non-Hodgkin lymphoma and cancer of the lung as well as bladder cancer are frequently described in patients with polymyositis. Asian patients with inflammatory myositis have a high incidence of nasopharyngeal cancer.

At a minimum, age-appropriate cancer screening is indicated for patients with dermatomyositis and polymyositis. Although no guidelines exist, some clinicians advocate additional screening, at least in certain circumstances. For example, pelvic ultrasonography and CA-125 are warranted in women with dermatomyositis, given the high incidence of ovarian cancer. Because the risk of ovarian cancer may be elevated for up to 5 years, some experts argue that screening should continue annually during this time.

MIMICKERS OF IDIOPATHIC RHEUMATIC DISEASES

Table 52–1 lists paraneoplastic syndromes that can mimic rheumatic syndromes.

Cancer-Associated Polyarthritis

 ESSENTIAL FEATURES

- *May precede or follow the diagnosis of malignancy.*
- *Asymmetric oligoarthritis or polyarthritis, often in the elderly and with abrupt onset.*
- *Frequent sparing of the wrists and hands.*
- *Usually rheumatoid factor negative.*

Cancer-associated polyarthritis is an uncommon paraneoplastic syndrome reported in association with carcinoma of the breast, carcinoma of the lung, and other solid tumors. There is a close temporal relationship be-

Table 52–1. Paraneoplastic syndromes
mimicking rheumatic disease.

Syndrome	Malignancy
Cancer-associated polyarthritis	Solid tumors
Jaccoud-like arthropathy	Carcinoma of the lung
Lupus-like syndromes	Thymoma; Hodgkin disease; carcinoma of the lung, breast, ovary
Small-vessel vasculitis	Myeloproliferative, lymphoproliferative disorders
Medium-vessel vasculitis	Hairy cell leukemia
Severe Raynaud phenomenon and digital necrosis	Various
Erythromelalgia	Myeloproliferative disorders
Reflex sympathetic dystrophy	Various
Erythema nodosum	Lymphoproliferative disorders
Scleroderma-like skin changes	Carcinoma of the stomach, lung, breast; melanoma; myeloma
POEMS syndrome[a]	Plasma cell dyscrasia

[a]POEMS syndrome is suggestive of scleroderma and is an
acronym for polyneuropathy, organomegaly, endocrinopathy,
monoclonal protein, and skin changes.

tween the development of the arthritis and detection of
malignancy (usually within 12 months). Characteristic
features of cancer-associated polyarthritis include the
abrupt onset of an asymmetric arthritis in an elderly patient (age greater than 65). The arthritis often involves
the lower extremities with sparing of the small joints of
the hands and wrists. Rheumatoid nodules are absent.
Less commonly cancer-associated arthritis presents as a
symmetric polyarthritis similar in appearance to rheumatoid arthritis. Serum rheumatoid factor is usually absent, and radiographs do not reveal erosions. Typically,
cancer-associated polyarthritis responds poorly to nonsteroidal anti-inflammatory drugs. Treatment of the underlying malignancy often results in resolution of the
arthritis.

REFERENCES

Fam AG. Paraneoplastic rheumatic syndromes. *Baillieres Best Pract Res Clin Rheumatol.* 2000;14:515. [PMID: 10985984]

Naschitz JE, et al. Rheumatic syndromes: clues to occult neoplasia. *Semin Arthritis Rheum.* 1999;29:43. [PMID: 10468414] (A thorough review of rheumatic associations and malignancy.)

Szendroi M, Deodhar A. Synovial neoformations and tumours. *Best Pract Res Clin Rheumatol.* 2000;14:363. [PMID: 10925750] (An excellent review of tumors that involve joints, tendon sheaths, and bursae.)

Amyloidosis

53

Paul S. Mueller, MD, MPH

Amyloidosis is a term used to describe a heterogeneous group of diseases caused by the extracellular deposition of insoluble fibrillar proteins in tissues and organs. These protein deposits derive from diverse and unrelated serum precursor proteins, yet share a beta-pleated sheet structural conformation. Furthermore, all forms of amyloid display apple green birefringence when stained with Congo red and viewed under polarized light. Indeed, this observation (via tissue biopsy) remains the gold standard for establishing the diagnosis of amyloidosis. Accumulation of amyloid deposits leads to tissue and organ dysfunction, which in turn causes clinical symptoms and, for some patients, death.

Amyloid diseases are classified by the biochemical composition of the serum precursor proteins that form the amyloid fibrils and deposits. To date, nearly 20 amyloid fibril precursor proteins and their associated diseases have been identified. Of these, the most common forms of amyloidosis are (1) primary or immunoglobulin light-chain protein-related (AL) amyloidosis, (2) secondary (AA) amyloidosis associated with chronic inflammatory disease, (3) dialysis-associated beta$_2$-microglobulin (β_2-m) amyloidosis, and (4) hereditary amyloidosis. The clinical manifestations of these forms of amyloidosis overlap but are not identical (Table 53–1).

AL AMYLOIDOSIS

ESSENTIALS OF DIAGNOSIS

- *AL amyloidosis should be suspected in all patients with unexplained heart failure, nephrotic syndrome, neuropathy, and hepatomegaly.*
- *Approximately 90% of patients with AL amyloidosis have detectable serum or urine monoclonal immunoglobulin light-chain protein.*
- *AL amyloid, like all forms of amyloid, displays apple green birefringence when viewed under polarized light after staining with Congo red.*
- *Bone marrow examination usually reveals a monoclonal population of plasma cells.*

- *In uncertain cases, immunohistochemical staining and other testing may be necessary to identify the light-chain origin of AL amyloid fibrils.*

General Considerations

AL amyloidosis is a plasma cell dyscrasia associated with multisystem involvement, rapid progression, and short survival. It is a rare disease with an incidence of 8 cases per 1 million persons per year. It usually affects people older than 40 years and men (65%) more than women. A monoclonal population of plasma cells in the bone marrow produces amyloidogenic immunoglobulin light-chain protein (λ more often than κ). Notably, only 10–15% of patients with multiple myeloma have AL amyloidosis, and it is unusual for multiple myeloma to develop in patients with AL amyloidosis. AL amyloidosis affects most organs and the vascular system.

Clinical Findings

A. SYMPTOMS AND SIGNS

The symptoms and signs of AL amyloidosis are nonspecific. For example, the most common symptoms are fatigue and involuntary weight loss. Other symptoms and signs of AL amyloidosis reflect the organs and tissues involved. Hence, clinicians should suspect AL amyloidosis when seeing patients with syndromes associated with the disease. The syndromes associated most commonly with AL amyloidosis are nephrotic syndrome, congestive heart failure, idiopathic peripheral neuropathy, hepatomegaly, and carpal tunnel syndrome (CTS).

One-third to one-half of patients with AL amyloidosis have symptoms related to kidney involvement. Nephrotic syndrome with hypoalbuminemia and edema is the most frequent initial manifestation of kidney involvement. Symptomatic cardiac involvement affects up to 40% of patients with AL amyloidosis. Amyloid involvement of the myocardium, intramural coronary arteries, and conduction system may cause congestive heart failure, ischemic syndromes (eg, angina, myocardial infarction), and rhythm disturbances. Nearly 20% of patients with AL amyloidosis have neuropathy. Lower extremity paresthesias usually present in these patients. Pain and temperature senses are lost before light touch

Table 53–1. Organ systems commonly involved clinically by various forms of amyloidosis.

Organ System	Primary (AL) Amyloidosis	Secondary (AA) Amyloidosis	Dialysis-Associated Beta$_2$-Microglobulin (β_2-m) Amyloidosis	Hereditary Amyloidosis[a]
Heart	X			X
Kidney	X	X		X
Vascular	X			
Peripheral nerves	X			X
Autonomic nerves	X			X
Liver	X			
Gastrointestinal tract	X	X		
Joints	X		X	

[a]Organ involvement varies according to the specific amyloid precursor protein mutation.

and vibratory senses. Motor neuropathy is rare. Patients may also have autonomic neuropathy, the manifestations of which include diarrhea, bladder control problems, impotence, and orthostatic hypotension. One-quarter of patients have hepatomegaly. Clinicians should consider AL amyloidosis in all patients who have nephrotic syndrome and unexplained heart disease, peripheral or autonomic neuropathy, or hepatomegaly.

Rheumatic manifestations develop in many patients with AL amyloidosis. For example, one-quarter of patients have CTS. Sensory abnormalities caused by amyloid neuropathy may lead to neuropathic joint destruction (Charcot joint). Joint disease resembling rheumatoid arthritis (RA) develops in some patients with AL amyloidosis. These patients have bilateral symmetric arthritis of the large and small joints characterized by pain, stiffness, swelling, and palpable nodules. However, unlike patients with RA, those with amyloid arthropathy do not experience fevers, joint tenderness on palpation, or evidence of inflammation on synovial fluid analysis. Patients with muscle involvement (amyloid myopathy) may complain of stiffness, weakness, and enlargement of muscles. Amyloid involvement of joints, muscles, and nerves may also lead to debilitating contractures. Finally, AL amyloidosis may masquerade as giant cell arteritis (GCA). Patients may have symptoms suggestive of GCA (eg, jaw claudication). However, rather than revealing GCA, temporal artery biopsy reveals amyloid involvement of the temporal artery.

Most patients with AL amyloidosis have vascular involvement. For some, this involvement may be symptomatic (eg, angina pectoris, orthostatic hypotension, and purpura). Pathologic enlargement of the tongue (macroglossia), commonly associated with AL amyloidosis, occurs in fewer than 20% of patients.

B. Laboratory Findings

No laboratory findings are pathognomonic of AL amyloidosis. Instead, laboratory abnormalities reflect the organs and tissues involved. For example, renal insufficiency, hypoalbuminemia, hyperlipidemia, and proteinuria suggest kidney involvement. Hematologic abnormalities are relatively uncommon. Amyloid infiltration of the spleen, however, may lead to functional hyposplenism and the finding of Howell-Jolly bodies on the peripheral blood smear.

Immunoelectrophoresis of the serum or urine detects a monoclonal immunoglobulin light-chain protein in 90% of patients with AL amyloidosis. For those who do not have detectable monoclonal light chain in the serum or urine (the "nonsecretory" form of AL amyloidosis), bone marrow examination usually reveals a monoclonal population of plasma cells.

C. Imaging Studies

In general, imaging studies do not reveal findings specific for AL amyloidosis. Some patients with kidney involvement may have enlarged kidneys when viewed by ultrasonography (most have normal-sized kidneys). Echocardiography usually reveals wall thickening (due to amyloid infiltration of the myocardium), evidence of diastolic dysfunction, and a misleadingly normal left ventricular ejection fraction. Reported radiographic findings in patients with AL amyloidosis include osteoporosis, pathologic fractures, osteonecrosis, soft tissue nodules and swelling, subchondral cysts and erosions, joint contractures, and neuropathic osteoarthropathy.

Quantitative scintigraphy with radiolabeled serum amyloid P (SAP) component is useful in determining the extent and total body burden of amyloid deposits in patients with AL amyloidosis. Serial studies reveal uptake of the radiolabeled SAP component that correlates with regression or progression of disease. This test, however, is not widely available.

D. Special Tests

Tissue biopsy is necessary to establish the diagnosis of amyloidosis. All forms of amyloid display apple green birefringence when viewed under polarized light after staining with Congo red. The least invasive method is aspiration of subcutaneous abdominal fat, which reveals amyloid in 70–80% of patients with AL amyloidosis. Bone marrow biopsy (usually done to evaluate a monoclonal protein) reveals amyloid in half of patients. Together, fat aspirate and bone marrow biopsy reveal amyloid in 90% of patients. If analyses of aspirated subcutaneous fat and bone marrow do not reveal amyloid, yet suspicion for amyloidosis remains high, other tissue biopsies must be obtained. One effective approach is to obtain tissue specimens from organs suspected of having amyloid involvement (eg, kidney, heart, liver). The presence of a monoclonal light-chain protein in a patient with biopsy-proven amyloidosis strongly suggests but is not absolutely diagnostic of AL amyloidosis. For example, because monoclonal gammopathies are reasonably common in the general population, the detection of a monoclonal protein in a patient with another form of amyloidosis (eg, hereditary amyloidosis) may be misleading. Some patients with AL amyloidosis do not have a detectable monoclonal protein. For these patients, further testing (eg, immunohistochemical staining, cellular studies with labeled antibodies for light chains) may be necessary to identify the light-chain origin of AL amyloid fibrils.

Treatment

The standard treatment of AL amyloidosis is the combination of melphalan and prednisone. This combination is superior to placebo and colchicine. Compared with placebo, treatment with melphalan and prednisone increases median survival time from 6 months to 12 months. This treatment, however, is less effective if the disease involves the heart or kidneys. High-dose melphalan and autologous blood stem cell support are a promising treatment for AL amyloidosis. In many patients who can tolerate this form of treatment, monoclonal light chains disappear from the serum and urine and the number of bone marrow plasma cells normalizes. Furthermore, the function of organs involved with amyloid may improve (eg, reduced proteinuria). Finally, organ transplantation (eg, heart) has been used successfully to treat organ failure in selected patients with AL amyloidosis. Organ transplantation, however, does not prevent amyloid deposition in other organs or in the transplanted organ.

In addition to treatment directed at the specific form of amyloidosis, most patients with amyloidosis, including those with AL amyloidosis, require supportive treatment (Table 53–2). The aims of supportive treatment are to relieve symptoms caused by amyloid involvement of various organ systems and to prolong survival.

When to Refer to a Specialist

Patients with AL amyloidosis should be referred to a hematologist who has experience managing this uncommon disease. Managing organ failure caused by amyloidosis can be challenging and often requires the assistance of subspecialists (eg, nephrologists, cardiologists). Furthermore, many patients with amyloidosis have daunting psychosocial and spiritual challenges. Under these circumstances, referral to an appropriate allied health colleague (eg, social worker, chaplain) or support group may be helpful.

Prognosis

The prognosis of AL amyloidosis is poor. Overall, the median survival of patients with this disease is 1–2 years. Survival depends on which organs and tissues are involved. Most deaths are attributable to cardiac involvement (congestive heart failure and sudden death). The median survival of patients with AL amyloidosis who have symptomatic cardiac involvement is only 6 months. However, patients with neuropathy but no involvement of the heart or kidney have a median survival of nearly 3 years. Patients with nephropathy but no involvement of the heart have a median survival of 21 months. Treatments, including melphalan and prednisone and organ transplantation, prolong life in selected patients.

AA AMYLOIDOSIS

 ESSENTIALS OF DIAGNOSIS

- *AA amyloidosis should be suspected in all patients with chronic inflammatory conditions in whom renal insufficiency, nephrotic syndrome, gastrointestinal (GI) tract symptoms, or other symptoms and signs of amyloidosis develop.*
- *AA amyloid, like all forms of amyloid, displays apple green birefringence when viewed under polarized light after staining with Congo red.*
- *Immunohistochemical staining identifies serum amyloid A protein from which AA amyloid fibrils derive.*

General Considerations

AA amyloidosis is an uncommon complication of chronic inflammatory diseases, including rheumatic

Table 53–2. Supportive measures for all forms of amyloidosis.

Organ System	Symptom	Treatment
Heart	Congestive failure	Salt restriction
		Diuretics
		ACE inhibitors
		Heart transplantation
		Avoidance of digoxin, calcium channel blockers, and β-blockers
	Heart block	Pacemaker
Kidney	Nephrotic syndrome	Salt restriction
		Elastic stockings
		Adequate dietary protein
		ACE inhibitors
	Kidney failure	Dialysis
		Kidney transplantation
Autonomic neuropathy	Orthostatic hypotension	Salt
		Elastic stocking
		Fludrocortisone
	Gastroparesis	Small, frequent meals low in fat
		Metoclopramide
		Jejunostomy tube
Peripheral neuropathy	Sensory neuropathy	Pain control (eg, amitriptyline, gabapentin)
		Avoidance of trauma
		Proper foot care
	Motor neuropathy	Physical therapy
		Braces, other devices
Gastrointestinal tract	Diarrhea	Psyllium
		Loperamide
		Somatostatin analogues
		Dietary changes
		Total parenteral nutrition
	Macroglossia	Maintenance of airway
Blood	Bruising	Avoidance of trauma
	Factor X deficiency	Factor replacement before surgery and other invasive procedures
	Hyposplenism	Vaccination
		Splenectomy for massive splenomegaly

ACE, angiotensin-converting enzyme.
Modified from Skinner M: Amyloidosis. In: Lichtenstein LM, Fauci AS eds. *Current Therapy in Allergy, Immunology, and Rheumatology,* 5th ed. Mosby, 1996.

conditions, infectious diseases, malignancies, and others. Amyloid fibrils derive from the acute phase reactant serum amyloid A protein. Serum amyloid A protein is made by the liver in response to inflammatory stimuli. Serum levels of this protein, which is involved in chemotaxis, cell adhesion, cytokine production, and other immune processes, often correlate with disease activity in inflammatory diseases. In fact, serum amyloid A protein levels may increase 1000-fold during an inflammatory response. Chronically elevated serum amyloid A protein levels precede AA amyloid fibril formation. Treating the underlying inflammatory disease suppresses the acute phase response, normalizes serum amyloid A protein levels, and prevents the development of AA amyloidosis. Indeed, the incidence of AA amyloidosis in the developed world has fallen in recent decades as a result of effective treatment of chronic infections (eg, tuberculosis) and other inflammatory diseases.

Of the cases of AA amyloidosis seen today, about two-thirds are caused by chronic rheumatic diseases, including RA, familial Mediterranean fever (FMF), psoriatic arthritis, ankylosing spondylitis, reactive arthritis (Reiter syndrome), adult-onset Still disease, juvenile chronic arthritis, systemic lupus erythematosus, Behçet disease, Takayasu arteritis, GCA/polymyalgia rheumatica, and polymyositis. Other chronic inflammatory diseases associated with AA amyloidosis include inflammatory bowel disease, bronchiectasis, cystic fibrosis, osteomyelitis, psoriasis, eosinophilic granuloma, and decubitus ulcers. The time from diagnosis of the underlying inflammatory disease to the diagnosis of AA amyloidosis is usually 10–20 years. Because chronic inflammatory illnesses afflict persons of all ages, AA amyloidosis may occur at any age.

Two diseases that cause AA amyloidosis, RA and FMF, warrant special attention. RA is the most common rheumatic cause of AA amyloidosis (75% of cases). However, AA amyloidosis does not develop in most patients with RA. The 15-year incidence of AA amyloidosis in RA was as high as 10% in older series. The incidence of AA amyloidosis in patients with RA has probably declined with the advent of more effective therapy. Patients in whom AA amyloidosis develops have had RA longer than those in whom amyloidosis did not develop. Continuously active RA or inadequately treated RA is a risk factor for the development of AA amyloidosis. FMF is characterized by recurrent attacks of fever, arthritis, pleuritis, peritonitis, or erysipelas-like erythema lasting 24–48 hours. FMF begins in childhood and usually affects persons of Mediterranean origin. AA amyloidosis develops in one-quarter of patients with FMF. Renal failure due to amyloid deposition usually occurs in the fifth decade of life.

Clinical Findings

A. SYMPTOMS AND SIGNS

The clinical manifestations of AA amyloidosis differ from those of AL amyloidosis in a number of ways. For example, renal and GI tract manifestations are common. More than 90% of people with AA amyloidosis have renal insufficiency, proteinuria, or both. Indeed, AA amyloidosis is the most common cause of nephrotic syndrome in people with RA. GI tract involvement affects 20% of patients; the manifestations include nausea, diarrhea, and poor nutritional intake. Unlike patients with AL amyloidosis, those with AA amyloidosis rarely have cardiac or peripheral nerve involvement. Macroglossia is not a feature of AA amyloidosis.

B. LABORATORY FINDINGS

No laboratory findings are pathognomonic of AA amyloidosis. Laboratory abnormalities reflect amyloid involvement of organs and tissues. For example, kidney involvement is common and is suggested by renal insufficiency and proteinuria.

C. IMAGING STUDIES

Imaging studies usually do not reveal findings specific for AA amyloidosis. Instead, they usually reveal findings associated with the underlying inflammatory condition (eg, RA). As with AL amyloidosis, however, quantitative scintigraphy with radiolabeled SAP component can be used in determining the extent and total body burden of amyloid deposits in patients with AA amyloidosis, as well as regression and progression of disease. However, this test is not widely available.

D. SPECIAL TESTS

Tissue biopsy is required to make the diagnosis of AA amyloidosis. Like other forms of amyloidosis, AA amyloid displays apple green birefringence when viewed under polarized light after staining with Congo red. Aspiration of subcutaneous abdominal fat reveals amyloid in 60–70% of patients with AA amyloidosis. If the fat aspirate does not reveal amyloid yet suspicion remains high, other tissue must be obtained. Notably, because AA amyloidosis commonly involves the kidney and GI tract, kidney and gastric mucosa biopsy specimens almost always reveal amyloid. Immunohistochemical staining of the specimen identifies the serum amyloid A precursor protein.

Treatment

The treatment of AA amyloidosis consists of treating the underlying inflammatory disease. This treatment results in reduced levels of serum amyloid A protein and prevents AA amyloid fibril formation and deposition. Treatment may also reverse organ dysfunction caused by amyloid deposits and improve survival, albeit large studies confirming this are not available. Remissions of nephrotic syndrome caused by AA amyloidosis have been reported with azathioprine and the combination of methotrexate and prednisolone. Colchicine, the drug of choice for treatment of FMF, prevents inflammatory attacks and the development of AA amyloidosis. Measuring serum C-reactive protein can assess response to treatment of the underlying inflammatory disease. Depending on the organs and tissues involved, patients with AA amyloidosis may require supportive treatment (Table 53–2).

When to Refer to a Specialist

Treating the underlying inflammatory disease may prevent or reverse AA amyloidosis. This treatment may require the assistance of a subspecialist (eg, rheumatologist). Treating the manifestations of AA amyloidosis (eg, kidney failure) may also require the assistance of a subspecialist (eg, nephrologist).

Prognosis

Having AA amyloidosis reduces survival. For example, RA patients without AA amyloidosis live nearly 8 years longer than RA patients with AA amyloidosis. Compared with AL amyloidosis, however, AA amyloidosis progresses slowly, and survival is often longer than 10 years.

Treating the underlying inflammatory disease improves survival of patients with AA amyloidosis. In addition, treating organ failure caused by amyloid involvement may improve survival. Dialysis or kidney transplantation improves survival of patients with AA amyloidosis in whom kidney failure develops.

DIALYSIS-ASSOCIATED β_2-M AMYLOIDOSIS

 ESSENTIALS OF DIAGNOSIS

- Beta$_2$-m amyloidosis should be suspected in all patients treated with long-term dialysis in whom rheumatic symptoms and signs, especially CTS, develop.
- Like all forms of amyloid, β_2-m amyloid displays apple green birefringence when viewed under polarized light after staining with Congo red.
- Aspiration of subcutaneous abdominal fat is of little value in detecting amyloid in patients with dialysis-associated β_2-m amyloidosis; hence, other tissue (eg, synovium) must be obtained to establish the diagnosis.
- Immunohistochemical staining identifies β_2-m precursor protein from which β_2-m amyloid fibrils derive.

General Considerations

Beta$_2$-m amyloidosis is a frequent complication of long-term dialysis (hemodialysis or peritoneal dialysis). Amyloid fibrils derive from β_2-m. Patients with renal failure have chronically elevated serum β_2-m levels because 95% of this protein is eliminated via glomerular filtration and is only partially cleared during dialysis. Indeed, β_2-m levels can be elevated 60-fold in anuric patients. Chronically elevated levels of this protein lead to the development of amyloidosis. Nearly all patients treated with dialysis for more than 15–20 years develop β_2-m amyloidosis. This form of amyloidosis may also develop in patients with chronic renal insufficiency not treated with dialysis.

Clinical Findings

A. SYMPTOMS AND SIGNS

Beta$_2$-m amyloidosis has a striking predilection for affecting the joints, especially synovial membranes. Although β_2-m amyloid deposits can be widespread, the principal clinical manifestations of β_2-m amyloidosis are rheumatologic: CTS, trigger finger, tendon rupture, joint pain and effusion, spondyloarthropathy, and cystic bone lesions.

CTS, caused by deposition of β_2-m amyloid in the synovium of the carpal tunnel, is the most common (and usually the first) manifestation of dialysis-associated β_2-m amyloidosis. Indeed, there is a direct relationship between development of CTS and duration of dialysis. In some patients, CTS develops after only 5 years of dialysis. The prevalence of CTS after 10 years of dialysis is 20%; after 15 years, 30–50%; and after 20 years, 80–100%.

Roughly half of patients treated with dialysis for more than 10 years experience persistent joint effusions accompanied by mild discomfort. Joint involvement is bilateral and includes large joints (eg, shoulders, knees, wrists, hips). Spondyloarthropathy is caused by destruction of the intervertebral disks and perivertebral erosions. Juxta-articular bone erosions and cystic defects have been described involving the femoral head, acetabulum, humerus, tibia, vertebral bodies, and carpal bones. These defects are not true cysts but rather eroded cavities. Furthermore, they are prone to pathologic fracture. Although β_2-m amyloid deposits have been found in visceral tissues and organs, this deposition usually does not manifest itself clinically.

B. IMAGING STUDIES

Imaging studies usually do not reveal findings specific for dialysis-associated β_2-m amyloidosis. The diagnosis is strongly suggested, however, in long-term dialysis patients in whom rheumatic symptoms develop and who have juxta-articular bone erosions or cystic defects on radiography or other imaging studies (eg, computed tomography).

C. SPECIAL TESTS

Unlike AL and AA amyloidosis, aspiration of subcutaneous abdominal fat is of little value in detecting amyloid in patients with dialysis-associated β_2-m amyloidosis. Hence, other tissue must be obtained to establish the diagnosis (usually from joints and synovial membranes). Beta$_2$-m amyloid displays apple green birefringence when viewed under polarized light after staining with Congo red. Immunohistochemical staining of the specimen identifies the β_2-m precursor protein.

Treatment

The treatment of dialysis-associated β_2-m amyloidosis is largely symptomatic. Rheumatic manifestations are treated with nonsteroidal anti-inflammatory drugs and local glucocorticoids (eg, intra-articular injections). Surgery (eg, carpal tunnel release, stabilization of areas of bone destruction) may be necessary.

Dialysis technology that clears β_2-m is improving. For example, high-flux hemodialysis with bicarbonate-buffered dialysate improves β_2-m clearance, is associated with fewer manifestations of β_2-m amyloidosis, and may improve survival. Kidney transplantation halts the progression of β_2-m amyloidosis. Serum β_2-m levels normalize and rheumatic symptoms lessen within days following transplantation. It is unclear, however, if kidney transplantation results in mobilization of β_2-m amyloid deposits.

When to Refer to a Specialist

Because this disease is associated with chronic renal failure and dialysis, nephrologists are almost always involved in the care of patients with dialysis-associated β_2-m amyloidosis. Rheumatic manifestations of this disease are common as well, and the assistance of other specialists (eg, rheumatologist, orthopedist) may be necessary.

Prognosis

Most patients treated with long-term dialysis develop β_2-m amyloidosis. Hence, the prognosis of this disease is determined, in part, by the underlying kidney disease and its cause (eg, diabetes mellitus). The rheumatic manifestations of this disease (eg, destructive spondyloarthropathy) may significantly impact patients' quality of life.

HEREDITARY AMYLOIDOSIS

ESSENTIALS OF DIAGNOSIS

- *Hereditary amyloidosis should be suspected in all patients with unexplained neuropathy, cardiomyopathy, or renal insufficiency, especially if there is a family history of these problems.*
- *Hereditary amyloid, like all forms of amyloid, displays apple green birefringence when viewed under polarized light after staining with Congo red.*
- *DNA analysis of blood and immunohistochemical staining of tissue specimens can be used to identify the mutant precursor protein.*

General Considerations

Hereditary amyloidosis consists of a group of autosomal dominant diseases in which amyloid fibrils derive from mutant serum proteins, including transthyretin, apolipoprotein A-I, lysozyme, and fibrinogen A α-chain. Gene mutations (eg, amino acid substitution) render the proteins amyloidogenic. Amyloid fibrils form (with consequent symptoms and signs) in middle age. A detailed family history may yield clues to the diagnosis of familial amyloidosis.

Many patients with hereditary amyloidosis are assumed mistakenly to have AL amyloidosis. In contrast to AL amyloidosis, patients with hereditary forms of this disease do not have associated monoclonal gammopathies. Because monoclonal gammopathies are relatively common in the general population, the detection of a monoclonal protein in a patient with hereditary amyloidosis may lead to the misdiagnosis of AL disease. Hence, it is important for clinicians to be certain of the origin of amyloid precursor protein in all patients with amyloidosis.

Clinical Findings

A. SYMPTOMS AND SIGNS

Peripheral neuropathy is the most common manifestation of the hereditary amyloidoses. Indeed, the term "familial amyloidotic neuropathy" was once used for these diseases. Cardiac involvement is also common, whereas kidney involvement is less common.

Transthyretin is the most commonly involved protein in hereditary amyloidosis. This protein is synthesized by the liver and choroid plexus and transports thyroxine and retinol-binding protein. More than 80 mutations (single amino acid substitutions) of transthyretin have been identified that cause amyloidosis. Peripheral and autonomic neuropathy is the most common manifestation of transthyretin-associated amyloidosis. Cardiac involvement is common but its severity varies according to the specific transthyretin mutation. Compared with AL amyloidosis, heart failure is less common and the prognosis is better among patients with familial variants. In addition, renal involvement is less common and macroglossia does not occur.

Kidney disease—but not neuropathy—usually develops in patients with hereditary amyloidosis caused by apolipoprotein A-I, lysozyme, and fibrinogen A α-chain mutations.

B. LABORATORY FINDINGS

No laboratory finding is pathognomonic of hereditary amyloidosis. Laboratory abnormalities reflect amyloid involvement of organs and tissues.

C. IMAGING STUDIES

Imaging studies usually do not reveal findings specific for hereditary amyloidosis. Like other forms of amyloidosis, quantitative scintigraphy with radiolabeled SAP component can be used to assess patients with transthyretin-associated amyloidosis. This test is not widely available, however.

D. SPECIAL TESTS

Amyloid deposits caused by the hereditary amyloidoses display apple green birefringence when viewed under polarized light after staining with Congo red. DNA analysis of blood and immunohistochemical staining of tissue specimens identify the mutant precursor protein.

Treatment

Liver transplantation has been used successfully to treat hereditary amyloidosis caused by mutant proteins synthesized by the liver. For example, liver transplantation to treat hereditary amyloidosis caused by mutations of transthyretin may result in disappearance of the mutant protein from the blood and improvement of neuropathy. Other manifestations of hereditary amyloidosis (eg, kidney failure) are treated with supportive measures (Table 53–2).

When to Refer to a Specialist

Relatives of patients affected by hereditary amyloidosis should undergo genetic counseling. Since liver transplantation has been used successfully to treat hereditary amyloidosis caused by mutant proteins synthesized by the liver, referral to a liver transplant subspecialist is warranted. Treating other manifestations of hereditary amyloidosis (eg, kidney failure) may also require the assistance of a subspecialist (eg, nephrologist).

Prognosis

Patients with hereditary amyloidosis caused by mutant proteins synthesized by the liver who undergo liver transplantation experience improvement in their symptoms and enjoy prolonged survival, especially if transplantation is done before irreversible organ failure has occurred. The rate of progression of hereditary amyloidosis caused by apolipoprotein A-I, lysozyme, and fibrinogen A α-chain mutations is usually slow. Patients with these forms of hereditary amyloidosis have kidney involvement and usually respond to supportive measures and, if necessary, kidney transplantation.

REFERENCES

Falk RH, et al. The systemic amyloidoses. *N Engl J Med*. 1997; 337:898. [PMID: 9302305] (Concise review of the clinical features, diagnosis, treatment, and prognosis of the most common systemic amyloidoses.)

Floege J, Ketteler M. Beta$_2$-microglobulin-derived amyloidosis: an update. *Kidney Int Suppl*. 2001;78:S164. [PMID: 11169004] (Detailed review of the clinical features, diagnosis, treatment, and prognosis of dialysis-associated β$_2$-m amyloidosis.)

Gertz MA, et al. Amyloidosis. *Hematol Oncol Clin North Am*. 1999;13:1211. [PMID: 10626146] (Detailed review of the clinical features, diagnosis, treatment, and prognosis of AL amyloidosis.)

Gertz MA, Kyle RA. Secondary systemic amyloidosis: response and survival in 64 patients. *Medicine (Baltimore)*. 1991;70:246. [PMID: 2067409] (Clinical features and outcomes of a large series of patients with AA amyloidosis from a single institution.)

Lachmann HJ, et al. Misdiagnosis of hereditary amyloidosis as AL (primary) amyloidosis. *N Engl J Med*. 2002;346:1786. [PMID: 12050338] (Amyloidogenic mutations consistent with hereditary amyloidosis in 34 of 350 patients in whom the diagnosis of AL amyloidosis was suggested by clinical and laboratory findings and the absence of a family history.)

Mueller PS, et al. Symptomatic ischemic heart disease resulting from obstructive intramural coronary amyloidosis. *Am J Med*. 2000;109:181. [PMID: 10974179] (Clinical and pathologic features of a series of patients with ischemic heart disease caused by AL amyloidosis.)

Relevant World Wide Web Sites

[Mayo Clinic]

http://www.mayoclinic.org/amyloidosis-rst/

[Boston University]

http://amyloid/bu.edu/amyloid/Amyloid1.htm

SECTION VIII

Disorders of Bone

Osteoporosis & Glucocorticoid-Induced Osteoporosis

54

Dolores Shoback, MD

Osteoporosis is a systemic skeletal disorder characterized by low bone mass, microarchitectural disruption of bone tissue, and compromised bone strength leading to an increased risk for fracture.[1]

Osteoporosis is commonly encountered in primary care settings in the management of postmenopausal women. It is often clinically silent until a fragility fracture occurs.

Osteoporotic fractures are common in postmenopausal women. Hip fractures are the most devastating osteoporotic fractures in terms of medical, psychosocial, and financial consequences. The lifetime probability of sustaining a hip fracture in a 50-year-old white woman is 14%; it is much lower (6%) in a 50-year-old African American woman.

Osteoporosis is being recognized with increasing frequency in older men with height loss, nontraumatic fractures, hypogonadism, and other risk factors. Fractures in men are an important public health problem. Approximately 150,000 hip fractures occur each year in men in the United States, accounting for about one-third of all hip fractures. The mortality from hip fractures in men at 1 year is 30%.

Patients receiving long-term glucocorticoid therapy are at risk for bone loss and should have prevention and treatment approaches implemented. It is important that the primary care provider decides whom to screen for osteoporosis. The decision should be based on an assessment of that individual's risk factors for bone loss and an understanding of disease pathogenesis.

---

[1]NIH Consensus Statement, Osteoporosis Prevention, Diagnosis, and Therapy, Office of the Director, Vol 17 (1), p.5, 2000.

■ CLASSIC PRESENTATIONS

POSTMENOPAUSAL OSTEOPOROSIS

  ESSENTIAL FEATURES

- *Altered microarchitecture.*
- *Decreased bone strength.*
- *Reduced bone mineral density.*

General Considerations

Clinically, osteoporosis is diagnosed when **bone mineral density** (BMD) is reduced and fractures occur due to skeletal fragility. The most common osteoporosis-related fractures occur in the thoracic and lumbar spine, hip, and distal radius.

Bone loss in women begins before the onset of menopause. Typically, women lose bone mass beginning in the late third and early fourth decades. The process accelerates for the 5 to 10 years around the menopause. Postmenopausal osteoporosis results from estrogen deficiency–induced changes in the production of several key cytokines. Ultimately, this leads to an imbalance between bone formation and resorption so that resorption is favored over formation. After the increased rates of bone loss immediately surrounding the menopause cease, a less aggressive phase of bone loss ensues that continues into the eighth and ninth decades. Estrogen deficiency as well as other factors related to aging (reduced osteoprogenitor population, nutritional deficiencies, malabsorption, etc) play a role in this phase of bone loss.

Osteoporosis can be diagnosed clinically with bone densitometry or by the presence of fragility fractures in a patient at risk for the disease. Bone densitometry has become widely available as a diagnostic tool in recent years. Several techniques for quantifying BMD have been developed. They include dual-energy x-ray absorptiometry (**DXA**), single-energy x-ray absorptiometry, quantitative computed tomography, quantitative ultrasound, and radiographic absorptiometry. DXA is, by far, the best standardized technique and is preferred for diagnosing osteoporosis and monitoring responses to therapy.

BMD by DXA has been used by the World Health Organization (WHO) to define **osteopenia** and **osteoporosis.** Their criteria are based on a large body of data on postmenopausal white women (Table 54–1).

In addition to age and BMD, a number of other clinical risk factors have been associated with an increased incidence of osteoporotic fractures (Table 54–2). The National Osteoporosis Foundation has categorized these factors as modifiable and nonmodifiable. Nonmodifiable risk factors include gender, ethnicity, age, and family and/or personal history of fracture. Modifiable risk factors include smoking, alcohol consumption, use of long-term glucocorticoid therapy, low dietary calcium intake, poor eyesight, and others. As described below, all treatment and prevention strategies for osteoporosis begin with risk factor modification.

Despite extensive information on risk factors for fracture and low BMD, no single combination—or

Table 54–1. WHO definition of osteoporosis for women based on DXA measurements.

	Definitions
T-score	Number of SD above or below peak bone mass ("young normal") according to gender and race
Z-score	Number of SD above or below age-matched bone mass according to gender and race
Normal	BMD T-score ≥ – 1
Low bone mass (osteopenia)	BMD T-score < – 1 and > – 2.5
Osteoporosis	BMD T-score ≤ – 2.5
Severe osteoporosis	BMD T-score ≤ – 2.5 with one or more fragility fractures

WHO, World Health Organization; DXA, dual-energy x-ray absorptiometry; SD, standard deviation; BMD, bone mineral density.

Table 54–2. Risk factors for osteoporotic fractures in women independent of bone density.

Nonmodifiable
History of fracture as an adult
Presence of fracture (especially of hip) in first-degree relative
White
Advanced age
Dementia and frailty
Immobilization

Modifiable
Alcohol and tobacco use
Low body weight (< 127 lbs for white, < 100 lbs for Asian)
Premature menopause
History of amenorrhea
Low dietary calcium intake
Frequent falls and poor eyesight
Low level of physical activity
Use of glucocorticoids
Vitamin D deficiency

Modified from National Osteoporosis Foundation. *Physician's Guide to Osteoporosis.* 1998; and Kanis JA. Excerpta Medica, Diagnosis of osteoporosis and assessment of fracture risk. *Lancet.* 2002; 359:1929.

weighting—of risk factors adequately predicts the prevalent BMD or fracture risk or can substitute for the measurement of BMD. Risk factor assessment in current practice is helpful in understanding the basis for ongoing bone loss and pointing to strategies for slowing it.

Despite the value of BMD measurements using DXA in assessing fracture risk, DXA instruments are not available everywhere, and testing can be expensive. This has led to the need for guidelines in recommending BMD testing. A variety of professional organizations have published guidelines on the use of BMD testing in postmenopausal women and in patients receiving long-term glucocorticoid therapy (Table 54–3). Most of these indications are based on clinical risk factors obtainable from the initial evaluation of the patient.

Clinical & Laboratory Evaluation

The evaluation of perimenopausal or postmenopausal women for osteoporosis or a low BMD begins with the clinical assessment. This includes the medical history with careful attention to the history of medication use (especially glucocorticoids), smoking, alcohol intake, dietary calcium intake, and family history of osteoporosis and fractures. The physical examination is focused on signs of bone pain or deformity, anemia, hyperthyroidism, hypercortisolism, malnutrition, or disorders that cause secondary forms of osteoporosis (Table 54–4).

Table 54–3. Indications for bone mineral density testing and medicare reimbursement.

National Osteoporosis Foundation guidelines[a]
- Women ≥ 65 years regardless of risk factor status
- Younger women after time of menopause with the following risk factors:
  - Positive family history for osteoporosis
  - History of fragility fracture at age 45 or older
  - Smoking
  - Low body weight (< 127 lbs)

US Preventive Services Task Force[b]
- Women ≥ 65 years should be screened
- Initiate screening at age 60 if increased risk of fractures is present:
  - Low body weight (< 70 kg)
  - Estrogen deficiency
  - Other risk factors

Medicare coverage of bone mineral density testing[c]
- Postmenopausal women at risk for osteoporosis
- Patients with vertebral abnormalities
- Patients receiving glucocorticoids long term (prednisone ≥ 7.5 mg/d)
- Patients with primary hyperparathyroidism
- Patients receiving approved therapy to monitor response

American College of Rheumatology Ad Hoc Committee on Glucocorticoid-Induced Osteoporosis[d]
- Obtain baseline bone mineral density measurement when initiating long-term (≥ 6 months) glucocorticoid therapy
- Repeat measurement at 12 months (or 6 months) to ascertain ongoing bone loss
- Monitor patients receiving therapy for osteoporosis annually

[a]Modified from National Osteoporosis Foundation. *Physician's Guide to Prevention and Treatment of Osteoporosis.* Excerpta Medica, 1998, www.nof.org/news/pressreleases/guide98.htm.
[b]Modified from US PSTF, *Ann Intern Med.* 2002;137:536, www.ahcpr.gov/clinic/uspstfix.htm.
[c]Modified from *Fed Reg.* 1998; 63:34320.
[d]Modified from *Arthritis Rheum.* 2001;44:1496, www.rheumatology.org/research/guidelines.

Table 54–4. Secondary causes of osteoporosis: men and women.

Rheumatologic disorders	Rheumatoid arthritis
	Ankylosing spondylitis
Connective tissue disorders	Marfan syndrome
	Ehlers-Danlos syndrome
	Osteogenesis imperfecta
Endocrine disorders	Primary hyperparathyroidism
	Hyperthyroidism
	Cushing syndrome
	Hypogonadism
	Anorexia nervosa with amenorrhea
	Hyperprolactinemia with amenorrhea or hypogonadism
	Insulin-dependent diabetes
Hematologic disorders	Multiple myeloma
	Systemic mastocytosis
	Lymphoma
	Leukemia
	Disseminated carcinoma
Gastrointestinal disorders	Malabsorption
	Celiac sprue
	Short bowel syndrome
	Crohn disease
	Chronic liver disease (especially cirrhosis)
	Primary biliary cirrhosis
	Postgastrectomy
Other conditions	Chronic obstructive pulmonary disease
	Post-transplantation
	Malnutrition
Drug therapy	Glucocorticoids
	Anticonvulsants
	Excessive thyroxine replacement
	Anticoagulants (heparin)
	Gonadotropin-releasing hormone agonists

In postmenopausal women, it is unusual to diagnose a secondary cause of osteoporosis. Most commonly estrogen deficiency is at fault. It has become apparent, however, that vitamin D deficiency and subtle forms of calcium malabsorption (eg, due to celiac sprue) are more common than previously thought and should be considered in patients with impressively low bone mass with or without fractures. In addition, multiple myeloma can be relatively "silent" clinically and present with osteoporosis, bone pain, pathologic fractures, or anemia. This diagnosis should be considered if BMD is remarkably low for age or an unexplained anemia or elevated erythrocyte sedimentation rate is present. Multiple myeloma can be easily excluded by a serum and urine protein electrophoresis. Establishing this diagnosis is important because it redirects therapy.

There has been considerable debate about what the appropriate and cost-effective laboratory work-up should be for postmenopausal women with low BMD or osteoporosis. There is no consensus. At a minimum, laboratory evaluation should include a complete blood cell count, serum chemistry panel, liver function tests, and serum thyroid-stimulating hormone and calcium determinations. Measurements of serum 25-hydroxyvitamin

D and urinary calcium and creatinine excretion can be extremely helpful. Subtle and overt vitamin D deficiency are relatively common in elderly patients and extremely difficult to diagnose on clinical grounds alone. Vitamin D deficiency is likely to contribute to bone loss because it interferes with the mineralization of bone matrix. High levels of urinary calcium excretion suggest idiopathic hypercalciuria. This can be associated with renal stones and low BMD. In addition, a urinary calcium measurement in a patient already taking calcium supplements can be informative as to the adequacy of therapy. If the urinary calcium excretion is low, then underlying malabsorption or an extremely low calcium intake must be considered. Postmenopausal women as a group are commonly affected by primary hyperparathyroidism (prevalence ~3 per 1000). A serum calcium determination adequately screens for this diagnosis. If it is elevated, serum intact parathyroid hormone should be measured.

It is estimated that 10–20% of postmenopausal women have additional secondary causes for their bone loss although this may be a conservative estimate. Given the costs and patient commitment required for years of treatment for osteoporosis, it is imperative that underlying causes—especially those that require different management approaches—be properly diagnosed.

Imaging Evaluation

The ideal study to assess BMD in a postmenopausal woman is a **DXA** measurement of the lumbar spine and hip. In many patients over age 65, spinal BMD measurements can be spuriously elevated due to aortic calcifications, arthritis, and degenerative disc disease. In such persons, only measurements of the total hip and femoral neck are reliable enough for diagnostic purposes.

BMD reports often include both T- and Z-scores (Figure 54–1). A **T-score** relates the BMD of the patient to peak bone mass for race and gender. A **Z-score** relates the BMD of the patient to persons of the same age, gender, and race. The T-score is the most useful determination clinically. Operationally, the lower of the two T-scores (spine or hip) is used for making the diagnosis. Typically, there is concordance between T-scores at both sites except if the spinal measurement is artifactually elevated, due to degenerative arthritis, disc disease, or aortic calcification, or if there is preferential bone loss at one site versus another.

Obtaining a BMD measurement allows the clinician not only to grade the severity of osteoporosis but also to predict fracture risk. Several studies have confirmed that the relative risk (RR) of fracture approximately doubles with each standard deviation (SD) below peak BMD (T-score) that a patient demonstrates.

The BMD measurement, along with the patient's age, is an even more powerful approach to predict fracture risk. The information in Figure 54–2 indicates that the 5-year risk of several types of osteoporotic fractures is strongly related to age and BMD T-score (in this case of the femoral neck). As is evident, there is a powerful interaction between these two variables. Advanced age (over 70 years) dramatically heightens the risks of vertebral and hip fractures.

Disease Course & Complications

Postmenopausal osteoporosis can progress silently over years to a dangerously low BMD and markedly reduced bone strength to a degree that the fracture threshold is reached. Osteoporosis in patients taking glucocorticoids long term is characterized by even more rapid bone loss. After this process progresses, fragility fractures can occur with minimal impact. Fractures are the dreaded complication of osteoporosis. Fractures of the spine cause pain but are generally self-limited. After multiple fractures, height is lost. With that can come reduced thoracic expansion capacity, difficulty with breathing, progressive spinal deformity called kyphosis, and ultimately increased frailty. As noted above, frailty is also a risk factor for fractures.

Hip fractures have a more dramatic course, and prognosis in the elderly osteoporotic patient is guarded. These fractures require hospitalization and surgery. Because of the underlying frailty of most of these patients, their comorbid conditions and advanced age, and the prolonged immobilization and rehabilitation required, patients who fracture their hips face decreased life expectancy. It is estimated that the overall mortality in the first year after a hip fracture is 20%. In men, the risk of death is three-fold greater than in women. Women fracture their hips at earlier ages and have fewer comorbidities than men. It has also been reported that men require longer hospitalizations and have more complicated courses after their hip fractures, mostly due to infections.

In addition to the medical and financial ramifications of the immediate treatment of the hip fracture, there are substantial long-term human consequences. It is estimated that 50% of patients who sustain a hip fracture do not live independently afterwards. Hip fractures are life-altering events for elderly people. Thus, it is imperative to recognize osteoporosis early and intervene with treatment strategies that reduce fracture risk. In view of the rapidly rising mean age of populations in the developed world, it is critical that interventions for osteoporosis be made expeditiously.

MALE OSTEOPOROSIS

General Considerations

In contrast to postmenopausal osteoporosis, the diagnosis of osteoporosis in men is often delayed. Osteo-

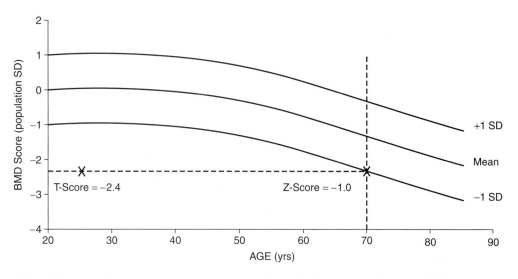

Figure 54–1. This graph shows the mean ± 1 standard deviation for bone mineral density (BMD). For a given femoral neck BMD value in a 70-year-old woman, her Z-score is –1 and her T-score (extrapolated back to the age of 20) is –2.4. (Reprinted with permission from Orwoll ES, Bliziotes M. *Osteoporosis: Pathophysiology and Clinical Management.* Humana Press, 2003:109.)

porosis in men, more often than in postmenopausal women, presents with fractures, height loss, or obvious stigmata of the secondary causes for bone loss.

In contrast to women, men do not experience a clear-cut, easily defined cessation of gonadal function that could serve to raise awareness of risks for bone loss. Clearly, testosterone production declines with age. There is controversy as to what the normal or accepted ranges of testosterone are for elderly men and how exactly age-related declines in testosterone contribute to age-related declines in BMD. It is clear, however, that replacing testosterone does not restore BMD to "normal" even in hypogonadal men and that there are other determinants of low BMD and fractures in men beyond hypogonadism.

Other issues that affect BMD in men are peak bone mass and the rate of bone loss. Men achieve higher peak bone mass than do women, and men lose bone mineral at different rates than do postmenopausal women. Once, however, the early rapid phase of post-menopausal bone loss ends, the rate of bone loss in women slows. Thereafter, the rates of bone loss in men and women are roughly equal (Figure 54–3). Because of the early rapid phase of menopause-related bone loss and the lower peak bone mass achieved by women, compared with men, women have lower BMDs at the same ages than do men. This leads to an earlier onset of the typical osteoporotic fractures (hip, vertebrae, Colles) in women compared with men (Figure 54–4). Men with low BMD, however, experience the same

fractures. They just occur at later ages—approximately 10 years later than they do in women. This means that osteoporotic fractures in men occur at times in their lives when they are likely to be more frail and less able to cope physically and emotionally with the loss of independence and the risks of hospitalization and fracture repair surgery. Hence, the morbidity and mortality of hip fractures are much greater in men than in women.

Many of the risk factors for osteoporosis and fractures are the same in men and women (Tables 54–2 and 54–5). Genetic factors play a key role in the acquisition of peak bone mass for both genders. A personal or family history of nontraumatic or fragility fractures is a risk factor in men and women—perhaps a clue that bone quality and rates of bone loss are genetically determined. Tobacco and alcohol use are important risk factors for bone loss in men as well as body habitus and underlying disease states.

Clearly, risk factors and secondary causes must be considered in the evaluation of men with osteoporosis. In fact, one of the most important aspects of osteoporosis in men is that 80% or more of these men have one or more secondary causes for bone loss. It is critical, therefore, that men with low BMD or fractures receive a thorough evaluation for secondary causes of osteoporosis (see Table 54–4).

Despite the emphasis on secondary causes for bone loss in men, there is still a subgroup of men who have primary osteoporosis. These men are often middle-aged with low BMD, height loss, and multiple fractures.

A

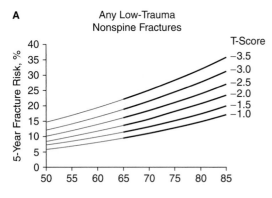

Any Low-Trauma
Nonspine Fractures

B

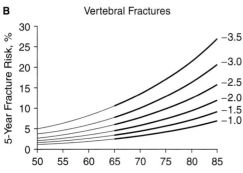

Vertebral Fractures

C

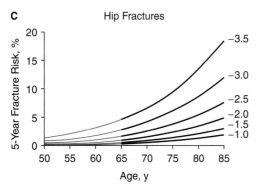

Hip Fractures

Figure 54–2. These figures show the influence of age and bone mineral density (BMD) on the 5-year fracture risk for any low-trauma fracture (**A**), vertebral fractures (**B**), and hip fractures (**C**). At approximately age 65, there is a steep increase in fracture risk at T-scores of −2.0 or −2.5 or greater in panels **B** and **C**. (Reprinted with permission from Cummings SR, et al. Clinical uses of bone densitometry: scientific review. *JAMA*. 2002; 288:1889.)

Even if all known secondary causes are carefully considered, there remains a group of men in whom no secondary diagnosis can be established. These patients constitute the other 10–20% of men with osteoporosis. Whether they have intrinsic abnormalities in bone remodeling—defects in formation or resorption—is unknown.

Clinical & Laboratory Evaluation

Because of the prominence of secondary forms of osteoporosis, the clinical and laboratory investigation of men with low BMD and fractures must be thorough. The history and physical examination should pay attention to underlying pulmonary, gonadal, adrenal, gastrointestinal, and hematologic disorders. Habits (alcohol and tobacco use) are important risk factors to pursue in men along with the signs and symptoms of diseases in Table 54–4.

What constitutes a complete, cost-effective laboratory evaluation of men with osteoporosis? This is still controversial. The initial evaluation in men should include a complete blood cell count, liver function tests, and determinations of serum chemistries, testosterone, thyroid-stimulating hormone, calcium, and 25-hydroxyvitamin D, and 24-hour urinary calcium and creatinine excretion.

Further testing should include serum and urine protein electrophoresis, if anemia is present and no other cause for osteopenia or osteoporosis has been demonstrated. Multiple myeloma is often cryptic, presenting only with osteopenia or osteoporosis, asymptomatic anemia, and renal insufficiency. Multiple myeloma should be carefully considered in older African American men with unexplained bone loss because of its predilection for that population. In addition, men with a history of prostate cancer should be asked about past (or current) use of long-acting gonadotropin-releasing hormone agonists and androgen blockers. These men lose bone at an accelerated rate and treating them to prevent bone loss is effective. Men with low testosterone levels should be evaluated for primary or secondary forms of hypogonadism. That includes additional laboratory studies (gonadotropin and prolactin measurements), possibly pituitary imaging, and referral to an endocrinologist.

Men with disorders such as ankylosing spondylitis, vasculitis, or inflammatory arthritides should be under the care of rheumatologists. In such persons, both the underlying disease and its treatment (glucocorticoids and other immunosuppressive drugs) are deleterious to bone. Optimal treatment of such patients requires a concerted approach by both internists and rheumatologists.

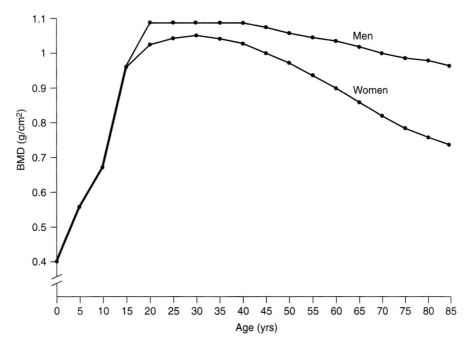

Figure 54–3. Mean bone mineral density (BMD) in men versus women from age 5 to 85 demonstrating the lower peak BMD values for women versus men, the rapid perimenopausal rates of bone loss in women, and the slow continuous phase of bone loss that continues into the eighth decade. (Reprinted with permission from Southard RN, et al. Bone mass in healthy children: measurement with quantitative DXA. *Radiology.* 1991;179:735; and from Kelly TL. Bone mineral reference databases for American men and women. *J Bone Miner Res.* 1990;5(Suppl 2):702.

Figure 54–4. The incidence of three common osteoporotic fractures in men and women over decades. (Reprinted with permission from Cooper C, Melton LJ III. Epidemiology of osteoporosis. *Trends Endocrinol Metab.* 1992;314:224.)

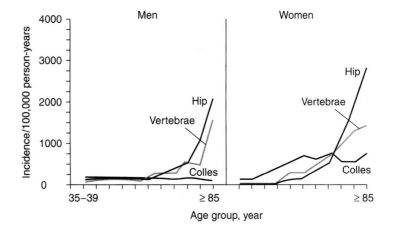

Table 54–5. Determinants of low bone mineral density in men.

Advanced age
Frailty
Low body weight
Alcohol intake
Smoking
Caffeine intake
Use of glucocorticoids
History of hyperthyroidism
History of peptic ulcer disease
History of chronic lung disease
History of rheumatoid arthritis
History of fracture after the age of 50
Height loss since age 20

Adapted from Orwoll ES, Bevan L, Phipps KR. Determinants of bone mineral density in older men. *Osteoporos Int.* 2000;11:815.

As noted above regarding postmenopausal women, measuring urinary calcium and creatinine excretion has the same diagnostic and therapeutic importance in men. In addition, hypercalciuria can often be treated successfully with thiazide diuretics.

While primary hyperparathyroidism is a key consideration in postmenopausal women, it is a less prominent cause of accelerated bone loss in men. Since it is a relatively common endocrine disorder, it should be considered if there is a history of renal stones or even a marginally elevated serum calcium value on screening laboratory studies.

Depending on the clinical situation, hypercortisolism should also be considered in the evaluation of men with unexplained osteoporosis and/or fractures. Cortisol excess states are admittedly rare, but bone loss may be the first clinical clue that cortisol excess is present. Cushing syndrome is easily excluded by a 24-hour urinary cortisol determination or overnight dexamethasone suppression testing.

Imaging Evaluation

The same imaging modalities are used to document loss of bone mineral content in men and women. DXA scanning of the spine is often affected by the presence of degenerative arthritis, disc disease, and aortic calcifications in elderly men. Instant vertebral assessment (IVA) can be helpful in assessing the presence of vertebral deformities and fractures, although dating such abnormalities is often very difficult. It is important to remember that men experience more traumatic fractures than do women (including fractures of the spine) at young ages.

The most important issue in using bone densitometry in men in the diagnosis of osteoporosis is the lack of sufficiently large databases compared with postmenopausal women. The WHO classification of osteoporosis and osteopenia (see Table 54–1) was developed on the basis of data from postmenopausal white women. While it is not rigorously defensible to apply the same DXA T-score cut-points to define osteoporosis and osteopenia in men, this is widely done. The few randomized trials of drugs to treat osteoporosis in men (summarized below) usually use a T-score of ≤ -2 and/or fractures to enroll patients. Experts in the field are moving toward using absolute BMD measurements and absolute fracture risk to make decisions about treatment in men and women. Ongoing studies with large cohorts of men should help better define BMD thresholds for treatment in men.

GLUCOCORTICOID-INDUCED OSTEOPOROSIS

General Considerations

Glucocorticoid therapy is associated with an array of potential side effects. The most serious and disabling of these are the skeletal complications osteonecrosis and osteoporosis. Skeletal adverse events are estimated to occur in approximately 50% of patients taking long-term glucocorticoid therapy. Although there is debate about the exact dose of prednisone required to increase the risk of bone loss and fractures, the weight of evidence supports the idea that oral doses of ≥ 7.5 mg/d (or its equivalent) are associated with an increased risk of both vertebral and hip fractures. In addition to drug dosage, the underlying disease often contributes in important ways to the pathogenesis of bone loss in patients taking glucocorticoids long term through changes in circulating hormones or inflammatory cytokines, concomitant drug therapy, nutritional issues, or inactivity. Men and women of all ages and even children can lose bone while taking long-term glucocorticoid therapy and deserve to be considered for the prevention and treatment strategies outlined below.

The pathogenesis of glucocorticoid-induced osteoporosis is complex. In the initial phase of such therapy (first few weeks), there is an increase in bone resorption. Within this phase, patients can lose considerable bone mass. In addition, glucocorticoids antagonize the actions of vitamin D, especially in the intestine, leading to reduced calcium absorption. This limits the amount of calcium available to form bone matrix properly. Glucocorticoids also promote calcium excretion by the kidney. In some cases, marked hypercalciuria can be seen. Glucocorticoids act on the pituitary to suppress gonadotropin production, rendering patients hypogonadal. Many women afflicted with the systemic illnesses that require chronic glucocorticoid therapy are amenorrheic secondary either to their underlying illness or its therapy. Impaired gonadal steroid production in both men and women, therefore, figures importantly in the pathogenesis of glucocorticoid-induced bone loss.

However, after a few months and continuing for years, the deleterious effects of glucocorticoids are on the lifespan and functional capacity of osteoblasts and osteocytes. Osteoblasts form new bone, and osteocytes are involved in mechanosensing. Apoptosis (programmed cell death) in these populations is promoted by long-term glucocorticoid therapy. This means that ongoing bone resorption is not answered by increased bone formation, and the sensing of normal mechanical forces and physical loading may be impaired. Overall, an imbalance in bone remodeling is favored, and in the end, resorption predominates. When glucocorticoids are discontinued, bone can recover. Whatever bone mineral has been lost, however, is unlikely to be fully restored. Hence, the prevention of bone loss is the ideal initial strategy.

Patients taking glucocorticoids long term are subject to an increased risk of fractures in the spine, hip, and other sites. It has been suggested that glucocorticoid-treated patients fracture at higher BMDs than other groups of patients, but this notion has been challenged. Needless to say, numerous patients who have had fractures while taking glucocorticoids have BMD measurements that are not extremely low. In such situations, it is important to recall that many of these patients may have had BMD values, prior to the onset of illness and glucocorticoid therapy, that were well above a T-score of −1. Since BMD determinations are often not done prior to the initiation of therapy, baseline BMD values are typically unknown.

The majority of patients receiving glucocorticoids are taking these drugs orally. Other routes of administration (inhaled, intranasal, or topical) are far less likely to have the deleterious skeletal consequences of oral therapy unless particularly high doses of long-acting glucocorticoid preparations are used. In addition, for unclear reasons, not all patients taking high doses of glucocorticoids suffer adverse skeletal consequences. As noted above, only 50% of patients receiving long-term glucocorticoid therapy experience bony complications. What protects the other patients remains unknown. It seems clear that the most vulnerable patients are postmenopausal women. Many of the diseases for which they receive glucocorticoids long term (eg, rheumatoid arthritis) are also especially deleterious to bone. Rheumatoid arthritis induces systemic as well as local (periarticular) bone loss. Therefore, the underlying disease is likely also to be an added risk to skeletal integrity.

Clinical, Laboratory, & Imaging Evaluation

Patients who are being given glucocorticoids for an illness that is likely to require long-term usage should have a careful history and physical examination performed to assess for any relevant skeletal risk factors. The menstrual and or menopausal status of women should be investigated historically. An evaluation of serum chemistries, calcium, and 25-hydroxyvitamin D is a reasonable initial laboratory work-up.

Most clinicians would agree that if long-term therapy is envisioned, a baseline BMD determination should be done to help decide whether preventive measures with drugs such as bisphosphonates need to be used and how aggressive the approaches should be. A baseline measurement also helps gauge when a repeat BMD determination is indicated. Menopausal status, other comorbid conditions, and clinical risk factors also influence the timing of repeat BMD measurements and the aggressiveness of the treatment plan.

In persons who are referred and already taking glucocorticoids long term, the baseline laboratory testing noted above is helpful along with a 24-hour urinary calcium and creatinine determination. The latter is used in much the same way as described above for postmenopausal women and men with osteoporosis. Because of the propensity of glucocorticoids to interfere with vitamin D action and enhance renal calcium excretion, this is a critical parameter to assess in long-term glucocorticoid-treated patients. In addition, a serum testosterone should be obtained in men due to the effects of glucocorticoids on pituitary release of gonadotropins. Many men taking glucocorticoids long term will often not complain of the typical symptoms of hypogonadism but will have frankly low testosterone levels.

BMD measurements are essential in evaluating patients taking glucocorticoids long term. They allow decisions to be made about whether drug therapy or watchful waiting is indicated. Any T-score that suggests that considerable bone loss has already occurred is a signal to treat aggressively if the other circumstances indicate this is appropriate. Young women of child-bearing age must be treated with great care since bisphosphonates accumulate in the skeleton and could potentially alter fetal skeletal development should pregnancy occur theoretically even within a few years of treatment for osteoporosis. None of the medications, especially bisphosphonates, are approved for use in pregnant or lactating women. Therefore, a careful clinical, laboratory, and densitometric evaluation of these patients is extremely helpful in determining the most safe and appropriate way to protect the skeleton and not expose the patient to undue risk.

In 2001, the American College of Rheumatology published its guidelines for BMD testing among patients taking glucocorticoids long term. Baseline BMD testing and testing patients already receiving treatment were recommended. Depending on the underlying disease, other concomitant risk factors, and the measurement itself, repeat BMD testing is recommended within 12 and sometimes even 6 months. The 6-month interval between repeat testing is appropriate if initial BMD is low, glucocorticoid dose is high, and the patient is not a candidate for the most effective therapies (such as bisphosphonates). Other scenarios could be envisioned in which knowing that bone loss has not progressed rapidly (within 6 months) is helpful in reassuring the patient or in confirming the need for aggressive therapy.

DIFFERENTIAL DIAGNOSIS

The differential diagnosis of low bone mass or a low BMD measurement is narrow. It is either due to osteoporosis or osteomalacia. Any primary or secondary form of osteoporosis described in this chapter could cause this picture. Osteomalacia causes low bone mass or low BMD because the mineralization of the matrix is defective. Mineral content of the skeleton (not the protein content) is reduced in osteomalacia. A host of different conditions cause osteomalacia. These need to be considered seriously if there is any abnormality in the levels of serum calcium, phosphorus, alkaline phosphatase, or 25-hydroxyvitamin D. Patients with osteomalacia may also have bone pain, pathologic fractures, muscle weakness, and difficulty walking, especially when osteomalacia is moderate or severe and the diagnosis has been delayed. Because the disease is difficult to detect early in its course, the astute clinician must be aware of the manifestations of this less common bone disease and not ignore subtle clinical and laboratory features that hint at the presence of osteomalacia.

TREATMENT

The essentials of management for most forms of osteoporosis include the following:

- Lifestyle modifications.
- Nutritional interventions.
- Pharmacologic therapies.

Nonpharmacologic

Lifestyle modifications are often introduced along with dietary and **nutritional interventions.** These approaches should be implemented in all patients in whom the prevention of bone loss is desired and in whom the goals are stopping bone loss and reducing

fractures. Initial efforts are directed at increasing the safety of the patient's immediate environment to prevent falls and fractures, eliminating habits that are deleterious to skeletal integrity and that can contribute to falls, and improving the calcium and vitamin D status of the patient. The latter strategy is absolutely essential if the pharmacologic therapies discussed below are to be successful.

The desired lifestyle modifications are straightforward in concept but not always in implementation. Patients should be encouraged to discontinue smoking and alcohol consumption. Both habits are injurious to bone. Patients should be prescribed a weight-bearing exercise program that emphasizes regular participation (5 times weekly if possible for at least 30 and preferably 45 or 60 minutes) and that is suitable for even frail elderly patients. Regular walking can provide benefits to the frail osteoporotic patient beyond positive changes in BMD. Exercise improves well-being and neuromuscular coordination, which can help condition reflexes to respond better to falls. In addition, although there is some controversy as to efficacy, hip protectors are a simple intervention that can help reduce the incidence of hip fractures in the frail elderly patient who is at risk for falls and is ambulatory.

In patients with inflammatory diseases who are receiving long-term glucocorticoid therapy and are at risk for osteoporosis, an exercise and physical therapy program is imperative. Such patients often suffer from glucocorticoid-induced myopathy as well as the disuse and deconditioning attendant to the joint pains, myalgias, and systemic inflammation caused by their underlying disorders (eg, rheumatoid arthritis, systemic lupus erythematosus, ankylosing spondylitis, and so forth).

Pharmacologic

Pharmacologic therapies have been intensively researched in recent years. Agents that are effective in preventing and treating osteoporosis and approved in the United States are (1) hormone replacement therapy (HRT), (2) selective estrogen response modulators (SERMs), (3) calcitonin, (4) bisphosphonates, and (5) teriparatide (parathyroid hormone [PTH] 1-34). A summary of the treatment strategies is outlined in Table 54–6.

A. HORMONE REPLACEMENT THERAPY

HRT refers to the combination of estrogen and progestin while estrogen replacement therapy (ERT) involves the use of an estrogen preparation exclusively, typically only in patients who have had a hysterectomy. A variety of estrogen preparations have been used in the prevention and treatment of postmenopausal osteoporosis. Perhaps the most popular and best studied has

Table 54–6. Management of postmenopausal and glucocorticoid-induced osteoporosis.

• Lifestyle modifications	Discontinue tobacco Discontinue alcohol intake Wear hip protector Exercise regularly
• Nutritional interventions	Increase calcium intake to 1000 mg elemental calcium per day for prevention of osteoporosis in premenopausal women and to 1000–1500 mg elemental calcium per day for postmenopausal women, men, and patients taking glucocorticoids long term; Vitamin D intake: 400 IU/d for men and postmenopausal women, 400–800 IU/d for patients taking glucocorticoids long term

• Pharmacologic therapies	• Hormone replacement therapy (various regimens)
	  Conjugated equine estrogens 0.3, 0.625, 0.9, or 1.25 mg + 2.5 or 5 mg medroxyprogesterone acetate per day
	  Transdermal estradiol 100 μg/day on days 1–21 + medroxyprogesterone acetate on days 11–31
	  Micronized estradiol 0.5 mg per day + progestin
	• SERMs
	  Raloxifene 60 mg/d
	• Calcitonin
	  Nasal spray calcitonin 200 IU intranasally daily
	• Bisphosphonates
	  Alendronate 5 mg/d or 35 mg/wk for prevention of osteoporosis; 10 mg/d or 70 mg/wk for treatment of postmenopausal, male, and glucocorticoid-induced osteoporosis
	  Risedronate 5 mg/d or 35 mg/wk for prevention and treatment of postmenopausal and glucocorticoid-induced osteoporosis
	• Parathyroid hormone
	  Teriparatide (PTH 1–34) 20 μg subcutaneous per day for postmenopausal and male osteoporosis

SERMs, selective estrogen response modulators.

been the combination of conjugated equine estrogens and medroxyprogesterone acetate in varying dosages. It has been well established that endometrial hyperplasia and carcinoma are prevented when unopposed estrogen is replaced with the combination because the latter does not permit continuous endometrial stimulation.

Studies like the PEPI (Postmenopausal Estrogen/ Progestin Interventions) trial established the efficacy of various HRT and ERT regimens to prevent postmenopausal bone loss at the spine and hip, based on DXA measurements after 36 months of therapy in 875 women. This study showed average +3 to 5% increases in lumbar spine BMD and +1.7% increases in hip BMD after treatment with a variety of ERT and HRT regimens for 36 months. Placebo-treated patients lost bone mineral (−1.8% and −1.7% in changes in BMD values in the lumbar spine and hip, respectively). However, what the PEPI trial and other studies of HRT/ERT in postmenopausal osteoporosis lacked was a direct quantification of antifracture benefit.

Despite the lack of documented fracture protection with HRT/ERT, these treatments remained popular preventive strategies for postmenopausal women until recently. HRT/ERT was believed to reduce the risks of coronary heart disease and its complications, based on epidemiologic studies, and to have little or no effect on breast cancer. Overall, HRT/ERT was thought to have an acceptable risk-benefit profile.

Publications from the HERS (Heart and Estrogen/ Progestin Replacement Study) trial and the WHI (Women's Health Initiative) have challenged those concepts fundamentally. HERS was a large secondary prevention trial in 2763 women with established coronary heart disease who were randomized to placebo or HRT (0.625 mg conjugated estrogens and 2.5 mg medroxyprogesterone acetate per day). This study failed to demonstrate a benefit of HRT on coronary heart disease outcomes in these patients.

The WHI further challenged any use of HRT in postmenopausal women. The WHI examined the risks and benefits of HRT (0.625 mg conjugated equine estrogens and 2.5 mg medroxyprogesterone acetate per day) in 16,608 women in the primary prevention of several postmenopausal health outcomes. There was a small but significant increased risk of invasive breast cancer in women receiving HRT compared with those receiving placebo after 5.2 years (HR [hazards ratio] 1.26; 95% confidence interval [CI] [1.00–1.59]) and a similar small increase in coronary heart disease end points due to HRT (HR 1.29; 95% CI [1.02–1.63]).

Ironically, this study did show a reduction in hip fractures (HR 0.66; [0.45–0.98]) due to HRT. Despite the salutary effect on fractures, the other negative outcomes from WHI (increased cardiovascular and breast cancer risks) have had a significant negative impact on the use of HRT in postmenopausal women. At present, it is recommended that HRT be used for as short a time as possible after menopause, in the lowest possible doses, and mainly for the control of vasomotor symptoms. Other approaches for the prevention and treatment of osteoporosis are recommended (see following sections).

B. RALOXIFENE

Raloxifene belongs to a growing class of drugs called SERMs. SERMs differ from estrogen biochemically and structurally, but they can act like estrogen agonists or antagonists depending on the specific target tissues. Raloxifene was developed with the goal of capitalizing on the benefits of estrogen in bone and eliminating or strongly diminishing the impact of estrogen-like compounds on cardiovascular and breast cancer risks. Results from studies with raloxifene suggest that it may be possible to achieve such outcomes.

The MORE (Multiple Outcomes of Raloxifene Evaluation) study was designed to assess the efficacy of raloxifene in postmenopausal women. Two groups of women were recruited: Group 1 had BMD T-scores at the lumbar spine or femoral neck of < −2.5; group 2 had reduced BMD and ≥ 1 moderate or severe vertebral fractures or ≥ 2 moderate fractures alone. The primary skeletal outcomes were changes in BMD and incident vertebral fractures. Secondary skeletal end points were nonvertebral fractures. Many other outcomes were also investigated including biochemical markers of bone turnover, cognitive function, breast cancer, and cardiovascular end points. MORE enrolled 7705 women who were treated with raloxifene (60 or 120 mg/d) or with placebo.

After 3 years of therapy, women treated with raloxifene (both doses) demonstrated +2.1 to 2.4% and +2.6 to 2.7% increases in lumbar spine and femoral neck BMD, respectively, which was significantly greater than the responses in placebo-treated women. After 3 years of treatment, the occurrence of vertebral fractures was significantly reduced by 45% (60-mg dose) and 40% (120-mg dose) in group 1 patients and by 30% (60-mg dose) and 50% (120-mg dose) in group 2 patients compared with the placebo group. The overall incidence of nonvertebral fractures (ankle, hip, wrist) was unchanged with raloxifene therapy (RR [relative risk] 0.9; 95% CI [0.8–1.1]), and there was no significant impact on hip fractures (RR 1.1; 95% CI [0.6–1.9]). Similar effects of raloxifene on vertebral and nonvertebral fractures persisted through a fourth year of the MORE trial.

Raloxifene was not associated with an increased risk of endometrial carcinoma, vaginal bleeding, or mastalgia. Venous thromboembolic events, however, were increased in women receiving raloxifene and were recorded in 25 patients (1%) and 24 patients (1%) of women taking 60 and 120 mg of raloxifene, respectively, compared with 8 (0.3%) women receiving placebo (RR 3.1; 95% CI [1.5–6.2]). This incidence of venous thromboembolic events was similar in frequency to that of patients receiving HRT or tamoxifen. Interestingly, the incidence of breast cancer was reduced in both groups of women treated for 40 months with either dose of raloxifene (RR 0.3; 95% CI [0.2–0.6]). Clearly, this SERM does not share the breast cancer risk of estrogen for up to 4 years of treatment, but longer trials are needed with breast cancer as a primary outcome. Additional adverse events that were increased in women taking raloxifene included hot flashes, leg cramps, edema, and a flu-like syndrome.

C. NASAL SPRAY CALCITONIN

Calcitonin in the form of a nasal spray is approved for the treatment of postmenopausal osteoporosis (200 U/d). Calcitonin, a 32-amino-acid peptide hormone, binds to receptors on osteoclasts, and this interaction inhibits osteoclast-mediated bone resorption.

The PROOF (Prevent Recurrence of Osteoporotic Fractures) trial established the efficacy of this agent by comparing the three different doses of calcitonin (100, 200, and 400 IU/d) with placebo in 1255 postmenopausal women. All patients received 1000 mg elemental calcium and 400 IU vitamin D daily. After 5 years of therapy, nasal spray calcitonin (200 IU/d) induced +1.0 to 1.5% increases in lumbar spine BMD that were accompanied by a 33% reduction in new spinal fractures compared with placebo. Hip BMD and hip fractures were not significantly affected by therapy with calcitonin. Adverse events included nasal irritation (congestion, discharge, or sneezing), which was significantly greater than in the placebo group. Despite its modest effects on spinal BMD and the absence of efficacy in reducing hip fractures, calcitonin is an agent that is selective for the skeleton with an excellent tolerability profile.

D. BISPHOSPHONATES

Two drugs in this class are approved for the prevention and treatment of osteoporosis in the United States: alendronate and risedronate. Both are approved for postmenopausal and glucocorticoid-induced osteoporosis, and alendronate is indicated to treat male osteoporosis. These drugs and the general category of bisphosphonates are discussed in detail in Chapter 56. The BMD changes observed with alendronate therapy in men and women treated with glucocorticoids for 24 months are shown in Table 54–7. Both men and women experience statistically significant increases in BMD by DXA measurements compared with placebo. Changes in BMD are larger if postmenopausal women are not taking HRT.

E. TERIPARATIDE

Teriparatide or parathyroid hormone (PTH) 1–34 was approved by the Food and Drug Administration in 2002 for the treatment of osteoporosis in postmenopausal women and men. This therapy capitalizes on the ability of PTH to produce anabolic effects on the skeleton to stimulate bone formation when it is administered in low doses and intermittently. Chronic infusions of PTH in animals and primary hyperparathyroidism in humans are "catabolic" to bone, causing excessive resorption and increased fracture risk. Thus, PTH as a therapy for osteoporosis must target the narrow therapeutic window between the anabolic and catabolic effects of PTH.

1. Indications—

a. Postmenopausal osteoporosis—The study that addressed the efficacy of teriparatide in postmenopausal women enrolled 1637 women with at least one moderate or two mild nontraumatic vertebral fractures by radiographic criteria (on average 2.3 to 2.7 vertebral fractures). Spinal or hip BMD T-scores were ≤ -1, indicating that this was a high-risk cohort for fractures. After 21 months of therapy with subcutaneous injections of

Table 54–7. Average BMD changes (%) due to alendronate (ALN) or placebo in patients on glucocorticoids after 24 months of therapy.

Parameter	Placebo	ALN 5 mg	ALN 10 mg
Lumbar spine BMD	−0.77	2.84	3.85
	(53)	(59)	(51)
Femoral neck BMD	−2.93	0.11	0.61
	(53)	(57)	(51)
Total hip BMD	−1.57	1.64	2.69
	(45)	(47)	(40)
Total body BMD	−0.36	0.77	1.09
	(40)	(44)	(41)
Lumbar spine BMD			
Men (N=17)	0.65	4.29	6.29
Premenopausal women (N=11)	−0.96	0.75	2.34
Postmenopausal women			
No HRT (N=18)	−0.73	1.95	3.91
HRT (N=7)	−3.98	5.36	1.4

BMD, bone mineral density; HRT, hormone replacement therapy. Adapted from Adachi JD et al. Two-year effects of alendronate on bone mineral density and vertebral fracture in patients receiving glucocorticoids. *Arthritis Rheum.* 2001;44:202.

teriparatide, dramatic increases in spinal BMD (+9.7% for 20 μg per day; +13.7% for 40 μg per day) occurred. Lesser but significant increases in femoral neck BMD (+2.8% for 20 μg per day; +5.1% for 40 μg per day) were noted compared with placebo-treated controls (−0.7% to +1.1 for femoral neck and lumbar spine BMD, respectively). The control group received placebo injections, and both groups of women took daily supplements of calcium (1000 mg) and vitamin D (400–1200 IU).

Therapy with teriparatide reduced the risk of new vertebral fractures by 65–69% (20- and 40-μg doses) and of nonvertebral fragility fractures by 53–54% (20- and 40-μg doses). This group of fractures included those of the hip, wrist, ankle, humerus, rib, and so forth. The number of hip fractures did not significantly differ in teriparatide- (4/1093) versus placebo-treated (4/544) patients. New moderate or severe vertebral fractures were substantially reduced by 78–90% in teriparatide- versus placebo-treated patients. This drug was not associated with an increase in nephrolithiasis or renal failure. Adverse events that were significantly more frequent in patients taking teriparatide (20 μg/d) included dizziness and leg cramps (both in < 10% of patients). Hypercalcemia (defined as serum calcium > 10.6 mg/dL) developed in 11% of patients receiving teriparatide (20 μg per day), compared with 2% of patients in the placebo group. Ninety-five percent of these serum calcium values were < 11.2 mg/dL and were managed by reducing calcium intake in most patients.

b. Osteoporosis in men—In a study of teriparatide in male osteoporosis, 437 men were enrolled with T-scores < −2 in the lumbar spine or hip (range: −2.0 to −2.7). Their average age was 59, and approximately 50% had low serum free testosterone levels. Men were treated for 11 months with 20 μg or 40 μg teriparatide subcutaneously per day or with placebo, and all patients received 1000 mg elemental calcium and 400–1200 IU vitamin D per day.

This trial was prematurely terminated because ongoing toxicology studies in rats found an increased incidence of osteosarcomas (see below). At study termination, Orwoll and colleagues found average increases in spinal BMD of +5.9 and +9.0% (20 and 40 μg per day, respectively), in femoral neck BMD of +1.5 and +2.9% (20 and 40 μg per day, respectively), and in total body BMD of +0.6 and +0.9% (20 and 40 μg per day, respectively). All of these changes were significantly greater than those in the placebo group. Teriparatide was found to be effective in men regardless of their gonadal status, age, or baseline BMD values. Biochemical markers of bone turnover showed what has come to be expected with an anabolic agent. Markers of bone formation increased within 1 month of therapy (bone-specific alkaline phosphatase and procollagen I carboxy terminal peptide). Markers of bone resorption (urinary N-telopeptide and deoxypyridinoline) increased at 1 month and remained above baseline throughout the study. The changes in BMD were impressive, given the short duration of the study. Both duration and number of subjects in this study render it underpowered for assessing fracture risk reduction.

2. Adverse effects—Both of the above studies were terminated early due to results from standard carcinogenicity studies in rats showing that lifelong daily injections of teriparatide induced osteosclerosis and a markedly increased incidence of osteosarcomas (48% of rats treated with teriparatide [75 µg/kg for 17 months]). These findings were carefully considered by the Food and Drug Administration. It was not thought that this outcome was a concern sufficient to block the use of this agent in humans, particularly under the recommended guidelines. These findings from animal testing, however, did lead the FDA to require a "Black Box Warning" in the package insert to inform practitioners and patients of this result.

3. Guidelines for use—Given the above findings, costs, and inconvenience of daily subcutaneous injections with this hormone, teriparatide is recommended to treat bone loss in the following groups: patients with severe osteoporosis, especially accompanied by fractures; patients intolerant to other therapies for osteoporosis; and patients who have not responded to other drugs for osteoporosis. Treatment is recommended not to exceed 2 years in duration and is approved for use in men and postmenopausal women. Teriparatide is *contraindicated* in growing children (with open epiphyses), patients with bone metastases or who have had skeletal irradiation, and patients with Paget disease or an unexplained elevation in the alkaline phosphatase value. Despite the above considerations, teriparatide still holds great promise for both building new bone and increasing the skeleton's biomechanical strength—outcomes that are highly desired to prevent ongoing osteoporotic fractures in high-risk patients.

How should teriparatide be best used to treat osteoporosis? It is anticipated that 2 years of therapy with this agent will be followed by long-term therapy with antiresorptive drugs in an effort to maintain the gains in BMD achieved with this anabolic agent. While this idea is at present intuitively sound, the exact nature and long-term efficacy of such regimens have not been evaluated in rigorous clinical trials. Many trials, however, are ongoing and should provide the data to support either sequential or combination regimens of anabolic and/or antiresorptive therapies.

F. COMBINATION AND SEQUENTIAL REGIMENS

A small number of trials combining approved agents for the treatment of osteoporosis, either together or in sequence, have been published. These studies include the combination of alendronate and HRT, risedronate and HRT, PTH and HRT, and alendronate and raloxifene, and the sequential use of PTH and alendronate. These studies are in general smaller than the pivotal trials reviewed above that established the efficacy of individual therapies in the treatment of osteoporosis and prevention of fractures. Nevertheless, there is typically a small additional increase in BMD that can be attained with the combination of two antiresorptive therapies—beyond the changes seen with one agent alone. None of the combination or sequential studies has had fracture reduction as an end point so a clear role for these approaches to prevent fractures is not yet established. Both costs and adverse events are potentially additive. There has been the additional concern that excessive blockade of resorption might produce so marked a degree of suppression of turnover that the ability to repair microdamage and microfractures and respond to the normal forces acting on the remodeling process would be blocked.

Sequential regimens that combine anabolic agents like teriparatide with potent antiresorptive drugs have theoretic appeal. There are, however, no data that firmly establish the superior efficacy of such regimens or that even point to the best technique for accomplishing anabolic effects followed by inhibition of resorption. In future years, clinicians will likely use more sophisticated approaches to the therapy of osteoporosis that will combine the unique features of the available drugs with a better understanding of how to manipulate the bone remodeling cycle to the best advantage.

■ WHEN TO REFER TO A SPECIALIST

The most ominous danger sign related to osteoporosis is the occurrence of multiple fractures in a patient receiving effective therapy. Decrements in BMD during therapy are also a cause for concern if they exceed the precision errors of DXA measurements. Noncompliance with therapy would be the first explanation to consider as the therapies discussed above are highly efficacious. None of them, however, completely prevents all fractures so the decision that the clinician must make is whether the fracture is to be expected or not in the context of the individual patient. The clinician must consider the length of therapy, underlying risk factors contributing to the patient's bone loss, baseline BMD values, degree of trauma if any, and other medications and conditions that may be exacerbating the fracture risk or bone loss. If a patient suffers a fracture while receiving therapy, the clinician must also decide whether the initial work-up was sufficient and whether all possible secondary causes were considered and properly eliminated. On many occasions, especially in postmenopausal women, this is the first opportunity for a thorough laboratory evaluation of the patient. Often, this type of evaluation will disclose additional disease states (eg, primary hyperparathyroidism, multiple myeloma, vitamin D deficiency, celiac sprue, etc) that were not diagnosed or even considered at the outset. If the clinician is inexperienced with the evaluation of secondary osteoporosis or deciding whether BMD determinations indicate adequate responses to treatment, then this is an excellent time to refer a patient with fractures or ongoing bone loss while receiving therapy to a specialist (rheumatologist or endocrinologist) experienced in the care of patients with osteoporosis.

REFERENCES

Cummings SR, et al. Risk factors for hip fracture in white women. Study of Osteoporotic Fractures Research Group. *N Engl J Med*. 1995;332:767. [PMID: 7862179]

Kanis JA. Diagnosis of osteoporosis and assessment of fracture risk. *Lancet*. 2002;359:1929. [PMID: 12057569]

Lane NE, Lukert B. The science and therapy of glucocorticoid-induced bone loss. *Endocrinol Metab Clin North Am*. 1998; 27:465. [PMID: 9669150]

Medicare program; Medicare coverage of and payment for bone mass measurement—HCFA. Interim final rule with comment period. *Fed Regist*. 1998;63:34320. [PMID: 10180295]

National Osteoporosis Foundation. *Physician's Guide to Prevention and Treatment of Osteoporosis*. Excerpta Medica, 1998.

Nelson HD, et al. Screening for postmenopausal osteoporosis: a review of evidence for the US Preventive Services Task Force. *Ann Intern Med*. 2002;137:529. [PMID: 12230356]

NIH Consensus Statement, Osteoporosis Prevention, Diagnosis, and Therapy, Office of the Director, Vol 17 (1), p.5, 2000.

Orwoll ES, et al. Determinants of bone mineral density in older men. *Osteoporos Int*. 2000;11:815. [PMID: 11199184]

Orwoll ES, Bliziotes M. *Osteoporosis: Pathophysiology and Clinical Management*. Humana Press, 2003.

Recommendations for the prevention and treatment of glucocorticoid-induced osteoporosis: 2001 update. American College of Rheumatology Ad Hoc Committee on Glucocorticoid-Induced Osteoporosis. *Arthritis Rheum*. 2001;44:1496. [PMID: 11465699]

Shoback D, et al. Mineral metabolism and metabolic bone disease. In: Greenspan F, Gardner D. *Basic & Clinical Endocrinology*. 6th ed. McGraw Hill, 2001:273–333.

US Preventive Services Task Force. Screening for osteoporosis in postmenopausal women: recommendation and rationale. *Ann Intern Med*. 2002;137:526. [PMID: 12230355]

Relevant World Wide Web Sites

[National Osteoporosis Foundation]
http://www.nof.org
[The American Society for Bone and Mineral Research]
http://www.asbmr.org
[Osteoporosiscme.org]
http://www.osteoporosiscme.org

Osteonecrosis

Carol M. Ziminski, MD

ESSENTIALS OF DIAGNOSIS

- *Pain is the most frequent presenting symptom of osteonecrosis.*
- *The most commonly affected sites are the proximal and distal femoral heads, resulting in hip or knee pain; ankle, shoulder, or elbow may also be affected.*
- *Groin pain is most common in patients with femoral head disease; thigh and buttock pain occur less often.*
- *Most patients have weight-bearing and motion-associated pain.*
- *Pain at rest occurs in two-thirds of patients; one-third report night pain.*
- *A small proportion of patients are asymptomatic, in which case the diagnosis is generally incidental.*

General Considerations

Osteonecrosis is a generic term that refers to cell death in the two components of bone, both hematopoietic fat marrow and osteocytes. Other terms frequently used for this condition are "ischemic necrosis, avascular necrosis, aseptic necrosis," and "osteochondritis dessicans."

Osteonecrosis is not a discrete disease but represents the final common pathway of several conditions, most of which result in impairment of the blood supply to the bone. Osteonecrosis may occur in a variety of clinical settings, in association with defined diseases (eg, infiltrative process such as Gaucher disease), medications (eg, glucocorticoids), physiologic or pathologic conditions (eg, pregnancy, thromboembolism, trauma), or without identifiable predisposing factors (idiopathic).

The real prevalence of osteonecrosis is unknown, but it is estimated that there are approximately 10,000 to 20,000 new cases annually in the United States, and osteonecrosis is the underlying diagnosis in approximately 10% of all total hip replacements. For the most part, osteonecrosis affects the epiphyses of the long bones, such as the femoral and humeral heads, but other bones (eg, carpal and tarsal) can also be affected. The disease occurs more frequently in males than females, with the overall male to female ratio in the range of 8:1. The age distribution is wide, although most patients are younger than age 50 at the time of diagnosis. The average age of female cases exceeds that of males by almost 10 years.

Pathogenesis

Osteonecrosis may be seen in association with a number of different conditions (Table 55–1). A definitive etiologic role has been established for some of these factors but most are probable relationships. Glucocorticoid use and excessive alcohol intake reportedly account for more than 90% of cases.

The pathogenesis of osteonecrosis remains controversial in current literature. Most clinicians believe that it results from the combined effects of metabolic factors, local factors affecting blood supply (such as vascular damage), increased intraosseous pressure, and mechanical stresses. It likely begins with interruption of the blood supply to bone; subsequently, the adjacent area becomes hyperemic, leading to demineralization, trabecular thinning, and if stressed, bony collapse. The process is usually progressive, resulting in joint destruction within 3 to 5 years if left untreated.

Trauma with fracture of the femoral neck, especially in the subcapital region, interrupts the major part of the blood supply to the femoral head and may lead to ischemia and osteonecrosis. The incidence of osteonecrosis in such cases is at least 30% and increases for badly displaced fractures, particularly in young adults. Dislocation and fracture-dislocation are much less common than hip fracture, but the incidence of osteonecrosis may be quite high if reduction is accomplished more than 6 hours after dislocation.

Osteonecrosis is common in patients with homozygous **sickle cell disease** because of red blood cell sickling and bone marrow hyperplasia. Osteonecrosis develops in about 50% of affected patients by age 35.

Gaucher disease is an autosomal recessive disorder of glucocerebroside metabolism that leads to the accumulation of cerebroside-filled cells within the bone marrow. This may result in compression of the vascula-

Table 55–1. Etiologic factors associated with osteonecrosis.

Osteonecrosis of Known Etiology
  Traumatic
    Femoral neck fracture
    Dislocation or fracture dislocation of the hip
  Nontraumatic
    Sickle-cell disease
    Gaucher disease
    Caisson disease (decompression sickness, diver's dis
      ease)
    Radiotherapy
Osteonecrosis with Probably Etiologic Relationships
  Traumatic
    Minor trauma
  Nontraumatic
    Glucocorticoids (exogenous and endogenous)
      Enteral, intra-articular, pulse intravenous
      Organ transplantation
      Cushing disease
    Alcohol use
    Connective tissue diseases (may occur independent of
      glucocorticoid use)
    Systemic lupus erythematosus
    Rheumatoid arthritis
    Systemic vasculitis
    Antiphospholipid antibody syndrome
    Other connective tissue diseases
    Metabolic disorders
      Hyperuricemia/gout
      Hyperlipidemia
      Chronic renal failure or hemodialysis
    Disorders associated with fat necrosis
      Pancreatitis
      Pancreatic cancer
    Hematologic disorders
      Intravascular coagulation
      Thrombophlebitis
    Pregnancy
    Cigarette smoking
    Tumors (infiltrative)
    Idiopathic

---

ture and subsequent osteonecrosis. Osteonecrosis has been reported in 60% of patients with Gaucher disease.

The increased pressure associated with **caisson disease (decompression sickness or diver's disease)** can lead to the formation of nitrogen bubbles, which may occlude arterioles and cause osteonecrosis. This may develop years after the exposure. The number of exposures, and the magnitude of depth or pressure, are important risk factors.

Many studies have related glucocorticoid use to the development of osteonecrosis, although many are small retrospective series and case reports with anecdotal evidence and inadequate controls. The overall incidence of developing osteonecrosis as a result of glucocorticoid therapy is very low.

The risk of osteonecrosis with glucocorticoid therapy appears to be dose-related. Patients treated with prolonged high doses of glucocorticoids seem to be at greatest risk for the development of osteonecrosis, although such patients often have multiple other risk factors. Osteonecrosis may develop in patients treated with physiologic glucocorticoid replacement for adrenal insufficiency. In comparison, osteonecrosis is a rare complication of short-term glucocorticoid use, including pulse therapy and intra-articular glucocorticoid injections.

Most studies have found that the risk is low (less than 3%) in patients treated with doses of prednisone less than 15–20 mg/d. In one series, the prednisone dose in the highest month of therapy exceeded 40 mg/d in 93%, and 20 mg/d in 100% of patients with osteonecrosis. The only clinical finding that distinguished patients with osteonecrosis from those without this complication was a Cushingoid appearance (86% vs 15%).

Osteonecrosis is a rare complication of **Cushing disease.** This probably reflects the lower glucocorticoid exposure than seen with high-dose glucocorticoid therapy.

Osteonecrosis is probably the most debilitating of the musculoskeletal complications following renal transplantation. In this setting, it is usually multifocal, with 50–70% of affected persons having more than one joint involved. The risk has decreased since the introduction of cyclosporine, with resultant decrease in glucocorticoid dose. It is not clear whether osteopenia and preexisting hyperparathyroidism are independent risk factors in this population.

Excessive alcohol use and the development of osteonecrosis have been linked for decades: fat emboli, venous stasis, and increased cortisol levels have all been implicated as etiologic factors. An elevated risk for regular drinkers and a clear dose-response relationship has been noted.

Osteonecrosis has been reported in 3–30% of patients with **systemic lupus erythematosus (SLE).** This range reflects the use of different techniques in defining the disorder (from the less sensitive radiograph to the very sensitive magnetic resonance imaging [MRI]), variations in glucocorticoid doses, and variable periods of follow-up. At greatest risk are patients with SLE who have taken glucocorticoids, although occasional cases have occurred in the absence of glucocorticoid treatment. Osteonecrosis often develops in patients with SLE a relatively short time after the initiation of glucocorticoid therapy. Other risk factors have been identified in patients with SLE, including Raynaud phenomenon, antiphospholipid antibodies, hyperlipidemia, regular doses of prednisone greater than 20 mg/d, and evidence of glucocorticoid-associated end-organ effects.

Clinical Findings

A. SYMPTOMS AND SIGNS

Many patients with osteonecrosis have had the disease for some time before symptoms are present. Initial symptoms are often felt during activity and include pain or aching in the affected joint. In some instances, the pain may begin quite suddenly. Osteonecrosis most frequently occurs in the anterolateral femoral head, although it may also involve the humeral head, femoral condyles, proximal tibia, and small bones of the hand and foot. Many patients have bilateral involvement at the time of diagnosis, including disease of the hips, knees, and shoulders.

Physical findings are largely nonspecific. In early stages, decreased range of motion is related primarily to pain, particularly with forced internal rotation and abduction. Bone remodeling allows some patients to remain functional for years, despite limited range of motion. As the disease progresses, the pain increases, associated with stiffness and restricted range of motion of the involved joint. Limping becomes common late in the course of lower extremity disease. The hip is the joint most frequently affected, and the pain is usually felt in the groin. The time from onset of symptoms to development of end-stage joint varies widely, from months to years.

MRI studies comparing symptomatic and asymptomatic joints in people at high risk for development of osteonecrosis have demonstrated a preclinical stage. Abnormalities in asymptomatic joints may predate clinical symptoms by weeks to months.

B. IMAGING STUDIES

1. Radiography—The diagnosis of osteonecrosis has been based on plain radiographs, which may identify advanced disease but are less helpful in early stages. The evaluation for suspected osteonecrosis of the femoral head should begin with anteroposterior and frog-leg lateral radiographs. Lateral views are necessary to evaluate the superior portion of the femoral head, where subchondral abnormalities may be seen. The plain radiograph may remain normal for months after onset of symptoms; the earliest findings are mild density changes followed by sclerosis and cysts as the disease progresses. The pathognomonic crescent sign (subchondral radiolucency) is evidence of subchondral collapse. Later stages evidence loss of sphericity or collapse of the femoral head. Eventually, joint space narrowing and degenerative changes in the acetabulum are apparent.

2. Radionuclide bone scan—Technetium-99m bone scanning is useful for patients with suspected disease who have normal radiographs, unilateral symptoms, and no risk factors. Increased uptake, either because of new bone formation or simply as a result of metabolic activity around the necrotic area, can be demonstrated. This technique has limitations, however:

- It is nonspecific except when a characteristic but rare decreased uptake is observed in the center of an uptake area within the femoral head ("cold in hot" image or doughnut sign).

- It should be judged by comparison with the contralateral joint, and so may be of little use in bilateral disease.

- It is relatively insensitive in the precollapse stages, where it gives a positive result in only 70% of cases.

3. Computed tomography—The introduction of computed tomography (CT) allowed considerable progress in imaging of osteonecrosis. CT images can display early sclerosis in the central part of the femoral head ("asterisk sign") and give an evaluation of the size of the sequestrum. Importantly, CT demonstrates well the anterior part that is preferentially involved in osteonecrosis of the femoral head, and slight anterior collapse is in some cases visible only on CT images.

4. Magnetic resonance imaging—MRI is much more sensitive than either plain radiographs or bone scanning, with a reported overall sensitivity of 91%. Changes can be seen early in the course of disease when other studies are negative.

In early osteonecrosis, there is an area of low-intensity signal in the medial aspect of the femoral head, particularly in the subchondral zone. The focal defect involving the anterosuperior aspect of the femoral head, but occasionally extending to the metaphysis, is the most common abnormality observed (96% of cases).

The most characteristic image, seen in 60–80% of cases, is a margin of low signal on T1- and T2-weighted images. An inner border of high signal associated with this low-signal line on T2-weighted images, the "double-line sign," is considered pathognomonic for osteonecrosis and has been described in 50–80% of cases. This high signal intensity on T2-weighted images is thought to result from an increased water content, either intravascular or in the interstitial spaces. It may also reflect the presence of mesenchymal tissue in the marrow surrounding the interface.

MRI is very sensitive; in fact, all cases of collapse of the femoral head demonstrate an identical MRI image, which is not necessarily useful. However, at early stages, before collapse, MRI has the best sensitivity and the best accuracy (75–100%) compared with other investigative techniques. Nevertheless, there have been reports of cases of osteonecrosis with normal MRI.

C. SPECIAL TESTS

Functional bone investigations (such as bone marrow pressure, stress tests with injection of saline, and intramedullary venography) have demonstrated that decreased blood flow and increased bone marrow pressure measurements with injection can occur even in the early stages of osteonecrosis. These tests are very sensitive but not specific and may be positive in processes such as osteoarthritis of the hip and transient osteoporosis of the hip. These studies have largely been replaced by MRI as a means of diagnosing osteonecrosis. However, caution must be exercised in interpreting MRI findings, particularly in asymptomatic patients. Treatment based on abnormal MRI findings alone, in the absence of symptoms, may result in overtreatment of some patients.

D. CLASSIFICATION AND STAGING

Classification of osteonecrosis has been based on pathologic findings, while staging is usually based on radiologic and histologic features. Several proposed systems of staging, based on the sequence of changes seen by radiography and by other investigative techniques, have been proposed since the initial description by Arlet and Ficat, which was based primarily on radiographic findings. Newer imaging modalities and the need for quantification of involvement have led to these revisions. Recently, the Subcommittee of Nomenclature of the International Association on Bone Circulation and Bone Necrosis (ARCO: Association of Research Circulation Osseous) has reassembled the results of these classifications to establish an internationally accepted system of classification of the various stages of osteonecrosis (Table 55–2). This standardized system is designed to enhance uniformity among comparative epidemiologic studies and to facilitate clinical trials of treatment strategies.

Differential Diagnosis

At stages 3 and 4, radiographic findings are specific, and no differential problem should occur. If late stages 5 and 6 are noted for the first time, is it impossible to diagnose osteonecrosis as the cause of destruction of the hip. The question is of no practical consequence, however, since total hip replacement is essentially the only therapeutic option.

The challenging differential diagnoses relate to stages 1 and 2. In stage 1, all diseases that may affect bone,

Table 55–2. Stages of osteonecrosis.

Stage 0
All diagnostic studies normal; diagnosis by histology, necrosis on biopsy. Thus, osteonecrosis can exist histologically without any associated clinical signs or symptoms.

Stage 1
Plain radiographs and computed tomography (CT) normal; radionuclide scan or magnetic resonance imaging (MRI) abnormal and biopsy positive, extent of involvement A, B, or C (less than 15%, 15–30%, and greater than 30%, respectively). The patient may or may not be symptomatic at this stage.

Stage 2
A variety of radiographic abnormalities that are signs of eventual bone death are evident within the femoral head. These may include areas of linear sclerosis, focal mineralization, or cysts in the femoral head or neck. The femoral head, however, is still spherical, as evidenced on both anteroposterior and lateral radiographs and on the CT scan. There is no subchondral lucency or collapse; extent of involvement A, B, or C.

Stage 3
The femoral head has begun to fail mechanically. The radiolucent "crescent sign" appearing just beneath the subchondral end plate is the hallmark of this stage; it indicates collapse of the subchondral cancellous trabeculae. The spherical configuration of the articular surface remains intact. The crescent sign does not always develop as the femoral head progresses from earlier to later stages of involvement. Because the femoral head remains spherical, it should theoretically be possible to preserve its integrity by surgical measures that allow the necrotic and collapsed bone to be replaced by viable tissue. Extent of involvement A, B, or C.

Stage 4
The first sign of stage 4 is any evidence of flattening of the femoral head with joint space narrowing. This has important therapeutic implications because the hip has now progressed to the point at which the changes are irreversible. The collapse usually occurs in the anterolateral or superior weight-bearing region. The distinction between stage 2 and stage 4 is best demonstrated by CT scan, which is more sensitive than plain radiographs. Extent of involvement is quantitated A, B, or C as above, with further characterization by amount of depression (in millimeters).

Stage 5
Any or all of the preceding radiographic changes may be seen, and in addition there is a decrease in the joint space. In this situation, there is osteoarthritis secondary to the mechanical collapse of the femoral head, with sclerosis, cysts of the acetabulum, and occasionally marginal osteophytes.

Stage 6
Extensive destruction of the femoral head following the degenerative process.

From the Subcommittee on Nomenclature of the International Association on Bone Circulation and Bone Necrosis (ARCO: Association of Research Circulation Osseous).

cartilage, or synovial tissue must be considered as possible explanation for the joint pain. In stage 2, nonspecific bone lesions on radiographs should prompt radionuclide scan or MRI if patients are thought to be at risk for osteonecrosis. The difficult differential diagnosis is transient osteoporosis of the hip or hip algodystrophy, in which the same osteopenia of the femoral head can be observed on radiographs, with the same radionuclide uptake and possibly the same low-signal area on T1-weighted MRI. The only difference is on the T2-weighted image, in which algodystrophy displays a high signal in contrast to the low signal seen in osteonecrosis.

Treatment

The management of osteonecrosis remains one of the most controversial topics in the orthopedic literature. The goal of treatment is to preserve the native joint for as long as possible. Conservative measures may be the only treatment needed for patients with stages 0 and 1 disease, although core decompression may provide some advantages in these cases. Total joint replacement in later-stage disease should ideally be performed before total collapse of the femoral head occurs.

A. CONSERVATIVE THERAPY

Stages 0, 1, and 2 may be treated by conservative measures or by core decompression. Conservative treatment includes bed rest, nonsteroidal anti-inflammatory drugs or other analgesics, physical therapy to maintain muscle strength and prevent contractures, and assistive devices to facilitate ambulation. This approach has generally been ineffective in halting the progression of disease.

Patients with osteonecrosis of non-weight-bearing joints may not require any intervention because they may have only mild to moderate pain, and minimal, tolerable functional limitation. Results of conservative therapy in non-weight-bearing joints may be more successful.

B. CORE DECOMPRESSION

The technique of core decompression was initially used as a diagnostic tool to measure bone marrow pressure and obtain biopsy specimens. It evolved into a treatment mode when it was observed that some patients had pain relief following the procedure.

The rationale for core decompression is to reduce intraosseous pressure, reestablish blood supply, and allow living bone adjacent to dead bone to contribute to the reparative process. Good to excellent results have been obtained in most of patients with stages 1 and 2 osteonecrosis, and in a significant proportion of patient with stage 3 disease. The results of this technique are still controversial, and the best results vary from

34–95% in early stages, but they are always better than simply discontinuing weight bearing.

C. OSTEOTOMY

Osteotomy has also been used as a joint-sparing technique. The stated goal of this procedure is to remove the diseased section of the femoral head from the region of major weight bearing, and to redistribute the weight-bearing forces to articular cartilage that is supported by healthy bone.

There are many reports in European and Japanese literature concerning the use of osteotomies for salvage of hips with stage 2 and 3 disease, with variable results. All of these osteotomies require a period of restricted weight bearing of 3 months to 1 year, and usually until there is radiographic evidence of healing of the osteotomy. One potential problem with the use of an osteotomy is that it may make it more difficult to obtain a good outcome if the hip in the future needs to be converted to an arthroplasty.

D. JOINT REPLACEMENT

Patients with persistent, intractable pain and progressive functional loss should be considered for arthroplasty. Ideally, this should be accomplished before total collapse of the femoral head occurs in patients with hip involvement. The usual treatment for late stage 3 or stage 4 disease has been total hip arthroplasty but results have been inconsistent. Most studies suggest a worse prognosis in this disease than for others, with a higher rate of early failures compared with age-matched patients with other diagnoses. Possible reasons for the higher failure rate in patients with osteonecrosis include poor bone quality (size of necrotic area and degree of bone collapse), bilateral disease, and presence of an underlying condition.

E. OTHER

A number of other treatment methods have been investigated, including the use of vascularized bone grafting with core decompression, and pharmacologic agents (such as naftidrofuryl oxalate, dihydroergotamine, and vincamine) aimed at reducing bone marrow pressure. None has yet met with great success. Some promising results have been reported with externally applied pulsing electromagnetic fields. This technique is still under study and development.

Complications

The optimal treatment for osteonecrosis has not yet been determined. Early diagnosis of osteonecrosis may lead to better outcomes. Unfortunately, the natural history of osteonecrosis is usually progressive disease with cortical collapse and joint dysfunction. The outcome is influenced by many factors, particularly the size and localization of the bone necrosis. Osteonecrosis is not a life-threatening process, but it can be a quite debilitating disease that frequently leads to destruction of the hip joint in patients in their third, fourth, or fifth decades of life. Early intervention, both surgical and nonsurgical, has improved the outcome, but still nearly 50% of cases of femoral head osteonecrosis require arthroplasty.

REFERENCES

Arlet J, Ficat RP. Diagnosis of primary femur head osteonecrosis at stage I (preradiologic stage). *Rev Chir Orthop Reparatrice Appar Mot.* 1968;54:637. [PMID: 4236312] (Early description of stages of osteonecrosis based on radiographs.)

Ficat RP. Idiopathic bone necrosis of the femoral head. Early diagnosis and treatment. *J Bone Joint Surg Br.* 1985;67:3. [PMID: 3155746] (Review and discussion of osteonecrosis.)

Mont MA, Hungerford DS. Non-traumatic avascular necrosis of the femoral head. *J Bone Joint Surg Am.* 1995;77:459. [PMID: 7890797] (Current concepts, extensive review of etiology, pathogenesis, staging, and treatment options, from a group with decades of interest and experience.)

Pavelka K. Osteonecrosis. *Ballieres Best Pract Res Clin Rheumatol.* 2000;14:399. [PMID: 10925752] (Thoughtful discussion of evidence-based diagnosis and treatment.)

Stulberg BN, et al. Making core decompression work. *Clin Orthop.* 1990;261:186. [PMID: 2245544] (Randomized, controlled study with compelling evidence for efficacy of core decompression.)

Zizic TM, et al. The early diagnosis of ischemic necrosis of bone. *Arthritis Rheum.* 1986;29:1177. [PMID: 3768054] (Postulated elevated intraosseous pressure as the common pathway of osteonecrosis.)

Relevant World Wide Web Sites

[The Center for Osteonecrosis Research and Education]
http://www.osteonecrosis.org
[The National Osteonecrosis Foundation]
http://www.nonf.org
[Support Group for Patients with Osteonecrosis]
http://members.aol.com/MarieS1520/2bkn.html

SECTION IX

Therapies

Medications

56

■ NONSTEROIDAL ANTI-INFLAMMATORY DRUGS

John B. Imboden, MD

MECHANISM OF ACTION

- Inhibition of prostaglandin synthesis: Nonsteroidal anti-inflammatory drugs (NSAIDs) inhibit cyclooxygenase (COX), which converts arachidonic acid to prostaglandins. Aspirin inhibits COX through the acetylation of the enzyme, a process that is irreversible. The other NSAIDs are competitive antagonists and reversible inhibitors. There are two isoforms of COX: COX-1, whose expression is constitutive and ubiquitous, and COX-2, which is not constitutively expressed by most tissues but can be induced by inflammatory stimuli. In general, it is thought that inhibition of COX-2 accounts for the anti-inflammatory, antipyretic, and analgesic effects of NSAIDs and that inhibition of COX-1 explains much of the toxicity of NSAIDs. Inhibition of COX-1 accounts for the inhibitory effect of NSAIDs on platelets, which do not express COX-2. Celecoxib, rofecoxib, and valdecoxib selectively inhibit COX-2; all other NSAIDs inhibit both COX-1 and COX-2.

OTHER ACTIONS

- Inhibition of COX may not explain all the effects of NSAIDs, but there is no consensus as to other pharmacologically relevant targets.

PHARMACOKINETICS

- Bioavailability: Very high.
- NSAIDs circulate tightly bound to plasma proteins (> 99% protein-bound for most; approximately 70% for aspirin).
- Metabolism: The liver converts NSAIDs to inactive metabolites. Some NSAIDs undergo extensive enterohepatic circulation.
- Half-life: Varies greatly among individual NSAIDs (Table 56–1). Longer half-lives permit once-daily dosing but lead to substantial delays in reaching steady-state levels of drug (eg, 7–12 days in the case of piroxicam).
- Aspirin and diflunisal exhibit concentration-dependent elimination kinetics with the result that small increases in doses can produce disproportionately large increases in plasma drug levels.
- Clearance: Renal excretion is the major means of elimination of metabolites. Usually only a small percentage of the parent drug is renally cleared.

USES IN RHEUMATIC DISEASE

NSAIDs are used in a wide range of rheumatic conditions. The Food and Drug Administration has approved most for use in osteoarthritis (OA) and many for rheumatoid arthritis as well. NSAIDs are used for treatment of the spondyloarthropathies, are effective in the management of acute flares of gout, and are prescribed widely for bursitis, tendinitis, and other soft tissue complaints.

Table 56–1. Selected nonsteroidal anti-inflammatory drugs.

Drug (trade name)	Half-life (h)	Dosing[a]	Comments
Arylcarboxylic acids			
Diflunisal (Dolobid)	8–12	250–500 mg bid	Concentration-dependent elimination kinetics
Arylalkanoic acids			
Diclofenac (Voltaren, Cataflam)	2	50–75 mg bid	
Ibuprofen (Motrin, Advil, Rufen)	2–2.5	200–800 mg qid	Available over the counter
Fenoprofen (Nalfon)	2–3	300–600 mg qid	
Naproxen (Naprosyn, Aleve, Anaprox, Naprelin)	12–17	250–500 mg bid	Available over the counter
Indomethacin (Indocin)	4.5	25–50 mg tid	
Sulindac (Clinoril)	16	150–200 mg bid	Converted by liver to an active metabolite
Enolic acids			
Piroxicam (Feldene)	50	10–20 mg qd	
Meloxicam (Mobic)	15–20	7.5–15 mg qd	
Nonacidic			
Nabumetome (Relafen)	24	1000 mg qd	Prodrug rapidly converted to an active metabolite by the liver
Selective COX-2 inhibitors			
Celecoxib (Celebrex)	11	100–200 mg bid	Sulfonamide hypersensitivity is contraindication
Rofecoxib (Vioxx)	10–17	12.5–25 mg qd	
Valdecoxib (Bextra)	8–11	10 mg qd	

[a]The dose and dosing interval differ for sustained-release formulations. COX, cyclooxygenase.

CHOICE OF NSAID

- A large number of NSAIDs are available in the United States. As a general rule, the NSAIDs are comparable in efficacy, but individual patients may exhibit different responses to particular NSAIDs. Physician and patient preferences, concerns regarding toxicity, and cost usually determine the choice of NSAID. See Table 56–1 for typical dosing ranges of selected NSAIDs in common use in the United States.

- Several factors should inform the choice between a nonselective NSAID (one that inhibits both COX-1 and COX-2) and a selective COX-2 inhibitor:
  - There is no evidence that these two classes of NSAIDs differ in efficacy.
  - The selective COX-2 inhibitors cost substantially more.
  - The selective COX-2 inhibitors have less clinically significant gastrointestinal toxicity than the nonselective NSAIDs. There is general agreement that selective COX-2 inhibitors should be used for patients who have one or more risk factors for the development of NSAID-induced gastrointestinal toxicity (Table 56–2).
  - There are no data to support the preferential use of selective COX-2 inhibitors for patients at risk for

NSAID-induced renal failure (Table 56–3). COX-2, which is constitutively expressed in the kidney, probably contributes to the production of prostaglandins that regulate renal blood flow.

- Patients on low-dose aspirin for primary or secondary cardiac protection present a complex problem. It is not certain whether NSAIDs that reversibly inhibit platelet COX-1 are cardioprotective and thus can

Table 56–2. Risk factors associated with development of NSAID-induced gastrointestinal toxicity.

- Age > 60 years
- Previous history of peptic ulcer or upper gastrointestinal bleeding
- Concomitant glucocorticoid therapy
- Anticoagulation
- Prolonged use of maximum doses of NSAID
- Comorbid conditions (cardiovascular disease, renal insufficiency, hepatic impairment, diabetes, hypertension)

NSAID, nonsteroidal anti-inflammatory drug.
Adapted from Wolfe MM, et al. *N Engl J Med.* 1999;340:1888; and Technology Appraisal Guidance No. 27 of the National Institute of Clinical Excellence, London, www.nice.org.uk.

Table 56–3. Risk factors for hemodynamically mediated renal failure induced by nonsteroidal anti-inflammatory drugs.

- Intrinsic renal disease
- Volume depletion
- Diuretic use
- Cirrhosis
- Heart failure
- Concomitant use of an angiotensin-converting enzyme inhibitor
- Advanced age

substitute for aspirin. Moreover, concomitant treatment with certain nonselective NSAIDs, such as ibuprofen and indomethacin, diminishes the effect of aspirin on platelet function, probably by limiting access of aspirin to the acetylation site of COX-1 (*N Engl J Med.* 2001;345:1809). Selective COX-2 inhibitors do not affect acetylation of platelet COX-1 by aspirin. Concomitant aspirin therapy, however, may reduce the advantage enjoyed by selective COX-2 inhibitors in terms of gastrointestinal toxicity.

INITIATING THERAPY

Complete blood cell (CBC) count, serum electrolytes and creatinine, and liver function tests should be obtained prior to initiating long-term therapy with NSAIDs.

MONITORING THERAPY

Although there are no firm guidelines for monitoring therapy, many clinicians check liver function tests 6–12 weeks after initiating NSAID therapy and periodically monitor the CBC count. Serum electrolytes and creatinine should be monitored closely if NSAIDs are started in a patient at risk for renal toxicity.

SPECIAL PRECAUTIONS

- The presence of one or more of the risk factors for gastrointestinal toxicity listed in Table 56–2 should prompt consideration of an alternative to NSAIDs (eg, acetaminophen) or the use of a selective COX-2 inhibitor.
- NSAIDs should be used cautiously, if at all, when one or more of the risk factors for NSAID-induced hemodynamically mediated renal failure are present (Table 56–3); NSAIDs should not be used when the creatinine clearance is less than 30 mL/min.
- Severe anemia places a patient at greater risk in the event of NSAID-induced gastrointestinal blood loss.

- The selective COX-2 inhibitors are safer for patients with thrombocytopenia or qualitative abnormalities of platelets.
- NSAIDs can worsen heart failure.
- NSAIDs can induce a modest elevation in blood pressure and can blunt the antihypertensive effects of β-blockers, angiotensin-converting enzyme inhibitors, and diuretics.
- NSAIDs can displace drugs from binding sites on plasma proteins, can alter their metabolism or excretion, and can interfere with their actions. The physician should determine whether there are any known interactions with coadministered medications (for example, by using the drug interaction search available at www.PDR.net).
- Patients should be cautioned that combining over-the-counter drugs (eg, aspirin, naproxen, ibuprofen, and ketoprofen) with prescription NSAIDs can increase toxicity.
- Aspirin should be discontinued 1–2 weeks before surgery because its effect on platelets is irreversible. Other NSAIDs should be discontinued for a period equal to 5 times their half-life prior to surgery.
- Aspirin and other nonselective NSAIDs can trigger attacks of severe asthma and marked nasal congestion, particularly in persons with a history of asthma and nasal polyposis. Up to 10% of asthmatic patients display aspirin sensitivity, which usually develops in the third or fourth decade. This reaction is due to inhibition of COX and is not an immune response to the drug. All nonselective NSAIDs are absolutely contraindicated for patients with known aspirin sensitivity. Currently, selective COX-2 inhibitors are also contraindicated although several small studies suggest that rofecoxib may be safe in this setting (*Chest.* 2002;121:1812).
- NSAIDs should be avoided during pregnancy if possible. Concerns regarding bleeding and premature closure of the ductus arteriosus preclude the use of NSAIDs in the final months of pregnancy.

COMPLICATIONS

Common

- Upper gastrointestinal toxicity: Dyspepsia, gastritis, peptic ulceration, hemorrhage, and perforation (*N Engl J Med.* 1999;340:1888; *Gut.* 2003;52:600). Dyspepsia is not a reliable indicator of patients at risk for ulceration, hemorrhage, or perforation; the majority of patients with serious gastrointestinal complications do not have antecedent dyspepsia. Coadministration of H_2-receptor antagonists is not recommended for the routine prevention or treatment of NSAID-induced dyspepsia. Although these agents reduce dyspepsia, they do not protect against, and may even increase, serious gastrointestinal complications. Proton pump inhibitors reduce NSAID-induced dyspepsia, are an effective treatment for NSAID-induced ulcers, and protect against ulcers detected endoscopically. There are as yet no direct comparisons of gastrointestinal toxicity of selective COX-2 inhibitors versus combinations of a nonselective NSAID and a proton pump inhibitor. Coadministration of misoprostol prevents ulcerations and reduces the rate of complications due to ulcers. However, side effects such as diarrhea and abdominal pain are common and limit the usefulness of misoprostol.

- Renal: Retention of sodium and fluid is common. Hemodynamically mediated acute renal failure is reversible and generally occurs when NSAIDs are administered to patients with risk factors for this complication (Table 56–3).
- Hepatic: Transient, modest (< two- to three-fold) elevations of serum aminotransferases are common and do not predict severe liver damage.
- Tinnitus and hearing loss: This frequent complication of high doses of aspirin also occurs with other NSAIDs.

Uncommon or Rare

- Renal: Interstitial nephritis, nephrotic syndrome, papillary necrosis.
- Acute liver injury.
- Lower gastrointestinal: Small bowel ulcers; strictures of the small or large bowel.
- Neutropenia.
- Central nervous system: aseptic meningitis, headaches, dysphoria, cognitive impairment.
- Hypersensitivity reactions.

■ SYSTEMIC GLUCOCORTICOID THERAPY: PREDNISONE, PREDNISOLONE, & METHYLPREDNISOLONE

John B. Imboden, MD

MECHANISM OF ACTION

- Bind to cytoplasmic receptors that then translocate to the nucleus and affect the transcription of target genes.
- Anti-inflammatory effects: The direct and indirect effects on inflammation are diverse and include reduc-

tion of arachnidonic acid release, inhibition of production of proinflammatory cytokines, decreased migration of neutrophils to sites of inflammation, impaired T-cell function, and decreased numbers of eosinophils.

PHARMACOKINETICS

- Bioavailability: 50–90%.
- Metabolism: Prednisone is biologically inactive until reduced to prednisolone in the liver. Prednisone, prednisolone, and methylprednisolone are converted to inactive metabolites by the liver.
- Half-life: 2–3 hours for prednisolone and methylprednisolone; 3–4 hours for prednisone
- Clearance: Metabolites are excreted in the urine.

USES IN RHEUMATIC DISEASE

Glucocorticoids are used for a wide variety of rheumatic diseases, but controlled studies documenting their efficacy in these conditions are few.

Rheumatoid Arthritis

Low-dose glucocorticoids (eg, prednisone or prednisolone 7.5–10 mg/d) are superior to placebo in controlling disease activity in short-term and medium-term studies (Criswell LA, et al. Moderate-term, low-dose glucocorticoids for rheumatoid arthritis [Cochrane Review]. In: The Cochrane Library, Issue 2, 2002. Oxford: Update Software; Gotzsche PC, Johansen HK. Short-term low-dose corticosteroids vs placebo and nonsteroidal antiinflammatory drugs in rheumatoid arthritis [Cochrane Review]. In: The Cochrane Library, Issue 1, 2003. Oxford: Update Software). The addition of low-dose prednisolone to standard care with disease-modifying antirheumatic drugs slowed radiographic progression relative to placebo in a 2-year study of patients with recent-onset rheumatoid arthritis (RA) (*N Engl J Med*. 1995;333:142). There is debate as to whether the benefits of therapy outweigh the risks of prolonged glucocorticoid therapy for chronic RA.

Systemic Lupus Erythematosus & Mixed Connective Tissue Disease

Despite a paucity of controlled trials, the efficacy of glucocorticoids is accepted. Glucocorticoids are a mainstay of regimens to treat acute flares of systemic lupus erythematosus (SLE) and to maintain remissions (see Chapter 19).

Vasculitis

High-dose glucocorticoids are often used in conjunction with cytotoxic drugs in the initial management of Wegener granulomatosis, microscopic polyangiitis, Churg-Strauss syndrome, and polyarteritis nodosa. Giant cell arteritis and Takayasu arteritis are often treated with glucocorticoids alone. (See Chapters 29–34.)

Polymyositis & Dermatomyositis

High-dose glucocorticoids are standard first-line therapy (see Chapter 25).

DOSAGE

- The doses of prednisone and prednisolone are equivalent. Methylprednisolone is slightly more potent (8 mg of methylprednisolone is equivalent to 10 mg of prednisone or prednisolone).
- High-dose oral glucocorticoids (eg, prednisone or prednisolone 1 mg/kg/d or 60 mg/d) are used in an attempt to control severe disease activity rapidly in cases of SLE, vasculitis, inflammatory myopathies, and the like. Because substantial toxicity is likely if high doses are maintained, the dose should be tapered as permitted by the activity of the disease or the use of glucocorticoid-sparing agents, or both.
- Intravenous "pulses" of methylprednisolone (eg, 500–1000 mg/d for 3 days) are sometimes used for severe complications of SLE, vasculitis, and the inflammatory myopathies. Pulses are infused over 1–2 hours (there are rare reports of sudden death and ventricular arrhythmias with rapid infusions).
- Generally only low-dose glucocorticoids (eg, prednisone or prednisolone ≤ 10 mg/d) are used in the treatment of RA. "Maintenance" doses in SLE are often somewhat higher (prednisone or prednisolone 10–15 mg/d).

INITIATING THERAPY

If prolonged therapy is contemplated, bone density should be determined, particularly for patients with risk factors for osteoporosis. Chapter 54 reviews the prophylaxis of glucocorticoid-induced osteoporosis.

MONITORING THERAPY

Serum glucose should be monitored closely when patients with diabetes are treated with systemic glucocorticoids. Routine laboratory studies otherwise are not necessary to monitor therapy but may be indicated to assess the underlying disease.

SPECIAL PRECAUTIONS

In the setting of active infection, diabetes, or osteoporosis, systemic glucocorticoids should be used only after very careful consideration of the indications for treatment, the risks of treatment, and the alternatives to glucocorticoids.

Renal failure does not affect dosing. Some clinicians argue that prednisone should not be used in the setting of severe liver disease, but delayed conjugation to inactive metabolites may offset impaired conversion of prednisone to prednisolone.

COMPLICATIONS

Virtually all complications of glucocorticoids are dose-dependent and increase with the duration of therapy.

- The risk of infection is substantial with prolonged high-dose therapy. The anti-inflammatory effects of systemic glucocorticoids can mask the signs and symptoms of infection, making diagnosis difficult. Systemic glucocorticoids cause the demargination of neutrophils, producing a peripheral leukocytosis in the absence of infection.
- Fat redistribution commonly produces a Cushingoid appearance (truncal obesity, "buffalo hump," and "moon facies") in patients treated with moderate to high doses for prolonged periods but is unusual with low-dose therapy. The complex effects of glucocorticoids on carbohydrate metabolism can exacerbate hyperglycemia in known diabetics or induce clinically apparent diabetes.
- Proximal muscle weakness without elevations of muscle enzymes is a common, reversible side effect of high-dose glucocorticoids (eg, prednisone ≥ 30 mg/d for several weeks).
- The hypothalamic-pituitary-adrenal axis is suppressed with glucocorticoid therapy. The dose, duration of therapy, and individual variation influence the onset and magnitude of this effect but, as a general guide, treatment with prednisone 7.5 mg daily for 3 weeks is sufficient to induce suppression.
- Patients who are receiving glucocorticoid therapy or were recently treated with glucocorticoids are at risk for adrenal insufficiency when stressed by surgery or intercurrent illness. Supplemental doses of glucocorticoids are usually not necessary for mild, nonfebrile illnesses (eg, a "cold"). Prednisone doses should be increased to 15 mg/d for patients undergoing minor surgical procedures or with uncomplicated febrile illnesses; the dose can be returned promptly to baseline with resolution of the event. Patients with severe medical illness or major trauma or facing major surgery should be treated with hydrocortisone 50 mg

intravenously or intramuscularly every 6 hours for several days; the dose can be tapered by 50% per day as the intercurrent event resolves. Patients with septic shock generally require a week of therapy before taper and may require supplementation with fludrocortisone as well (*N Engl J Med.* 1997;337: 1285; 2003;348:727).

- Osteoporosis: See Chapter 54.
- Osteonecrosis: See Chapter 55.
- The risk of peptic ulcer disease is increased in patients receiving systemic glucocorticoids and concomitant nonsteroidal anti-inflammatory drugs.
- Striae, acne, and ecchymoses.
- Hypertension.
- Cataracts.
- Insomnia and mood disturbances are common. Severe side effects (eg, psychosis) can occur with high doses of glucocorticoids.
- Pseudotumor cerebri and pancreatitis are rare side effects.

DISCONTINUING THERAPY

The nature of the underlying disease, the activity of that disease, the use of glucocorticoid-sparing agents, the presence of comorbidities, and practice styles influence the rate at which glucocorticoid therapy is tapered; guidelines for tapering, therefore, are only approximate. For SLE and other diseases that require prolonged treatment with glucocorticoids, high doses (eg, 60–80 mg of prednisone daily) should be continued no longer than necessary and in general should be reduced to moderate levels (eg, 30 mg/d) after 6–10 weeks. Tapering from moderate levels to low doses (10–15 mg/d) can occur at a rate of 2.5 mg every week or 5 mg every other week. Most clinicians taper very slowly (1 mg per month) when the daily dose is 10 mg or less.

Patients treated with long-term glucocorticoids often experience a "steroid withdrawal syndrome" of myalgias, fatigue, and malaise that can at times mimic a flare of the underlying disease.

Following discontinuation of glucocorticoids, the time to recovery of the hypothalamic-pituitary-adrenal axis varies widely (from days to 1 year).

KEY POINTS

- Glucocorticoids are widely used in the treatment of rheumatic disease.
- Toxicity is substantial and increases with dose and duration of treatment.

■ METHOTREXATE (MTX)

John B. Imboden, MD

MECHANISM OF ACTION

- Inhibits dihydrofolate reductase (DHFR) and other folate-dependent enzymes. Inhibition of DHFR accounts for its antineoplastic effects (fully reduced folate is required for DNA synthesis) and much of its toxicity (eg, mucositis, cytopenias).
- Mechanism of action in rheumatoid arthritis (RA) is unclear but may relate to the ability of polyglutamates of MTX to cause the release of extracellular adenosine, which has anti-inflammatory and immunomodulatory properties.

PHARMACOKINETICS

- Bioavailability of low-dose oral MTX: Generally high (mean 70%) but there is considerable individual variability (40–100%).
- 50–60% of MTX is bound to plasma proteins and can be displaced by aspirin and nonsteroidal anti-inflammatory drugs—not clinically significant for low-dose regimens used in rheumatology but very important in high-dose chemotherapy.
- Metabolism: Can be metabolized to polyglutamated derivatives that are active and are retained intracellularly longer than MTX (a monoglutamate).
- Half-life: 3–10 hours for low-dose MTX.
- Clearance: MTX and metabolites are renally cleared (filtered and secreted).

USES IN RHEUMATIC DISEASES

Rheumatoid Arthritis

Randomized controlled trials comparing MTX with placebo established that MTX has substantial clinical benefit in the treatment of the signs and symptoms of RA (*Ann Intern Med.* 1985;103:489; *N Engl J Med.* 1985;312:818). Compared with auranofin, MTX slows the rate of radiographic changes (joint space narrowing and erosions) (*Arthritis Rheum.* 1993;36:613).

Psoriasis

Although widely used for the treatment of psoriatic arthritis, low-dose weekly MTX has been studied in only one randomized controlled study (*Arthritis Rheum.*

1984;27:376), which showed a trend in favor of MTX compared with placebo. High-dose MTX is efficacious in psoriatic arthritis (Jones G, Crotty M, Brooks P. Interventions for treating psoriatic arthritis [Cochrane Review]. In: The Cochrane Library, Issue 1, 2003. Oxford: Update Software). MTX has been used to treat the skin disease of psoriasis since the 1950s.

Other Spondyloarthropathies

Although sometimes used in the treatment of reactive arthritis and ankylosing spondylitis, MTX has not been rigorously studied in these diseases.

Juvenile Chronic Arthritis

MTX is the most widely used DMARD for juvenile chronic arthritis, but data from controlled trials are limited (Takken T, Van der Net J, Helders, PJM. Methotrexate for treating juvenile idiopathic arthritis [Cochrane Review]. In: The Cochrane Library, Issue 1, 2003. Oxford: Update Software).

Polymyositis & Dermatomyositis

MTX, sometimes in doses higher than generally used in the treatment of RA, appears to be effective as an adjunct to glucocorticoid therapy and as a glucocorticoid-sparing agent. The combination of MTX and azathioprine probably has efficacy in refractory disease (*Arthritis Rheum.* 1998,41:392).

Systemic Lupus Erythematosus

MTX is superior to placebo in the management of articular and cutaneous manifestations of the disease and may have glucocorticoid-sparing effects (*J Rheumatol.* 1999;26:1275; *Lupus.* 2001;10:162).

Vasculitis

In an effort to minimize toxicity due to prolonged exposure to cyclophosphamide, MTX has been used to maintain remissions induced in antineutrophil cytoplasmic antibody (ANCA)-associated vasculitis by cyclophosphamide (*Arthritis Rheum.* 2002;47:326).

DOSING

- Given *weekly* as a single dose (can split dose over 24 hours if gastrointestinal symptoms occur).
- Usual starting dose is 7.5 mg orally every week.
- Dose can be increased by increments of 2.5–5 mg every 4–8 weeks until (1) there is a therapeutic effect, (2) the maximal dose is attained (generally 15–20 mg/wk in RA; higher doses are sometimes used in inflammatory diseases of muscle and psoriasis), or (3) toxicity develops. Some clinicians increase the dose to 15 mg/wk at week 4 and, if there is no response, then to 20 mg/wk at week 8. Clinical responses generally occur after a lag of 3–6 weeks in RA.
- Because there is individual variability in bioavailability, many clinicians switch to parenteral administration (usually subcutaneous injection) of MTX before discontinuing for lack of efficacy.
- Use oral folate concomitantly (1 mg/d) to reduce side effects.

INITIATING THERAPY

- Before initiating therapy, the following laboratory tests should be obtained: CBC with platelets; serum electrolytes and creatinine; liver function tests (LFTs), including serum albumin; and tests for hepatitis B and C.
- Chest radiograph (particularly important for patients with underlying pulmonary disease).
- Pretreatment liver biopsy if the patient has (1) a prior history of excessive alcohol consumption, (2) persistently abnormal levels of transaminases, or (3) chronic hepatitis B or C infection (*Arthritis Rheum.* 1994;37: 316).
- Document the mode of contraception, if applicable.

MONITORING THERAPY (ADAPTED FROM *ARTHRITIS RHEUM.* 1994;37:316)

- CBC (including platelets) and LFTs 2–4 weeks after starting, then every 4 weeks, and then every 4–8 weeks **as long as patient is taking MTX.**
- Perform liver biopsy if 5 of 9 (or 6 of 12, if determined monthly) aspartate aminotransferase (AST) levels are abnormal **or** there is an unexplained drop in the serum albumin below the normal range. The extent of fibrosis on liver biopsy dictates whether MTX can be continued. Discontinue MTX if patient refuses liver biopsy.

SPECIAL PRECAUTIONS

- Pregnancy is an absolute contraindication because MTX is an abortifacient and teratogenic. Adequate contraception (for male as well as female patients) is absolutely necessary while taking MTX. Women should not breastfeed while taking MTX.
- Cytopenias (except due to Felty syndrome), active liver disease, alcoholism, and active infections are contraindications to the use of MTX.

- Renal insufficiency reduces the clearance of MTX and its active metabolites and substantially increases the risk of toxicity. Other factors that predispose patients to MTX toxicity include dosing errors, advanced age, untreated folate deficiency, and the use of drugs that block tubular secretion (eg, probenecid, salicylates). Major surgery often leads to transient decreases in renal function and may predispose patients to toxicity.
- MTX should not be given to anyone with a history of "MTX lung" or any other allergic reaction to MTX.
- MTX therapy requires ongoing monitoring and should be used cautiously, if at all, in patients with records of poor compliance.
- Patients taking MTX should not receive live virus vaccines.

COMPLICATIONS

- Common toxicities (likely due to inhibition of DHFR) include gastrointestinal disturbances (nausea, vomiting, diarrhea, anorexia), stomatitis, and cytopenias (especially leukopenia). An elevated mean corpuscular volume (MCV) may presage hematologic toxicity. The incidence of these common toxicities is reduced by daily folate therapy.
- MTX lung is a hypersensitivity reaction that can develop at any time during therapy but occurs most often within the first year (50% within 32 weeks; *Arthritis Rheum.* 1998;42:1327). The onset is usually subacute (weeks) but can be acute (days) or chronic (months). Dyspnea, cough, fever, headache, and malaise are common complaints. Bilateral interstitial infiltrates are the classic radiographic findings, but alveolar infiltrates are not rare. The major diagnostic issues are (1) recognition of MTX as cause of the symptoms and (2) ruling out infectious causes. MTX should be discontinued; most patients receive glucocorticoids.
- Hepatotoxicity correlates with total cumulative dose and manifests as fibrosis of increasing severity, culminating in cirrhosis. The mechanism is unknown. Clinically significant MTX-induced liver disease in appropriately selected patients with RA is very rare in the absence of abnormalities of either transaminases or albumin **when monitoring is performed regularly** (every 4–8 weeks).
- Other toxicities include reversible oligospermia, rash (including urticaria and cutaneous vasculitis), alopecia, accelerated nodulosis, dysphoria and headache, infections (localized and disseminated zoster, opportunistic infections), and low-grade lymphomas.

- Overdoses should be treated as quickly as possible with leucovorin.

KEY POINTS

- MTX has established efficacy in RA and is commonly used in the treatment of other rheumatic diseases.
- MTX should only be administered in the form of weekly pulses; regular monitoring of CBC and LFTs is mandatory during therapy.

■ LEFLUNOMIDE (ARAVA)

John B. Imboden, MD

MECHANISM OF ACTION

- Activity requires conversion to the active metabolite, M1.
- M1 inhibits dihydroorotate dehydrogenase, the rate-limiting enzyme for de novo pyrimidine synthesis, and thereby inhibits B and T lymphocytes, whose proliferation depends on the de novo pathway of pyrimidine synthesis.

PHARMACOKINETICS

- Bioavailability: 80%.
- Metabolism: Rapid metabolism to M1 following oral administration.
- Half-life: The half-life of M1 is approximately 2 weeks.
- Clearance: M1 is eliminated by biliary excretion (about 40%) and further metabolism and renal excretion (about 40%).

USES IN RHEUMATIC DISEASE

Rheumatoid Arthritis

In its ability to improve clinical outcomes and to delay radiographic progression, leflunomide is superior to placebo and comparable to sulfasalazine and methotrexate (Osiri M, et al. Leflunomide for treating rheumatoid arthritis [Cochrane Review]. In: The Cochrane Library, Issue 1, 2003. Oxford: Update Software).

DOSING REGIMEN

- Loading dose: 100 mg/d × 3 days. (Without a loading dose, steady-state levels are not reached for 2 months due to the long half-life. However, because some patients experience gastrointestinal toxicity during loading, many physicians forego loading and begin therapy with 20 mg/d.)

- Maintenance dose: 20 mg/d (may be reduced to 10 mg/d if not tolerated).

INITIATING THERAPY

- Laboratory evaluation prior to initiating leflunomide should include CBC, serum creatinine, LFTs, tests for hepatitis B and C, and urinalysis.
- The possibility of pregnancy must be excluded prior to starting leflunomide.

MONITORING THERAPY

Recommendations call for monthly monitoring of LFTs initially and then as determined by the individual clinical situation. In view of the possible link with serious liver toxicity, however, regular monitoring of LFTs throughout treatment is prudent.

SPECIAL PRECAUTIONS

- Pregnancy is an absolute contraindication. Mothers should not breastfeed. Adequate contraception is required for female and male patients.
- Preexisting liver disease, excessive consumption of alcohol, and infection with hepatitis B or C viruses are contraindications.
- Because renal excretion is an important mechanism of drug elimination, leflunomide should be used cautiously, if at all, in patients with renal insufficiency.
- Leflunomide should not be used in the setting of severe immunodeficiency, active infection, or bone marrow dysplasia.
- Patients taking leflunomide should not receive live vaccines.

COMPLICATIONS

- Gastrointestinal toxicity is common, especially within the first 2 weeks of therapy and may manifest as nausea and vomiting, abdominal pain, and diarrhea.
- Mild elevations (< twofold) in serum transaminases are common and often resolve on therapy. Elevations > threefold occurred in 2–4% of patients in initial clinical trials and reversed with discontinuation of leflunomide. There are postmarketing reports of severe liver disease temporally associated with leflunomide (see www.fda.gov).
- Rash and allergic reactions (including, rarely, Stevens-Johnson syndrome and toxic epidermal necrolysis).

- Reversible alopecia.
- Cytopenias appear to be rare.

DISCONTINUING THERAPY

Because of the unusually long half-life of leflunomide, drug elimination therapy with cholestyramine is recommended for (1) serious toxicity (eg, hypersensitivity reactions) and (2) women of child-bearing age who have stopped taking leflunomide. Serum levels of M1 should be documented to be < 0.02 mg/L prior to attempts to become pregnant; unless cholestyramine elimination therapy is used, it can take up to 2 years for M1 levels to reach this level after the drug has been discontinued.

LONG-TERM CONCERNS

The risk of developing malignancy with long-term treatment is unknown but is increased with several other immunosuppressive therapies.

KEY POINTS

- Leflunomide is comparable in efficacy to methotrexate and sulfasalazine in the treatment of rheumatoid arthritis.
- Because of the uncertainties regarding the risk of severe liver disease, many physicians reserve leflunomide for patients with rheumatoid arthritis who have not responded to methotrexate.

■ SULFASALAZINE (SSA)

John B. Imboden, MD

MECHANISM OF ACTION

- SSA consists of salicylic acid joined to sulfapyridine (SP) by an azo bond.
- The mechanism of action is not certain; SSA may affect inflammatory mediators and may have immunomodulatory activity.

PHARMACOKINETICS

- Bioavailability: < 15% of SSA is absorbed as intact drug. SSA undergoes cleavage by intestinal bacteria, releasing 5-aminosalicylic acid (5-ASA), which is poorly absorbed (bioavailability 10–30%), and SP, which is well absorbed (bioavailability 60%).
- Half-life: Serum levels of SP peak 10 hours after ingestion of SSA. SP, which is metabolized by acetyla-

tion, has a half-life of 10–15 hours depending on acetylation status.

- Clearance: SP and its metabolites are excreted in the urine.

USES IN RHEUMATIC DISEASE

Rheumatoid Arthritis

SSA is superior to placebo in control of disease activity (*J Rheumatol.* 1992;19:1672; *Arthritis Rheum.* 1993;36:1501). In short-term studies, SSA appears comparable to leflunomide and methotrexate. In long-term studies, leflunomide is superior to SSA in terms of clinical responses (*J Rheumatol.* 2001;28:1983), and the drop-out rate is higher for SSA than for methotrexate. The combination of SSA, hydroxychloroquine, and methotrexate appears to be superior to methotrexate alone in patients with suboptimal responses to methotrexate (*N Engl J Med.* 1996; 334:1287).

Spondyloarthropathies

The superiority of SSA over placebo in the management of psoriatic arthritis and reactive arthritis has been demonstrated in controlled studies (*Br J Rheumatol.* 1996;35:664; *Arthritis Rheum.* 1996;39:2013; (*Arthritis Rheum.* 1996;39:2021). In ankylosing spondylitis, SSA does not have efficacy in the treatment of the disease of the axial skeleton but is superior to placebo in controlling the activity of peripheral arthritis (*Arthritis Rheum.* 1996;39:2004). SSA is widely used in the treatment of inflammatory bowel disease.

DOSING REGIMEN

- 1 g twice daily.

INITIATING THERAPY

- Prior to initiating therapy: CBC, electrolytes, and creatinine; LFTs should be obtained. Screen for glucose-6-phosphate-dehydrogenase (G6PD), especially in persons at risk for G6PD deficiency (eg, males of African or Mediterranean descent).
- Start with low dose (0.5 g/d or 0.5 g twice daily) and increase by 0.5-g increments at intervals of a week or more in order to reduce gastrointestinal side effects.
- Treatment for 4–12 weeks required before benefit is observed.

MONITORING THERAPY

- CBC and LFTs every 2 weeks for the first 3 months of therapy; monthly for the next 3 months of therapy; and then every third month. Periodic urinalysis and determinations of serum creatinine.

SPECIAL PRECAUTIONS

- Contraindicated for patients with a history of allergies to sulfonamides, aspirin sensitivity, or hypersensitivity to SSA.
- Should be used cautiously, if at all, in patients with blood dyscrasias, liver disease, renal insufficiency, or severe asthma.
- Patients with G6PD deficiency are at risk for hemolytic anemia.

COMPLICATIONS

- Gastrointestinal side effects (nausea, vomiting, dyspepsia, anorexia, abdominal discomfort), headache and dizziness, and reversible oligospermia are common.
- Rash and pruritus.
- Leukopenia (usually in the first few months but can occur at any time), thrombocytopenia, and hemolytic anemia.
- Hepatitis.
- Rare toxicities include aplastic anemia, agranulocytosis, and Stevens-Johnson syndrome.

KEY POINTS

- SSA has proved effective in the treatment of rheumatoid arthritis and the spondyloarthropathies.

■ ANTIMALARIAL DRUGS: HYDROXYCHLOROQUINE (PLAQUENIL) & CHLOROQUINE

John B. Imboden, MD

MECHANISM OF ACTION

- Raise the pH of acidic intracellular compartments such as endosomes and lysosomes.
- The mechanism of action of antimalarial drugs in treating rheumatic disease, however, is not clear.

PHARMACOKINETICS

- Bioavailability: Both drugs are well absorbed.
- Half-life: The drugs concentrate in tissues and, as a result, have a long terminal half-life (50 days).
- Clearance: Approximately 50% of drug is excreted unchanged in the urine; another 25–30% is metabolized prior to renal clearance.

USES IN RHEUMATIC DISEASE

Discoid Lupus

Hydroxychloroquine and chloroquine have been used for decades in the treatment of discoid lupus and are considered effective.

Systemic Lupus Erythematosus

Hydroxychloroquine is widely used for the treatment of systemic lupus erythematosus (SLE). A controlled, double-blinded study demonstrated that withdrawal of hydroxychloroquine led to flares of disease (*N Engl J Med.* 1991;324:150).

Rheumatoid Arthritis

Hydroxychloroquine is superior to placebo for the treatment of relatively mild rheumatoid arthritis (*Am J Med.* 1995;98:156; *Arthritis Rheum.* 1995;38:1447) but is generally considered to be less effective than other commonly used disease-modifying antirheumatic drugs (DMARDs), such as methotrexate. The onset of action may be slow (up to 6 months). Hydroxychloroquine may be useful in combination with other DMARDs. For example, the combination of hydroxychloroquine, sulfasalazine, and methotrexate appears to be superior to methotrexate alone in patients with suboptimal responses to methotrexate (*N Engl J Med.* 1996;334:1287).

DOSING REGIMEN

- Hydroxychloroquine: Initial therapy 400 mg/d; maintenance therapy 200–400 mg/d.
- Chloroquine: Initial therapy 500 mg/d; maintenance therapy 500 mg every other day.

INITIATING THERAPY

- Baseline ophthalmologic examination should be performed.

MONITORING THERAPY

- Ophthalmologic examination for retinal toxicity every 6 months.

SPECIAL PRECAUTIONS

- Hydroxychloroquine and chloroquine are contraindicated in persons with retinopathy due to any cause.

COMPLICATIONS

- In general, antimalarials are well tolerated and have the lowest incidence of side effects of DMARDs.
- Rash.
- Gastrointestinal side effects (dyspepsia, nausea, vomiting).
- Headache, insomnia.
- Ocular toxicity:
  - Retinal toxicity: Irreversible retinal damage has occurred with long-term therapy and has been reported more with chloroquine than hydroxychloroquine. With regular ophthalmologic examinations and appropriate dosing, irreversible retinal damage should be rare.
  - Extraocular muscle palsy producing diplopia.
  - Corneal deposits.
- Neuromuscular syndrome (uncommon) presents with proximal lower extremity weakness and can mimic steroid myopathy.

KEY POINTS

- Antimalarial drugs are commonly used to treat discoid lupus and appear to be useful adjunctive therapy for SLE. In rheumatoid arthritis, they are generally reserved for mild disease or used in combination with other DMARDs.
- Although antimalarials are well tolerated relative to other DMARDs, regular monitoring for retinal toxicity is required. There are fewer reports of retinopathy associated with hydroxychloroquine, which, as a result, is preferred by many clinicians over chloroquine.

■ CYCLOPHOSPHAMIDE (CYC; CYTOXAN)

John H. Stone, MD, MPH

MECHANISM OF ACTION

- Alkylates various cellular constituents, leading to DNA cross-linking and disruption of transcription and translation.
- Depletes both B and T cells (with perhaps a greater effect on B cells), impacting both humoral and cellular immunity.
- Affects both proliferating and resting cells.

PHARMACOKINETICS

- Bioavailability: Oral CYC is rapidly absorbed and has a bioavailability of greater than 75%.
- Metabolism: Metabolized in the liver to 4-hydroxy-cyclophosphamide and aldophosphoramide. Aldophosphoramide is then converted to phosphoramide mustard (the active metabolite) and the nonalkylating metabolite acrolein (which often leads to bladder toxicity). Phosphoramide mustard, which is highly protein-bound, is distributed to all tissues (including the central nervous system). This active metabolite of CYC is secreted in breast milk and assumed to cross the placenta.
- Half-life: 2–10 hours; 95% is excreted by the kidney.
- Elimination: Both active and inactive metabolites are excreted unchanged in the urine, with elimination complete by 48 hours.

USES IN RHEUMATIC DISEASE

CYC is a lifesaving intervention in some patients with organ- or life-threatening rheumatic disease. Its therapeutic index is narrow, however, so the drug must be used with great caution and strict monitoring. Systemic vasculitis and systemic lupus erythematosus (SLE) are the diseases in which CYC is used most consistently. With some exceptions, there are no unequivocal data favoring one schedule (daily or intermittent) or route of administration (oral or intravenous) over another in a particular disease.

Systemic Vasculitis

For most forms of systemic vasculitis, daily CYC is the preferred regimen of choice, principally because of studies in Wegener granulomatosis suggesting that daily regimens are more likely to lead to sustained remissions (*Arthritis Rheum.* 1997;40:2099). However, intermittent CYC regimens (eg, every month) are probably equally effective in the induction of remission in systemic vasculitis (*Nephrol Dial Transplant.* 2001;16:2018). There has never been a sufficiently powered, head-to-head comparison of these treatment approaches in vasculitis. Other considerations in the choice of administration schedule and route are discussed under Dosing Regimen.

A. WEGENER GRANULOMATOSIS

In the 1970s, CYC converted severe Wegener granulomatosis from an invariably fatal condition to one that can be controlled in most cases, albeit with risk of substantial toxicity and a high likelihood (> 50%) of eventual flares following remission. The usual starting dose in young patients with normal kidney function is 2 mg/kg/d. Dose adjustments for renal dysfunction and advanced age are important (see below).

B. MICROSCOPIC POLYANGIITIS

Because of the high frequency of major organ involvement in microscopic polyangiitis (alveolar hemorrhage, rapidly progressive glomerulonephritis, mononeuritis multiplex, mesenteric vasculitis), CYC is usually indicated from the start of therapy.

C. CHURG-STRAUSS SYNDROME

Eosinophils are typically exquisitely sensitive to glucocorticoids. Nevertheless, at least 50% of patients with Churg-Strauss syndrome eventually require CYC as well. Patients with severe disease manifestations, such as vasculitic neuropathy, should be treated with CYC immediately.

D. IDIOPATHIC POLYARTERITIS NODOSA

Approximately half of all patients with polyarteritis nodosa not associated with hepatitis B may be treated with glucocorticoids alone. The other half usually require CYC. Patients with severe disease features should be treated with CYC immediately.

E. RHEUMATOID VASCULITIS

Patients with rheumatoid vasculitis who have scleritis, peripheral ulcerative keratitis, mononeuritis multiplex, significant cutaneous ulcerations, digital gangrene, evidence of mesenteric vasculitis, or other serious disease manifestations should be treated with CYC. Although CYC is effective in treating the synovitis of rheumatoid arthritis, the potential adverse effects profile of this medication serves as a contraindication to its use in this disease except in the setting of vasculitis (or severe ocular manifestations, which often correlate with vasculitis).

F. BEHÇET DISEASE

Posterior uveitis (retinal vasculitis) and significant central nervous system disease are usually indications for CYC.

Systemic Lupus Erythematosus

In contrast to systemic vasculitis, evidence-based data favoring the use of intermittent CYC do exist in SLE (*N Engl J Med.* 1986; 314:614; *Ann Intern Med.* 1996;125:549). CYC is particularly important in the treatment of proliferative glomerular lesions of SLE nephritis (eg, World Health Organization [WHO] class 4 disease, diffuse proliferative glomerulonephritis). (Mycophenolate mofetil [MMF] is now often used for this indication, too, however.) The traditional National Institutes of Health (NIH) protocol for the treatment of lupus nephritis with intermittent CYC calls for

6 monthly pulses, followed by 18 months of "consolidation" therapy in which the patient receives intravenous CYC every 3 months (times 6), for a total duration of therapy of 24 months. Because of the potential hazards associated with this regimen, shorter courses of CYC are often used now, followed by MMF.

Inflammatory Myopathy

CYC is rarely the initial treatment of choice for inflammatory myopathies but is sometimes required for patients whose disease is refractory to such second-line agents as azathioprine, methotrexate, and intravenous immune globulin.

Scleroderma

CYC is often used in the treatment of interstitial lung disease that occurs as a complication of diffuse scleroderma (*Curr Rheumatol Rep.* 2002;4:108).

DOSING REGIMEN

Under most circumstances, daily administration corresponds to oral use and intermittent therapy to intravenous administration. For patients who cannot take oral medications, however, such as intubated patients in the intensive care unit, CYC may be administered in small daily doses equivalent to what the would be given orally.

- Daily use: In the setting of normal renal function, the usual starting dose for CYC is 2 mg/kg/d. Adjustments for both renal dysfunction and advanced age are essential. Table 56–4 shows an algorithm for the adjustment of CYC dose according to creatinine clearance.
- Intermittent use: The NIH protocol for the use of pulse intravenous CYC is shown in Table 56–5. Patients who undergo hemodialysis but who require intravenous CYC should receive 500 mg/m^2 BSA and

Table 56–4. Algorithm for adjusting CYC dose based on creatinine clearance.

Creatinine Clearance[a] (mL/min)	CYC Dose (mg/kg/d)
> 100	2.0
50–99	1.5
25–49	1.2
15–24	1.0
< 15 or on dialysis	0.8

[a]Creatinine clearance calculated by the Cockroft equation: CL_{cr} = [120 − age]/serum Cr in mg/dL *(multiplied by a factor of 0.8 for women).* CYC, cyclophosphamide.

Table 56–5. National Institutes of Health pulse intravenous CYC protocol.

Dosage
Creatinine clearance > 30 mL/min: initially 750 mg/m^2 BSA.
May increase to a maximum of 1000 mg/m^2 BSA if tolerated.
Creatinine clearance < 30 mL/min: initially 500 mg/m^2 BSA.

Monitoring of WBC count after CYC administration (between days 8 and 12)
If WBC nadir < 1500/μL, reduce subsequent dose by 25%.
If WBC nadir > 4000/μL, increase subsequent doses to a maximum of 1000 mg/m^2 BSA.

Preparation and infusion
Mix in 150 mL normal saline or D5W.
Infuse over 60 minutes.

MESNA administration
Each MESNA dose is 20% of the CYC dose.
Infuse MESNA immediately before CYC and every 3 hours thereafter, for a total of 4 doses[a].

Antiemetic regimen
Dexamethasone 10 mg orally 3–4 hours after CYC.
Ondansetron 4–8 mg intravenously or orally starting 4 hours after CYC, then every 4 hours × 3.
Granisetron 10 μg/kg intravenously 30 minutes before CYC.

Diuresis
In patients with normal cardiac function, hydration with $D_5 1/2NS$ at 150–200 mL/h for a total of 2–4 L.
Bladder irrigation may be used if patient unable to tolerate intravenous fluids.

[a]This is sometimes decreased to a total of two doses.
WBC, white blood cell; CYC, cyclophosphamide; MESNA, 2-mercaptoethane sulfonate.

undergo dialysis 12 hours after CYC. Patients with creatinine clearances < 30 mL/min should also receive 500 mg/m^2 BSA. Finally, those with creatinine clearances > 30 mL/min may receive 750 mg/m^2 BSA, with subsequent upward adjustments of the monthly dose if tolerated to a maximum of 1000 mg/m^2 (see below).

MONITORING THERAPY

In theory, with regard to infection, daily CYC should be safer than intermittent CYC because of the "titration" of the dose that is possible with careful monitoring of the white blood cell count. However, compared with intermittent CYC administered for the same length of time, daily CYC results in substantially more total CYC. In practice, infectious complications with daily CYC appear to be at least as common (if not more so) than with intermittent CYC. The reality of CYC is that neither route is "safe"; **both** routes are potentially hazardous, and patients receiving either route of administration must be monitored carefully.

Guidelines for using daily CYC safely are shown in Table 56–6. The most critical point in monitoring patients on CYC is checking a complete blood cell count not less often than every 2 weeks. Patients with cell counts that are borderline (eg, white blood cell counts in the range of 4000/μL) may need to have the counts checked more frequently. Even if patients appear to tolerate daily CYC well for several months, there is usually a gradual decline in the white blood cell count that eventually requires dose adjustments.

For patients receiving intermittent CYC, white blood cell counts are checked about 10 days after the pulse of treatment. If the white blood cell count is $< 1.5 \times 10^6$/L, the next dose should be decreased by 25%. If the white blood cell count nadir is $> 4.0 \times 10^6$/L, the next dose may be increased (but should not exceed 1000 mg/m^2).

SPECIAL PRECAUTIONS

- Pregnancy and breastfeeding are strictly contraindicated.
- Daily CYC should be administered in the morning, to reduce the likelihood of adverse bladder effects. The risk of bladder toxicity is heightened if the metabolite acrolein is permitted to reside in the bladder over night.

Table 56–6. Guidelines for the safe use of daily CYC.

Limit duration of CYC use (ideally 6–12 months or less, followed by a conversion—if appropriate—to a less toxic second-line agent).
Instruct patients to take CYC in the morning.
Instruct patients to drink eight 8-oz glasses of water daily.
Adjust dose to maintain the total white blood cell count greater than 3500/μL.
Decrease the dose in the setting of renal dysfunction (including the elderly, whose glomerular filtration rate is lower than that of younger patients).
Check complete blood cell counts (with differential) and serum creatinine levels every 2 weeks (more frequently for those with borderline counts). Urinalyses should be performed monthly.
Monthly urinalyses. Patients should notify their physicians immediately if dysuria develops (unfortunately, not all cases of CYC-induced bladder injury are symptomatic).
Long-term surveillance for CYC-induced bladder injury.
Always use *Pneumocystis jiroveci* prophylaxis.

CYC, cyclophosphamide.

- 2-Mercaptoethane sulfonate (MESNA) should be administered to patients receiving intermittent CYC (see Table 56–5).
- Patients taking CYC daily should drink eight 8-oz glasses of water a day. Those receiving intermittent CYC should receive pre- and post-CYC intravenous hydration (see Table 56–5).
- Prophylaxis against *Pneumocystis jiroveci* pneumonia (PCP) is important for all patients taking CYC daily. Single-strength trimethoprim-sulfamethoxazole (1 tablet daily), dapsone (100 mg/d), and other strategies may be appropriate. The consensus about the need for PCP prophylaxis among patients with SLE who are receiving intermittent CYC is not as strong, but such infections occur occasionally in SLE patients treated in this fashion, as well. Because allergies to trimethoprim-sulfamethoxazole are more common in SLE, dapsone may be the more appropriate choice for prophylaxis.
- Some data suggest that the subcutaneous administration of gonadotropin-releasing hormone agonists (eg, lupron) 10–14 days before the administration of intermittent CYC may be useful in preserving the ovulatory status of young women (*Ann Oncol.* 2002; 13[Suppl 1]:138).

COMPLICATIONS

In the longitudinal study from the NIH involving 158 patients with Wegener granulomatosis, 42% of those treated with daily CYC (for a mean period of 2 years) suffered permanent treatment-related morbidity (*Ann Intern Med.* 1992;116:488). The common complications of CYC include the following:

- Bone marrow suppression: Neutropenia is the most common adverse effect of CYC on the bone marrow, followed by thrombocytopenia and anemia.
- Infection: Opportunistic infection is believed to correlate with the degree and duration of neutropenia.
- Gastrointestinal effects (eg, anorexia, nausea, and vomiting): The gastrointestinal side effects of CYC are more common with intermittent dosing but can usually be controlled adequately with the aggressive use of antiemetics.
- CYC-induced cystitis: Can occur as early as within several weeks of CYC use. Many patients (but not all) complain of severe dysuria. The development of CYC-induced cystitis is an indication for the immediate cessation of this drug and is a contraindication to the use of CYC in any form.
- Malignancy: A long-term risk, correlated with the overall quantity of CYC exposure. Hematopoietic malignancies (eg, leukemia and lymphoma) and

bladder cancers are the most common types of CYC-associated cancers.

- Infertility: 57% of women of child-bearing age became infertile on the NIH regimen of CYC administration. Males are also at risk for infertility, although the risk has not been quantified precisely. Among women, age and duration of CYC use are strong predictors of the development of anovulation/early menopause, with an 18-year-old woman being substantially less likely than a 36-year-old woman to suffer this complication.
- Hepatitis: A reversible form of hepatocellular injury with cholestasis occurs in a minority of patients with CYC.
- Pneumonitis: Interstitial pulmonary inflammation and fibrosis are rare complications of CYC.
- Hypersensitivity reactions occur rarely in CYC, but are reported to occur. These are associated with fever, "drug rash," myalgias, liver function test abnormalities, gastrointestinal symptoms, and hypotension and may sometimes be confused with the underlying disease.

DISCONTINUING THERAPY

For most patients, CYC should not be viewed as a long-term medication for the maintenance of remission. The aim of therapy should be to discontinue CYC in favor of a less toxic therapy after 3–6 months of treatment. The exception to this is SLE nephritis, in which longer courses (up to 2 years, according to the NIH protocol) are sometimes prescribed. Tolerance of the long-term treatment regimens is poor, even in SLE. When it is time to discontinue CYC, no tapering is required.

LONG-TERM CONCERNS

- Malignancy: Daily CYC use is associated with a 33-fold increase in the risk of bladder cancer (*Ann Intern Med.* 1996;124:477). Moreover, cases of bladder cancer may occur a decade or more after discontinuation of the medication. Thus, continued surveillance of the urine is essential. Urine cytologies are not sensitive for cancer. The best method of screening is with annual or semiannual urinalyses screening for nonglomerular hematuria. The long-term risk of malignancy is also increased among patients treated with CYC.

KEY POINTS

- CYC remains an essential medication in the treatment of many severe forms of rheumatic disease.
- Because of its multiple potential short- and long-term side effects, patients on CYC must be monitored

closely and the medication should be discontinued in favor of a less toxic agent as soon as possible.

CHLORAMBUCIL (CHL; LEUKERAN)

John H. Stone, MD, MPH

Because of its narrow therapeutic window, the short-term risk of significant bone marrow dysfunction, and the long-term risk of lymphoproliferative disease, CHL is now employed in the treatment of rheumatic disease only in patients who cannot take cyclophosphamide (CYC). The usual reason for CHL use is the development of CYC-induced cystitis. Because of its uncommon use in rheumatic diseases, most of the literature on this agent and rheumatic illnesses is several decades old.

MECHANISM OF ACTION

- An alkylating agent. Cross-links DNA, leading to the disruption of transcription and translation.

PHARMACOKINETICS

- Bioavailability: Rapidly absorbed orally, with a bioavailability of > 80%. Peak plasma concentrations occur 30–70 minutes after ingestion.
- Metabolism: Converted to phenylacetic acid mustard and other metabolites.
- Half-life: 1.5–1.7 hours.
- Clearance: The active metabolite phenylacetic acid mustard is excreted nearly entirely by the kidney.

USES IN RHEUMATIC DISEASE

CHL is used occasionally in systemic vasculitis (Wegener granulomatosis, polyarteritis nodosa, and Behçet disease), systemic lupus erythematosus (SLE), and (very rarely now) refractory rheumatoid arthritis. CHL is generally a default treatment in rheumatic disease, used only in patients who cannot take cyclophosphamide.

DOSING REGIMEN

- The usual starting dose is between 0.1 and 0.2 mg/kg/d (ie, in the range of 6–10 mg/d).

INITIATING THERAPY

- Patients who get as far down in the treatment algorithm to warrant consideration for CHL therapy have usually been treated with ample quantities of other immunosuppressive agents before that time.

Consequently, they may be more susceptible to CHL-associated bone marrow toxicity, and additional caution is advised.

MONITORING THERAPY

Complete blood cell counts should be obtained on a weekly basis for patients taking CHL. Bone marrow aplasia may develop very rapidly in these patients, justifying this frequent interval of monitoring. Thrombocytopenia may be a particular problem with CHL.

SPECIAL PRECAUTIONS

Pregnancy and breastfeeding are strictly forbidden in patients taking CHL.

COMPLICATIONS

Most of the potential adverse effects of CHL are very similar to those observed in cyclophosphamide. The major exception is that CHL, unlike cyclophosphamide, does not have a propensity to induce bladder injury.

- Bone marrow suppression: May occur more suddenly in comparison to CYC.
- Infection: *P jiroveci* prophylaxis and vigilance for other possible opportunistic infections are essential.
- Gastrointestinal effects (eg, anorexia, nausea, and vomiting).
- Infertility.
- Malignancy: The risk of malignancy, particularly of acute myelocytic leukemia, is even higher than with cyclophosphamide.

DISCONTINUING THERAPY

CHL should be prescribed for as short a time as possible. Once it has achieved its intended effect of controlling a refractory disease manifestation, it should be replaced by another safer medication designed to maintain disease control.

LONG-TERM CONCERNS

- Malignancy: The long-term concerns about the induction of bone marrow malignancies are greater with CHL than with cyclophosphamide.

KEY POINTS

- The principal role currently for CHL in the treatment of rheumatic disease is as a fallback position for patients who cannot take cyclophosphamide.

- CHL is effective in many rheumatic conditions, but its substantial toxicity profile greatly limits its use.

■ AZATHIOPRINE (AZA; IMURAN)

Philip Seo, MD, & John H. Stone, MD, MPH

MECHANISM OF ACTION

- Inhibits the proliferation of B and T lymphocytes.
- Reduces antibody production.
- Decreases interleukin-2 secretion.
- Inhibits purine synthesis through its metabolite, 6-mercaptopurine (6-MP).

PHARMACOKINETICS

- Bioavailability: 60% (oral).
- Metabolism: Metabolized by glutathione in red blood cells to 6-MP.
- Half-life: 3 hours.
- Clearance: Inactivated in the liver, gastrointestinal tract, and red blood cells by several enzymes, including xanthine oxidase and thiopurine methyltransferase (TPMT). The metabolites are excreted in the urine.

USES IN RHEUMATIC DISEASE

AZA is commonly used as a second-line agent in rheumatic disease, particularly in glucocorticoid- or cyclophosphamide-sparing roles, and only rarely used as a first-line agent.

Lupus Nephritis

The efficacy of AZA for the maintenance of remission in lupus nephritis was shown in a prospective study in which 20 patients with membranous lupus nephritis were treated with prednisolone and oral cyclophosphamide for 6 months, followed by 6 months of prednisolone and AZA (*Lupus* 1999;8:545). At the end of 12 months, 85% of patients were in complete or partial remission.

This regimen may be efficacious for other forms of lupus nephritis as well. In a retrospective study of 55 patients with diffuse proliferative glomerulonephritis, 89% of patients treated with the sequential use of cyclophosphamide and AZA were in complete or partial remission at the end of 12 months. Sixty-three percent remained in remission after 5 years (*Arthritis Rheum.* 2002;46:1003).

Cyclophosphamide-containing regimens were shown to be slightly superior to a regimen that used AZA in a longitudinal study from the National Institutes of Health (*N Engl J Med.* 1986;314:614).

Systemic Lupus Erythematosus (SLE)

Although AZA is used as a glucocorticoid-sparing agent for the treatment of other manifestations of SLE (including arthritis, serositis, anemia, and neuropsychiatric lupus), it has not been studied rigorously in these indications.

Inflammatory Myopathy

AZA ranks with methotrexate as the glucocorticoid-sparing agent of choice in inflammatory myopathy. Treatment of polymyositis with AZA and glucocorticoids led to better long-term function than treatment with glucocorticoids alone in one randomized controlled trial. (*Arthritis Rheum.* 1981;24:45).

Rheumatoid Arthritis

AZA is more effective than placebo in the treatment of rheumatoid arthritis; however, because of its associated toxicity and the availability of alternatives, it is not used for this indication.

Scleroderma

Anecdotal reports suggest that AZA slows disease progression in scleroderma (*Immun Infekt.* 1979;7:165), but its role in the treatment of this disease, if any, remains unclear.

Vasculitis Associated with Antineutrophil Cytoplasmic Antibodies (ANCAs)

The efficacy of AZA for the maintenance of remission in patients with ANCA-associated vasculitis was examined in a prospective, randomized controlled trial involving patients with Wegener granulomatosis and microscopic polyangiitis. Patients were treated with oral cyclophosphamide and prednisolone for 3 months (after which more than 90% were in remission). They were then randomized to continued therapy with cyclophosphamide or to AZA, and their prednisolone dose was tapered to 5 mg/d for the remainder of the trial. After 18 months of follow-up, there was no difference in the rate of relapse (*Curr Opin Rheumatol.* 2001;13:48).

Behçet Disease & Other Vasculitides

The addition of AZA to glucocorticoid treatment in patients with Behçet disease was shown to preserve vision better than glucocorticoids alone in a double-blind, placebo-controlled trial (*Arthritis Rheum.* 1997;40:

769). In other forms of vasculitis, eg, polyarteritis nodosa, AZA is commonly used as a second-line agent to maintain disease remissions and diminish patients' requirements for glucocorticoids.

Spondyloarthropathies

AZA resulted in improvement in overall disease activity compared with placebo in a study of six patients with psoriatic arthritis (*Arthritis Rheum.* 1984;27:376). With the emergence of methotrexate and, more recently, biologic agents for the treatment of inflammatory arthritis, the role of AZA in the spondyloarthropathies is quite limited.

DOSING REGIMEN

- 100–200 mg daily.

INITIATING THERAPY

- Genotype patients for TPMT alleles before starting AZA therapy (see Special Precautions, below). Genotyping can now be performed through a commercially available blood test (http://www.prometheus-labs.com).
- Start with low doses (eg, 50 mg/d orally for several days) to monitor for violent gastrointestinal intolerance.
- If the patient is not TPMT-deficient and tolerates the low dose without gastrointestinal upset, AZA may be increased quickly to the target dose.

MONITORING THERAPY

Complete blood cell counts and liver function tests should be checked every 2 weeks until a stable dose is achieved, then every 4–6 weeks thereafter.

SPECIAL PRECAUTIONS

- Homozygosity for the absence of TPMT alleles is an absolute contraindication to the use of AZA, because patients completely deficient in TPMT cannot metabolize the drug. Approximately 1 individual in 300 is deficient in both TPMT alleles. However, 11% of the general population are heterozygotes (ie, are absent one TPMT allele), placing them at increased risk for many of the toxicities commonly associated with AZA (eg, bone marrow suppression, hepatotoxicity, and gastrointestinal intolerance). For such patients, lower doses and great caution are required (*Ann Intern Med.* 1998;129:716). When possible, patients who are heterozygous for the TPMT mutation should be treated with alternative agents.

- Sulfasalazine may inhibit TPMT and should be used cautiously in patients receiving AZA. The use of other agents that contain sulfa moieties, such as trimethoprim-sulfamethoxazole, is not contraindicated.

- AZA is not teratogenic and, when necessary, can be used in pregnant women. However, its use during pregnancy has been associated with premature births and low birth weight.

- Allopurinol, an inhibitor of xanthine oxidase, slows the elimination of AZA and can lead to life-threatening myelosuppression. As a rule, these two drugs should not be used in the same patient.

- In renal failure (ie, a creatinine clearance of less than 10 mL/min), the dosage of AZA should be decreased by 50%.

COMPLICATIONS

- Bone marrow suppression is dose-dependent. AZA frequently causes leukopenia or, less commonly, thrombocytopenia, both of which generally resolve with dose reduction. In SLE, distinguishing cytopenias related to the disease from those induced by therapy can be challenging. A short course of glucocorticoids (eg, 20 mg/d) may help resolve the issue.

- Gastrointestinal effects (eg, anorexia, nausea, and vomiting) are common and may be ameliorated by splitting the dose, reducing the dose, or taking the medication with meals.

- Hepatitis and pancreatitis may occur with AZA use. Both of these side effects are reversible following cessation of the drug. Cholestasis may require dose modification.

- Hypersensitivity reactions (which are associated with fever, rash, myalgias, liver function test abnormalities, gastrointestinal symptoms, and hypotension) are occasionally seen during the first few weeks of therapy, and may be mistaken for a flare of the underlying rheumatic illness.

DISCONTINUING THERAPY

AZA should be discontinued in patients in whom severe leukopenia, thrombocytopenia, or gastrointestinal intolerance develops.

LONG-TERM CONCERNS

- The association between AZA and secondary cancers is controversial. Renal transplant recipients treated with AZA seem to have an increased risk of malignancy (including non-Hodgkin lymphoma, Kaposi sarcoma, and skin carcinoma), but an increased risk of cancer has

not been reported in patients receiving AZA for rheumatoid arthritis or inflammatory bowel disease (*Aliment Pharmacol Ther.* 2002;16:1225).

- AZA is known to decrease spermatogenesis and sperm viability in rats. Its effect on male fertility in humans is not known.

- Patients treated with AZA may experience more frequent bacterial and viral infections.

KEY POINTS

- AZA is useful in the treatment of lupus nephritis and vasculitis, particularly following cyclophosphamide as a remission maintenance agent.

- It is also useful as an adjunctive medication in the long-term therapy of polymyositis.

- AZA has an increasingly limited role in the treatment of spondyloarthropathies.

- Because of the availability of better medications, AZA is not used in the treatment of rheumatoid arthritis.

■ MYCOPHENOLATE MOFETIL (MMF; CELLCEPT)

Philip Seo, MD, & John H. Stone, MD, MPH

MECHANISM OF ACTION

- Lymphocytes are dependent on the de novo synthesis pathway of purine nucleotides, which is catalyzed by inosine monophosphate (IMP) dehydrogenase.

- MMF reversibly inhibits the type II isoform of IMP dehydrogenase, an enzyme expressed in activated lymphocytes.

- Inhibits the proliferation of B and T lymphocytes.

- Decreases antibody production.

PHARMACOKINETICS

- Bioavailability: 94% (oral).

- Metabolism: Hydrolyzed to mycophenolic acid in the gastrointestinal tract almost immediately after absorption.

- Half-life: 11.6 hours.

- Clearance: Mycophenolic acid is conjugated in the liver to a glucuronide, an inactive metabolite that is excreted in the urine and feces.

USES IN RHEUMATIC DISEASE

Lupus Nephritis

A 12-month course of MMF and prednisolone proved effective in achieving remission in patients with diffuse proliferative lupus nephritis in a randomized controlled trial (*N Engl J Med.* 2000;343:1156). MMF has been used successfully to treat other forms of lupus nephritis as well.

Systemic Lupus Erythematosus (SLE)

Treatment with MMF reduced disease activity (and significantly decreased oral glucocorticoid dose) in a prospective study of patients with manifestations of SLE refractory to other immunosuppressive agents (including cyclophosphamide, azathioprine, and methotrexate) (*Rheumatology.* 2002;41:876).

Inflammatory Myopathy

There are three case reports of patients with polymyositis or dermatomyositis successfully treated with MMF (*Neurology.* 2001;56:94; *Dermatology.* 2001;202:341; *Muscle Nerve.* 2002;25:286). In a case series of four patients, MMF was effective in controlling the cutaneous manifestations of dermatomyositis (*J Rheumatol.* 2000; 27:1542).

Vasculitis

MMF was used to maintain remission in nine patients with Wegener granulomatosis and two patients with microscopic polyangiitis in an unrandomized, open-label study. (*J Am Soc Nephrol.* 1999;10:1965). Another case series described three patients with refractory Takayasu arteritis who responded well to treatment with MMF (*Ann Intern Med.* 1999;130:422).

OTHER USES

MMF is being studied for the treatment of the cutaneous manifestations of scleroderma. There is some limited evidence that MMF may be efficacious in the treatment of rheumatoid arthritis, although it is not used for this indication.

DOSING REGIMEN

- 1.5–3.0 g/d in divided doses.

INITIATING THERAPY

- Start with lower doses at first (eg, 500 mg orally at bedtime for several days), which may promote tolerance to the gastrointestinal side effects, then rapidly increase to the target dosage.

- Most patients will tolerate twice-daily dosing of MMF. Some patients experience fewer gastrointestinal side effects if the total daily dose is split among three or four smaller doses.

MONITORING THERAPY

- Complete blood cell counts should be performed after the first 2 weeks of therapy, then once a month for the first year of therapy.

SPECIAL PRECAUTIONS

- MMF may be teratogenic. Women should have a pregnancy test before starting therapy and use contraception during therapy.
- Aluminum and magnesium hydroxide antacids and iron supplements decrease absorption of MMF.
- The maximum dose of MMF in patients with chronic renal failure (glomerular filtration rate < 25 mL/min) should not exceed 2 g/d. Dose adjustment for hepatic insufficiency is not necessary.
- Attenuated vaccines should be avoided during therapy. Killed vaccines (including influenza and pneumococcal vaccines) are not contraindicated.

COMPLICATIONS

- Leukopenia and gastrointestinal effects (such as anorexia, nausea, vomiting, and diarrhea) are not uncommon. Leukopenia usually responds to dose reductions. Gastrointestinal side effects may improve with increasing the dosing frequency (while maintaining the same total daily dose) but may also require reductions in the total dose.
- In four randomized, controlled trials of MMF in renal allograft transplant recipients, none of the patients treated with MMF developed *P jiroveci* infection (*Clin Infect Dis.* 2002;35:53). When used in conjunction with high doses of glucocorticoids, however, the use of *P carinii* prophylaxis is prudent.

DISCONTINUING THERAPY

- Contraception should be continued for 6 weeks after MMF has been stopped.

LONG-TERM CONCERNS

- In the transplant literature, immunosuppression with MMF has been associated with an increased incidence of opportunistic infections (especially cytomegalovirus) and lymphoproliferative disease.
- The long-term risk to patients with rheumatic illnesses treated with MMF is less clear.

KEY POINTS

- MMF is effective in the treatment of diffuse proliferative lupus nephritis and may allow patients to avoid cyclophosphamide altogether for this indication.
- There are some data supporting the use of MMF in the treatment of other manifestations of SLE, as well.
- Although used for a wide variety of indications, there are few data supporting the use of MMF in the treatment of inflammatory myopathies, vasculitis, or scleroderma. MMF is not used in the treatment of rheumatoid arthritis.

■ ALLOPURINOL

David B. Hellmann, MD

MECHANISM OF ACTION

- Blocks the production of uric acid by inhibiting the enzyme xanthine oxidase, which catalyzes the conversion of hypoxanthine to xanthine and of xanthine to uric acid. Thus, allopurinol reduces the level of uric acid in serum and urine.

PHARMACOKINETICS

- Bioavailability: High (80–90%) for oral allopurinol.
- Serum uric acid levels begin to fall slowly 24–48 hours after starting allopurinol.
- Metabolism: Metabolized to oxypurinol.
- Half-life: 1–3 hours for allopurinol and 18–30 hours for oxypurinol.
- Clearance: Allopurinol and metabolites are cleared by the kidney.

USES IN RHEUMATIC DISEASES

Gout

Allopurinol can help prevent recurrent attacks of gout by reducing serum uric acid levels (*N Engl J Med.* 1996;334:445). Since allopurinol has no anti-inflammatory effects, it has no role in the treatment of acute gouty arthritis. Allopurinol is indicated for treating patients who have the following: (1) recurrent gout attacks not prevented by or amenable to treatment with uricosuric agents, (2) tophi, or (3) renal uric acid stones. Because of its possible serious side effects, allopurinol is not indicated in the treatment of asymptomatic hyperuricemia.

DOSING

- Because abrupt changes in serum urate levels can provoke gout, allopurinol is usually initiated at 100 mg orally each day, and increased by 100 mg weekly until the serum uric acid level falls below 6 mg/dL or until the maximum recommended daily dose (800 mg) is reached.
- Colchicine (0.6 mg/d orally) is often administered during the first 6 months of allopurinol treatment to reduce the chance of provoking a gout flare when serum urate levels fall.
- After months or years of treatment, a smaller dose of allopurinol may be required to achieve the target serum uric acid level.
- The usual maintenance dose of allopurinol in most patients with normal renal function is 300 mg/d administered as a single daily dose.
- In the absence of side effects, allopurinol should be continued indefinitely. Intermittent use of allopurinol is a major cause of treatment failure.
- Doses greater than 300 mg should be given in divided doses.
- Because allopurinol is chiefly renally excreted, the dose must be reduced for renal insufficiency. Recommended maintenance doses of allopurinol are 200 mg/d for a creatinine clearance of 10–20 mL/ min, and no more than 100 mg/d for a creatinine clearance less than 10 mL/min. Indeed, some clinicians recommend reducing allopurinol to 100 mg every 3 days when the creatinine clearance is 0 mL/min.

INITIATING THERAPY

- CBC with platelets, serum electrolytes, and creatinine; LFTs; and serum uric acid should be performed.

MONITORING THERAPY

- CBC counts, LFTs, and renal function tests should be monitored periodically, especially during the first few months of treatment.
- Serum uric acid level should be checked periodically during the first months of therapy to determine the dose of allopurinol needed to reduce the serum uric acid to less than 6.0 mg/dL.

SPECIAL PRECAUTIONS

General

- Allopurinol is contraindicated in persons who have had a previous severe hypersensitivity reaction.

- Hypersensitivity to allopurinol can cause life-threatening or fatal cutaneous reactions (including toxic epidermal necrolysis, vasculitis with desquamatous and exfoliative dermatitis accompanied by multiorgan failure). Allopurinol hypersensitivity may also cause severe hepatic reactions including elevations of LFTs accompanied by fever, eosinophilia, and rash. Allopurinol should be stopped immediately if a hypersensitivity reaction is suspected.

Drug Interactions

- The simultaneous use of allopurinol and azathioprine or mercaptopurine should be avoided or approached with great caution. Allopurinol inhibits the catabolism of azathioprine and mercaptopurine by xanthine oxidase and thereby increases their effect on bone marrow suppression. If concomitant use of allopurinol and azathioprine cannot be avoided, then the usual azathioprine dose should be reduced by 75% and the patient's CBC count should be monitored carefully.
- By an unknown mechanism, allopurinol can increase the risk of cytopenia from cyclophosphamide.
- Concomitant use of allopurinol and ampicillin or amoxicillin increases the risk of developing rash.
- Allopurinol increases the half-life of dicumarol.
- Concomitant use of diuretics and allopurinol may increase the risk of allopurinol toxicity.

COMPLICATIONS

- Approximately 2% of patients experience minor reactions to allopurinol (*N Engl J Med.* 2003;349: 1647). More severe hypersensitivity reactions chiefly affecting skin and liver occur rarely but can be life-threatening (see above).
- The most common complication of allopurinol is a maculopapular rash. Nausea, vomiting, diarrhea, or other gastrointestinal effects develop more infrequently in the absence of hypersensitivity reactions. Hematologic effects are rare except in patients taking myelosuppressive drugs (see above).
- Management of all hypersensitivity reactions includes immediately stopping allopurinol. The drug cannot be restarted in patients who have had severe hypersensitivity reactions. About half the patients with mild hypersensitivity reactions can be desensitized to allopurinol. The desensitization protocol involves reintroducing minute doses of allopurinol orally and increasing the dose gradually while monitoring the patient closely (*N Engl J Med.* 2003;349: 1647).

KEY POINTS

- Allopurinol is effective in preventing reoccurrence of gout by inhibiting the production of uric acid.
- Because of (rare) fatal hypersensitivity reactions, allopurinol should be used cautiously in patients with gout and should not be used to treat asymptomatic hyperuricemia.

■ COLCHICINE

David B. Hellmann, MD

MECHANISM OF ACTION

- Colchicine inhibits phagocytosis of urate crystals by neutrophils by impairing microtubule function.
- Colchicine has other broader anti-inflammatory effects: The drug impairs neutrophil metabolism, chemotaxis, and motility, and inhibits the release of chemotactic factor.
- In addition, colchicine interferes with the secretion of serum amyloid A protein, which is found in amyloid deposits in patients with familial Mediterranean fever (FMF).
- Toxic effects of colchicine may be related to its ability to inhibit cell division by interfering with the mitotic spindle.

PHARMACOKINETICS

- Orally administered colchicine is absorbed from the gastrointestinal system, partially metabolized by the liver, secreted in bile, and then partially reabsorbed. This enterohepatic circulation of colchicine helps account for the frequent gastrointestinal toxicity of orally administered colchicine.
- Colchicine is concentrated in leukocytes, where the half-life of the drug is 60 hours.
- Colchicine is eliminated chiefly in feces and to a lesser degree in urine.

USES IN RHEUMATIC DISEASES

Colchicine is approved by the Food and Drug Administration for the treatment of gout. However, it is not approved for FMF, sarcoidosis arthropathy, pseudogout, Behçet disease, and other uses in rheumatic diseases.

Gout

Colchicine has two uses in gout. First, colchicine in high doses (see below) is an effective treatment for acute gouty arthritis. Second, colchicine in lower doses (see below) is frequently used as prophylaxis against recurrent attacks of gout (*N Engl J Med.* 1996;334: 445).

Familial Mediterranean Fever

Colchicine helps prevents recurrent attacks of FMF. Daily colchicine therapy also reduces the risk of systemic amyloidosis, a common complication of untreated FMF (*N Engl J Med.* 2001;345:1748).

Sarcoidosis Arthropathy

Acute arthritis from sarcoidosis may respond to colchicine (*N Engl J Med.* 1960;263:778; *Arch Intern Med.* 1963;112:924).

Pseudogout

Colchicine is inconsistently effective in treating pseudogout.

Behçet Disease

In doses of 0.5–1.5 mg/d orally, colchicine has been effective as first-line therapy for the following manifestations of Behçet disease: oral ulcers, genital ulcers, and pseudofolliculitis (*N Engl J Med.* 1999;341:1284).

Other Uses in Rheumatic Diseases

Colchicine has been used to treat cutaneous manifestations of scleroderma, primary biliary cirrhosis, Sweet syndrome, and palmar fibromatosis.

DOSING

For prophylaxis against gout:

- Given as 0.6 mg orally once per day.
- Some patients may require 1.2–1.8 mg/d in divided doses to prevent recurrent gouty arthritis.
- The daily dose should not exceed 0.6 mg for those with renal insufficiency.

For treatment of acute gout:

- Usually given orally as 1 mg initially, followed by 0.5–0.6 mg orally every 1–2 hours until the patient improves or until abdominal discomfort or diarrhea develops or a total dose of 8 mg has been administered.

- Can be administered intravenously if oral dosing not possible, but intravenous administration requires special precautions (see below).
- The usual initial intravenous dose is 2 mg diluted in 20–50 mL of normal saline and administered over 20 minutes through a well-functioning catheter (to avoid extravasation). Subsequent doses of 0.5–0.6 mg every 6 hours may be administered until the patient improves or until a cumulative dose of 4 mg is reached.
- Because of the risk of toxicity, intravenous colchicine should be avoided in a patient taking oral colchicine.
- Colchicine should never be administered subcutaneously or intramuscularly because doing so causes severe local irritation.

MONITORING THERAPY

- Serum creatinine and liver function tests should be checked before starting colchicine.

SPECIAL PRECAUTIONS

- Colchicine is contraindicated in patients with serious gastrointestinal, cardiac, or renal disease.
- Colchicine is contraindicated in patients with both renal and liver disease or failure.
- Colchicine is contraindicated in patients with blood dyscrasia or with a history of hypersensitivity reactions to the drug.
- Intravenous colchicine should be avoided or used with extreme caution because it can result in fatal bone marrow and multiorgan failure, especially when the recommended doses are exceeded or when the patient has renal and/or liver insufficiency.
- Oral daily colchicine should not exceed 0.6 mg in patients who are over the age of 60 and/or have an elevated serum creatinine. Colchicine-induced neuromyopathy occurs most frequently in patients with renal insufficiency. Oral colchicine should generally be avoided in patients requiring hemodialysis.
- Fertile women should avoid colchicine unless they are using effective contraception. Colchicine is teratogenic in animals and may be unsafe during pregnancy for humans.

COMPLICATIONS

- Oral colchicine most commonly causes abdominal discomfort, nausea, and diarrhea. If these side effects develop, the drug should be stopped; once the gastrointestinal symptoms have resolved, the drug can be cautiously restarted at a lower dose. Gastrointestinal manifestations do not usually develop after the recommended dose of intravenous colchicine.

- Neuromyopathy may complicate long-term daily colchicine use. The clinical presentation resembles polymyositis with proximal muscle weakness and creatinine kinase (CK) enzyme elevations. Neuromyopathy requires stopping colchicine.
- Intravenous colchicine, especially at higher than recommended doses, can cause pancytopenia.

KEY POINTS

- Low-dose, daily colchicine effectively reduces recurrent episodes of gout.
- The high risks of intravenous colchicine limit its usefulness.

■ INTRAVENOUS IMMUNE GLOBULIN (IVIG)

Fiona A. Donald, MD

DEFINITION

- Pooled immune globulin from human plasma, 3000–10,000 donors per batch.
- Contains 95% IgG, < 2.5% IgA, and trace IgM.
- IgG antibodies are directed against a wide variety of antigens.
- Contains trace amounts of soluble CD4, CD8, and HLA molecules.

MECHANISMS OF ACTION

Multiple mechanisms are likely, including the following:

- Modulation of Fc receptor function.
- Suppression of antibody synthesis.
- Direct inhibition of cytokines by naturally occurring anticytokine antibodies.
- Inhibition of superantigen-mediated T-cell activation.
- Inhibition of complement component binding and activation.

PHARMACOKINETICS

- Serum levels of IgG increase immediately postinfusion (fivefold increase with dose of 2 g/kg) and then decrease by 50% after 72 hours due largely to equili-

bration between the intravascular and extravascular spaces.

- In-vivo half-life: Approximately 3 weeks.

USES IN RHEUMATIC DISEASE

Kawasaki Disease

Administration of IVIG within 10 days of onset reduces coronary artery involvement according to well-controlled trials (*N Engl J Med.* 1991;324:1633; *N Engl J Med.* 1986;315:341).

Inflammatory Myopathy

IVIG has demonstrated benefit in refractory adult dermatomyositis (DM). Uncontrolled trials suggest benefit in refractory adult polymyositis (PM) and juvenile DM. A double-blind, placebo-controlled trial of 15 patients with refractory adult DM demonstrated improvement in neuromuscular symptoms, muscle power, and rash in treated patients after one or two infusions. No patients in the placebo group showed improvement. (*N Engl J Med.* 1993;329:1993). Ten patients with PM and 5 with DM demonstrated improvement in muscle strength and creatinine kinase in an open trial of IVIG in 14 patients with PM and 6 with DM. Improvement occurred after two infusions, with maximum benefit after four infusions (*Am J Med.* 1991;91:162-168). Due to cost considerations, it is unlikely that IVIG will become a first-line therapy for inflammatory myositis.

Systemic Lupus Erythematosus

The addition of IVIG to a standard treatment regimen for class III or IV lupus nephritis did not result in improvement in creatinine clearance or proteinuria according to a small randomized trial (*Lancet.* 1999;354:569). An uncontrolled trial of IVIG in 20 patients with SLE reported clinical benefit in 17 of 20 patients. Improvements were seen in arthritis, thrombocytopenia, fever, and neuropsychiatric manifestations (*Semin Arthritis Rheum.* 2000;29:321). Many case reports suggest that thrombocytopenia, psychosis, pleural effusions, carditis, and vasculitis due to SLE may respond to IVIG.

Other Vasculitides

Beneficial effects of IVIG in Wegener granulomatosis, Churg-Strauss syndrome, and microscopic polyangiitis have been suggested by case reports and small open studies. However, the only prospective randomized controlled trial of IVIG in Wegener granulomatosis and microscopic polyangiitis failed to show benefit in terms of reduced disease activity at 3 months versus placebo (*Q J Med.* 2000;93:433).

Rheumatoid Arthritis

IVIG is ineffective in adult rheumatoid arthritis. Two randomized controlled trials (*Arthritis Rheum.* 1996;39: 1027; *Arthritis Rheum.* 1993,36[Suppl]:S57) failed to show benefit of IVIG over the placebo arm.

Antiphospholipid Antibody Syndrome

For recurrent fetal loss, the addition of IVIG to a standard regimen of aspirin plus heparin did not achieve statistical benefit compared with placebo in a randomized double-blind controlled trial of 16 patients (*Am J Obstet Gynecol.* 2000;182:122).

Other Uses

Efficacy of IVIG in managing idiopathic thrombocytopenic purpura, Guillain-Barré syndrome, and chronic inflammatory demyelinating polyneuropathies has been demonstrated in controlled clinical trials.

COMPLICATIONS

- Nonanaphylactic reactions (5–10%): Fever, chills, dyspnea, back pain, and modest hypotension. Treatment includes nonsteroidal anti-inflammatory drugs, antihistamines, and glucocorticoids.
- Aseptic meningitis: Occurs in up to 10% of patients 48–72 hours postinfusion; unrelated to underlying disease.
- Acute renal failure: Due to acute tubular necrosis; diabetes, preexisting renal disease, and advanced age are risk factors.
- Other (rare): Thromboembolic events due to increased serum viscosity.

SPECIAL PRECAUTIONS

- Contraindicated in patients with selective IgA deficiency due to the risk of anaphylaxis.

KEY POINTS

- IVIG is effective in the treatment of Kawasaki disease and refractory dermatomyositis and may have efficacy in polymyositis.
- IVIG has been used in a wide variety of rheumatic diseases. While its use may be warranted in patients with SLE and severe thrombocytopenia, the evidence to date does not support routine use of IVIG for SLE, rheumatoid arthritis, vasculitis other than Kawasaki disease, or the antiphospholipid antibody syndrome.

■ ANTI-TUMOR NECROSIS FACTOR AGENTS: ETANERCEPT (ENBREL), INFLIXIMAB (REMICADE), AND ADALIMUMAB (HUMIRA)

Jonathan Graf, MD

STRUCTURE

- Etanercept is a recombinant, dimeric fusion protein consisting of the soluble human p75 tumor necrosis factor (TNF) receptor coupled to the Fc fragment of human IgG1 lacking the C_H1 domain.
- Infliximab is a "humanized" monoclonal antibody in which the antigen-binding regions of a mouse anti-TNF monoclonal antibody have been placed in the framework of a human IgG1κ antibody.
- Adalimumab is a recombinant, fully human monoclonal IgG1κ antibody.

MECHANISM OF ACTION

- The cytokines TNF-α and TNF-β bind cell-surface TNF receptors and regulate a wide array of biologic functions necessary for normal inflammatory and immune responses.
- TNF-α mediates many of the proinflammatory processes implicated in inflammatory arthritis.
- Etanercept binds soluble TNF-α and TNF-β and prevents their association with TNF receptors.
- Both infliximab and adalimumab bind soluble as well as membrane-bound TNF-α and block cell signaling through TNF receptor pathways.

PHARMACOKINETICS

- Bioavailability: Etanercept (subcutaneous) 60% and adalimumab (subcutaneous) 64%. Infliximab is administered intravenously.
- Average half-life: Etanercept, 4.25 days; infliximab, 8–12 days; and adalimumab, 14 days.
- Clearance: The exact mechanisms of clearance for etanercept, infliximab, and adalimumab have not been definitively determined, although the reticuloendothelial system may play a role. No formal studies have been done to determine the effects of hepatic or renal impairment on clearance.

USES IN RHEUMATIC DISEASE

Rheumatoid Arthritis

Etanercept has been studied in diverse populations of adult patients with active rheumatoid arthritis (RA), including patients with active RA despite previous therapy with at least one disease-modifying antirheumatic drug (DMARD) (*N Engl J Med.* 1997;337:141; *Ann Intern Med.* 1999;130:478) and DMARD-naïve patients with early RA (*N Engl J Med.* 2000;343:1586). Etanercept is superior to placebo as either monotherapy or add-on therapy with methotrexate (*N Engl J Med.* 1999; 340:253) in relieving many of the signs and symptoms associated with RA.

In patients with active RA despite treatment with methotrexate, infliximab is superior to placebo in reducing the signs and symptoms of disease when given in concert with methotrexate (*N Engl J Med.* 2000; 343:1594).

Adalimumab has been studied as monotherapy and in combination with methotrexate (*Arthritis Rheum.* 2003;48:35) and other DMARDs. It has also been studied in patients who did not respond to at least one previous DMARD, remained on stable doses of current DMARD therapy, or were DMARD-naïve. In all populations, adalimumab is superior to placebo in controlling the signs and symptoms of RA.

Etanercept (*Arthritis Rheum.* 2002;46:1443), infliximab (*N Engl J Med.* 2000;343:1594), and adalimumab (*Ann Rheum Dis.* 2002;61:311) have been shown to slow or inhibit the radiographic progression of joint destruction in RA.

Psoriatic Arthritis

Etanercept is the only anti-TNF agent approved by the Food and Drug Administration for the treatment of psoriatic arthritis, and it has demonstrated efficacy as monotherapy in a randomized, placebo-controlled study (*Lancet.* 2000;356:385). Other anti-TNF agents, such as infliximab, are thought to provide similar benefits but have only been evaluated in smaller trials (*Ann Rheum Dis.* 2000;59:428).

Ankylosing Spondylitis

The efficacy of etanercept (*N Engl J Med.* 2002;346: 1349) and infliximab (*Lancet.* 2002;359:1187) in managing the signs and symptoms of ankylosing spondylitis has been demonstrated in several studies.

Other Spondyloarthropathies

The effectiveness of infliximab in the treatment of undifferentiated spondyloarthropathy (*J Rheumatol.* 2002;

29:118) and the axial and peripheral arthritis associated with inflammatory bowel disease (*Lancet.* 2000;356: 1821) has been suggested in small, open studies. The anti-TNF agents have not been rigorously studied in reactive arthritis.

Juvenile Idiopathic Arthritis

Etanercept is the only anti-TNF agent to be approved by the Food and Drug Administration for the treatment of juvenile idiopathic arthritis. It has been rigorously studied in both short- and long-term clinical trials and has been found to be efficacious when used as monotherapy or as an addition to treatment with methotrexate (*N Engl J Med.* 2000;342:763).

Adult Still Disease

A small open-label study suggests that etanercept may reduce the signs and symptoms of adult Still disease (*Arthritis Rheum.* 2002;46:1171).

Vasculitis

Adding etanercept to standard therapy for Wegener granulomatosis is not beneficial.

DOSING

- Etanercept: Given as a single, 25-mg subcutaneous injection twice weekly; must be refrigerated and reconstituted in sterile solution before being administered.

- Infliximab: Infusion is given in a doctor's office or infusion center and takes approximately 2–3 hours to complete. Administered as an intravenous infusion beginning with a loading dose of 3 mg/kg at 0, 2, and 6 weeks. Dosing is usually maintained at 3 mg/kg every 8 weeks. Flexibility in dosing allows for the dose to be increased up to 10 mg/kg and/or the interval decreased to as little as every 4 weeks, depending on response to therapy.

- Adalimumab: Given as a single, 40-mg subcutaneous injection once every other week. Medication comes preloaded in a syringe, does not need to be reconstituted, and should be refrigerated before use. Dosing flexibility allows the medication to be given as often as 40 mg every week as clinical conditions warrant.

INITIATING THERAPY

- The risk of reactivation of latent tuberculosis should be assessed and should include, at a minimum, a

baseline test for reactivity to purified protein derivative (PPD) prior to initiation of therapy.

- The risk of reactivation of latent infection with histoplasmosis and coccidioidomycosis should be considered in patients from endemic regions.
- No baseline or routine laboratory testing is officially
recommended.
- Age-appropriate cancer screening, while not officially
recommended, may be of benefit prior to initiating
therapy.
- Patients are recommended not to receive live vaccinations after initiating or continuing therapy.
- Patients should be monitored for injection site or infusion reactions while receiving therapy.
- Anti-TNF agents should not be used in patients with
a history of multiple sclerosis or any other demyelinating disease.

SPECIAL PRECAUTIONS

- TNF antagonists should not be used in patients with
a history of latent tuberculosis unless they have completed an adequate course of prophylactic therapy.
- The TNF antagonists are contraindicated in patients
with active acute or chronic infections.
- Patients receiving infliximab should have baseline
screening for infection, including temperature and
symptom assessment, prior to each infusion.
- Patients should be instructed to contact their physician if any symptoms of acute infection develop.
- The anti-TNF agents should not be used in patients
with active or suspected malignancies.
- Hypersensitivity to an anti-TNF agent is a contraindication to its use.
- Patients with previous allergies to mouse-derived
products should not receive infliximab.
- All anti-TNF agents are pregnancy category B.
- The use of anti-TNF agents in the setting of hepatic
disease or renal failure has not been studied.
- Infliximab is specifically contraindicated in patients
with moderate or severe congestive heart failure; extreme caution should be exercised for the other anti-
TNF agents in this setting.

COMPLICATIONS

- Postmarketing surveillance of these agents has reported hospitalizations and deaths from serious infections, although randomized trials have not demonstrated an increased frequency of serious infections.

- Blockade of TNF poses a theoretic risk of increased
malignancy. There are postmarketing reports of lymphomas developing in patients treated with either
etanercept or infliximab, but it remains to be determined whether there is an actual increase in the incidence of malignancy.
- Etanercept and adalimumab are associated with a
high degree of mild to moderate injection site reactions, including erythema, pruritus, pain, and/or
swelling, which are commonly self-limited early in
the course of therapy.
- Infliximab is associated with a significant incidence
of infusion reactions within 1–2 hours after receiving
the therapy, including fever, chills, urticaria, and cardiopulmonary symptoms.
- Infliximab has been linked to a serum-sickness type
of syndrome.
- The use of the anti-TNF agents, especially infliximab, can lead to the development of antibodies to
the agent. Whether these antibodies influence efficacy or adverse reactions is uncertain.
- The use of TNF antagonists can be associated with
the development of antinuclear antibodies and other
autoantibodies and, rarely, a lupus-like syndrome.
- Use of anti-TNF agents may worsen symptoms of
congestive heart failure.
- Rarely, a demyelinating syndrome has been observed
in patients using anti-TNF agents.
- Cytopenias and aplastic anemia have been reported
in sporadic cases of patients taking anti-TNF agents.

DISCONTINUING THERAPY

- TNF antagonists should be discontinued if active
infection, malignancy, or a serious adverse event develops.
- Because of their relatively long half-lives, the immunosuppressive effects of infliximab and adalimumab should be considered when evaluating and
treating those patients who have recently discontinued therapy.

KEY POINTS

- The TNF antagonists reduce the signs and symptoms
and inhibit structural joint damage of moderate or
severe RA. They are of proven efficacy in controlling
the signs and symptoms of ankylosing spondylitis
and psoriatic arthritis.
- Lack of long-term safety data, need for parenteral administration, and high cost should be considered
when tailoring this therapy to specific patients.

■ BISPHOPHONATES: ETIDRONATE (DIDRONEL), PAMIDRONATE (AREDIA), ALENDRONATE (FOSAMAX), RISEDRONATE (ACTONEL), AND ZOLEDRONIC ACID (ZOMETA)

Dolores Shoback, MD

MECHANISM OF ACTION

- Bind to bone matrix at sites of active resorption and are thus considered antiresorptive agents.
- Inhibit bone resorption by two mechanisms: (1) All bisphosphonates enhance osteoclast apoptosis; and (2) aminobisphosphonates (eg, pamidronate, alendronate, risedronate, zoledronic acid) interfere with osteoclast function by blocking the mevalonate pathway and the geranylgeranylation of low-molecular-weight guanyl nucleotide (GTP) binding proteins (GTPases). Such proteins are involved in the formation of the ruffled border of the osteoclast—a cellular structure that allows the osteoclast to adhere tightly to bone matrix and allow resorption.
- Adhere avidly to bone and remain there for days, months, and even years. In vivo, this translates into a long half-life for biologic action.

PHARMACOKINETICS

- Bioavailability: Poorly absorbed from the gastrointestinal tract—less than 1% of the administered dose even on an empty stomach (www.pdr.net; *Arch Intern Med.* 2001;161:353).
- Metabolism: Not substantially metabolized in vivo.
- Half-life: Depends on duration of therapy, specific compound, total amount administered, and rate of bone remodeling.
- Clearance: Renally without significant in vivo metabolism.

USES IN RHEUMATIC DISEASES

Postmenopausal Osteoporosis

The efficacy of oral bisphosphonates alendronate (10 mg/day) and risedronate (5 mg/d) in treating postmenopausal osteoporosis and the preventing vertebral and hip fractures has been confirmed in several randomized, double-blind, placebo-controlled trials. (*N Engl J Med.* 1995;333:1437; *Lancet.* 1996;348:1535; *JAMA.* 1999;282:1344; *N Engl J Med.* 2001;344:333). Alendronate (5 mg/d) has also been approved for the prevention of postmenopausal bone loss (*N Engl J Med.* 1998;338:485; *Ann Intern Med.* 1998;128:253).

Alendronate and risedronate reduce the incidence of new vertebral fractures by 40–50% and hip fractures by approximately the same percentage for alendronate, compared with placebo. With risedronate, statistically significant reductions in hip fractures were seen in postmenopausal women aged 70–79 in whom osteoporosis was diagnosed by low bone mineral density measurements. Women aged 80 years or older, enrolled on the basis of clinical risk factors for fracture (eg, poor eyesight, history of smoking, fall-related injury, etc), did not experience an improvement in hip fracture risk after 3 years of risedronate therapy.

Glucocorticoid-Induced Osteoporosis

The oral bisphosphonates alendronate and risedronate have been approved in the United States for the treatment and prevention of glucocorticoid-induced bone loss in men and women. These double-blind, placebo-controlled, multicenter trials included patients with a variety of rheumatologic, gastrointestinal, pulmonary, and dermatologic conditions. Patients were receiving either initial glucocorticoid therapy (*N Engl J Med.* 1998;339:292; *Arthritis Rheum.* 1999;42:2309) or maintenance therapy with glucocorticoids long term (*N Engl J Med.* 1998;339:292; *J Bone Miner Res.* 2000;15:1006). The dose of glucocorticoids administered to patients enrolled in these trials was 7.5 mg of prednisone equivalents per day or more. Therapy with bisphosphonate or placebo was for 12 months, and in one case was followed by a 12-month, open-label extension (*Arthritis Rheum.* 2001;44:202). Primary outcomes were changes in lumbar spine bone mineral density. Secondary outcomes were changes in proximal femur bone mineral density, vertebral fractures, and changes in biochemical markers of bone turnover. Therapy with either bisphosphonate significantly increased bone mineral density at the lumbar spine and femoral neck compared with placebo-treated persons. Although the incidence overall of vertebral fractures was low in these trials, there were fewer patients with vertebral fractures (0.7%) who had been treated with alendronate at any dose (5 or 10 mg/d for 24 months or 2.5 mg/d for 12 months followed by 10 mg/d for 12 months) compared with those patients treated with placebo for 24 months (6.8%) (*Arthritis Rheum.* 2001;44:202). Similarly, patients treated with risedronate (5 mg/d for 12 months) experienced a statistically significant reduction in new vertebral fractures of 70% compared with placebo-treated patients (*Calcif Tissue Int.* 2000; 67:277).

Osteoporosis in Men

Alendronate (10 mg/d) has been approved for the treatment of low bone mass in men. This drug is effective at increasing bone mineral density at the spine, femoral neck, and total body and decreasing the vertebral fracture incidence (*N Engl J Med.* 2000;343:604).

Paget Disease of Bone

Both alendronate and risedronate are approved for the treatment of this disease (*J Bone Miner Res.* 2001;16: 1379). Risedronate improves both the elevated alkaline phosphatase and the pain due to Paget disease after 3 months of therapy (30 mg/d) (*Bone.* 1998; 22:51; *J Clin Endocrinol Metab.* 1998;83:1906). In one series, risedronate was also shown to enhance radiologic healing of Pagetic lesions (*Bone.* 2000;26:263). In a randomized, double-blind trial comparing risedronate (30 mg/d for 2 months) to etidronate (400 mg/d for 6 months), a higher percentage of patients normalized their alkaline phosphatase values on risedronate (73%) versus etidronate (15%). The maintenance of a normal alkaline phosphatase at 6 months after therapy was more common in patients treated with risedronate (77%) versus etidronate (15%). Patients on risedronate were also noted to have greater reduction in skeletal pain. Alendronate has also been successfully used to treat Paget disease. In a randomized, double-blind trial comparing alendronate (40 mg/d for 6 months) with placebo, there was a mean decline in alkaline phosphatase levels of 73%, which was markedly greater than placebo-treated patients who experienced no significant change in this parameter (*Am J Med.* 1996;171:341). In this same study, approximately 50% of patients showed a normalization of alkaline phosphatase levels and a radiologically documented improvement in their bone lesions. In a double-blind, randomized trial comparing alendronate (40 mg/d) with etidronate (400 mg/d) for 6 months, alendronate was shown to be superior. Alkaline phosphatase activity decreased to a greater extent (by 79% with alendronate compared with 44% with etidronate) (*J Clin Endocrinol Metab.* 1996;81:961). In addition, alendronate was able to normalize alkaline phosphatase activity in 63% of patients, which was significantly greater than the efficacy of etidronate—only 17% of patients normalized this parameter with 6 months of therapy.

OTHER USES

Bisphosphonates have been successfully used in the prevention of skeletal complications (bone pain, pathologic fractures, spinal cord compression, and hypercalcemia) in patients with solid tumors and multiple myeloma (pamidronate: *J Clin Oncol.* 1998;16:593; zoledronic acid: *Cancer.* 2001;91:1191; *Cancer Pract.* 2002;10: 219). Although skeletal-related complications are reduced with this therapy in multiple myeloma, no survival advantage over placebo has been observed (*J Clin Oncol.* 2002;20:719).

Intravenous bisphosphonates are the treatment of choice for hypercalcemia of malignancy (pamidronate: *Am J Med.* 1993;95:297; zoledronic acid: *J Clin Oncol.* 2001;19:558).

DOSING REGIMEN

- Alendronate: 70 mg once weekly for osteoporosis (*J Bone Miner Res.* 2002; 17:1998). Weekly alendronate (35 mg/wk) has also been approved for the prevention of postmenopausal bone loss (*J Bone Miner Res.* 2002;17:1998).
- Risedronate: 35 mg once weekly for osteoporosis (*Calc Tissue Int.* 2002;71:103).
- Oral bisphosphonates are best absorbed on an empty stomach, 30–60 minutes before breakfast, with 8 oz of water and while remaining upright.

INITIATING THERAPY

- Weekly oral alendronate or risedronate is preferred in combination with adequate daily calcium and vitamin D supplementation in treating and preventing osteoporosis. Therapy can be initiated on the basis of bone mineral density measurements or the history of fragility fractures in a patient at high risk for bone loss.

MONITORING THERAPY

- The efficacy of bisphosphonate therapy to increase bone mineral density can be monitored on an annual or semiannual basis in patients with osteoporosis.
- A reduction in bone resorption can also be assessed by measuring biochemical markers of bone turnover (eg, urinary excretion of N-telopeptide, deoxypyridinolines, and pyridinolines). The latter measurements, however, are subject to variation. Most patients with osteoporosis do not demonstrate elevated rates of bone turnover by these measurements.
- In treating Paget disease of bone, regular monitoring of alkaline phosphatase is advised along with periodic skeletal radiologic evaluation to assess the response to therapy.

SPECIAL PRECAUTIONS

- Because these drugs have a long half-life in bone and significantly reduce skeletal remodeling, their use is strongly discouraged in growing children (except in very unusual circumstances) and in women of child-bearing age.

- These drugs should be used with great care, if at all, in patients with renal insufficiency.

COMPLICATIONS

- Daily, long-term alendronate and risedronate therapy for glucocorticoid-induced or postmenopausal osteoporosis may potentially cause gastrointestinal irritation, especially abdominal pain and, less commonly, esophagitis, ulceration, and bleeding (*N Engl J Med.* 1996;335:1016). Weekly administration of both alendronate and risedronate has obviated most concerns regarding gastrointestinal adverse events. Additional minor adverse events have included headache, nausea, and body pain, which have generally been mild.

- Patients receiving intensive, higher-dose daily oral bisphosphonates (alendronate and risedronate) for Paget disease of bone should be closely monitored for upper gastrointestinal adverse events.

- Acute phase reactions, characterized by joint pains, myalgias, and fever within 24–48 hours of the infusion, can develop in patients receiving intravenous aminobisphosphonates. Such reactions occur in approximately 10% of patients receiving these therapies and are self-limited.

- Patients with mild renal insufficiency (serum creatinine < 2.5 mg/dL) do not need doses of bisphosphonate adjusted for renal function. Long-term oral bisphosphonates are not recommended in patients with serum creatinine > 2.5 mg/dL.

- Alendronate is not recommended for use in patients with renal insufficiency (creatinine clearance < 35 mL/min) (www.pdr.net).

- Intravenous zoledronic acid (4 mg infused over 15 minutes) has the potential for inducing renal failure, and patients with significant renal insufficiency (serum creatinine ≥ 3.0 mg/dL) should not receive this medication. Renal function should be assessed before each dose of zoledronic acid or other intravenous bisphosphonate.

- Although oral bisphosphonates are not contraindicated for use with nonsteroidal anti-inflammatory agents, the potential for increased upper gastrointestinal adverse effects with such a combination suggests that careful clinical monitoring is indicated.

- Second- and third-generation bisphosphonates (alendronate, risedronate) used in established treatment regimens have not been associated with the development of osteomalacia by bone biopsy studies. Older first-generation bisphosphonates (eg, etidronate), when used in high doses for conditions like Paget disease, must be used with care. There is the potential for the accumulation of such agents in bone over time with the subsequent induction of a mineralization defect, low bone turnover, and frank osteomalacia (*J Clin Endocrinol Metab.* 1996;81:961).

LONG-TERM CONCERNS

- It is unclear how long women at risk for postmenopausal bone loss or men with idiopathic or hypogonadism-induced osteoporosis should be treated. Therapy for years with oral alendronate or risedronate leads to a large skeletal reservoir of these drugs that may have long-term effects—yet unknown—on the repair of microdamage to the skeleton. Thus far, excessive clinical fracture risk with 7 years of therapy with alendronate has not been observed (*J Clin Endocrinol Metab.* 2000;85:3109).

KEY POINTS

- Bisphosphonates are the most skeletally selective agents currently available for the treatment of a variety of metabolic bone diseases including osteoporosis, Paget disease, and the skeletal complications of malignancy. They demonstrate excellent therapeutic efficacy and can be used in both oral and intravenous formulations depending on the disease state.

Practical Guide to the Use of Assistive Devices, Physical Therapy, & Occupational Therapy

57

David I. Daikh, MD, PhD

Rehabilitation therapy, which is a critical component in the overall care of the patient with rheumatic disease, seeks to prolong, promote, or restore function. In the absence of normal use, joints and muscles rapidly lose function. The effectiveness of even the most up-to-date medical treatment, therefore, may be significantly limited if physical and occupational therapies are not also undertaken. The goal of "therapy" in this context is not to control the disease process but rather to minimize the adverse effects of the disease on mobility, dexterity, and in general, the complex activities required for the normal range of human activities.

EVALUATION OF THE PATIENT

Determination of functional status is critical when evaluating a patient's need for physical or occupational therapy. The classification of functional status developed by the American College of Rheumatology (Table 57–1) describes the important levels of functional limitation and emphasizes the impact of these limitations on normal activities of daily living. In the evaluation of a patient with arthritis or other rheumatic disease, it is essential to determine how a given symptom impacts that person's function. Important functional limitations require appropriate rehabilitation therapy. Such therapy may range from simple home exercises prescribed by the clinician to a formal referral to a physical or occupational therapist. The need for therapy occurs not only among patients with chronic conditions, such as rheumatoid arthritis, but also among patients with acute or subacute musculoskeletal injury and in postoperative patients. In addition to restoring function, therapy is often required to maintain a patient's current level of function and to prevent loss of function. Therefore, the assessment of a patient for the need for physical or occupational therapy should also anticipate future loss of function.

SPECIFIC INTERVENTIONS

Effective interventions are individualized, practical, economical, and valued by the patient. Initiation of the rehabilitation early in the disease process encourages compliance because the patient identifies rehabilitation therapy as part of the overall treatment plan. Physical and occupational therapists play an important, but underappreciated role in patient education, which in turn is an important determinant of the effectiveness of a therapeutic plan.

Goals of Therapy

The goals of therapy can generally be classified as prevention, restoration, or maintenance. **Prevention** requires early diagnosis and institution of a treatment program to prevent loss of function. Such a program includes an assessment of activities, advice on joint preservation, and encouragement of energy conservation for patients with systemic disease. **Restoration** of lost function requires a physical therapy program to recover lost muscle strength and range of motion and, often, the provision of biomechanical or assistive devices that allow for more effective or less painful activity. The goal of **maintenance therapy** is to prevent further decline in the patient's functional level. The therapist meets these general goals by designing interventions that specifically address a number of key issues (Table 57–2). In general, the physical therapist addresses issues of strength, mobility, and range of motion, and the occupational therapist deals with issues that arise from the activities of daily living or vocation, including provision of assistive devices. The therapist usually applies local therapy to improve strength, to preserve and increase range of motion, to maintain or improve joint stability, to improve stamina, to increase the efficacy of motion, or to decrease pain and swelling.

Table 57–1. American College of Rheumatology classification of global functional status in rheumatoid arthritis.

Class	Functional Status
I	Completely able to perform usual activities of daily living (self-care, vocational, and avocational).[a]
II	Able to perform usual self-care and vocational activities but limited in avocational activities.
III	Able to perform usual self-care activities but limited in vocational and avocational activities.
IV	Limited in ability to perform usual self-care, vocational, and avocational activities.

[a]Usual self-care activities include dressing, feeding, bathing, grooming, and toileting. Avocational includes recreational and leisure, and vocational includes work, school, and homemaking. Activities are patient-desired and age- and sex-specific.

Important examples of these therapies are described below.

Rest & Exercise

Rest and exercise are both beneficial and problematic for many patients with rheumatic disease. While rest can decrease inflammation, excessive rest and avoidance of activity can hasten disability. Similarly, although exercise increases strength and endurance, it can also exacerbate joint inflammation. Thus, optimal therapy requires the judicious and balanced use of both rest and exercise. Rest can be applied locally to specific joints in the form of splints. Rest of involved joints or tendons is of clear benefit for a number of use-related conditions, such as tendinitis or carpal tunnel syndrome. There is little evidence, however, that splinting affects the progression of joint deformity. For some patients with early or reducible deformities, however, splinting of in-

Table 57–2. Functions commonly addressed by physical and occupational therapy.

Strength
Range of motion
Mobility
Joint stability
Stamina
Activities of daily living
Vocational level
Self-image
Communication skills
Sexuality
Education

dividual finger joints can restore mechanical advantage for specific functions. There also can be a cosmetic benefit of splinting of certain joints. Generalized rest improves symptoms and inflammation in rheumatoid arthritis. However, because the benefit is temporary and largely symptomatic and because of adverse effects of generalized rest (eg, loss of conditioning, strength, range of motion, and bone mass), disease-modifying medical therapy has been emphasized in recent years over prolonged systemic rest.

Exercise is a critical component of physical therapy because of its ability to increase strength, stamina, and range of motion. Exercise of specific muscle groups in the setting of disuse atrophy can improve the biomechanical function of joints. Exercise can be **passive, active,** or **active-assistive.**

Passive exercise is used to increase range of motion and is used in situations in which a patient is unable to move and, therefore, at risk for contracture. Passive exercise is particularly important for patients with weakness due to neurologic conditions or inflammatory myopathy. Because passive exercise can increase inflammation in a significantly inflamed joint, it should be avoided in acute inflammatory arthritis, such as the crystalline-induced arthropathies or a severely inflamed rheumatoid joint.

Active exercise increases strength and endurance. Various forms of strengthening exercises may be used. Isometric or static contraction develops maximal muscle tension and strength without muscle shortening. Isometric exercise increases the period of time that a specific force can be generated by a muscle. This form of exercise uses no joint motion and, therefore, is preferred for patients with inflammatory arthritis. Isotonic or dynamic contraction produces muscle shortening or lengthening with tension applied to a joint throughout its range of motion. In addition to strengthening, isotonic exercise improves cardiovascular endurance. For arthritis patients, the preferred exercise progression initially involves isometric exercise to build strength and static endurance. Once adequate strength is obtained and joint inflammation and pain are adequately controlled, the patient progresses to isotonic exercise to further increase strength and cardiovascular stamina. During dynamic exercise, repetitive motions should be under low resistance to avoid excessive joint stress. Exercise in therapy pools warmed to 90 °F can be more comfortable and allow for more effective exercise for many arthritis patients. The local chapter of the Arthritis Foundation usually can provide information regarding the location and use of such pools.

Because rheumatic disease is generally chronic and because referrals to therapists are often limited by third-party payers, patients are usually instructed in proper exercise technique during a few sessions with a physical therapist and then given a program for home exercise. Reinforcement of the importance of this program by both the therapist and physician is important for long-term compliance.

Physical Modalities

Therapists use physical modalities, such as the application of heat or cold, to lessen symptoms and improve function. By providing temporary relief of pain, these modalities can help prepare the patient with arthritis or soft tissue musculoskeletal injuries for exercise or physical therapy. Heat therapy and cryotherapy may be used by the physical or occupational therapist before a therapy session, or by patients at home for symptomatic pain relief.

Heat therapy is generally used to reduce pain and increase flexibility. Superficial heat is applied by hot packs, paraffin oil baths, hydrotherapy, warmed air, or infrared radiation, generally for 15–20 minutes at a time. Paraffin wax heating baths are now widely available to the general consumer. Deep heat generated by ultrasound or by short-wave diathermy warms tissues below the submucosa. Heat is thought to reduce pain through a combination of increased blood flow, reduction of muscle spasm, and elevation of the pain threshold. Heat may improve flexibility by increasing the viscous properties of collagen and by reducing pain. It has been difficult to clearly establish a benefit of heat therapy in controlled trials; an exception is a report that the combination of exercise and paraffin wax baths increased hand function. The therapeutic efficacy of either form of deep heating has not been established. Nonetheless, heat therapy generally improves patient global assessments.

While the therapist usually decides whether to use heat and determines the specific heating modality, the clinician should be aware that heat may be used and inform the therapist about specific medical conditions for which heat is contraindicated. Heat should not be used on patients with impaired sensation (eg, a peripheral neuropathy affecting the involved joint or region) or severely impaired judgment. Heat modality is also not recommended for acute inflammatory arthritis. Special precautions apply to deep heating. Because tissues are heated below the skin, there is less stimulation of cutaneous temperature-sensing neurons. Patients therefore perceive less intense heat, despite elevations in temperature sufficient to cause tissue burns. In addition, because it is applied to a large tissue area, short-wave diathermy can cause systemic heating and activation of thermoregulatory responses. This modality is contraindicated for patients with cardiac insufficiency, impaired circulation, and rheumatoid arthritis.

Cryotherapy is used primarily to decrease the pain and swelling of inflammation. Cold is applied by ice pack, cold bath, or vapor coolant spray, generally for 10–15 minutes. The mechanism of its beneficial effects is thought to be through a combination of vasoconstriction, decreased nerve conduction velocity, and possibly, inhibition of proinflammatory mediators. Cold therapy is effective in relieving pain in uncontrolled studies. The same precautions for heat therapy also apply to cold therapy. In addition, cryotherapy is contraindicated for patients with Raynaud phenomenon, and therapists should be forewarned of the presence of this condition.

Transcutaneous Electrical Nerve Stimulation

Transcutaneous electrical nerve stimulation (TENS) is used for the temporary relief of joint or muscle pain, or muscle spasm. The rationale for TENS is based on the gate theory of pain, in which stimulation of local sensory nerves is thought to block the conduction of pain to the ascending spinal tract by small C fibers. The most commonly used TENS modes are high-frequency TENS, low-frequency TENS, and burst-mode, which delivers low-frequency bursts of high-frequency TENS. High-frequency TENS stimulates sensory nerves and is applied to affected joints for immediate and short-term pain relief. Low-frequency TENS stimulates the motor end plate and is applied to involved areas of muscle, such as an area of spasm or a trigger point, or to the muscles around a painful joint. Both low-frequency and burst-mode TENS are believed to produce longer-lasting pain relief, but burst-mode is more comfortable for the patient. TENS may also decrease stiffness for short periods of time. Placebo-controlled trials of TENS indicate that the analgesia produced by TENS is comparable to that produced by placebo. However, other studies suggest that the duration of its analgesic effects may be longer than that produced by placebo in some patients. TENS should not be used near the heart of patients with pacemakers or cardiac rhythm problems.

ASSISTIVE DEVICES & ENVIRONMENTAL MODIFICATION

Assistive devices can provide the critical difference between functional independence and the inability to perform simple or complex tasks. For patients with significant or refractory functional limitations, an occupational therapist can be extremely helpful in assessing the need for specific devices and instructing the patient on their use. Although a device may solve a functional problem, there may be a psychological barrier to its use, and the therapist can also be very useful in helping the patient overcome this obstacle as well. In general, assistive devices function by providing leverage, allowing a patient to generate increased force with less effort; extending reach beyond the limit imposed by impaired joints; or supporting and maintaining joints in a stable anatomic position. An amazing array of assistive devices are available through suppliers of medical devices.

For many patients, significant modifications to their home or work environment may be necessary to accommodate the functional disability that results from rheumatic disease or to prevent progression of a musculoskeletal problem. Functional and ergonomic assessment by an occupational therapist can discover and remedy significant environmental obstacles.

SELECTED PROBLEMS

Gait Problems

Falls are an overwhelmingly important problem in the elderly population; estimates are that one-third of all people over the age of 65 fall at least once a year. Ten percent of these falls result in injury and approximately 5% them result in fracture. Hip fracture is the most common and the most devastating injury. Hip fracture is the leading cause of injury-related admissions to American hospitals and is a contributing factor in up to 40% of all admissions to nursing homes. Gait problems resulting from arthritis in the lower extremities are an important contributing factor in many falls. Balance and joint function depend on lower extremity strength, which is frequently diminished among patients with hip or knee arthritis. Thus, in addition to medical therapy to minimize arthritis, physical therapy aimed at improving strength and balance is an important part of the therapeutic approach to improving gait and reducing the risk of falls for patients with lower extremity arthritis.

Many patients with gait instability find that a **cane** improves their feeling of stability. The major role of the cane, however, is pain reduction. A single prong cane can support up to 25% of body weight. Proper cane function requires that the patient carry the cane in the hand opposite that of the involved leg. The cane is extended and placed in parallel with the involved leg. To go upstairs and downstairs with a cane, the saying "up with the good, down with the bad" should be taught. Proper cane length should be such that the arm is slightly flexed 15–30 degrees with the cane touching the ground. A simple rule of thumb is that the top of the cane should be level with the proximal wrist crease with the patient standing.

Osteoarthritis of the Knee

Osteoarthritis of the knee is a common cause of long-term disability. Medial compartment disease generally begins first and progresses more rapidly than degeneration of either the lateral compartment or patellofemoral joint. As a result, there is a progressive varus deformity of the knee and pronation of the foot. A recent controlled trial of lateral wedge insoles in patients with knee osteoarthritis demonstrated that this intervention reduces varus knee strain and improves symptoms. Weakness of the muscles that move the knee joint is an early and progressive condition that accompanies knee arthritis. Furthermore, by exacerbating the biomechanical abnormalities associated with knee arthritis, weakness of the leg muscles contributes to pain and progressive damage of articular cartilage. Physical therapy combined with an exercise program can improve symptoms and functional status of patients with knee arthritis. An ideal treatment program for osteoarthritis of the knee should include the following: exercises to promote range of motion and leg strengthening, correction of foot pronation with supportive insoles, and appropriate use of a cane. Weight reduction should also be strongly encouraged for the overweight patient because obesity is an established risk factor for the development and progression of knee osteoarthritis.

A typical prescription for quadriceps strengthening exercises includes non-weight-bearing isometric holding of the leg in extension—10 repetitions of 5 seconds each. This exercise should be done 3 to 4 times a week at first, progressing to daily and then slowly to 3 sets of 10–15 repetitions each day. Isotonic exercise of the quadriceps also begins with 10 repetitions without weight resistance, then also progresses to 3 sets of 15 repetitions, followed by progressive addition of weight resistance. These same exercises can be used for hamstring strengthening.

Foot Care in Patients with Rheumatoid Arthritis

Rheumatoid arthritis affects joints of the foot and ankle in up to 90% of patients, and foot pain is extremely common among patients with rheumatoid arthritis. Pain may result from active synovitis, from structural or biomechanical changes, from secondary degenerative joint disease, or from a combination of these processes. Although medical therapy may control pain due to inflammation, improvement in pain due to abnormal biomechanical function requires the use of proper shoes, internal bracing, and foot orthotics. Patients with rheumatoid arthritis frequently experience forefoot pain (metatarsalgia) due to inflammation of the metatarsophalangeal joints and, in severe disease, to the anterior dislocation of the fat pad cushion and subluxation of the metatarsal heads. Normally, non-weight-bearing portions of the foot become painful as they assume a greater weight-bearing role. Semirigid foot orthotics aimed at distributing weight equally over the plantar surface of the foot are effective for relief of metatarsalgia. In addition, a shoe with an adequately sized toe box and substantial heel counter is essential. Individualized, custom-made shoes with appropriate internal bracing can be of benefit for difficult cases.

Hand Arthritis

Arthritis of the small joints of the hand results in pain, stiffness, and loss of function in patients with either osteoarthritis or rheumatoid arthritis. Both conditions can cause hand deformities that result in further functional loss. While an increasing body of evidence indicates that aggressive medical therapy can slow the progression of joint damage in rheumatoid arthritis, there is little convincing evidence that occupational therapy impacts the progression of joint damage in rheumatoid arthritis. Occupational therapy, however, clearly can improve functional status. Joint contractures develop rapidly and subtly, especially in joints that retain partial motion. Active or passive joint motion stretches the joint capsule and associated ligaments and muscles. Normal joint motion can be maintained with as little as five repetitions of full joint motion daily. Therefore, range of motion exercises for all affected joints should be part of the daily therapy for patients with arthritis. Such exercises can be taught or reinforced by an occupational therapist. Even in the setting of severe deformities of the hand, the provision of assistive devices improves functional status and the ability to undertake many activities of daily living. An experienced occupational therapist can provide a wide range of devices, such as mechanical reachers, utensils with enlarged handles, enhanced gripping materials, and button hooks. Splinting also can improve the function of specific joints by restoring biomechanical advantage.

WHEN TO REFER FOR PHYSICAL OR OCCUPATIONAL THERAPY

Referral of a patient with rheumatic disease for physical or other rehabilitative therapy requires specific attention on the part of the clinician. Because patients with chronic rheumatic disease commonly have specific and unique problems, it is important to identify therapists and other allied professionals who have experience and interest in treating these specialized problems. If such persons are not available, then it is incumbent upon clinicians to develop a close working relationship with therapists and teach them about the specific medical problems of their patients. When a patient is referred for physical or other therapy, therapists should be provided with the primary diagnosis for the problem they are being asked to treat and information about the specific problem for which the patient is being referred. Pain and inflammation should be under optimal control at the time of referral so that the patient can participate to the fullest possible extent in the rehabilitative therapy and so that symptoms and disease will not be aggravated by overuse. The therapist should be explicitly notified of active areas of inflammation so that excessive exercise of these joints can be avoided. If the physician has identified a specific functional deficit in a patient, it should be noted along with specification of the desired functional outcome. The efficacy of the therapist in patient education may also be enhanced if relevant supporting information, such as reports of radiographic findings, is included in the referral. After the patient has been referred for therapy, the clinician should determine whether the therapy has been effective and provide appropriate feedback to the therapist through regular communication. This communication can help develop a rapport between physician and therapist that will foster increased knowledge on the part of the therapist about rheumatic diseases, and that will also ultimately benefit the patient.

REFERENCES

Clark BM. Physical and occupational therapy in the management of arthritis. *CMAJ.* 2000;163:999. [PMID: 11068573]

Lorig K, Fries JF. *The Arthritis Help Book.* 5th ed. Perseus Publishing, 2000.

Robbins L, Burckhardt CS, Hannan MT, eds. *Clinical Care in the Rheumatic Diseases.* 2nd ed. Association of Rheumatology Health Professionals. American College of Rheumatology, 2001.

Relevant World Wide Web Sites

[Association of Rheumatology Health Professionals]
http://www.rheumatology.org/arhp/index.html
[An online catalog of assistive devices for people with arthritis]
http://www.aidsforarthritis.com/

Complementary & Alternative Therapies

58

Sharon L. Kolasinski, MD

The majority of patients with chronic rheumatic diseases seek adjunctive care outside the medical mainstream. Although patients usually continue to see medical physicians and to take prescription medications, most will add some form of complementary and alternative therapy at some point during the course of their illness. Patients' choices reflect their cultural and ethnic background, financial resources, and the availability of alternative providers. Not all interventions have yet been studied in a scientifically rigorous manner, but a considerable number of well-designed clinical trials have been published in several areas relevant to patients with rheumatic diseases.

GENERAL CONSIDERATIONS

Definition

Complementary and alternative medicine (CAM) has been defined as that which is not traditionally taught in US medical schools and not traditionally available in US hospitals. With the recognition of its widespread use and the provision of services like acupuncture within academic medical centers, however, defining the limits of alternative medicine has become more difficult. The National Center for Complementary and Alternative Medicine, established by Congress in 1998 as one of the centers within the National Institutes of Health, has divided CAM therapies into (1) alternative medical systems (traditional Chinese medicine, Ayurvedic medicine, naturopathy, homeopathy, etc), (2) mind-body interventions (meditation, spiritual healing, etc),(3) biologic-based therapies (herbal medicines, dietary supplements, special diets, etc), (4) manipulative and body-based therapies (chiropractic, massage, osteopathy, etc), and (5) energy therapies (reiki, therapeutic touch, magnets, etc). Furthermore, with the increasing number of randomized controlled trials examining these therapies, practitioners have increasing resources with which to evaluate the usefulness of CAM therapies, provide advice to patients, and consider incorporating CAM into standard treatment plans.

Epidemiology

Initial epidemiologic work suggested that overall about 35% of the general public seeks alternative care in a given year. Demographic data showed that these patients were more likely to be between the ages of 25 and 49, have some college education, be in higher income brackets, and live in the western United States, and were less likely to be African American. Patients with rheumatic disease who seek alternative care, however, appear to be a more diverse group. Use correlates with pain and over 90% of patients with diagnoses like fibromyalgia and osteoarthritis (OA) may seek alternative care. Similarly, a variety of ethnic and racial groups and the elderly with musculoskeletal complaints have higher rates of CAM use than average American populations. However, patients with rheumatic diseases are unlikely to discuss their CAM use with their physician, similar to patients in general, unless the physician specifically asks.

Quality & Safety Issues

Practitioners have a responsibility to help inform patients regarding their choices of alternative therapies, particularly where medical data exist. However, in this developing field, data may be lacking and patients often hold strong beliefs that alternative products are effective and safe. Despite this, only about 10% believe that CAM therapies will cure arthritis.

Efforts to study aspects of traditional Chinese and Ayurvedic medicine and many herbal therapies have been hampered by the passage of the Dietary Supplement and Health Education Act (DSHEA) by the US Congress in 1994. This legislation permitted the classification of numerous over-the-counter products with pharmacologic activity as dietary supplements. As such, they were exempted from the safety and efficacy requirements that must be met by prescription drugs. In fact, this legislation mandated that the US Food and Drug Administration (USFDA) assume the burden of proof when a product is considered for removal from the market as unsafe. Furthermore, consumers may

457

make certain assumptions about testing, quality, and efficacy since DSHEA permits labeling claims regarding "structure and function" that may suggest to the consumer that the products being sold have been proved to have health benefits.

Recently, a number of safety considerations concerning herbal remedies were reviewed. A variety of herbs may themselves have toxic side effects (Table 58–1). They may also have important interactions with prescription medications. Garlic and gingko may increase bleeding risk in patients on warfarin, whereas ginseng may reduce the ability of warfarin to lead to appropriate anticoagulation. St. John's wort may reduce the plasma levels of numerous medications, including antidepressants, antiviral agents, and immunosuppressive drugs. Thus, even if a patient is not taking an herbal product to address arthritis symptoms, he or she should be questioned about all over-the-counter product use since medication interactions may be significant.

Adulterants and contaminants in herbal preparations have been reported, including heavy metals, microorganisms and their toxins, and pesticides. Unsuspected botanicals other than those identified on the label may be present. One such case involved contamination of a weight loss preparation with the root of *Aristolochia fangchi,* resulting in interstitial renal fibrosis, renal failure and, in some, urothelial carcinoma. Pharmaceuticals may be present as well. A number of reports have detailed the presence of glucocorticoids and nonsteroidal anti-inflammatory drugs (NSAIDs) in herbal arthritis preparations, with resultant side effects including gastrointestinal bleeding and hepatotoxicity.

To date, the USFDA has issued specific warnings about a number of alternative products. These include an April 1996 warning to consumers to avoid products containing botanical ephedrine (ma huang, ephedra) due to reports of myocardial infarction, cerebrovascular accidents, seizures, psychosis, and death after use; a June 2002 warning to certain manufacturers of synthetic ephedrine alkaloid products regarding illegal labeling of nonherbal ephedra as a dietary supplement; a July 2001 warning to manufacturers to remove comfrey from the market due to hepatotoxicity and possible car-

Table 58–1. Potential adverse effects of herbal remedies and their major constituents.

Cardiotoxicity	*Alocasia macrorrhiza* root tuber
Aconite root tuber	*Artemisia* sp. rich in santonin
Herbs rich in cardioactive glycosides	Essential oils rich in ascaridole
Herbs rich in colchicine	Essential oils rich in thujone
Leigongteng	Gingko seed or leaf
Licorice root	Herbs rich in colchicine
Ma huang	Herbs rich in podophyllotoxin
Pokeweed leaf or root	Indian tobacco herb
Scotch broom	Kava rhizome
Squirting cucumber	Ma huang
Hepatotoxicity	Nux vomica
Certain herbs rich in anthranoids	Pennyroyal oil
Certain herbs rich in protoberberine alkaloids	Star fruit
Chaparral leaf or stem	Yellow jessamine rhizome
Germander sp.	**Renal toxicity**
Green tea leaf	β-Aescin (saponin mixture from horse chestnut leaf)
Herbs rich in coumarin	Cape aloes
Herbs rich in podophyllotoxin	Cat's claw
Herbs rich in toxic pyrrolizidine alkaloids	Certain essential oils
Impila root	Chaparral leaf or stem
Kava rhizome	Chinese yew
Kombucha	Herbs rich in aristolochic acid
Ma huang	Impila root
Pennyroyal oil	Jering fruit
Skullcap	Squirting cucumber
Soy phytoestrogens	Star fruit
Neurotoxicity, convulsions	
Aconite root tuber	

From De Smet PA. Herbal remedies. *N Engl J Med.* 2003;347:2046.

cinogenesis; a March 2002 warning to consumers of the risk of hepatotoxicity due to kava; a June 2002 recall of products containing PC SPES and SPES because of undeclared prescription drug adulterants; and an August 2002 warning to the public about Chinese weight loss pills (Chaso [Jianfei] Diet Capsules and Chaso Genpi) containing fenfluramine and phentermine. The USFDA encourages the reporting of adverse events by consumers, physicians, and manufacturers via their web site (www.fda.gov/medwatch) or telephone (consumers: 1-800-MEDWATCH; physicians: 1-800-FDA-1088).

There has been a long-standing interest in systematic investigation and regulation of herbal medications in Germany. The Federal Health Agency Commission E was formed in 1978 and has amassed over 400 monographs on herbal medicines that provide a resource for practitioners attempting to inform themselves and advise patients. An additional up-to-date guide with references regarding herbal and other alternative therapies has recently been published.

The American College of Rheumatology has issued a position paper on the use of CAM therapies. The College acknowledges that CAM use is widespread among patients with rheumatic diseases. It notes that all therapies must meet the same rigorous standards of scientific scrutiny using scientific methods and that those proven safe and effective can be integrated into the therapeutic armamentarium. It further suggests that rheumatologists should be informed about CAM therapies and be able to knowledgeably discuss them with their patients. Many studies show that little discussion about CAM occurs in the office visit setting, however. Several authors have offered advice to physicians on what information should be discussed in order to facilitate the dialogue, particularly when patients are using herbal products (Table 58–2).

Blumenthal M, et al, eds. The complete German Commission E monographs: therapeutic guide to herbal medicine. Integrative Medicine Communications, 1998. (This compendium has been the standard source of information on herbal medicine for many years and reflects an accumulation of data from studies and anecdotal experience, analysis, and recommendations.)

De Smet PA. Herbal remedies. N Engl J Med. 2003;347:2046. [PMID: 12490687] (This review article summarizes the current state of knowledge on quality and safety issues regarding herbal products.)

Ernst E, ed. The Desktop Guide to Complementary and Alternative Medicine. An Evidence-Based Approach. Mosby, 2001. (This up-to-date encyclopedia of alternative therapies is edited by one of the foremost authorities on evidence-based analysis of CAM. The format includes listing of herbal medicines, physical interventions, and other therapeutic methods and beliefs with cross-references by diagnosis or condition.)

Rao JK, et al. Use of complementary therapies for arthritis among patients of rheumatologists. Ann Intern Med. 1999;131:409.

Table 58–2. Obtaining and providing information about CAM therapies.

Questions for patients

1. Are you taking any vitamins, supplements, or herbal remedies? If so, which ones?
2. How much are you taking of each? How often do you take each? How long have you been taking each?
3. What are the symptoms you want to treat?
4. Do you have a prescription medication for the same symptoms? If so, are you still taking it?
5. Have you noticed any improvement or worsening of symptoms since taking the remedy?

Information for patients

1. Natural does not always mean safe.
2. Commercial availability does not guarantee safety and efficacy. Manufacturers are not legally required to back their claims with scientific studies.
3. The quantity and quality of active ingredients may vary from product to product and from time to time in the same product.
4. Herbal products are not regulated like prescription drugs, and contamination can occur.
5. Supplements or remedies may interact with prescribed medication or with each other with possible serious consequences.
6. Some products are safe for short-term use but long-term studies with appropriate controls are generally lacking.
7. Infants, children, pregnant women, women trying to conceive, and the elderly should not use any CAM therapy without medical supervision.

CAM, complementary and alternative medicine.
From Kolasinski SL: Complementary and alternative therapies for rheumatic disease. Hosp Prac 2001;36:31. [PMID 11327343].

[PMID: 10498556] (Consecutive patients in academic and private rheumatology offices were asked about CAM use and the investigators found that 56% currently used CAM and > 90% regularly used CAM or had done so in the past. Despite high use rates, patients noted that they rarely discussed CAM use with their physicians because the physicians never asked.)

HERBAL MEDICINES

Avocado/Soybean Unsaponifiables

A very popular treatment for OA in Western Europe is an extract of unsaponifiable oils of avocado and soybean in a one-third avocado to two-thirds soybean mixture. A large body of in vitro and animal data suggests this mixture possesses anti-inflammatory actions. A prospective, randomized, double-blind, placebo-controlled multicenter clinical trial of patients with knee and hip OA showed promising results. After 6 months of treatment with 300 mg of the extract, patients experienced significant reductions in pain and functional disability. Many required less NSAIDs. No significant side effects were reported. Patients with hip OA seemed to benefit more than those with knee OA. Avocado/soybean unsaponifiables may achieve these benefits through structural effects on cartilage, as suggested by a subsequent study. This 2-year trial showed that avocado/soybean unsaponifiables may reduce cartilage loss in patients with hip OA and advanced joint space narrowing at baseline.

Capsaicin

The American College of Rheumatology Subcommittee on Osteoarthritis identifies topical capsaicin cream as an option for treatment of OA symptoms. It may be used as an adjunct to systemic therapy or as monotherapy in those who wish to avoid oral medications. The cream should be applied 4 times daily. It initially results in a burning sensation but judicious and repeated use lessens the severity of the burning, which rarely results in discontinuation of therapy.

Capsaicin is one of a number of pharmacologically active substances found in the *Capsicum* red pepper. It is known to initially induce the release of the neurotransmitter substance P from skin sensory C fibers when applied topically. Repeated application leads to specific blockade of transport and de novo synthesis of substance P, resulting in desensitization to pain by raising the pain threshold. A number of randomized trials have suggested that capsaicin is useful in the treatment of neurogenic pain, including the pain of diabetic neuropathy, as well as low back pain and pain due to OA.

Ginger

Extracts of members of the Zingiberaceae family have been used in Chinese traditional medicine and Ayurvedic tradition for millennia. Over a hundred species have been tested and a number have been found to have anti-inflammatory effects, including inhibition of the actions of cyclooxygenase and lipoxygenase, synthesis of leukotrienes, and rat paw edema in an animal model of inflammation. As with other herbal products, ginger is pharmacologically complex and may contain salicylate (though in amounts that are not thought to account for all of its anti-inflammatory effect), gingeroles, β-carotene, capsaicin, caffeic acid, and curcumin.

Fifty-six patients in Copenhagen with radiographically verified OA of the knee participated in a study in which they received either a ginger extract (Eurovita Extract 33, 170 mg orally 3 times a day), ibuprofen 400 mg orally 3 times a day, or placebo in each of three treatment periods of 3 weeks each. Overall, the investigators could demonstrate no differences between ginger and placebo. A larger, more recent multicenter study included 247 patients with radiographically confirmed knee OA. Participants were required to have visual analog scores between 40 mm and 70 mm on a 100-mm scale for pain on standing during the 24 hours preceding the baseline visit. They received either placebo or ginger extract (Eurovita Extract 77, 255 mg orally twice daily) for 6 weeks in this double-blind, randomized trial. Patients in both placebo- and ginger-treated groups had improvement in pain on standing, but the ginger group had a higher percentage of responders (63% vs 50%), a greater degree of response on average (8.1 mm more in ginger group), and a greater percentage of participants with large responses. Pain after walking and overall functioning measured by the Western Ontario and McMaster Universities OA composite index (WOMAC) were also significantly improved in the ginger group. Gastrointestinal side effects (eructation, dyspepsia, nausea) were more common in the ginger group (45% vs 16%), but none were serious. The investigators concluded that ginger has efficacy for pain management in knee OA, but that a future dose finding study would be of benefit as would long-term investigation of side effects.

Thundergod vine

Extracts of *Tripterygium wilfordii* Hook F (TWHF) have been used in traditional Chinese medicine to treat a variety of autoimmune and inflammatory disorders, including rheumatoid arthritis, systemic lupus erythematosus (SLE), ankylosing spondylitis, psoriasis, and idiopathic IgA nephropathy. Traditional use dates back centuries, and while the Chinese literature has been uncontrolled, it does represent observations made on thousands of patients for time periods as long as a decade. In addition, several preliminary controlled trials have suggested that use of thundergod vine represents a promising herbal therapy for a number of rheumatic diseases. Laboratory data suggest that active ingredients include triptolide and tripdiolide and that they inhibit laboratory models of inflammatory arthritis, delayed type hypersensitivity reactions, and primary antibody responses.

Uncontrolled reports from China on a total of about 250 patients have shown that TWHF can be of benefit in treating SLE. Subjects have experienced improvements in fatigue, arthralgias, fever, skin rash, lymphadenopathy, hepatomegaly, and laboratory abnormalities including proteinuria, renal function, thrombocytopenia, and the presence of antinuclear antibodies. Reports have suggested that glucocorticoid doses can be reduced and, sometimes, eliminated.

The Chinese experience with TWHF has also been considerable with rheumatoid arthritis patients. An early placebo-controlled trial of 70 patients with rheumatoid arthritis had a crossover design. The majority of subjects improved in parameters of disease activity and laboratory abnormalities. Peripheral blood mononuclear cells from those receiving active treatment produced less IgM rheumatoid factor than cells from placebo-treated persons. Adverse effects gleaned from the Chinese experience include dry mouth, loss of appetite, nausea or vomiting, abdominal pain, diarrhea, leukopenia, thrombocytopenia, rash, skin pigmentation changes, and amenorrhea.

The safety and efficacy of TWHF have been most recently examined in a small, double-blind, placebo-controlled trial of patients with rheumatoid arthritis seen at the National Institutes of Health and at the University of Texas Southwestern. Twenty-one participants completed the 20-week study. They received either placebo or an oral dose of TWHF of 180 mg/d or 360 mg/d. Eighty percent of those receiving the high dose, 40% of those receiving the low dose, and none of those receiving placebo had at least a 20% improvement in the criteria for a clinical response (as established by the American College of Rheumatology). In this trial, the most common side effect was diarrhea and no person withdrew due to an adverse event. Investigations into the role of thundergod vine extract in the treatment of rheumatoid arthritis are continuing.

Altman RD, Marcussen KC. Effects of a ginger extract on knee pain in patients with osteoarthritis. *Arthritis Rheum.* 2001;44:2531. [PMID: 11710709] (Two hundred forty-seven participants were evaluated in a double-blind, randomized, placebo-controlled trial over 6 weeks. There were statistically significant differences between the ginger extract used and placebo for pain on standing and WOMAC scores with more gastrointestinal side effects in the ginger group.)

American College of Rheumatology Subcommittee on Osteoarthritis Guidelines. Recommendations for the medical management of osteoarthritis of the hip and knee; 2000 update. *Arthritis Rheum.* 2000;43:1905. [PMID: 11014340] (This position statement outlines current best practices in the management of symptoms due to osteoarthritis of the hip and knee.)

Bliddal H, et al. A randomized, placebo-controlled, crossover study of ginger extracts and ibuprofen in osteoarthritis. *Osteoarthritis Cartilage.* 2000;8:9. [PMID: 10607493] (Fifty-six participants were evaluated in a double-blind, randomized, placebo-, and NSAID-controlled trial. Participants sequentially received placebo, ibuprofen, or a ginger extract for 3 weeks each in random sequence and the effects of ginger could not be distinguished from those of placebo.)

Fusco BM, Giacovazzo M. Peppers and pain. The promise of capsaicin. *Drugs.* 1997;53:909. [PMID: 9179523] (This summary article gives an overview of the mechanism and action of topical products containing capsaicin.)

Lequesne M, et al. Structural effect of avocado/soybean unsaponifiables on joint space loss in osteoarthritis of the hip. *Arthritis Rheum.* 2002;47:50. [PMID: 11932878] (This prospective, multicenter, randomized, parallel group, double-blind,

placebo-controlled trial of 2 years included 108 patients with hip OA. In those most severely affected, there was a significant reduction in joint space loss in those who received avocado/soybean unsaponifiables compared with those who received placebo.)

Maheu E, et al. Symptomatic efficacy of avocado/soybean unsaponifiables in the treatment of osteoarthritis of the knee and hip. *Arthritis Rheum.* 1998;41:81. [PMID: 9433873] (This prospective, randomized, double-blind, placebo-controlled, multicenter clinical trial treated 85 OA patients with avocado/soybean unsaponifiables for 6 months and compared them to 79 patients receiving placebo. Participants in the treatment group experienced reductions in pain, functional disability, and NSAID use.)

Puett DW, Griffin MR. Published trials of non-medicinal and noninvasive therapies for hip and knee osteoarthritis. *Ann Intern Med.* 1994;121:133. [PMID: 8017727] (This review article outlines the current state of knowledge and the directions for future research on interventions such as capsaicin, laser therapy, acupuncture, transcutaneous electrical nerve stimulation, and pulsed electromagnetic fields.)

Tao X, et al. Benefit of an extract of *Tripterygium wilfordii* hook F in patients with rheumatic arthritis. *Arthritis Rheum.* 2002;46:1735. [PMID: 12124856] (This is the most recent clinical publication addressing the specific effects of thundergod vine extract in subjects with rheumatoid arthritis. Patients with treatment-refractory rheumatoid arthritis benefited and tolerated the preparation well.)

Tao X, Lipsky P. The Chinese anti-inflammatory and immunosuppressive herbal remedy *Tripterygium wilfordii* hook F. *Rheum Dis Clin North Am.* 2000;26:29. [PMID: 10680192] (This review article outlines the studies of the chemical composition and active ingredients in thundergod vine extracts. It reviews mechanistic studies of effects on cellular immune responses in vitro and anti-inflammatory effects in animal models. It also summarizes the available worldwide literature, including information about side effects.)

DIETARY SUPPLEMENTS

Dehydroepiandrosterone

The wild Mexican yam is a natural source of diosgenin, an inactive prohormone of dehydroepiandrosterone (DHEA). However, wild yam products do not contain DHEA and require chemical treatment to yield usable hormone. DHEA is widely available without prescription in pharmacies and health food stores. However, before passage of DSHEA, DHEA was considered a drug and was banned from over-the-counter sales since the 1980s. DHEA is a weak androgen and increases testosterone and estrogen levels as well as altering cytokine production.

The observations that there is a striking female predominance among SLE patients, that there are low circulating levels of DHEA in lupus patients, and that DHEA is beneficial in a mouse model of lupus have fueled interest in DHEA as a treatment for SLE. Several human trials have now been published and offer intriguing findings.

Fifty female patients with mild to moderate SLE were studied in an uncontrolled year-long longitudinal trial. Patients received 200 mg/d of oral DHEA in addition to their usual medications and monthly follow-up visits. The SLE disease activity index (SLEDAI) and patient and physician global assessments improved over the 12-month period in those who completed the trial. However, 58% of the persons discontinued the medication, 30% due to lack of efficacy, and 16% due to androgenic or other side effects.

Several placebo-controlled trials have been published. A double-blind, randomized trial monitored 191 patients with SLE for 7–9 months. The investigators found that a significantly greater proportion of persons who took oral DHEA (at the 200-mg/d dose but not at the 100-mg/d dose) were able to reduce their prednisone dose to ≤ 7.5 mg/d orally and sustain disease quiescence for 2 months than were those persons receiving placebo. However, differences between groups were small. Forty-one percent of the placebo-treated group responded, compared with 44% of the low-dose DHEA group and 51% of the higher-dose group. Furthermore, 65% of those with SLEDAI scores of 0 or 1 were responders and the percentage of responders decreased progressively and rapidly as baseline SLEDAI score increased. The most common side effect was acne, occurring in twice as many DHEA-treated patients as those receiving placebo. High-density lipoprotein cholesterol and C3 levels were reduced, and serum levels of testosterone and estrogen were increased.

A second multicenter, randomized, double-blind, placebo-controlled trial was published later in 2002 that monitored 120 female patients with SLE in Taiwan. Participants took either placebo or 200 mg/d of oral DHEA for 6 months. These investigators found no difference between the clinical status of patients in the two groups as measured by the systemic lupus activity measure (SLAM) or SLEDAI. However, the number of disease flares were significantly lower in the DHEA group, and this group had a significant improvement in the patient global assessment. Serious adverse events were mostly characterized as disease flares and were increased in the placebo group. Increased levels of testosterone and increased incidence of acne were noted in the DHEA group. C3 and C4 levels declined in the DHEA group in this study as well.

None of the trials published to date, however, is large enough to answer questions about the possible contribution of this hormone to risk of myocardial infarction or cerebrovascular accidents due to accelerated atherogenesis, altered cholesterol profile, or increased insulin resistance. In addition, concern has been raised because consequent elevations in sex hormones levels could result in increases in breast, ovarian, uterine, and prostate cancer risk.

Glucosamine Sulfate & Chondroitin Sulfate

Glucosamine sulfate and chondroitin sulfate are likely the most commonly used over-the-counter alternative therapy for arthritis. Their tremendous popularity in the United States results in part from the best selling book, *The Arthritis Cure*, by Jason Theodosakis, MD, who drew on decades of use and study in Europe in making his recommendations. While not a cure, glucosamine and chondroitin are of interest because they occur naturally in connective tissue and are, therefore, intrinsically appealing as "nutraceuticals" for OA. In vitro work suggests a multitude of potential mechanisms, including inhibitory effects on cartilage-damaging agents like lysosomal enzymes, oxygen free radicals, matrix metalloproteinases, and aggrecanase, as well as dose-dependent increases in proteoglycan synthesis.

Glucosamine is available in a sulfate and a hydrochloride form, but studies have been carried out most often with the sulfate form. Most studies have been small and short in duration. Meta-analyses suggest that an analgesic benefit can be obtained from an oral dose of 1500 mg/d in a majority of those who take it. The effect is similar in magnitude to that of NSAIDs but is delayed in onset. The duration of the analgesic benefit is not known.

Considerable interest was raised by the single long-term glucosamine study that has been published to date because it suggested that glucosamine could halt radiographic progression of OA. In a 3-year Belgian trial, 212 patients received either 500 mg of oral glucosamine sulfate 3 times daily or placebo. Radiographs obtained at baseline, 1, and 3 years of follow-up suggested that no radiographic progression occurred in those taking glucosamine while those receiving placebo had 0.34-mm joint space narrowing detectable after 3 years. However, the radiographic technique used and its ability to detect the very small differences noted have been questioned. An ongoing National Institutes of Health study will examine whether or not glucosamine can prevent radiographic progression, as well as be the first long-term study to compare the combination of glucosamine and chondroitin, although the two are widely sold together.

Trials suggest that chondroitin has analgesic benefit in OA as well. An oral dose of 1200 mg/d has generally been used. Studies of chondroitin are subject to the same criticisms as those of glucosamine; namely, they involve small numbers of participants and are of short duration, in addition to often being industry-sponsored.

The side effect profiles of glucosamine and chondroitin have been indistinguishable from that of placebo in many of the short-term studies that have been carried out. Occasionally, gastrointestinal intolerance leads to discontinued use. Some have hypothesized that since glucosamine readily participates in the hexosamine biosynthesis pathway, it could induce insulin resistance and should be avoided by diabetics. However, no cases of such an occurrence have been reported in the medical literature.

Methylsulfonylmethane

Methylsulfonylmethane (MSM) is a commonly used ingredient in over-the-counter topical and oral preparations for the treatment of a vast variety of conditions, including musculoskeletal pain, inflammation, asthma, allergies, headaches, cancer prevention, gastrointestinal complaints, and parasitic infections. Despite considerable popularity and millions of dollars in sales annually, few data support its use as an arthritis treatment. MSM is naturally present in a variety of foods including grains, meat, eggs, and fish as well as raw broccoli, peppers, brussels sprouts, onions, and cabbage. When taken as a dietary supplement, doses of 1000–6000 mg/d are generally recommended.

MSM is a metabolite of dimethyl sulfoxide (DMSO), which was itself popular as a topical arthritis treatment throughout the last century. However, the pungent odor and occasional skin irritation associated with use of DMSO have likely contributed to its decline and the increase in popularity of MSM. Until recently, few toxicologic data were available on MSM. A study in rats showed no toxicity from a dose 5–7 times higher than the recommended human dose when given as a single gavage dose nor from long-term use of a 1.5 g/kg dose over 90 days.

Evidence that MSM is of benefit in arthritis treatment is largely anecdotal and published in the lay press. Celebrity endorsements and a best-selling volume by two physician proponents have enhanced public awareness of this substance, but rigorous trials and convincing evidence that it might have a specific role in thwarting pathophysiologic processes in arthritis are lacking.

Vitamins

Vitamins are among the most popular and readily accessible supplements that patients might choose to treat their arthritis symptoms. There are a number of possible mechanisms through which vitamins could be of benefit, particularly in the pathogenesis of OA. It is thought, for example, that oxidative stress is a major contributor to the progression of OA and antioxidant vitamins like C and E might, therefore, have a role in slowing progression. The current concept of OA is that it is a disease of not only the articular cartilage, but also of the subchondral bone and that the nature of the

bone response to OA determines outcome. Vitamin D appears to play an important role in bone mineralization, in proteoglycan synthesis by chondrocytes, and in reduction of degradative matrix metalloproteinases that could be protective from OA progression. Epidemiologic surveys have suggested that there may be a role for optimizing vitamin intake, but prospective intervention trials have not yet emerged.

A 1996 study analyzing Framingham data was the first to suggest that vitamin D intake could have an impact on OA progression. Participants had been followed for more than 40 years and have had radiographs performed in the early 1980s and again in the early 1990s. Serum 25-hydroxyvitamin D levels had been obtained in the late 1980s, along with a dietary questionnaire. The investigators analyzed 788 normal and 126 osteoarthritic knees and found that the risk of progression of prevalent OA at baseline was markedly increased in those in the middle and lower tertiles for both intake and serum levels of vitamin D.

The importance of dietary vitamin D was again addressed in a more recent study of hip OA. A subset of participants in the Study of Osteoporotic Fractures was randomly selected for further investigation of the biochemical antecedents of fractures. Serum 1,25-dihydroxyvitamin D and 25-hydroxyvitamin D levels were measured and radiographs of the hip were obtained. Participants were women with a mean age of 71 years. The investigators found that in those with low serum 25-hydroxyvitamin D—but not 1,25-dihydroxyvitamin D—levels there was a three-fold increase in the incidence of hip OA characterized by joint space narrowing rather than osteophyte formation. This result supported the hypothesis that the action of vitamin D was likely to be through effects on cartilage metabolism.

Data have also appeared regarding the role of dietary antioxidant vitamins and the risk of OA. Framingham data were analyzed for a relationship between knee OA and intake of vitamins B_1, B_6, C, E, β-carotene, niacin, and folate as assessed by food frequency questionnaire. Six hundred forty participants were available for analysis and incident and progressive OA developed in 81 and 68 knees, respectively. The investigators found a threefold reduction in risk of OA progression for the middle and highest tertiles of vitamin C intake. This finding correlated predominantly with a reduced risk of cartilage loss. Interestingly, those with high vitamin C intake also had a reduced risk of developing knee pain. A less consistent reduction in risk of OA progression was also seen for β-carotene and vitamin E.

Chang DM, et al. Dehydroepiandrosterone treatment of women with mild-to-moderate systemic lupus erythematosus. A multicenter randomized, double-blind, placebo-controlled trial. *Arthritis Rheum.* 2002;46:2924. [PMID: 12428233] (This multicenter randomized, placebo-controlled trial followed 120 patients with SLE over 6 months and found a reduction in the number of disease flares and an improvement in the patient global assessment with only expected androgenic side effects.)

Horvath K, et al. Toxicity of methylsulfonylmethane in rats. *Food Chem Toxicol.* 2002;40:1459. [PMID: 12387309] (This report details the only public information on the toxicology of MSM.)

Kolasinski SL. Dimethylsulfoxide (DMSO) and methylsulfonylmethane (MSM) for the treatment of arthritis. *Alternate Medicine Alert.* 2000;3:115. (This review article summarizes the history and current use of MSM for musculoskeletal complaints.)

Lane NE, et al. Serum vitamin D levels and incident changes of radiographic hip osteoarthritis. A longitudinal study. *Arthritis Rheum.* 1999;42:854. [PMID: 10323440] (This subset analysis of participants in a trial examining osteoporosis quantified the risk of incident hip OA as threefold greater in those with low serum 25-hydroxyvitamin D levels.)

McAlindon TE, et al. Glucosamine and chondroitin for treatment of osteoarthritis: a systematic quality assessment and meta-analysis. *JAMA.* 2000;283:1469. [PMID: 10732937] (This report is the most authoritative meta-analysis of data on glucosamine and chondroitin for osteoarthritis symptom reduction. Careful selection of trials for analysis and assessment of their design and findings result in the conclusion that these substances are likely modestly effective and safe.)

Petri M, et al. Effects of prasterone on corticosteroid requirements of women with systemic lupus erythematosus. *Arthritis Rheum.* 2002;46:1820. [PMID: 12124866] (This multicenter, randomized, placebo-controlled trial monitored 191 patients with SLE over 7–9 months and found a modest benefit of 200 mg/d of oral DHEA in that it permitted reduction in prednisone dose to 7.5 mg/d orally while maintaining disease stability over 2 months.)

Reginster JY, et al. Long-term effect of glucosamine sulphate on osteoarthritis progression: a randomized, placebo-controlled clinical trial. *Lancet.* 2001;357:251. [PMID: 11214126] (This is the longest study to date to assess the benefit of glucosamine in knee OA. It remains controversial because of the type of radiographic assessment that was performed.)

PHYSICAL INTERVENTIONS

Acupuncture

Acupuncture is a centuries old practice of inserting needles into predetermined locations. In the traditional Chinese explanation for the efficacy of acupuncture, the movement of chi, or vital energy, along channels called meridians is influenced by the placement of the needles. An imbalance in the flow of chi can be redressed by certain needle placements depending on the ailment being treated and improve health and well being. In the Western medical tradition, it is recognized that one explanation, although incomplete, of the efficacy of acupuncture is analgesia in that needle placement stimulates the production of endogenous opioids. Inadequate understanding of the mechanism of action of acupuncture, however, is not as much of an impedi-

ment to systematic study as is the very nature of the intervention. Deciding what an appropriate control is (Can an intervention that does not use needles provide an adequate control? Where should the control needles be placed? How many? For how long?) has an important bearing on interpretation and comparison of trials. Regardless of the availability of scientific appraisal of acupuncture, about 1 million consumers in the United States seek treatment each year.

No individual trials have been adequately designed to address the efficacy of acupuncture in pain control in rheumatic diseases. The National Institutes of Health compiled a consensus statement in 1998 on the use and efficacy of acupuncture in a variety of medical conditions. The statement concluded that acupuncture might be useful for analgesia in tennis elbow, fibromyalgia, myofascial pain, OA, low back pain, and carpal tunnel syndrome but that there was a paucity of high-quality research from which to draw conclusions.

A recent best evidence synthesis of seven trials regarding the use of acupuncture for knee OA included results from 393 participants. Meta-analysis of these trials could not be performed due to the variability of control groups and insufficient reports of data. However, the authors were able to conclude that there was strong evidence that acupuncture was more effective than sham acupuncture for control of pain. For function, however, the evidence was inconclusive. There was limited evidence that acupuncture was more effective than being on a waiting list or receiving treatment as usual. Evidence was insufficient to draw conclusions about comparisons of acupuncture and other treatments.

Acupuncture has been used in several trials as a therapy for the pain of fibromyalgia. As with OA, no single trial is able to definitively establish the place of acupuncture in the treatment regimen for fibromyalgia. However, the systematic review of one high-quality and six lower-quality studies provides some assistance. This clinical review concluded that the high-quality study suggested acupuncture was more effective than sham acupuncture for relieving pain, increasing pain thresholds, improving global ratings, and reducing morning stiffness. It was unclear how long-lasting the benefits were. Some patients received no benefit, and others had an exacerbation of pain. The lower-quality studies were in agreement with these results.

Few trials have addressed the use of acupuncture in rheumatoid arthritis. However, available evidence suggests no improvement in parameters of inflammation. Methodologic limitations need to be taken into account in the interpretation of the data.

Adverse events due to acupuncture have been documented and include serious consequences such as pneumothorax, cardiac tamponade, spinal injuries, and septic complications. However, considerable evidence supports the safety of acupuncture. A survey was conducted of preceptors and interns at a Japanese national medical facility at which about 60% of the patients undergo acupuncture. Results were compiled on over 55,000 acupuncture treatments and 64 adverse events were identified. The most frequent was failure to remove the needle after the procedure was completed. Almost as common were dizziness, discomfort, and perspiration thought to be associated with a transient vasovagal episode. Less common side effects were burn injuries due to moxibustion, ecchymoses, and needling site reactions. A systematic review of the literature revealed a similar safety record. Nine prospective surveys encompassing over 250,000 acupuncture treatments were reviewed. Minor side effects were common. These included pain at the site of needling and pain due to aggravation of the presenting condition that occurred in up to half of those undergoing acupuncture. Post-procedure fatigue was noted in up to about 40%; an unusual feeling of relaxation (characterized by some as necessary for efficacy) was seen in over 80%. Minor bleeding was seen in up to about 40% as well. Fainting was reported in less than 0.2%. Serious side effects reported included two cases of pneumothorax and two cases in which needles needed to be retrieved surgically after they fractured.

Tai chi

Tai chi is a centuries old Chinese form of conditioning exercise based in martial arts traditions and consisting of slow, flowing movements, relaxation, and deep breathing. The aim of the practice is balance of mind and body by stimulating chi. Tai chi involves cognitive, cardiovascular, and musculoskeletal responses that evoke physiologic and psychological changes including maximum oxygen consumption, muscular strength, and flexibility. Early studies encouraged enthusiasm for tai chi as an intervention for geriatric patients since these small trials suggested that improvements in balance and fall prevention could follow training in tai chi. A more recent study of 54 patients with OA showed that a 12-week program held twice weekly improved arthritis self-efficacy outcomes measures. Participants reported being better able to manage general arthritis symptoms, control fatigue, deal with the frustration of arthritis, and regulate pain during activities. Yet while subjects reported improved satisfaction with their general health status, the investigators were unable to demonstrate significant changes in lower extremity functional mobility.

No serious side effects of tai chi have been reported.

Yoga

Yoga derives from a more than 2000-year-old Indian tradition based on eight branches of practice, including postures (asanas), breathing, and meditation. The aim of hatha yoga, or the practice of asanas, is to prepare the practitioner for the spiritual experience of purifying the body. The ultimate goal of this practice is the achievement of harmony in body, mind, and spirit. A number of studies have attempted to quantify physiologic effects of yoga and found reductions in oxygen consumption, minute ventilation, and heart rate after exercise in persons participating in regular yoga practice.

Small studies have suggested that yoga may be efficacious for a variety of musculoskeletal conditions, but all studies to date have methodologic limitations that reduce their generalizability. Nonetheless, the trials that have been carried out support a role for yoga in reducing pain and increasing function. Persons with carpal tunnel syndrome participated in an 8-week yoga program and had significant improvements in grip strength and pain. A study of the effects of a 10-week course of yoga for symptoms of OA of the hands showed reductions in finger joint tenderness and range of motion and hand pain during activity. A more recent trial has suggested that yoga represents an exercise alternative for even obese patients with OA of the knee who are not regular exercisers. Reductions in pain and functional disability were demonstrated in a group who completed an 8-week yoga program.

No serious side effects have been reported in the trials assessing yoga for musculoskeletal complaints. There have been rare reports of reversible compression neuropathy after 6 hours of kneeling and very rare instances of vertebral and basilar artery occlusion after neck standing and prolonged flexion of the cervical spine.

Berman BM, et al. The evidence for acupuncture as a treatment for rheumatologic conditions. *Rheum Dis Clin North Am.* 2000; 26:103. [PMID: 10680198] (This is a very readable overview that provides a wealth of references and analysis of the use of acupuncture for a broad range of rheumatologic conditions.)

Ernst E, White AR. Prospective studies of the safety of acupuncture. A systematic review. *Am J Med.* 2001;110:481. [PMID: 11331060] (A review of nine surveys from the literature detailing acupuncture side effects in an attempt to get a more realistic assessment of acupuncture safety than is available from the anecdotal, case report literature. It concludes that serious adverse events are rare.)

Ezzo J, et al. Acupuncture for osteoarthritis of the knee. A systematic review. *Arthritis Rheum.* 2001;44:819. [PMID: 11315921] (The most up to date and rigorous examination of the data on acupuncture for knee OA.)

Hartman CA, et al. Effects of t'ai chi training on function and quality of life indicators in older adults with osteoarthritis. *J Am Geriatr Soc.* 2000;48:1553. [PMID: 11129742] (This is the best designed trial in the literature to address the role of tai chi for management of OA symptoms.)

Kaptchuk TJ. Acupuncture: theory, efficacy and practice. *Ann Intern Med.* 2002;136:374. [PMID: 11874310] (A scholarly discussion of the traditional concepts and theoretical underpinning of acupuncture in the context of current practice.)

Kolasinski SL. Acupuncture for arthritis. *Alternative Medicine Alert.* 2002;5:37. (This review article provides an overview of methodologic considerations, mechanism of action, and trials in OA and rheumatoid arthritis. Side effects of acupuncture are reviewed.)

Kolasinski SL. Yoga for degenerative joint disease. *Alternative Medicine Alert.* 2001;4:28. (This review outlines the pathophysiologic effects of yoga as an exercise and the clinical trials performed using yoga as an intervention for arthritis symptoms.)

SECTION X

Special Topics

Legal Issues

Victor R. Cotton, MD, JD

The practice of medicine is an increasingly complex endeavor in which errors, omissions, and miscommunications are not entirely preventable. In addition, a variety of societal changes have combined to make it easier to sue a physician for malpractice. Practicing "good medicine" is no longer a guarantee that one will not be sued, and an understanding of the origins of lawsuits, along with how to manage them once they occur, is essential.

Although the field of rheumatology is not particularly laden with malpractice concerns, the potential for difficulty in diagnosis and the complex and potentially debilitating nature of the disease processes combine to create a legitimate level of risk.

FACTORS IN MALPRACTICE LAWSUITS

The medical malpractice problem is multifactorial in nature. The increasing incidence and financial impact of this problem can be linked to a variety of medical, societal, and legal phenomena. The exact contribution of each factor is the subject of some debate and probably varies by location and situation.

Medical

Although scientific advancement has greatly enhanced the ability to care for patients, the practice of medicine is more difficult than it has ever been. The number of diseases, tests, and treatments that must be managed can be overwhelming. The challenge is made greater by the financial pressure to see more patients in less time, and the barriers that are often created by formulary and managed care requirements.

The increased mobility of physicians and greater role that large corporations have taken in the practice of medicine have attenuated the interpersonal aspects of medicine. Unfortunately, the impact on the doctor-patient dynamic hurts not only the diagnostic and treatment capabilities but also the patient's tolerance of mistakes.

Finally, medical training has traditionally provided little instruction on the legal process and how risk can be reduced. Although physicians are well trained in science, they receive little guidance when it comes to cultivating the doctor-patient relationship and avoiding situations that increase the risk of malpractice litigation.

Societal

A generation ago, the advice that physicians gave was referred to as "doctor's orders," and given a degree of respect that was almost never questioned. Today, patients are more willing to question the accuracy of their physician's decisions and often second-guess what has been done. In addition, most of the stigma associated with bringing a lawsuit has disappeared, eliminating a barrier that previously provided a reasonable amount of physician protection.

Relying on what they have heard in the lay press or read on the Internet, many patients enter the medical system with enormous, unrealistic expectations. When these expectations are not met, disappointment occurs, and blame sometimes follows. There is often little tolerance for what are unpreventable side effects and unavoidable consequences.

Finally, there is no question that the possibility of financial enrichment leads many patients to bring a medical malpractice lawsuit. The regularity with which enormous sums of money are awarded for intangible damages like pain and suffering leads many patients to seek compensation through litigation.

Legal

The increased number of attorneys drawn to the field by the potential for lucrative reward has certainly contributed to the medical malpractice risk. In conjunction with this, advertising by attorneys, a phenomenon that was prohibited until the late 1980s, has made some plaintiff attorneys into household names and undoubtedly has led more patients to seek their services.

The widespread availability of physicians who are willing to serve as expert witnesses against other physicians has increased the legal risk for all physicians. The law contains few penalties for physicians who testify in a manner that may skew the facts, and the financial reward for doing so often makes this an irresistible temptation.

Geography

Physicians who practice in large metropolitan areas are much more likely to be sued than physicians who practice in smaller towns. There are more law firms in larger towns, patient expectations are often higher, and the anonymity of living in a city helps the plaintiff avoid any stigma that might otherwise be associated with bringing a lawsuit. In addition, juries in metropolitan areas are more willing to find physicians liable for malpractice and generally award larger amounts of money when they do so.

Patient Age

Younger patients are associated with a greater medical-legal risk. Although most debilitating and fatal illnesses generally spare young people, rheumatologic disease does not, and it can have devastating consequences. When this occurs, patients and their families can suffer enormous physical, emotional, and financial burdens. These burdens are often accompanied by a strong urge to look for answers and an explanation. In the end, what started as a search for answers often becomes a means of blaming someone, and this occasionally is the physician.

Type of Illness

Every lawsuit begins with an accident or illness that results in injury to a patient. The injury is usually physical in nature but can be psychological or financial. Although any patient who suffers an injury may choose to sue for medical malpractice, injuries that are severe, occur with suddenness, or are unexpected are more likely to result in a lawsuit.

Nearly 40% of all medical malpractice lawsuits arise because of errors or perceived errors that occur in the course of a procedure. Many rheumatologic patients undergo procedures to alleviate the functional and cosmetic impact of their disease. Because it is not possible to guarantee a perfect result, time should be taken to ensure that patient expectations are not unrealistically high.

Approximately one-third of medical malpractice lawsuits arise as a result of a "failure to make a timely diagnosis." Although cancer and heart disease are the usual culprits, any disease state that presents a challenging diagnosis contributes to this phenomenon. Because rheumatologic disease can present with vague, seemingly unrelated complaints accompanied by nonspecific laboratory abnormalities, any patient situation that eludes diagnosis should be considered for referral. This is especially true for patients who repeatedly seek medical attention for the same complaint or who become progressively ill despite treatment.

A large number of lawsuits are directly or indirectly related to the treating physician's level of recent experience with the disease process and its treatment. The threshold for referral should be lower when the patient has an uncommon disease or requires an unusual treatment. Although many rheumatologic diseases can be managed by nonrheumatologists, the medical-legal risks associated with the potential for the sudden onset of blindness from giant cell arteritis or severe joint deformity caused by progressive rheumatoid arthritis should not be underestimated. It is worth noting that no physician has ever been sued for making a referral to a specialist, while many have been sued for not doing so. The medical and medical-legal value of a properly timed second opinion should not be underestimated.

Patient Motive

Some patients see medical malpractice lawsuits as a way to obtain a monetary windfall. Driven primarily by a desire to "get rich," these persons can be best viewed as plaintiffs looking for defendants. In the worst cases, no amount of due care, communication, and documentation will be sufficient to insulate the physician from an allegation of medical malpractice. The only lawsuit avoidance strategy that works in such a case is termination of the doctor-patient relationship prior to occurrence of an adverse outcome.

On occasion, physicians encounter patients with whom it is not possible to develop the proper relationship of trust and open communication. These patients may be confrontational, manipulative, dishonest, accusatory, or argumentative. To some degree, this type of behavior can be accepted, but it occasionally reaches the point of undermining the ability to properly care for the patient.

Physicians should be attentive to patients who are not approaching the doctor-patient relationship in an appropriate manner. If these relationships cannot be rehabilitated, they should be terminated. As a general rule, physicians have the right to unilaterally terminate virtually any doctor-patient relationship at any time. The only requirements are that the patient must be given notice of the physician's choice to end the relationship, and afforded sufficient time to establish a relationship with a new physician. The exact amount of time is not written in any law or regulation but is generally regarded to be 30 days.

Degree of Empathy

A perception that the physician did not "care" is the most common reason cited by patients who sue for medical malpractice. Despite all of the changes that have occurred in the medical field, the majority of patients are still looking for a physician who "cares." As has been taught for many years, a strong doctor-patient relationship remains the most valuable lawsuit prevention technique.

Patients are generally more willing to forgive mistakes when they perceive that their physician put his heart into the case and tried his best. On the other hand, patients are often led to suspicion and open dissatisfaction when they believe that their physician approached the situation with anything less than a caring, fully committed attitude. Answering questions, explaining the disease process, and clarifying the goals of treatment are all valuable in this regard. In a sense, being sued has more to do with what the physician says than what the physician actually does.

Family Discord

Serious illness can bring out both the best and the worst in the patient's family. Although a patient may be fully satisfied with the care that he or she is receiving, a member of the family will occasionally express dissatisfaction. The family member is generally not directly involved in the patient's care and is often driven by factors that are totally unrelated to the care at hand. Nonetheless, physicians can be caught in the middle of what is primarily family discord and are occasionally blamed as a result.

In dealing with family discord, it is important to make clear that the physician's obligation is to the wishes of the patient, and that disagreement with these wishes is between the patient and his or her family. In addition, the family should be asked to designate one person as the point of contact with the physician, so as to improve efficiency and decrease confusion. In those unfortunate cases where the family is unmanageable, consideration to termination of the doctor-patient relationship should be given. Although the circum-

stances may not be the patient's "fault," the consequences of an unmanageable clinical and medical-legal situation are the same.

Miscommunication

Errors in communication are at the root of many, if not the majority, of medical malpractice cases. Effective patient care requires the coordination of responsibilities among treating physicians, other health care providers, and the patient. Although physicians regularly comanage patients, it is generally undesirable to comanage a given aspect of a patient's disease process. Because the risk of miscommunication and error is greatly multiplied when two or more persons are responsible for the same issue, clear delineation of roles should exist.

Anytime that a new physician becomes involved in a patient's care, everyone who is also involved, including the patient, should have a working understanding of their respective roles. This is especially important in the outpatient setting, where there are less opportunities to review one another's progress notes and treatment plans.

Proper communication with the patient is also essential. Many patients suffer adverse consequences as a result of not understanding or remembering their physician's instructions. What may seem routine and simple to a physician is often new and complex to the patient, and patients regularly make mistakes with medications and other treatments. Although this is often the patient's own "fault," some patients use the legal system to try to hold their physician responsible.

In order to provide the best possible patient care and also prevent the possibility of legal entanglement, it is imperative that every reasonable effort be made to ensure that the patient knows what he or she is to do. When feasible, verbal instructions should be accompanied by a written summary. Although written instructions are not legally required, they make sense when the patient is being asked to undertake a new or complex endeavor. If the patient receives both verbal and written instructions, the chance of error is reduced and the likelihood of a favorable outcome is increased. In addition, the probability that the treating physician can be held responsible should the patient choose to do otherwise is virtually eliminated.

PREVENTION

Like most problems in medicine, the best approach to a medical-legal problem is prevention. Recognizing cases where the patient's condition is worsening, eludes diagnosis, or is not responding to treatment and making a timely referral are paramount. Drawing limits in terms of the type of patient and family conduct that will be permitted, and rehabilitating or ending those relationships that fall outside these boundaries are things that most physicians are not accustomed to doing but are necessary nonetheless. When comanaging a patient with another physician, time should be dedicated to the communication of the scope of one another's responsibilities.

Most importantly, it is not possible to spend too much time answering patients' questions, addressing their concerns, and ensuring that they understand what their role will be in the diagnostic or treatment plan. In the event that the patient is unwilling to go along with the physician's recommendation, the risks of making this choice should be discussed in terms that the patient can understand. Although physicians are not required to persuade the patient into submitting to the recommended treatment, clinicians should be sure that patients understand the potential consequences of any decision.

In cases where the patient chooses an option other than the physician's suggestion, an entry noting the physician's recommendation, the resulting discussion, and the patient's choice should be made in the medical record. In making this entry, it is not necessary nor desirable to note every word that was said. However, some notation should be made. It is also helpful to have the patient sign the medical record entry. Although it is not legally required, the patient's act of signing reinforces the seriousness of the decision and also decreases the viability of a later claim of misunderstanding or miscommunication.

MANAGEMENT OF ADVERSE OUTCOMES

The majority of adverse outcomes are not caused by medical malpractice. They arise because medical science is not perfect and the human body is mortal. Physicians cannot control these variables and are not legally expected to do so. Other adverse outcomes are the result of medical malpractice, medical care that falls below recognized standards. These events are within the control of physicians.

Regardless of their cause, adverse outcomes are the reason that patients sue doctors. Put another way, all lawsuits begin with a "bad" outcome. Sometimes the adverse event is caused by a physician's mistake. In others, physicians are sued despite the fact that the adverse event was not their fault. Although most of these latter cases will be dismissed or otherwise successfully defended, the experience is unpleasant and something that most physicians want to avoid. Because adverse outcomes of any cause are inherently linked to the risk of litigation, they must be effectively managed.

Patient Care

The most important aspect of managing an adverse outcome is taking care of the patient's medical needs. This alleviates the patient's suffering, demonstrates attentiveness, and reduces any ongoing medical-legal injury that the patient has suffered. The sooner that a patient can regain function and return to normal activities, the less likely it is that he or she will have a viable lawsuit. Plaintiff attorneys work on a contingency basis, receiving a percentage of any verdict or settlement. Adverse events that have minimal injury and quick recovery are unappealing to a plaintiff attorney, and most will never result in a lawsuit.

Communication

Communication with the patient is the next most important function. When an unexpected outcome, adverse event, or treatment error occurs, malpractice literature suggests that aggrieved patients want three things: to learn what happened, to receive acknowledgement of their suffering, and to know that lessons have been learned and corrective steps taken. These discusssions are an important part of the practice of medicine and a valuable medical-legal strategy. They require a measured, well-timed, and empathic approach that avoids both self-criticism and blame of others.

Documentation

Documentation is the final consideration in the management of an adverse outcome. The medical record is a powerful legal document. It is entirely admissible as evidence and almost uniformly believed by judges and juries. Most physicians understand the need for documentation, but many are unfamiliar with the manner in which adverse outcomes should be handled in the medical record.

No amount of documentation can change a bad outcome, undo a mistake, or alter a test result. Whatever happened is over and done. It is a mistake to attempt to use documentation to recharacterize or change events that have already occurred. Efforts to do so invariably create inconsistency and might even be interpreted as attempting to hide the truth. At best, the additional documentation draws attention to the matter. This, too, is undesirable.

Physicians must also resist the urge to make "heat of the moment" entries in the medical record. Efforts to document the physician's thought process and explain why a certain choice was made are among the most harmful entries that are ever made. Once these items are recorded in the patient's chart, the physician is legally bound to them. The problem is that the pressure of the situation may result in a poorly worded explanation that omits critical facts. This creates a compromised medical-legal situation that is best avoided. Explanations and thought processes should be saved for a time when they can be carefully measured.

Self-criticism should never be present in a medical record. Physicians, as a group, are very self-critical. To an extent, this criticism is a necessary part of molding one's skills to the highest possible level. However, when self-criticism becomes a part of the medical record, it becomes an unmanageable liability. The appearance in a medical record of self-criticism of any type or degree is inappropriate. It does not advance the care of the patient in any way, and renders the physician indefensible in any subsequent legal action. When a physician openly blames himself for the plaintiff's condition, there is little likelihood of convincing a judge and jury otherwise.

The legal tragedy of self-criticism is deepened by the fact that much of it results from physicians holding themselves to an inappropriately high and unachievable standard.

Physicians can raise their awareness of self-criticism by exercising care when using the pronoun "I" in the medical record. As a general rule, the word "I" should appear very infrequently in the medical record. Because self-criticism can be subtle with statements like "I did not have a chance to look at the lab report," one must always be careful when using the word "I."

The only thing worse in a medical record than self-criticism is criticism of other health care providers. Unfortunately, there exists a potentially devastating misperception that it is possible to cover oneself by documenting the shortcomings of others. The extent to which this occurs between physicians, nurses, pharmacists, and other hospital staff is sometimes alarming.

There is no question that pointing the finger at another health care provider is likely to bring his or her conduct under scrutiny. However, if a lawsuit arises, the plaintiff usually looks for as many potential defendants as he can find. The conduct of everyone who was involved with the case will eventually be brought under scrutiny. This will usually include the person who did the original finger-pointing along with the person against whom the criticism was levied. Regardless of the facts, this type of case is inherently compromised from a defense perspective and most can never be won.

Unless there is a desire to express appreciation or agreement, references to the conduct of another provider should not be made in the medical record. Any concern for the care that has been delivered by someone else should be expressed directly and in person. Once the matter is resolved, the medical record can reflect that an agreement has been reached.

Exclamation points or big, block letters should generally not be used in the medical record. The presence of these notations in a patient's chart suggests frustration or dissatisfaction. This draws attention to the events and can serve as a nidus for additional scrutiny. Although these feelings can be normal, it is better if they are left out of the medical record.

When an adverse outcome occurs, the patient should be treated and apprised of the situation. An entry should be made in the medical record that objectively describes the patient's condition and the treatment plan. Explanations, second-guessing, and any type of criticism should be avoided. From both a patient care and a liability perspective, it is better to spend any extra time with the patient rather than with the chart.

It is worth noting that physicians are not sued over documentation. Patients do not care about documentation. Patients want proper care, communication, and empathy.

MANAGEMENT OF LITIGATION

Litigation is a difficult and unrewarding experience for most physicians. There is limited satisfaction even when the case has been successfully defended. There are virtually no means by which physicians can obtain compensation for the loss of their practice time and financial expenditures. The litigation process should be viewed as something that must be avoided if possible and endured when necessary. There is simply no way for a physician defendant to truly "win" a medical malpractice case.

Lawsuits begin with service of the court-related documents. This is done in person at the physician's office or residence by a sheriff, deputy, or officer of the court. A physician who is served with a lawsuit should immediately contact his malpractice insurance carrier. Most carriers require immediate notification as a condition of coverage. Any instructions that the carrier gives should be followed.

The relevant medical records should be located and secured. From a litigation perspective, the only way to deal with a lost record is to find it. Lost records create the appearance of sloppiness or concealment, neither of which is desirable. Cases that involve lost records are generally considered to be severely compromised from a defensive perspective.

Nothing should be added to or subtracted from the record. This includes modifications, addendums, and clarifications. The patient and his attorney probably obtained a copy of the record months earlier, and any type of modification creates suspicion. At the least, modifications draw attention to an area of concern of which the plaintiff may not have been aware. Nothing should be written in any other log, diary, or journal about the case. The discovery process that accompanies litigation generally gives the parties access to any documents or records relating to the case. The fact that notes are not in the patient's "official" medical record will not protect them from discovery, nor will it prevent the plaintiff from using those notes against the physician.

The only writings and communications that are protected from the plaintiff's discovery are those that occur between the physician and his attorney. With rare exception, communication between attorney and client is protected from discovery. Physicians can record their thoughts, recollections, or strategy insights on paper, but the writing must be part of a confidential communication between attorney and client. Any such document should be addressed to one's attorney and, as an added measure, be prefaced with the words "Confidential, Attorney-Client Privilege."

Nothing should be said about the case to anyone other than the physician's attorney or the physician's spouse. Although spouses are not part of the attorney-client privilege, spousal immunity generally limits the ability of spouses to testify against one another. Physicians who are facing litigation have an understandable desire to seek reassurance from colleagues, but this must be avoided. Other physicians may also be involved as defendants or be serving as witnesses for the plaintiff. Even when they are not involved, any conversation that takes place is not protected from discovery.

The patient should not be contacted. Once litigation has been initiated, there is no longer an opportunity to clarify a misunderstanding or miscommunication. Apologies should be strictly avoided, and hostility must be contained. Sometimes the patient will want to continue to see a physician whom he has sued for malpractice. Physicians should not see see such an individual. The purpose is not to punish the person, but simply to avoid the possibility of further conflict. The patient should be asked to find another physician and should be assisted in doing so if the need is acute or emergent.

Most lawsuits involve depositions as part of the discovery process. These generally occur even in cases that are eventually dropped or settled before trial. A deposition is a question and answer session that is conducted under oath. For the defendant physician, most of the questions will come from the plaintiff's attorney. Depositions are not conducted in front of a judge or jury. There are no scorekeepers at a deposition, and it is impossible to win a deposition. For a physician defendant, the only goal is to keep from losing. Depositions are lost when major discrepancies about the patient's care are uncovered, when the physician repeatedly contradicts himself or herself, and when the physician loses his or her composure.

Demeanor and candor are everything. It is imperative that the physician be himself or herself. Jurors are ordinary people who function at the level of most patients. They are asked to solve a complex problem and are generally not permitted to take notes. They are much better at assessing credibility and candor than they are at engaging in a complex analysis of the therapeutic options. If the defendant physician's testimony is logical and the delivery is respectful, then the story is credible. Malpractice cases are not about technical minutia. They are about whether a witness is believable. Personable, patient, and respectful witnesses are the most believable. The ability to demonstrate these characteristics at a deposition and at trial are as important as the facts of the case.

Tennenhouse DJ, Kasher MP. *Risk Prevention Skills.* PMSLIC Press, 1996.

INDEX

NOTE: Page numbers in **boldface** type indicate a major discussion. A *t* following a page number indicates tabular material, and *f* following a page number indicates a figure. Drugs are listed under their generic names. When a drug trade name is listed, the reader is referred to the generic name.